Endocrinology of Breast Cancer

CONTEMPORARY ENDOCRINOLOGY

P. Michael Conn, SERIES EDITOR

19. ***Human Growth Hormone:*** *Research and Clinical Practice,* edited by *ROY G. SMITH AND MICHAEL O. THORNER,* 1999
18. ***Menopause:*** *Endocrinology and Management,* edited by *DAVID B. SEIFER AND ELIZABETH A. KENNARD,* 1999
17. ***The IGF System:*** *Molecular Biology, Physiology, and Clinical Applications,* edited by *RON G. ROSENFELD AND CHARLES ROBERTS,* 1999
16. ***Neurosteroids:*** *A New Regulatory Function in the Nervous System,* edited by *ETIENNE-EMILE BAULIEU, MICHAEL SCHUMACHER, AND PAUL ROBEL,* 1999
15. ***Autoimmune Endocrinopathies,*** edited by *ROBERT VOLPÉ,* 1999
14. ***Hormone Resistance Syndromes,*** edited by *J. LARRY JAMESON,* 1999
13. ***Hormone Replacement Therapy,*** edited by *A. WAYNE MEIKLE,* 1999
12. ***Insulin Resistance:*** *Epidemiology, Pathophysiology, and Nondiabetic Clinical Syndromes,* edited by *GERALD M. REAVEN AND AMI LAWS,* 1999
11. ***Endocrinology of Breast Cancer,*** edited by *ANDREA MANNI,* 1999
10. ***Molecular and Cellular Pediatric Endocrinology,*** edited by *STUART HANDWERGER,* 1999
9. ***The Endocrinology of Pregnancy,*** edited by *FULLER W. BAZER,* 1998
8. ***Gastrointestinal Endocrinology,*** edited by *GEORGE H. GREELEY, JR.,* 1999
7. ***Clinical Management of Diabetic Neuropathy,*** edited by *ARISTIDIS VEVES,* 1998
6. ***G Proteins, Receptors, and Disease,*** edited by *ALLEN M. SPIEGEL,* 1998
5. ***Natriuretic Peptides in Health and Disease,*** edited by *WILLIS K. SAMSON AND ELLIS R. LEVIN,* 1997
4. ***Endocrinology of Critical Diseases,*** edited by *K. PATRICK OBER,* 1997
3. ***Diseases of the Pituitary:*** *Diagnosis and Treatment,* edited by *MARGARET E. WIERMAN,* 1997
2. ***Diseases of the Thyroid,*** edited by *LEWIS E. BRAVERMAN,* 1997
1. ***Endocrinology of the Vasculature,*** edited by *JAMES R. SOWERS,* 1996

ENDOCRINOLOGY OF BREAST CANCER

Edited by

ANDREA MANNI, MD

The Pennsylvania State University College of Medicine, Hershey, PA

HUMANA PRESS
TOTOWA, NEW JERSEY

999 Riverview Drive, Suite 208
Totowa, New Jersey 07512

For additional copies, pricing for bulk purchases, and/or information about other Humana titles, contact Humana at the above address or at any of the following numbers: Tel: 973-256-1699; Fax: 973-256-8341; E-mail: humana@humanapr.com or visit our website at http://humanapress.com

This publication is printed on acid-free paper. ∞
ANSI Z39.48-1984 (American National Standards Institute)
Permanence of Paper for Printed Library Materials.

Printed in the United States of America. 10 9 8 7 6 5 4 3 2 1

Library of Congress Cataloging-in-Publication Data

Endocrinology of breast cancer / edited by Andrea Manni
p. cm. —(Contemporary endocrinology; 11)
Includes index.
ISBN 0-89603-591-3
1. Breast—Cancer—Endocrine aspects. I. Manni, Andrea. II. Series: Contemporary endocrinology (Totwa, N. J.); 11.
[DNLM: 1. Breast Neoplasms—physiopathology. 2. Breast Neoplasms—etiology. 3. Breast Neoplasms—therapy. 4. Hormones. WP 870E565 1999]
RC280.B8E54 19999
616.99'449—dc21
DNLM/DLC 98-33989
for Library of Congress CIP

PREFACE

Breast cancer is the most common malignancy affecting women in developed countries. It is estimated that one in eight women will develop this disease in her lifetime. Close to 200,000 new cases are diagnosed each year in the United States alone. Breast cancer frequently affects women during the most productive and interactive years of their lives, thus having major financial, social, and psychological consequences. The importance of hormones in the development and growth of human breast cancer has been recognized for over a century, when Beatson in 1897 reported the therapeutic efficacy of ovariectomy in women with advanced disease. More recently, over the last couple of decades, considerable evidence has indicated that estrogens are the predominant hormones involved in the biology of human breast cancer. With the advent of molecular biology techniques, an enormous wealth of new information has been generated on a variety of cellular mechanisms by which hormones influence breast cancer development and proliferation. Concomitantly, on the clinical side, improved antihormonal agents have been and are being developed with the goal of introducing them not only in the treatment, but also in the prevention of breast cancer. This explosion of new information covers a wide spectrum of basic and clinical disciplines ranging from endocrinology to tumor biology, genetics, medical oncology, surgery, and pathology. The major object of *Endocrinology of Breast Cancer* is to integrate this wealth of multidisciplinary information into a single volume that will constitute a highly useful reference for all those basic scientists and clinicians from diverse backgrounds who share an interest in breast cancer.

Section 1 focuses primarily on the hormonal mechanisms controlling normal breast development and growth. Special emphasis is placed on reviewing the roles of estrogens, progesterone, insulin-like growth factors, and their binding proteins.

Section 2 addresses possible derangements in the hormonal milieu of the host that can lead to mammary carcinogenesis. The likely importance of local estrogen production, mediated by overexpression of the aromatase enzyme, is emphasized. This section also contains an updated review of the genetic changes implicated in breast cancer development. This is a topic of major importance, since growth factor signaling activated by various oncogenes is likely to interact with the "classic" estrogen receptor pathway in inducing the transformed phenotype. Although estrogens are likely to be involved in the genesis of virtually every breast cancer, transition to hormone independence and to a more aggressive phenotype inevitably occurs in every case, leading to the patient's demise. Considerable research efforts are being devoted to elucidating the steps involved in such tumor progression, since they can be targeted for therapy. Updated information on this important area of breast cancer biology is summarized in Section 3. The roles of oncogenes and tumor suppressor genes, stromal–epithelial interactions, angiogenesis, the IGF system, and polyamines are reviewed. An updated summary of the prognostic value of expression of related factors in clinical breast cancer is also provided.

Although estrogens are the predominant hormones affecting human breast cancer biology, other hormones may be exerting an important influence. Section 4 summarizes the roles of progesterone, prolactin, and their receptors. In parallel with the increased awareness of the importance of estrogens in human breast cancer, major efforts have been made to introduce methods for the inhibition of estrogen biosynthesis and action into clinical practice. This important area is covered in Section 5, which provides an updated review of the clinical use of LHRH superagonist/antagonists, aromatase inhibitors, and antiestrogens. Finally, Section 6 covers important aspects of benign breast disease with emphasis on their treatment and potential for malignant transformation.

By providing an integrated overview of the most significant basic and clinical developments related to the hormonal aspects of breast cancer, *Endocrinology of Breast Cancer* will constitute an invaluable broad-ranging resource for all basic scientists, clinicians, students, and fellows-in-training. Our thanks go to the many contributors to this volume who are leading experts in their fields and without whose major efforts this book would not be possible.

Andrea Manni, MD

CONTENTS

CONTRIBUTORS

ELS M. J. J. BERNS, *Dr. Daniel den Hoed Cancer Center, Rotterdam Cancer Institute, Rotterdam, The Netherlands*
RICHARD E. BLACKWELL, *Department of Obstetrics and Gynecology, Reproductive Biology and Endocrinology, The University of Alabama at Birmingham School of Medicine, Birmingham, AL*
FLORENCIA BULLRICH, *Jefferson Cancer Center, Jefferson Medical College, Thomas Jefferson University, Philadelphia, PA*
ROBERT CALLAHAN, *Laboratory of Tumor Immunology and Biology, National Cancer Institute, National Institutes of Health, Bethesda, MD*
PASQUALE CARACI, *Universita di Torino, Dipartimento di Scienze Cliniche e Biologiche, Torino, Italy*
CARLO M. CROCE, *Jefferson Cancer Center, Jefferson Medical College, Thomas Jefferson University, Philadelphia, PA*
KEVIN J. CULLEN, *Division of Hematology/Oncology, Vincent T. Lombardi Cancer Research Center, Washington, DC*
LUIGI DOGLIOTTI, *Universita di Torino, Dipartimento di Scienze Cliniche e Biologiche, Torino, Italy*
MITCHELL DOWSETT, *Department of Biochemistry, Royal Marsden Hospital, London, UK*
HEATHER SPENCER FEIGELSON, *Norris Cancer Center, University of Southern California, Los Angeles, CA*
JOHN A. FOEKENS, *Dr. Daniel den Hoed Cancer Center, Rotterdam Cancer Institute, Rotterdam, The Netherlands*
WILLIAM J. GRADISHAR, *Breast Cancer Research Progam, Robert H. Lurie Cancer Center, Northwestern University Medical School, Chicago, IL*
GEOFFREY L. GREENE, *The Ben May Institute for Cancer Research, The University of Chicago, Chicago, IL*
ANNE GUIOCHON-MANTEL, *Unité de Recherches Hormones et Reproduction, Faculté de Medicine de Bicetre, Université Paris-Sud, Le Kremlin-Bicetre, France*
KAREN R. HAMMOND, *Department of Obstetrics and Gynecology, Reproductive Biology and Endocrinology, The University of Alabama at Birmingham School of Medicine, Birmingham, AL*
HAROLD A. HARVEY, *Division of Hematology/Oncology, Pennsylvania State University College of Medicine, Hershey, PA*
BRIAN E. HENDERSON, *Norris Cancer Center, University of Southern California, Los Angeles, CA*
V. H. T. JAMES, *Editor-in-Chief, Endocrine-Related Cancer, Bristol, UK*
ROY A. JENSEN, *Pathology Tumor Biology Research Laboratories, Vanderbilt University School of Medicine, Nashville, TN*
V. CRAIG JORDAN, *Director, Breast Cancer Research Progam, Robert H. Lurie Cancer Center, Northwestern University Medical School, Chicago, IL*
SAHANA S. KAUP, *Division of Hematology/Oncology, Vincent T. Lombardi Cancer Research Center, Washington, DC*

Francis G. Kern, *Department of Biochemistry and Molecular Biology, Vincent T. Lombardi Cancer Center, Washington, DC*

David L. Kleinberg, *Department of Medicine, New York University Medical Center, VA Medical Center, New York, NY*

Jan G. M. Klijn, *Dr. Daniel den Hoed Cancer Center, Rotterdam Cancer Institute, Rotterdam, The Netherlands*

Adrian Lee, *Division of Medical Oncology, The University of Texas Health Science Center at San Antonio, San Antonio, TX*

Paul Mainwaring, *Department of Biochemistry, Royal Marsden Hospital, London, UK*

Andrea Manni, *Section of Endocrinology, Diabetes, and Metabolism, Department of Medicine, The Milton S. Hershey Medical Center, Pennsylvania State University School of Medicine, Hershey, PA*

Pierre Mauvais-Jarvis, *Department of Reproductive Endocrinology, Necker Faculty of Medicine, Paris, France*

Edwin Milgrom, *Unité de Recherches Hormones et Reproduction, Faculté de Medicine de Bicetre, Université Paris-Sud, Le Kremlin-Bicetre, France*

Mark D. Pegram, *Division of Hematology/Oncology, UCLA School of Medicine, Los Angeles, CA*

Richard J. Pietras, *Division of Hematology/Oncology, UCLA School of Medicine, Los Angeles, CA*

Geneviève Plu-Bureau, *Department of Reproductive Endocrinology, Necker Faculty of Medicine, Paris, France*

Audrey A. Rasmussen, *Division of Hematology/Oncology, Vincent T. Lombardi Cancer Research Center, Washington, DC*

Monica M. Richert, *Department of Neuroscience and Anatomy, Pennsylvania State University College of Medicine, Hershey, PA*

Richard J. Santen, *Clinical Research, University of Virginia Health Sciences Center, Charlottesville, VA*

Rajeshwar Rao Tekmal, *Division of Research, Department of Obstetrics/Gynecology, Emory University School of Medicine, Atlanta, GA*

Philippe Touraine, *Department of Reproductive Endocrinology, Necker Faculty of Medicine, Paris, France*

Maria Luisa Veronese, *Jefferson Cancer Center, Jefferson Medical College, Thomas Jefferson University, Philadelphia, PA*

Barbara K. Vonderhaar, *Molecular and Cellular Endocrinology Section, Laboratory of Tumor Immunology and Biology, National Cancer Institute, National Institutes of Health, Bethesda, MD*

Teresa L. Wood, *Department of Neuroscience and Anatomy, Pennsylvania State University College of Medicine, Hershey, PA*

Douglas Yee, *Division of Medical Oncology, The University of Texas Health Science Center at San Antonio, San Antonio, TX*

I

Hormonal Control of Mammary Development and Growth

1 Hormonal Control of Normal Breast Morphology and Function

Richard E. Blackwell, PhD, MD
and Karen R. Hammond, MSN, CRNP

INTRODUCTION

As a result of selective pressures, apocrine sweat glands evolved into milk producing organs in various species. The milk-products vary among these species, and the variation is probably due to nutritional demands and environmental restrictions placed on the female. The mammary gland is unique in the animal kingdom in that only 4,200 species of mammals possess the organ, most of them (95%) belonging to the subclass Eutheria. The only other mammals that possess mammary glands belong to the subclass Monotremata, which includes the primitive egg-laying mammals such as the duckbill platypus and the subclass Methatheria, which contains the single order Marsupialia (the kangaroo) *(1)*. Nevertheless, throughout history the breast has assumed a prominent role in art and literature and has been identified as an object of beauty and sexuality. As such, its role goes far beyond its primary function of lactation. Because of the importance attached by society to the breast, any pathology of the organ is viewed by the patient with alarm. Fortunately, with the exception of carcinoma, disorders of the breast are not life threatening; however, any deviation from normal size and appearance must be thoroughly evaluated. Therefore, an understanding of the endocrine physiology of the breast is essential to meet this goal.

Historical Milestones

The treatment of breast disease is recorded from Egyptian history in the Edwin Smith Papyrus. This manuscripts dates to 1600 BC and contains 48 cases, the 45th being dedicated to a description of the treatment of breast cancer. Its physiology is mentioned in the aphorism of Hippocrates, who stated that when the pregnant uterus contained twins, if one breast became flaccid one of the twins was expelled. If the right breast became flaccid the male was expelled, but if it was the left breast the female was expelled. Regarding menstrual function, it was stated that the woman who was neither pregnant nor had lately delivered and who had milk in her breast labored under obstructive menstruation. Furthermore, breasts were linked to mood lability, in that blood originating from the breast of females was considered to denote an attack of mania.

From: *Contemporary Endocrinology: Endocrinology of Breast Cancer*
Edited by: A. Manni © Humana Press Inc., Totowa, NJ

During the late 18th to 19th centuries, controversy existed as to the origin of milk. Many of the original drawings by Leonardo De Vinci showed the uterus and the mammary glands to be connected by a system of ducts. Such an idea may have arisen because of the observation that uterine cramping is often associated with nursing. However, Haller in 1765 was the first to conclude that milk was derived from blood. This idea became firmly entrenched by the 19th century:

> *The secretion of milk would appear to illustrate, even more fully and clearly than do other glands, the truth on which we have so often insisted, that is secretion is eminently the result of the metabolic activity of the secretory cell. The blood is the ultimate source of milk, but it becomes milk only through the activity of the cell, and that activity consists largely in a metabolic manufacture by the cell and in the cell of the common things brought by the blood to the special things present in the milk.*

The relationship of blood and milk production was further investigated by Sir Astley Cooper, the English surgeon, who in 1845 described the lobular alveolar anatomy of the breast, its blood supply and innervation. He first described the very early physiologic occurrences in milk let-down and lactogenesis. In 1930, Peterson showed by means of pressure monitoring the separation of milk secretion and injection *(2)*. In 1928, Riddle et al. *(3)* extracted prolactin and showed it to be separate from other pituitary hormones. In 1940, Meites and Turner *(4)* proposed that in pregnancy, estrogen and progestogen promote full mammary growth, and progesterone inhibits estrogen stimulation and prolactin secretion, and that at parturition an increase in circulating prolactin and cortisol is accompanied by fallen estrogen and progesterone, which brings about the onset of menstruation. Although incorrect in many aspects, the Turner/Meites hypothesis has remained intact for more than 40 years. These observations were challenged by Clifton and Furth *(5)*, who implanted pituitary mammotropic tumors which secreted prolactin, growth hormone, and corticotropin in the adrenal ectomized rat. Mammary growth occurred in the absence of steroid hormones. Testing their own hypothesis, Chen and Meites *(6)* also showed that estrogen stimulates the secretion of prolactin. While partially inhibiting the response, progesterone further suppressed prolactin secretion below the baseline level. Finally, Kuhn *(7)* proposed that elevated prolactin levels during pregnancy prevented the secretion of milk and that withdrawal of this hormone after parturition is partially responsible for lactogenesis. Thus, a concept of multihormonal control of lactation evolved.

The knowledge of anatomy and surgery of the breast proceeded at a similar pace. Camper, in the mid-1700s, described the internal mammary lymph nodes. Dran *(8)* and Petit in France, determined that breast cancer spread by metastasis and they advocated removal of the breast, underlying pectoralis muscles, and axillary lymph nodes. The introduction of anesthesia by Morton and Crawford Long, and the concept of anesepsis by Joseph Lister allowed surgery of the breast to undergo exponential growth. However, progress did not occur without setbacks. James Paget *(9)* in 1856 reported an operative mortality rate of 10% in 235 patients with 100% recurrence rate in eight years. Samuel D. Gross, in the United States, performed simple mastectomy and removed lymph nodes only if they were grossly involved. His son, Samuel W. Gross, however, removed the entire breast and skin covering the mammary, fat, fascia, pectoralis muscle, and lymph nodes. However, William Stuart Halsted *(10)* in the early 1900s introduced contemporary radical mastectomy. He recommended the removal of tissue in one piece including the skin and en bloc resection of the pectoralis muscle. His successor, Thomas Cullen *(11)*, working with William Henry Welch at Johns Hopkins University, was the first to use frozen sections in the diagnosis of breast lesions in 1891. Five years later, Grubbe first irradiated a breast cancer patient, and by 1898 Erlich had isolated the first alkylating agents that would serve as early chemotherapies.

The history of breast physiology is forever bound up with the history of prolactin biology. Chiari *(12)* and Frommel *(13)* in 1885 and 1882, respectively, described two cases of puerperal atrophy of the uterus associated with persistent lactation after pregnancy. It is of interest that neither investigator knew of the other's work, and the original report, which appeared in German, consisted of one page. The structure of this classic work should give contemporary authors cause to consider the virtue of brevity in scientific writing. Subsequently, Argonz and DelCastillo *(14,15)* described the clinical nature of persistent lactation occurring independent of pregnancy, yet associated with a hyposecretion of estrogen. Forbes and Albright *(16)* described a syndrome of galactorrhea, amenorrhea, and associated low urinary follicle-stimulated hormone levels in 1954. They noted that 25% of these patients had what appeared to be a tumor of the pituitary gland. These clinical observations suggested an association between menstruation and lactation, but it was not until the iodination of growth hormone by Greenwood and Hunter *(17)* and the development of the first radioimmonoassay techniques by Bersen and Yalow *(18)* that small quantities of circulating peptide could be measured. It was not until the 1970s that human prolactin was purified and shown to be different from growth hormone when specific and sensitive radioimmunoassays were developed that allowed measurement of prolactin, both in vitro and in vivo *(19,20)*.

PHYSIOLOGY OF PROLACTIN SECRETION

Prolactin is an ancient molecule that influences numerous functions of the vertebrate organism. These extend from luteal support and maintenance of lactation to regulation of free fatty acid metabolism in mammals, to salt and water metabolism in amphibians, and the regulation of sexual behavior in the bony fish. Comparative physiology of this hormone is extensive as with the octapeptides and neuropeptides. Prolactin consists of a single polypeptide containing 198 amino acid residues with a molecular weight of 22,000. The structure is folded into a globular form with the folds being connected by three disulfide bonds. There is great similarity between the structure of human placental lactogen, human growth hormone, and prolactin. The gene for human prolactin was cloned in the early 1980s and it is thought that this gene was derived from a common somatomammotropic precursor. The prolactin gene is positioned on chromosome 6 and located near the human leukocyte antigen *(21)*. Prolactin exists in at least five forms, the most active being a 22,000 molecular weight monomeric variant *(22)*. Big prolactin with a 50,000 molecular weight is a mixture of diametric and trimetric forms. Big big prolactin has a molecular weight of 100,000 with little biologic activity, and iso-B prolactin which has been isolated by isofocusing, is thought to be biologically active. Glycosylated prolactin has a molecular weight of approximately 25,000. Apparently all the forms reside in the human lactotrope, which is located in the anterior pituitary. The lactotrope arises from a common stem cell and gives rise to both the somatotropes and lactotropes. The lactotrope is found in the lateral aspect of the pituitary gland and makes up at least 20% of the cell population. The cellular concentration of prolactin varies considerably, reflecting the fact this is a dynamic hormone released by a variety of agents. Prolactin shows some variations throughout the menstrual cycle, being highest before ovulation in the middle of the luteal phase. The studies of Neill et al. *(23)*, using the reverse hemolytic plaque assay, evaluated several populations of cells including ones that showed little biologic activity and secreted a small amount of prolactin and others that secreted large amounts of prolactin. It has been suggested that some lactotropes are less responsive to the inhibitory influence of dopamine than others, and pituitary tumors have been described that are devoid of D2 receptors *(24)*.

It was originally thought that prolactin was unique among the pituitary hormones in that its release was regulated solely by inhibitory influences from the hypothalamus. It was observed that prolactin secretion persisted when the pituitary gland was transplanted in vivo to sites removed from the base of the brain such as the pneumoderma pouch or the kidney capsule, or maintained in vitro in organ or cell culture. The prolactin inhibiting factor was at one time thought to be a polypeptide, but numerous attempts to isolate it have failed. Prolactin appears to be regulated by a host of chemicals that both stimulate and inhibit the hormone secretions. Dopamine appears to be the principle inhibitor of prolactin secretion, yet γ-aminobutyric acid (GABA) may play a physiologic role. When L-dopa is administered to test subjects, it crosses the blood-brain barrier and decreases prolactin secretion within about $2^1/_2$ h. A rebound response occurs that is greater in women than in men. In the stalk-transected monkey, the inhibitory effect of dopamine on plasma prolactin level varies as a function of estrogen concentration. Furthermore, in the estrogen-treated stalk-transected monkey, the infusion of dopamine at 0.1 mg/kg/min, in pulses ranging from 2.5 to 7.5 min, produces a dose-dependent inhibition of prolactin secretion. Likewise, it has been demonstrated in vivo in the rodent that the infusion of dopamine into animals pretreated with the inhibitor of dopamine synthesis α-methyl tyrosine, accounts for 70% of prolactin inhibiting activity *(25)*. The rest appears to arise from factors produced in the neurohypophysis. Such studies have been confirmed in the monkey model but not the human: infusion of 0.02–8 mg/kg/min dopamine results in a dose-dependent suppression of prolactin secretion. Although dopamine is thought not to cross the blood-brain barrier, the median eminence and adenohypophysis lie outside this hypothetical barrier. Furthermore, it has been shown that dopamine isolated from stalk portal blood is approximately 0.8 ng/mL which is eightfold greater than that found in the peripheral plasma of the rhesus monkey. A physiologic role for GABA is supported by the fact that it is secreted into the portal system, and receptors for this peptide have been isolated on human lactotropes. GABA is, in fact, a more potent inhibitor of prolactin secretion than dopamine; however, the two agents seem to produce different effects on the lactotrope *(26)*.

In addition to the study of dopamine physiology and prolactin secretion, great interest has been shown in various prolactin stimulating factors. It was shown in the early 1970s that thyrotropin-releasing hormone (TRH) could acutely release prolactin both in vitro and in vivo *(27)*. Vasoactive intestinal peptide (VIP) and angiotensin-II have also been shown to stimulate both the synthesis and release of prolactin. The injection of hormones such as TRH causes the release of thyroid-stimulating hormone (TSH). This response is regulated by circulating tri-iodothyronine (T3) and thyroxin (T4). This accounts for the fact that prolactin secretion occurs independent of TSH, for instance, following suckling.

VIP was originally derived from porcine duodenal ducts. It is found throughout the central nervous system and in fact can be measured in hypothalamic blood samples. Infusion of VIP into stalk-transected monkeys at 20 μg/kg induces an acute rise in prolactin secretion. VIP is also produced in the pituitary gland and appears to serve as an autocrine regulator of prolactin secretion *(28)*.

Angiotensin-II has been shown to stimulate prolactin secretion both in vitro and in vivo. Angiotensin-II receptors are found on the lactotrope, and injection of this compound results in the rapid release of prolactin. In fact, it appears to have greater releaser effect than a comparable injection of TRH *(29)*. Furthermore, other neurotransmitters modify prolactin secretion; these include serotonin (which stimulates prolactin secretion), the opioids (which inhibit dopamine turnover), histamine, a hypothalamic neurotransmitter that stimulates prolactin release by acting on the H1 receptor, and neurotensin (a tridecapeptide) and substance P, (an undecapeptide), both of which stimulate prolactin. Furthermore, whether any of these compounds play a physiologic role in the regulation of prolactin secretion is unclear *(30)*.

It appears that prolactin is controlled by endocrine, autocrine, and paracrine mechanisms. Retrograde flow in the hypothalamic portal system has been demonstrated, and prolactin appears to effect its own secretion via a short feedback loop *(31)*. The interventricular injection of prolactin results in an increased dopamine turnover in the median eminence, and a high rate of turnover has been demonstrated, both during lactation and pregnancy. This is decreased by both hypophysectomy or treatment with dopamine. Intrahypophyseal mechanisms appear to be involved in the regulation of prolactin secretion as VIP has been demonstrated to be synthesized in the lactotrope from radiolabeled amino acids that have been shown to stimulate prolactin secretion *(28)*. A number of reports also suggest that gonadotropes may exert regulatory influences on prolactin secretion. For instance, in vivo and in vitro studies have shown that synthetic gonadotropin-releasing hormone (GnRH) will release prolactin in the rat using a superfusion model, and also in vitro using a human pituitary monolayer system *(32)*. The incubation of GnRH with lactotropes separated from large gonadotropes fails to increase prolactin secretion, whereas coaggregation of these two cell types restores the secretory effect of GnRH on prolactin *(33)*. In addition, coincubation of GnRH antagonists with GnRH inhibits the release of prolactin, whereas coincubation of the same antagonist with synthetic TRH fails to alter prolactin release *(32)*. Likewise, incubation of the α-chain of luteinizing hormone (LH) has been shown to stimulate the differentiation of rat fetal lactotropes, and the incubation of β-LH or follicle-stimulating hormone (FSH) with human pituitary cells in vitro fails to stimulate prolactin secretion, whereas coincubation of antiserum to LH or FSH inhibits the GnRH-mediated release of prolactin *(34)*. Likewise, GnRH-associated peptide (GAP), a precursor to GnRH, has been reported to increase prolactin secretion in the rat.

HYPERPROLACTINEMIA

Dysfunctional Prolactin Secretion

Hyperprolactinemia can be caused by numerous divergent lesions and insults. These include central nervous system injury at birth, encephalitis, meningitis, central nervous system trauma, granulomatous forming lesions such as syphilis and tuberculosis, acute arteritis, cavernous sinus thrombosis; infiltrative disorders such as histiocytosis X; various forms of head trauma; central dopamine dysfunction; lactotrope hyperplasia; prolactinomas; endocrinopathies such as primary hypothyroidism; chest trauma and thoracotomy; breast augmentation or reduction; breast biopsy; herpes zoster; metabolic disorders such as renal failure; hysterectomy or oophorectomy; and the injection of a myriad of pharmaceutical products including birth control pills, tranquilizers, antidepressants, antihypertensives, isoniazid, and cimetidine *(35)*.

Fortunately, most of these causes of hyperprolactinemia are quite rare. The most common etiologies are functional hyperprolactinemia, prolactinomas, drug intake, and hypothyroidism. The latter disorder, while often discussed and frequently found in women, infrequently presents with hyperprolactinemia. These patients will usually have an elevated TSH level and a low-normal T4 level, indicative of compensated hypothyroidism. On rare occasions, patients with this disorder may present with a markedly enlarged pituitary gland, which may be mistaken for a macroadenoma *(36)*. Drugs are frequently associated with hyperprolactinemia; however, care must be taken to rule out other etiologies. At times, the absolute prolactin level can be of use as it has been demonstrated that levels of 100 ng/mL are associated with the findings of pituitary tumors some 47% of the time, and levels of 200 ng/mL are diagnostic of the presence of pituitary tumors *(37)*. Unfortunately, one will find a pituitary lesion 27% of the time when imaging is carried out in all patients. Therefore, there is a one in three probability of finding an "incidentaloma" on radiography *(38)*. Despite this frequency, the prolactinoma is thought to be the most common lesion of the central nervous system. These tumors are classified as microadenomas if they are <1 cm in size, and macroadenomas if they are >1 cm. The behavior of these two types of tumors differs markedly, and their management is different *(39)*. Probably the most likely cause of hyperprolactinemia is a functional disorder, found in individuals who do not have pituitary tumors demonstrated by either computed tomography (CT) or magnetic resonance imaging (MRI) (usually <2 mm in size, its limit of resolution). Patients with these lesions are thought to have some decrease in the delivery of dopamine into the hypothalamic portal system resulting in an escape of the lactotrope from suppressive control. A number of papers have described functional disorders of dopamine metabolism in patients with pituitary tumors, and at times this overall condition may self-correct, for instance, after pregnancy *(40–44)*.

Hyperprolactinemia and Menstrual Dysfunction

It has been demonstrated that menstrual dysfunction usually precedes the appearance of galactorrhea by about 5 years. The mechanism by which hyperprolactinemia results in menstrual dysfunction was an enigma until recently. It has been suggested that any mechanism that increases hypothalamic portal vessel prolactin levels might increase central dopamine secretion. Dopamine is a known inhibitor of GnRH, which might account for menstrual disturbances. On the other hand, prolactin appears to have a direct effect at the level of the ovary *(45–50)*. In the rat ovarian interstitial cell, a single class of specific high-affinity receptors has been isolated, and prolactin acts as the potent inhibitor of LH-mediated androgen synthesis. Androgens serve as substrates for estrogen production in the ovary, and the hypoestrogenism seen with hyperprolactinemic syndromes may be at least in part of ovarian origin. In addition, high-affinity prolactin receptors have been demonstrated on granulosa cell surfaces. These receptors are located near the basal lamina. Granulosa cells contain the aromatase enzyme that metabolizes androgens to estrogens. Estrogen-induced aromatase activity has been shown to be blocked by coincubation of granulosa cells with levels of prolactin exceeding 100 ng/mL. Although the role of prolactin in the ovary of the rodent appears clear-cut, evidence for similar mechanisms in humans is less clear. It has been shown that prolactin is seques-

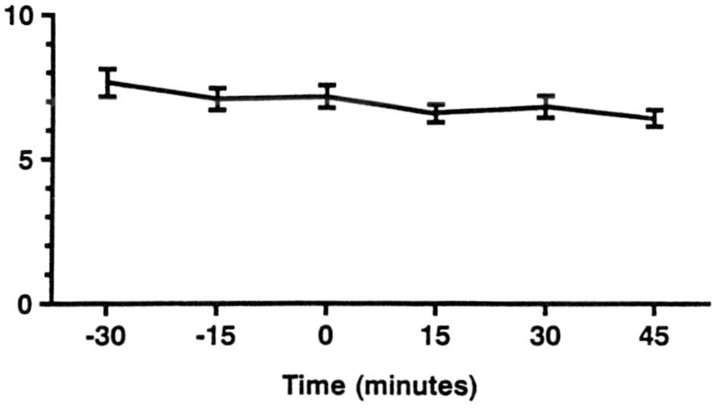

Fig. 1. The effect of breast examination on prolactin levels in normal cycling reproductive age women ($n = 12$).

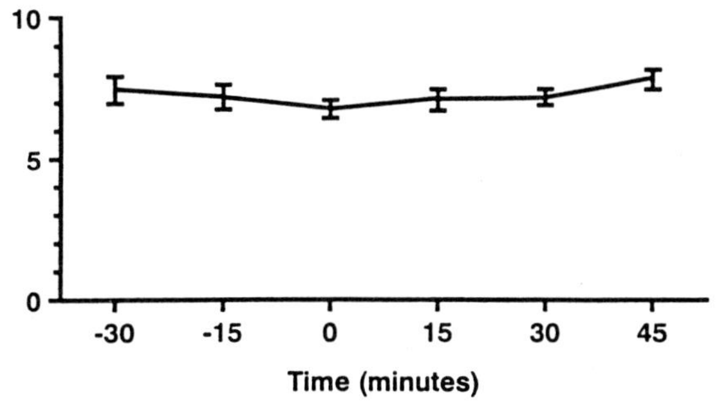

Fig. 2. The effect of protein ingestion (foods rich in arginine, tyrosine, and tryptophane) on prolactin levels in normal cycling reproductive age women ($n = 12$).

tered in the microenvironment of the human follicle four- to sixfold against a gradient. Follicles found to have high concentrations of prolactin are usually noted to have low concentrations of estradiol. Atretic follicles generally contain prolactin levels exceeding 100 ng/mL. Furthermore, prolactin has been shown to stimulate and to inhibit the corpus luteum. Prolactin appears to be necessary for complete luteinization, and high levels have been shown to inhibit progesterone and estradiol synthesis in vitro. Despite this evidence, the recent observation that delivery of pulsatile GnRH induces complete folliculogenesis, which can result in ovulation in the hyperprolactinemic patient, would seem to suggest that the central mechanism is more important in the creation of ovulation disturbance *(51)*.

Patient Evaluation

Prolactin is a dynamic hormone that is involved in many aspects of metabolism. Prolactin varies throughout the menstrual cycle and has a sleep-entrained rhythm. Physical examination, stress, and food intake will stimulate prolactin secretion; however, recent studies have demonstrated that breast examination does not elevate prolactin levels in normal cycling reproductive age women, nor does the intake of food sources with high levels of tyrosine, tryptophane or arginine, stimulate prolactin secretion (Figs. 1 and 2). Historically, blood samples have been obtained for prolactin measurement in the later morning or early afternoon, avoiding both food intake and examinations. This precaution may not be warranted in view of these recent reports. It is suggested that,

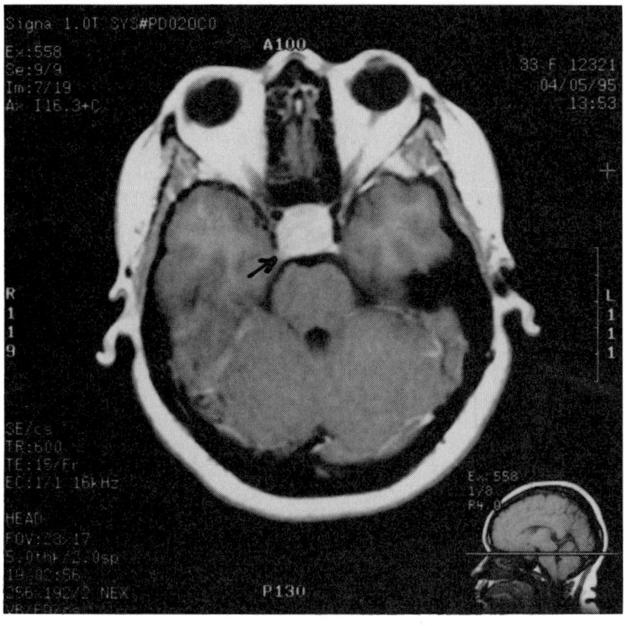

Fig. 3. MRI of patient with macroadenoma.

once prolactin is found to be elevated, it would be prudent to repeat the test in view of the volatile nature of the hormone secretion and the fact that the American College of Pathologists assayed reference standard in 1987 showed a mean prolactin level of 95 ng/mL, yet 300 laboratories had a variance on this assay between 5 ng/mL (normal) and 150 ng/mL (markedly elevated). Furthermore, radioimmunoassays using heterologous serum may be more likely to measure hyperprolactinemia than those using a hybridoma assay. Our own group has found a number of patients with markedly elevated prolactin levels when evaluated by chemiluminescence assays, yet multiple radioimmunoassays failed to demonstrate hyperprolactinemia. Once hyperprolactinemia has been determined on multiple occasions, it is advisable to measure a T4 and TSH to rule out compensated hypothyroidism and, depending on the prolactin level, proceed with some radiographic imaging. There is a difference of opinion regarding when imaging should be utilized. Some endocrinologists would image with any sustained elevated prolactin level, others at 50 ng/mL, and all at 100 mg/mL. The choice of radiographic imaging is debatable; both CT and MRI can image at 2-mm intervals, yet CT scanning costs about four times less than MRI (Figs. 3 and 4). In the era of managed care this is important, and when one considers that the object of imaging is to separate a lesion > or <1 cm, it seems irrelevant which technique is chosen. Visual field examinations likewise should be carried out in patients who have macroadenomas as supracellar involvement produces superior bitemporal hemianopia about 68% of the time. The routine use of visual field examinations in the patient with a microadenoma is unwarranted.

Therapy

The treatment of hyperprolactinemia is generally tailored to whether a patient wishes to be pregnant or not, the extent of her symptoms, her age, whether she has a pituitary

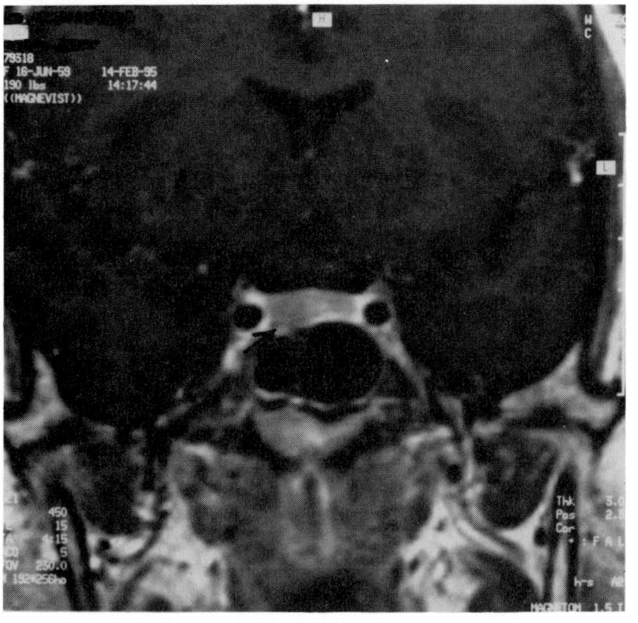

Fig. 4. MRI of patient with microadenoma.

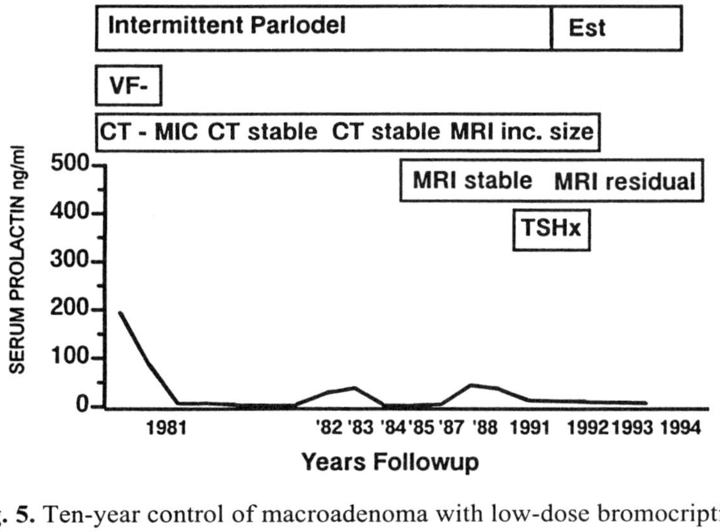

Fig. 5. Ten-year control of macroadenoma with low-dose bromocriptine.

tumor and of what size, and whether bone loss is an issue *(52,53)*. The patient who is contemplating pregnancy has a choice between medical or surgical therapy. Surgery, while first employed for the treatment of these lesions, is more successful in resolving the presence of a tumor if it is <10 mm. Unfortunately, there is a discordance between removal of tumor and resolution of the endocrinopathy, and many patients, whether they have micro- or macroadenomas, require drug therapy after surgery. Medical therapy is quite successful in the management of large or small pituitary tumors and is certainly the treatment of choice in the patient with functional hyperprolactinemia (Figs. 5 and 6) *(54)*.

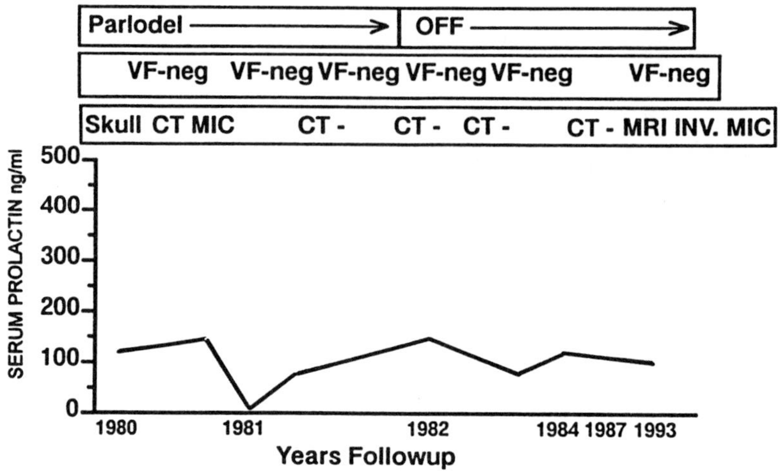

Fig. 6. Long-term suppression of microadenoma with bromocriptine after discontinuing therapy.

Transsphenoidal resection of microadenomas usually results in persistent hyperprolactinemia approximately 50% of the time, whereas the failure rate with a macroadenoma can reach 70% *(55,56)*. Surgery is frequently used in patients with tumors that do not secrete prolactin. Dopamine agonist therapy is frequently used as the first order of therapy, even by neurosurgeons.

It was noted during the middle ages that women who ate bread made from rye flour contaminated with the fungus *Claviceps purpurea* developed gangrenous ergotism and failure to lactate. The disease, called St. Anthony's fire, resulted from the ingestion of ergot alkaloids (ergot peptines). These substances were extracted for obstetrical use, and in the mid-1970s bromocriptine (Parlodel, Sandoz), was introduced for the treatment of hyperprolactinemia, and subsequently pituitary tumors. This compound acts on the D2 receptor, inhibits prolactin secretion and synthesis, both in vivo and in vitro, and normalizes prolactin levels in the vast majority of patients affected with hyperprolactinemia *(57)*. Bromocriptine is administered orally in doses ranging from 1.25 mg up to 160 mg in patients with Parkinson's disease *(58)*. Most patients with hyperprolactinemia will respond effectively to doses between 2.5 and 15 mg/d. The ingestion of bromocriptine is not without side effects, and the vast majority of patients develop gastrointestinal complaints such as nausea. Some patients have hypersensitivity to the drug, and intractable vomiting develops. Likewise, nasal stuffiness, dysphoria, and lethargy are common side effects, and in extremely high doses, psychosis and fatal tachyarrhythmias have been reported. To maximize the effectiveness of bromocriptine and minimize the side effects, it should be taken at bedtime; nausea can be limited by its vaginal administration *(59)*. The ingestion of the drug is usually begun at a 1.25-mg dose at bedtime, and increased until it suppresses prolactin levels over the next 4 weeks.

Patients who are unable to tolerate bromocriptine ingestion or who fail to respond to it may be treated with pergolide mesylate (Permax, Eli Lilly) *(60)*. This drug is a nonergoline dopamine agonist, is three times more potent than bromocriptine, and is taken once a day. Its active dose range is 50–100 μg, and it is highly effective in suppressing hyperprolactinemia in patients with and without pituitary tumors. The drug is currently approved by the Food and Drug Administration (FDA) for the treatment of

Parkinson's disease, but it is used for the treatment of hyperprolactinemia in Canada and throughout Europe *(61)*.

CV-205-502 is a drug that was developed by Sandoz for the treatment of hyperprolactinemia *(62)*. It is effective in suppressing the release of prolactin in a 60–80 μg dose range and has a better side effect profile than does bromocriptine. Like bromocriptine or pergolide mesylate, patients can still have dysphoria, lethargy, nasal stuffiness, and at times nausea. It is unclear whether this drug will be approved by the FDA; however, it is sold in Europe under the trade name Norprolac.

Recently, cabergoline (Dostinex) has been introduced by Pharmacia/Upjohn. Cabergoline is a dopaminergic ergoline derivative with a molecular formula of C26H35N502 and has a molecular weight of 451.62. It is a white crystalline powder with a melting point of 101–108°C. Because cabergoline is a base, it dissolves rapidly in the gastrointestinal tract. The drug is a dopamine receptor agonist and it selectively binds to the D2 receptor on the lactotrope. Cabergoline crosses the placenta in animal models, but studies have failed to demonstrate teratogenicity. The drug is metabolized after oral administration via hydrolysis to the acylurea bond or the urea moiety of the side chain. Seventy-two percent of the compound is excreted in the feces, 18–20% in the urine within 10 days of administration. Cabergoline has a long half-life; therefore patients are treated with 0.5 mg twice a week. Kinetic studies have shown that cabergoline reduces prolactin secretion between 74 and 95% of the time. Patients do have side effects, consisting of nausea, headache, dizziness, abdominal pain, and fatigue. Twenty-nine percent of the patients versus 43% of the patients on bromocriptine had the side effect of nausea *(63,64)*.

Finally, radiation therapy is highly effective in the treatment of all prolactinomas. Therapy of course is generally divided into four to five fractions over 5 weeks with doses ranging between 35 and 155 rads at the 95% isodose line *(65)*.

MORPHOLOGY AND BREAST DEVELOPMENT

The mammary gland is derived from ectoderm and can be identified 6 weeks after fertilization. At this point in gestation, the ectodermal ridge forms from an ectodermal pit and begins to penetrate the mesenchyme, producing the mammary primordium. At 20 weeks gestation, 16–24 primitive lactiferous ducts invade the mesoderm. The ectodermal projections continue to branch and go deeper into the tissue. Canalization occurs near term, and it should be noted that although the central lactiferous duct is present at birth, differentiation of the gland does not occur until it receives the appropriate hormonal signals. Mammary tissue remains unresponsive until pregnancy, yet it will respond to systemic hormonal administration during fetal life. In the third trimester when fetal prolactin levels increase, terminal differentiation of ductal cells occur. After birth these cells revert to a more primitive state *(66)*. The mammary gland is quiescent during puberty; however, once ovulatory menstrual cycles are established, breast development proceeds according to the descriptions of Marshall and Tanner. Although the hormonal regulation of mammogenesis is unclear, estrogen given in utero appears to bring about ductal proliferation *(67)*. In vitro, estrogens have not been shown to promote mammary growth, and it has been suggested that various epidermal growth factors may be involved in the process *(68)*. Progesterone, when administered in vivo, produces lobuloalveolar development *(69)*. The administration of both estrogen and progesterone to hypophysectomized animals fails to promote mammogenesis alone *(70)*. This strongly suggests that other hormones play a central role in mammogenesis. For instance, if the pituitary and adrenal glands are removed from oophorectomized rats, the addition of estrogen plus corticoids in growth hormone restores ductal growth *(71)*. This is comparable to the events seen during puberty.

Before pregnancy occurs, breast lobules consist of ducts lined with epithelium that are embedded in connective tissue. The majority of tissues in the gland are connective and adipose type. There is a scant contribution of glandular parenchyma and a few sacculations arise from the duct. The entire gland consists of the lactiferous system. Breasts undergo cyclic changes associated with normal ovulation, and the premenstrual breast engorgement noted by most women is secondary to tissue edema and hyperemia *(72)*. After conception, mammary glands undergo remarkable augmentation. The lobular alveoli units differentiate during the first trimester, and it is possible to induce mammary development either with placental lactogens or prolactin in the absence of steroids. This has been demonstrated both in vivo and in vitro *(73)*. Placental lactogen and prolactin increase throughout pregnancy, and data suggest that either of these hormones is capable of stimulating mammogenesis. The role of estrogen in mammogenesis is secondary, as lactation has been reported in pregnancies with placental sulfatase enzyme deficiencies *(74)*. Progesterone, while stimulating lobular alveolar development, appears to antagonize the terminal effects induced by prolactin, at least in vitro. Cortisol, while potentiating the action of prolactin on mammary differentiation, is unnecessary for either ductal or alveolar proliferation *(75)*. A strong case can be made for the involvement of both insulin and other growth factors in stimulating mammogenesis. For instance, insulin is required for the survival of postmammary tissue in vitro *(76)*. It is possible that insulin-like molecules such as the somatomedins may be involved in the process. However, studies have also suggested that epidermal growth factor may be involved in mammogenesis and, together with a group of corticoids, may facilitate the accumulation of type 4 collagen and components of the basal lamina in which epithelial cells are supported.

The mature mammary gland lies on the pectoralis fascia and the musculature of the chest wall over the upper anterior rib cage. It is surrounded by layers of fat and encased in skin. The tissue extends into the axilla, where it forms the tail of Spence. The mammary gland consists of 12–20 glandular lobules that are connected by a ductal system. The ducts are surrounded by connective and periductal tissues that are hormonally responsive, as described previously. The lactiferous ducts enlarge as they approach the nipple and are surrounded by a pigmented areola. The ducts contain contractile smooth muscle fibers. The ductal tissue is lined by epithelial cells and fibroseptum that run from the lobules to the superficial fascia. Cooper's ligament (suspensory ligament) allows for mobility of the breast. The major blood supply of the breast comes from the lateral thoracic and internal thoracic arteries, although components have been identified from the anterior intercostal vessels. The breast is enervated chiefly by the intercostal nerves carrying both sensory and autonomic fibers. The areola and nipple are enervated by the inferior ramus of the fourth intercostal nerve. Seventy-five percent of the lymphatic drainage involves axillary pathways, although the pectoral and apical lymph nodes are also involved, as are the parasternal nodes.

HORMONAL CONTROL OF MILK SECRETION AND LACTATION

Lactogenesis can be divided into two stages. Stage I occurs prepartum, and stage II occurs at the time of parturition. Milk letdown occurs abruptly during the second to fourth days postpartum in humans, although colostrum production progresses to milk secretion gradually. This process can take up to a month and coincides with a fall in plasma progesterone levels and a rise in serum prolactin, at least intermittently. Twelve weeks after parturition, changes in milk composition occur. One finds an increased production of lactose, proteins, and immunoglobulins and a decrease in sodium and chloride. There is an increase in blood flow, oxygen, and glucose uptake as well *(77)*. There is an increase in the amount of citrate present in the breast at about the time of parturition. Milk secretion occurs in the third trimester and the composition of milk remains fairly stable into term. This is exemplified by the stable production of alkalic albumin and milk-specific protein. At parturition there is a fall in placental lactogen production, and progesterone levels reach the nonpregnant range within several days. Estrogen falls to baseline levels in 5 days, whereas prolactin decreases over approximately 14 days. A fall in progesterone seems to be the most important event in the establishment of lactogenesis *(78,79)*. This was confirmed by the observation in the late 19th century that milk secretion would not occur until removal of the placenta. The administration of exogenous progesterone prevents lactose and lipid synthesis after oophorectomy in the pregnant rat and in ewes *(80)*. Furthermore, progesterone administration inhibits casein and lactalbumin synthesis in vitro.

At least in the human, lactation is maintained by the interaction of numerous hormones including prolactin, corticoids, thyroxin, growth hormone, insulin, estradiol, and progesterone. Removal of either the pituitary or adrenal gland from a number of animal species terminates milk production *(81)*. The species dictates the type of replacement therapy that is required to reinstitute milk production. For instance, in the rabbit and the sheep, prolactin is effective alone. In ruminants milk secretion is restored by the addition of corticoids, thyroxin, growth hormone, and prolactin. Prolactin appears to be the key hormone in the maintenance of lactation because the administration of bromocriptine, a dopamine agonist, inhibits prolactin secretion and blocks lactogenesis *(82)*. This effect varies with the species as inhibition of prolactin in ruminants shows very little effect on the establishment of lactation, especially in the ovine species. The role of thyroid hormones in lactation is unclear. Thyroidectomy inhibits lactation, and replacement therapy with thyroxin increases milk yield. It has been suggested that growth hormone and thyroxin synergize to alter milk yield, and tri-iodothyronine has been shown to act directly on mouse mammary tissue in vitro to increase its sensitivity of prolactin.

Suckling and Milk Release

During pregnancy the integrated baseline of serum prolactin is elevated when compared with the nonpregnant state. Either suckling or manipulation of the breast leads to an elevation in prolactin within about 40 minutes *(83)*. The response can be duplicated by the application of electrical stimulation to rat mammary nerves *(84)*. Growth hormone and cortisol are also released by this stimulus. The response appears to be greatest in the immediate postpartum period and is attenuated over 6 months. The application of lidocaine to the nipple blocks nerve conduction and obliterates the response of prolactin to the stimuli. Furthermore, if two infants suckle simultaneously, the rise in prolactin is amplified. Suckling increases the secretion of prolactin as well as oxytocin. After application of the stimulus, there is an 8–12 h delay before milk secretion is fully maximized. This response correlates with the frequency and duration of suckling. There is no correlation between the amount of prolactin released and milk yield. Suckling of the breast results in an increase in intramammary pressure bilaterally. This occurs secondary to contraction of myoepithelial cells in response to oxytocin, an octapeptide. This occurs after application of a stimulus to the nipple, which activates sensory receptors, transmitting impulses to the spinal cord and hypothalamus. Oxytocin is produced in neurons located in the superoptic and paraventricular nucleus. It is estimated that 2 ng of oxytocin are released per 2–4 s pulse intervals *(85)*. Oxytocin is synthesized in the hypothalamus as part of a large prohormone that is cleaved and packaged into secretory granules. It is transmitted by exoplasmic flow and further cleaved into the native hormone and a neurophysin-like binding protein. The synthesis and release of oxytocin is rapid, and 1.5 h after injection of a radioactive amino acid tracer into the cerebrospinal fluid, labeled oxytocin is released by exocytosis. Electrical pulse activity has been measured in oxytocic neurons 5–15 s before milk ejection in the rat model system. The response is continuous because the cry of an infant or various other perceptions associated with nursing can trigger activity in the central circuits.

Milk letdown may be conditioned to the cry of an infant or various other perceptions associated with nursing. When nursing women are allowed to hold their infants but not to breast feed, serum prolactin concentrations are not increased despite the occurrence of milk letdown. Prolactin levels rise only with nursing. The increase in prolactin when nursing is apparently sufficient to maintain lactogenesis and an adequate milk supply for the next feeding. This accounts for the ability to breast feed infants for years once lactation is established.

OVARIAN FUNCTION IN THE PUERPERIUM

Whether a mother nurses or not does not appear to be a major factor in determining the timing of first ovulation *(86,87)*. The frequency of breast feeding and the addition of solid food supplementation to the infant's diet are important *(88)*. A study in Mexico indicated that in the absence of bleeding and supplementation, 100% of breast-feeding mothers remained anovulatory for 3 months postpartum, and more than 95% remained anovulatory for 6 months *(89)*. The mean delayed ovulation after delivery is approximately 45 days in nonbreast-feeding women, but may occur as soon as 3 weeks postpartum *(90)*. Presumably, as a result of pituitary suppression persisting from pregnancy, the lower levels of estradiol present after delivery do not result in an increase in serum FSH concentrations until about 2 weeks postpartum. Immunoreactive LH may appear to be increased for the first several days postpartum because of crossreactivity with human chorionic gonadotropin, but in fact they are suppressed. Basal prolactin levels fall to normal, and ovarian secretion of estradiol begins to rise. As referred to previously, perhaps prolactin interferes directly or indirectly with gonadal steroidogenesis. The relationship of prolactin, lactation, and gonadal function is dramatically illustrated by studies of the Kung hunter gathers in Africa *(91)*. Coitus is initiated within days after delivery yet contraception is not used. The average interval between births in this population is 44.1 months. It is suggested that the long birth spacing is attributable to nursing patterns. These mothers nurse briefly but frequently, and infants are kept by their mothers until 2 years of age and nursed at about 13 min intervals. The infants sleep with their mothers and are allowed to nurse at night as desired.

CONCLUSIONS

As has been demonstrated, the breast, which is possessed by a limited number of mammals, has been the object of study, art, and concern for more than 3,000 years. It is perceived in many cultures as the symbol of womanhood and fertility. Alterations in size, shape, consistency, or function of the breast assume great importance to the patient and the society in general. Dysfunction of the organ results in a huge number of office visits, diagnostic studies, and surgeries. Breast cancer, as described by Rowland Grant nearly 25 years ago, "is the foremost of cancers, . . . the most fatal cancer in women in the United States and the most feared cancer, . . . the most self-discovered cancer, the cancer that has given rise to the largest number of articles in medical journals, etcetera." Virtually all women experience dysfunction of the organ that is the result of either primary or secondary pathology. One in eight women by the age of 85 years will bear the diagnosis of breast cancer. Subsequent chapters will deal with the biology of the breast and its pathologies, both benign and malignant.

REFERENCES

1. Mepham T (1983) Physiological aspects of lactation, In: Biochemistry of Lactation (McPhan T, ed.), Elsevier, New York, p. 3.
2. Peterson LV (1944) Lactation. Physiol Rev 24:340.
3. Riddle O, Bates R, Dykshorn S (1933) The preparation, identification and assay of prolactin-A hormone of the anterior pituitary. Am J Physiol 105:191.
4. Meites J, Turner C (1942) Studies concerning the mechanism controlling the initiation of lactation at parturition II: why lactation is not imitated during pregnancy. Endocrinology 30:719.
5. Clifton K, Furth J (1960) Ducto-alveolar growth in mammary glands of adreno- gonadectomized male rats bearing mammotropic pituitary tumors. Endocrinology 66:893.
6. Chen C, Meites J (1969) Effects of estrogen and progesterone on serum and pituitary levels in ovariectomized rats. Endocrinology 86:503.
7. Kuhn N (1969) Progesterone withdrawal as the lactogenic trigger in the rat. J Endocrinol 44:39.
8. Le Dran F (1757) Mémoire avec un précis de plusieurs observations sur le cancer. Mem Acad Chir, Paris 3:1–546.
9. Paget J (1856) On the average duration of life in patients with scirrhosus cancer of the breast. Lancet 1:62–63.
10. Halsted WS (1907) The results of radical operations for cure of cancer of the breast. Am Surg 46:1–19.
11. Cullen TS (1895) A rapid method of making permanent specimens from frozen sections by the use of formalin. Bull J Hopkins Hosp 6:67–73.
12. Chiari J, Braun C, Spaeth J (1855) Report of two cases of puerperal atrophy of the uterus with amenorrhea and persistent lactation, In: Klinik der Geburtshilfe and Gynaekologie, Erlangen, Enke, p 371.
13. Frommel R (1882) Ueber puerperale Atrophie des Uterus. Gynakologe 7:305.
14. Argonz J, DelCastille E (1953) A syndrome characterized by estrogenic insufficiency, galactorrhea and decreased urinary gonadotropins. J Clin Endocrinol Metab 13:79.
15. Ahumada J, DelCastillo E (1932) Amenorrhea/galactorrhea. Bol Soc Obstet Ginecol (Buenos Aires) 11:64.
16. Forbes A, Henneman P, Griswold G, Albright F (1954) Syndrome characterized by galactorrhea, amenorrhea and low urinary FSH: comparison with acromegaly and normal lactation. J Clin Endocrinol Metab 14:265.
17. Greenwood FC, Hunter WM (1963) The preparation of ^{131}I-labelled human growth hormone of high specific radioactivity. Biochem J 89:114.
18. Berson SA, Yalow RS, Bauman A, Rothschild MA, Newerly K (1956) Insulin -I^{131} metabolism in human subjects: demonstration of insulin binding globulin in the circulation of insulin treated subjects. J Clin Invest 35:170.
19. Hwang P, Guyda H, Friesen H (1971) A radioimmunoassay for human prolactin. Proc Natl Acad Sci USA 68:1902.
20. Guyda H, Hwang P, Friesen H (1971) Immunologic evidence for monkey and human prolactin. J Clin Endocrinol Metab 32:120.
21. Owerbach D, Rutter WJ, Cooke NE, et al. (1981) The prolactin gene is located on chromosome 6 in humans. Science 212:815–916.

22. Sinha YN (1995) Structural variants of prolactin. Occurrence and physiological significance. Endocr Rev 16:354.
23. Neill JD, Luque EH, Mulchahey JJ, Nagy G (1987) Regulation of prolactin secretion, In: Prolactin-Related Disorders (Blackwell RE, Chang RJ eds.), McMillan Healthcare Information, New York pp. 5–14.
24. Pellegrini I, Rasolonjanahary R, Gung G, et al. (1989) Resistance to bromocriptine in prolactinomas. J Clin Endocrinol Metab 60:500–501.
25. Gibbs OM, Neill JD (1978) Dopamine levels in hypophyseal stalk blood in the rat are sufficient to inhibit prolactin secretion in vitro. Endocrinology 102:1895.
26. Matsushita N, Kato Y, Shimatsu A, et al. (1983) Effects of VIP, TRH, GABA and dopamine on prolactin release from superfused rat anterior pituitary cells. Life Sci 32:1263.
27. Vale W, Blackwell R, Grant G, Guillemin R (1973) TRF and thyroid hormones on prolactin secretion by rat anterior pituitary cells *in vitro*. Endocrinology 93:26.
28. Hagen TC, Arnaout MA, Scherzer WJ, et al. (1986) Antisera to vasoactive intestinal polypeptide inhibit basal prolactin release from disbursed anterior pituitary cells. Neuroendocrinology 43:641.
29. Aguilera G, Hyde CL, Catt KJ (1987) Angiotensin-II receptors and prolactin release to pituitary lactotrophs. Endocrinology 111:1045.
30. Knigge U, Dejgaard A, Wollesen F et al. (1982) Histamine regulation of prolactin secretion through H_1-H_2-receptors. J Clin Endocrinol Metab 55:118.
31. Bergland R, Page R (1978) Can the pituitary secrete directly to the brain? (Affirmative anatomical evidence). Endocrinology 102:1325.
32. Blackwell RE, Rogers-Neame NT, Bradley EL, et al. (1986) Regulation of human prolactin secretion by gonadotropin releasing hormone in vitro. Fertil Steril 46:26.
33. Denef C, Andries M (1983) Evidence for paracrine interaction between gonadotrophs and lactotrophs in pituitary cell aggregates. Endocrinology 112:813.
34. Blackwell RE, Garrison PN (1987) Inhibition of prolactin secretion by antiserum to the alpha- and beta-subunits of gonadotropin. Am J Obstet Gynecol 156:863–868.
35. Blackwell RE (1988) Diagnosis and management of prolactinomas, In: Modern Trends in Infertility and Conception Control, vol. 4 (Wallach EE, and Kempers RD, eds.), Year Book Medical Publications, Chicago, pp. 197–208.
36. Yamamoto K, Saito K, Takai T, et al. (1983) Visual field defects and pituitary enlargement in primary hypothyroidism, J Clin Endocrinol Metab 67:283–287.
37. Blackwell RE, Boots LR, Goldenberg RL, et al. (1970) Assessment of pituitary function in patients with serum prolactin levels greater than 100 ng/ml. Fertil Steril 32:177.
38. Reincke M, Allolio B, Saeger W, et al. (1990) The 'incidentaloma' of the pituitary gland. Is neurosurgery required? JAMA 263:2772.
39. Newton DR, Witz S, Norman D, Newton TH (1983) Economic impact of CT scanning on the evaluation of pituitary adenomas, AJR 140:576.
40. Camanni F, Ghigo E, Ciccareli E, et al. (1983) Defective regulation of prolactin secretion after successful removal of prolactinomas. J Clin Endocrinol Metab 57:1270.
41. Ho PJ, Jaffe CA, Friberg RD, et al. (1994) Persistence of rapid growth hormone (GH) pulsatility after successful removal of GH-producing pituitary tumors. J Clin Endocrinol Metab 78:1403.
42. Genazzani AR, de leo V, Murru S, et al. (1982) Dynamic tests of prolactin secretion in hyperprolactinemic states: carbidopa-L-dopa and indirectly acting dopamine agonists. J Clin Endocrinol Metab 43:429.
43. Crosignani PG, Ferrari C, Malinverni A, et al. (1980) Effect of central nervous system dopaminergic activation on prolactin secretion in man: evidence for a common central defect in hyperprolactinemic patients with and without radiological signs of pituitary tumors. J Clin Endocrinol Metab 51:1068.
44. Ho KY, Smythe GA, Duncan M, et al. (1984) Dopamine infusion studies in patients with pathological hyperprolactinemia: evidence of normal prolactin suppressibility but abnormal dopamine metabolism. J Clin Endocrinol Metab 58:128.
45. Magoffin DA, Erickson GF (1982) Prolactin inhibition of LH stimulated androgen synthesis in ovarian interstitial cells cultured in defined medium: mechanism of action. Endocrinology 111:2001.
46. McNatty KP (1979) Relationship between plasma prolactin and the endocrine microenvironment of the developing human antral follicle. Fertil Steril 32:433.
47. Kauppila A, Martikainen H, Puistola U, et al. (1988) Hypoprolactinemia and ovarian function. Fertil Steril 49:437.
48. Lane TA, Chen TT (1991) Heterologous down-modulation of luteinizing hormone receptors by prolactin: a flow cytometry study. Endocrinology 128:1833.

49. Adashi EY, Resnick CE (1987) Prolactin as an inhibitor of granulosa cell luteinization: implications for hyperprolactinemia-associated luteal phase dysfunction. Fertil Steril 48:131.
50. Martikainen H, Ronnberg L, Puistola U, et al. (1989) Prolactin suppression by bromocriptine stimulates aromatization of testosterone to estradiol in women. Fertil Steril 52:51.
51. Matsuzaki T, Azuma K, Irabara M, et al. (1994) Mechanism of anovulation in hyperprolactinemic amenorrheic deficiencies by pulsatile gonadotropin-releasing hormone injection combined with hCG. Fertil Steril 62:1143.
52. Weiss MH, Teal J, Gott P, Wsycoff R, et al. (1983) Natural history of microprolactinomas: six year follow-up. Neurosurgery 12:180.
53. Klibanski A, Need RM, Bettins IZ, et al. (1980) Decreased bone density in hyperprolactinemic women. N Engl J Med 303:1511.
54. Molitch M, Elton R, Blackwell RE, et al., and the Bromocriptine Study Group (1985) Bromocriptine as primary therapy for prolactin secreting macroadenomas: results of a prospective multicenter study. J Clin Endocrinol Metab 60:698.
55. Faria MA, Tindall GT (1982) Transsphenoidal microsurgery for prolactin-secreting pituitary adenomas: results in 100 women with the amenorrhea-galactorrhea syndrome. J Neurosurg 56:33–43.
56. Serri O, Rasio E, Beauregard H, Hardy J, Somma M (1983) Recurrence of hyperprolactinemia after selective transsphenoidal adenomectomy in women with prolactinoma. N Engl J Med 309:280–283.
57. Barbiere RL, Ryan KJ (1983) Bromocriptine: endocrine pharmacology and therapeutic applications. Fertil Steril 39:72.
58. Soto-Albors CE, Walters CA, Riddick DH, Daly DC (1984) Titrating the dose of bromocriptine when treating hyperprolactinemic women. Fertil Steril 41:58.
59. Katz E, Weiss BE, Hassell A, et al. (1991) Increased circulating levels of bromocriptine after vaginal compared with oral administration. Fertil Steril 55:882.
60. Blackwell RE, Bradley EL Jr, Kline LB, et al, (1983) Comparison of dopamine agonists in the treatment of hyperprolactinemic syndromes: a multicenter study. Fertil Steril 39:744.
61. Lamberts SWJ, Quik RFP (1991) A comparison of the efficacy and safety of pergolide and bromocriptine in the treatment of hyperprolactinemia. J Clin Endocrinol Metab 72:635.
62. Vance ML, Cragun JR, Reimnitz C, et al. (1989) CV205-502 treatment of hyperprolactinemia. J Clin Endocrinol Metab 68:336.
63. Ferrari C, Barbieri C, Caldara R, et al. (1986) Long-lasting prolactin-lowering effect of cabergoline, a new dopamine agonist, in hyperprolactinemic patients. J Clin Endocrinol Metab 63:941.
64. Melis GB, Gambacciani M, Paoletti AM, et al. (1989) Reduction in the size of prolactin-producing pituitary tumor after cabergoline administration. Fertil Steril 52:412.
65. Kjelberg R, Kliman B (1979) Proton radiosurgery for functioning pituitary adenomas, In: Clinical Management of Pituitary Disorders (Tindall GE, Collins WF, eds.), Raven Press, New York, p. 315.
66. McKiernan J, Coyne J, Canglone S (1988) History of breast development in early life. Arch Dis Child 63:136.
67. Cowie AT (1978) Backward glances, In: Physiology of Mammary Glands (Yokoyama A, Mizuno H, Nagasawa H, eds.), University Park Press, Baltimore, p. 43.
68. Toneli G, Sorof S (1980) Epidermal growth factor: requirement for development of cultured mammary glands. Nature 285:250.
69. Ichimose R, Nandi S (1966) Influence of hormones on lobulo-alveolar differentiation of mouse mammary glands in vitro. J Endocrinol 35:331.
70. Cowie A, Tindal J, Yokoyama A (1966) The induction of mammary growth in the hypophysectomized goat. J Endocrinol 34:154.
71. Lyons WR (1958) Hormonal synergism in mammary growth. Proc R Soc Biol 149:303.
72. Going JJ, Anderson TJ, Battersby S, et al. (1988) Proliferative and secretory activity in human breast during natural and artificial menstrual cycles. Am J Pathol 130:193.
73. Talwalker P, Meites T (1961) Mammary lobulo-alveolar growth induced by anterior pituitary hormones in adreno-ovariectomized-hypophysectomized rats. Proc Soc Exp Biol Med 107:880.
74. France J, Seddon R, Liggins G (1973) A study of a pregnancy with low estrogen production due to placental sufatase deficiency. J Clin Endocrinol Metab 36:19.
75. Topper Y, Freeman C (1980) Multiple hormone interactions in the developmental biology of the mammary gland. Physiol Rev 60:1049.
76. Elias J (1959) Effect of insulin and cortisol on organ cultures of adult mouse mammary gland. Proc Soc Exp Biol Med 101:500.

77. Fleet J, Goode J, Harmon M, et al. (1975) Secretory activity of goat mammary glands during pregnancy and the onset of lactation. J Physiol (Lond) 251:763.
78. Vonderhaar BK (1977) Studies on the mechanism by which thyroid hormones enhance α-lactalbumin activity in explants from mouse mammary glands. Endocrinology 100:1423.
79. Martin R, Glass M, Wilson G, Woods K (1973) Human -lactalbumin and hormonal factors in pregnancy and lactation. Clin Endocrinol 13:323.
80. Hartmann P, Trevethan P, Shelton J (1973) Progesterone and oestrogen and the initiation of lactation in ewes. J Endocrinol 59:249.
81. Hearn J (19713) Pituitary inhibition of pregnancy. Nature 241:207.
82. Brun F, del Re R, del Pozo E, et al. (1973) Prolactin inhibition and suppression of puerperal lactation by a Br-ergocriptine (CB 154): a comparison with estrogen. Obstet Gynecol 41:884.
83. Gross B, Eastman C, Bowen C, McEldruff A (1979) Integrated concentration of prolactin in breast-feeding mothers. Aust N Z J Obstet Gynaecol 19:150.
84. Tyson J (1977) Nursing and prolactin secretion principal determinants in the mediation of puerperal infertility, In: Prolactin and Human Reproduction (Crosignani P, Robyn C, eds.), Academic Press, Orlando, FL, p. 97.
85. Lincoln O, Wakerley J (1974) Electrophysiological evidence for the activation of supraoptic neuronics during the release of oxytocin. J Physiol 242:533.
86. Rolland R, Lequin RM, Schellekens LA, De Jong FH (1975) The role of prolactin in the restoration of ovarian function during the early postpartum periods in the human female. I. A study during physiological lactation. Clin Endocrinol (Oxf) 4:15.
87. Rebar RW (1989) The breast and physiology of lactation, In: Maternal-Fetal Medicine: Principles and Practice (Creasy RK, Resnick R, eds.), WB Saunders, Philadelphia, p. 153.
88. Stern JM, Konner M, Herman TN, Reichlin S (1986), Nursing behavior, prolactin and postpartum amenorrhea during prolonged lactation in American and Kung mothers. Clin Endocrinol (Oxf) 15:247.
89. Rivera R, Kennedy KI, Oritz E, et al. (1988) Breast-feeding and the return to ovulation in Durango, Mexico, Fertil Steril 49:780.
90. Gray RH, Campbell OM, Zacur HA, et al. (1987) Postpartum return of ovarian activity in nonbrestfeeding women monitored by urinary assays. J Clin Endocrinol Metab 64:645.
91. Konner M, Worthman C (1980) Nursing frequency, gonadal function, and birth spacing among Kung hunter-gatherers, Science 207:788.

2

Interactions Between Estradiol and Progesterone in Normal Breast

Implications for Mammary Carcinogenesis

Geneviève Plu-Bureau, MD, PHD,
Philippe Touraine, MD, *and*
Pierre Mauvais-Jarvis, MD

INTRODUCTION

Breast cancer in developed countries represents the major cause of cancer mortality in women *(1)*, and the lifetime risk in the early 1990s is estimated to be 1:8 women *(2)*. Despite considerable therapeutic and screening efforts, no decrease in mortality has been observed over the last 10 years.

Breast cancer appears to be a multifactorial disease. Although the mechanisms of mammary carcinogenesis remain unclear, the role of hormonal factors appears essential. By the late 1970s, on the basis of both experimental animal and in vitro studies using human breast cells, it was commonly accepted that estrogen was the major hormonal determinant of breast pathology, whereas progesterone appeared to oppose the estrogen effects on the breast epithelial cells both locally at the breast level and centrally at the hypothalamic–pituitary level by its antigonadotropin effect *(3)*. Many controversies have arisen in the last few years about progesterone action in the breast *(3–6)*. They are related to the possibility that an unopposed estrogen effect due to a defect in progesterone secretion during the luteal phase might be a promoting factor in human breast cancer genesis. The fact that this hypothesis remains controversial is due to lack of knowledge on the antiestrogenic activity of progesterone and progestins in human breast cells. Whereas the information has been well documented for the endometrium *(7,8)*, only a few data are available regarding the human mammary gland. Difficulties in collecting normal breast tissue, unlike endometrial tissue, have drastically limited the studies of hormonal control on the normal human mammary gland.

Only a clear pathophysiologic understanding could lead to a efficient policy of hormonal breast cancer prevention and decrease in the mortality due to this cancer. This review is an attempt to collect available information about experimental data from animal, biochemical, and human studies, as well as epidemiologic data on estradiol and progesterone interactions in the normal breast.

From: *Contemporary Endocrinology: Endocrinology of Breast Cancer*
Edited by: A. Manni © Humana Press Inc., Totowa, NJ

EXPERIMENTAL DATA IN ANIMALS

Action of Estradiol and Progesterone

Experimentally, many indirect data suggest an antagonism between estradiol and progesterone at the level of breast tissue. Many investigators have shown that the mammary gland of different species responds differently to estrogens according to its administration either at physiologic or supraphysiologic doses or in combination with progesterone or alone *(9–12)*.

High doses of estrogen administered for a prolonged period to castrated female rats induce proliferation and dilatation of the lobules in the glandular tissue with formation of cysts and overgrowth of the epithelium *(13)*. Administration of estradiol to female rats results in a cascade of mammary alterations, i. e., proliferation of tubular system secretion, dilatation of ducts, formation of cysts, and fibrosis. These changes observed with supraphysiologic doses of estrogen could be related to human fibrocystic disease *(13,14)*. By contrast, when estradiol is administered in combination with progesterone, complete and proper development of the mammary gland with an extensive alveolar proliferation is observed provided the ratio between estrogen and progesterone is adequate *(9,10)*. Cowie et al. *(11)* found that a combination of estrogen and progesterone in castrated goats resulted in uniform development and secretion when the dose of estrogen remained low (0.25 mg/d). This suggests that the existence of a harmonious ovarian cycle function is important for perfect mammary development. A coherent organization of both the ductal system and the adjacent connective tissue depends on the monthly occurrence of a corpus luteum secreting a proper amount of progesterone for a sufficient period of time *(13)*.

Which ovarian steroids stimulate normal human mammary epithelial cell proliferation is an important issue that can be addressed using the athymic nude mice model. McManus and Welsch *(15)* and more recently Laidlaw et al. *(16)* have analyzed the effects of estradiol and progesterone on normal human breast tissue implanted into athymic nude mice. They showed that estradiol appears to be sufficient to stimulate human breast epithelial cell proliferation at physiologically relevant concentrations and that progesterone does not affect proliferation either alone or after estradiol priming. They also demonstrated a dose-response relationship between proliferation and serum estradiol concentrations. Longman and Buehring *(17)* showed that progesterone or progestins when added alone did not stimulate cell growth in explants of normal mammary tissue. When added to ethinylestradiol, progestins slow down cell growth.

Experimental Mammary Carcinogenesis

Hormone-dependent mammary tumors can be induced in animal models (in particular, rodents) by chemical carcinogens or radiation *(8)*. The protective action of progesterone against the carcinogenic induction of mammary tumors was first shown by Segaloff et al. *(18)* in an interesting experiment on estrogen- and X-ray-induced mammary carcinogenesis in female rats. The continuous administration of progesterone protected these animals from the synergism between estrogen and radiation. In addition, it also appeared that progesterone had an overall protective effect against the individual carcinogenic agents, since fewer tumors occurred on the opposite side as well as on the radiated side.

In the same way, Grubbs et al. *(19)* have clearly demonstrated that stimulation of the mammary gland to a highly differentiated state early in life can provide protection against future carcinogen exposure. In the Sprague-Dawley rat model the authors administered immediately after puberty either nitromethylurea (NMU) alone, or estradiol or progesterone, or both, followed by NMU exposure, to determine whether prevention of NMU-induced tumors was possible. They showed that pretreatment of rats with 17β-estradiol and progesterone resulted in 88% reduction in cancer incidence.

In these different experiments the protective effect of progesterone against various carcinogens was dependent on the time of administration relative to the carcinogen and was generally related to stimulation by progesterone of terminal duct differentiation, thus protecting lobuloalveolar glands from carcinogens *(20)*.

BIOCHEMICAL DATA

Synergistic Action of Estradiol and Progesterone

In most target cells of the female genital tract, cell differentiation involves the successive and synergistic action of estradiol and progesterone. It is now well established that estrogen priming increases progesterone receptor (PR) titers in the target cell. Estrogenic induction of progesterone receptor synthesis would seem to provide a basis for the priming effect of estrogen in the preparation of the target cell for subsequent progesterone action. The increase of PR synthesis by estrogen action involves the stimulation of RNA and protein synthesis, and this response seems to be regulated by the estradiol receptor (ER) system *(21)*. These different sequences in receptor synthesis and inactivation first primed by estradiol have been essentially observed in the uterus of cycling animals and also in women. In the breast, the presence of PR has been demonstrated in human mammary tumors, and it has been proposed that these receptors might serve as markers of estrogen action in breast cancer *(22)*. However, a few data suggest that estradiol and progesterone act synergistically in the normal breast. Estradiol is the hormone initially responsible for the differentiation and development of the ductal epithelium, increasing mitotic activity of the cylindral cells of the internal layer of the ducts. Progesterone acts synergistically with estrogens on the distal part of the duct, enabling differentiation into acini. Generally, in those species in which the cycle consists mainly of a follicular phase, the mammary gland primarily contains a ductal system. Well-developed alveoli, on the other hand, are found for the most part only in species that have a definite luteal phase.

Recently, the genes coding for the receptors for both the estrogen *(23)* and the progesterone receptors *(24)* have been mutated by knockout. In both cases, mice were sterile, and the inability to support pregnancy made it impossible to investigate the role of these hormone receptors in mammary development. However, the role of the PR in mammary gland development has been investigated by chronic treatment of the mice bearing the PR knockout (PRKO), with estrogen and progesterone. Treatment of wild-type mice with these hormones caused stimulation of ductal growth and lobuloalveolar development. PRKO mice exhibited a significant reduction in ductal branching and a failure in lobuloalveolar differentiation. Moreover, it has been shown that wild-type mammary epithelia grew in the presence of PRKO stroma and vice versa *(25)*.

These experiments demonstrate that progesterone is important for mammary stromal regulation of ductal development and that the PR is required for alveolar development.

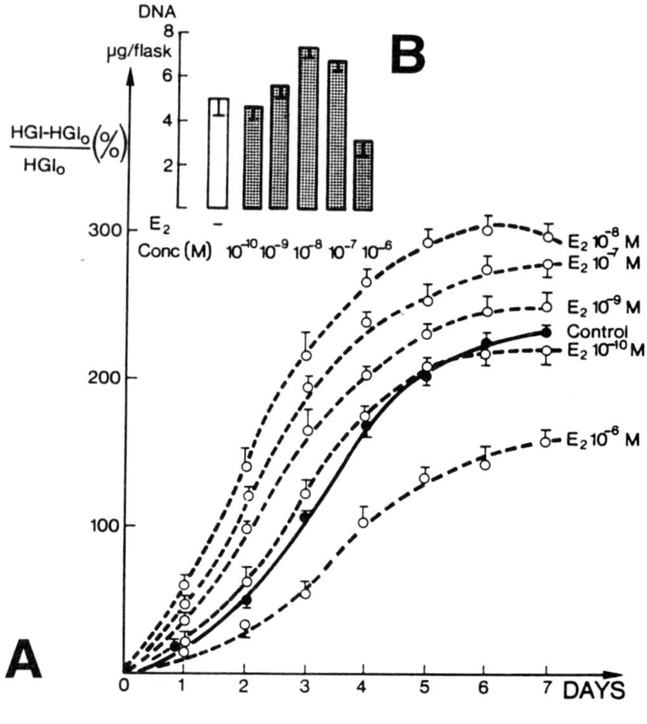

Fig. 1. a: Stimulatory dose-dependent effect of estradiol (E2) on the growth of normal human breast epithelial cells in secondary culture. The study of cell growth was based on daily cell counting and determination of a histometric growth index (HGI). The results are expressed as percentage increase in HGI compared with the value on day 0 (HGI_0). **b:** DNA values on day 7 (mean of triplicate flasks; bars, SD) (From ref. *26*, with permission.)

Antiestrogen Action of Progesterone in Normal Human Breast Epithelial Cells

In our laboratory, we routinely obtain cultures of normal human breast cells established from samples obtained during reductive mammoplasty. In these cultures, it is possible to conduct separate studies of epithelial cells and fibroblasts. Ultrastructural characteristics of normal human breast epithelial (HBE) cells have been examined by scanning (SEM) and transmission (TEM) electron microscopy. Under SEM, cells exhibit a homogeneous pattern: they are large, polygonal, and flattened. Microvilli are short and rare. Following estradiol treatment, cells appear young and show extensive protrusions with numerous bunches. Microvilli increase markedly in number and density, indicating intense replicative activity. However, the addition of progestin promegestone (R5020) causes the cell to appear flattened; they are similar to control cells with sparse microvilli. Parallel TEM reveals an extensive Golgi apparatus and secretory activity under R5020 treatment.

Growth of these HBE cells was evaluated using daily cell counting and DNA assay. Growth was stimulated by estradiol in a dose-dependent manner and inhibited by the progestin R5020, also in a dose-dependent manner (Figs. 1 and 2). Progesterone itself inhibits cell growth. [^{3}H]Thymidine incorporation after 4 d of treatment was higher following estradiol treatment than in control cells. Incorporation decreased when either

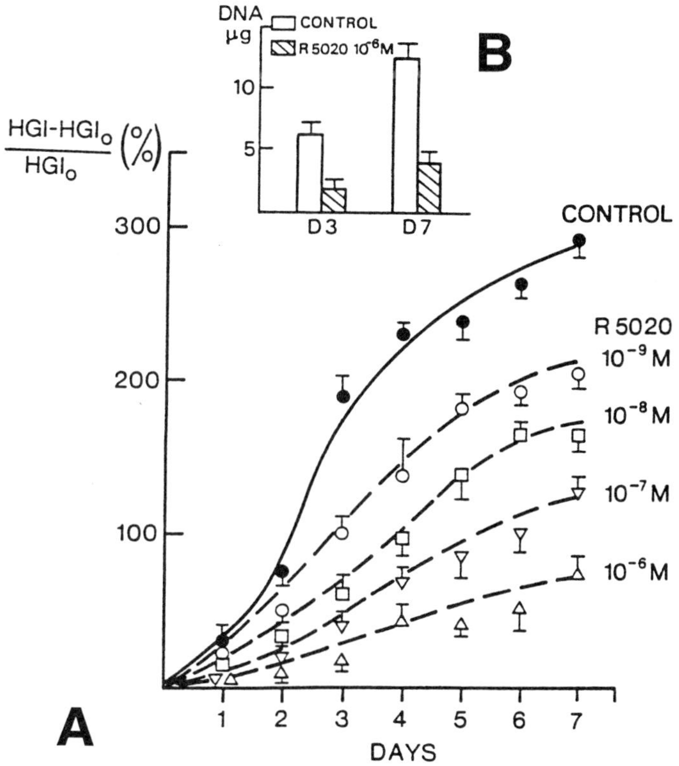

Fig. 2. a: Inhibitory effect of the progestin promegestone (R5020) on the growth of normal HBE cells in culture. The study of cell growth was based on daily cell counting and determination of a histometric growth index (HGI). The results are expressed as percentage HGI compared with the value on day 0 (HGI_0). **b:** DNA values on day 3 and 7 in control cell cultures (no hormone addition) and cells cultured in the presence of R5020 (10^{-6} mol/L) (mean ± SD of determinations in triplicate flasks). (From ref. *26*, with permission.)

progesterone or R5020 was added to estradiol in a dose-dependent manner. The action of the antiprogesterone RU486 was also studied in HBE cells. It is interesting to note that RU486 also has an inhibitory effect on cell growth but to a lesser extent than R5020, thus exhibiting a potential progesterone agonistic effect *(26)*.

On the other hand, Musgrove et al. *(27)* have performed in vitro studies demonstrating that cancerous breast cells in the late phase of cell cycle activity are initially driven to the S phase of DNA synthesis by progestins. This effect is transient, and further application of progestins suppresses the cycling and then halting the breast cell division in early G_1 phase.

Mechanisms of Estradiol and Progesterone Antagonism in Normal Human Breast Cells

Two mechanisms underlying the progesterone regulation of estradiol action have been characterized in fibroadenomas and normal HBE: (1) progesterone stimulates the enzyme 17β-dehydrogenase (E2DH), which converts estradiol, the active estrogen, into estrone, its less active metabolite *(28)*; and (2) progesterone decreases the ER content.

E2DH Activity

This was measured as the production of estrone by cells incubated with [^{3}H]estradiol. E2DH activity was high and stimulated by progestins in epithelial cells but low and not stimulated by progesterone in fibroblasts. Consequently, E2DH was proposed as a marker of epithelial cells, of progesterone dependency, and also of PR operativity. In HBE cells, progestin treatment lowered DNA content and stimulated E2DH activity. It thus slows down cell multiplication while favoring cell differentiation.

Steroid Receptors

Most effects of estrogens and progestins are mediated via intracellular proteins; the classical model for the interaction of these two classes of hormones is that estrogens increase both ER and PR and thereby increase sensitivity to progestins. Progestins downregulate both PR and ER. However, even if this model is applicable to breast tumors, data concerning the normal breast are sometimes less obvious *(29)*. Early reports, based on limited sample numbers, indicated more ER and PR *(30)* in the first half of the menstrual cycle, whereas little change seems to occur for PR through the menstrual cycle *(31)*. Indirect information of the cyclic changes in the content of ER and PR was obtained in our laboratory from studies of fibroadenomas removed in young women at different times of the menstrual cycle. In these tumors, cyclic changes in the distribution of cytosolic and nuclear receptors—ER and PR—are very similar to those noted in the human endometrium *(7)*. Indeed, during the follicular phase, the increase of ovarian secretion seems to be responsible for a progressive increase in the ER content since estradiol stimulates synthesis of its own receptor *(32)*. During the luteal phase, the decrease of ER probably reflects the action of the secreted progesterone since progesterone is known to inhibit ER synthesis. Moreover, variations in PR give valuable information on the hormone dependency of PR. The decrease of PR during the luteal phase probably reflects the inhibition by progesterone of its own receptor. Finally, the moderate increase of PR at the end of the luteal phase might be explained either by the decrease of progesterone levels at this stage of the menstrual cycle or by the insufficient progesterone levels frequently observed in patients with fibroadenomas and luteal insufficiency *(33)*. Indeed, correction of luteal insufficiency in patients with fibroadenomas induces a translocation of the PR from cytosol to nucleus, which is more important than what is noted in fibroadenomas removed during the luteal phase.

ER and PR studies are more difficult in cultured normal breast epithelial cells, owing to their lower levels compared with cancer cells. Large number of cells are therefore required when using the classical biochemical methods for receptor assay. However, immunocytochemical studies using monoclonal antibodies have enabled the characterization of ER and PR in these cells. Immunostaining specific for ER has been observed in epithelial cells; it is nuclear and varies from cell to cell in positivity and intensity. Moreover, it is enhanced in estradiol-treated cells and decreases after addition of the progestin R5020. PR was also detected with monoclonal antibodies *(34)*. It is also hormone modulated—increased by estradiol exposure and decreased by R5020.

Therefore, in normal HBE cells, E2 stimulates both its own receptor and PR, whereas the progestin R5020 lowers the number of both ER and PR (Table 1). ER and PR are also present in fibroblasts, but at a lower level than in epithelial cells, and they are only weakly hormone dependent.

Table 1
Variations in Estrogen Receptor Immunostaining in Human Breast Epithelial Cells[a]

Estrogen receptor immunostaining (% of7 stained cells)	*Positive (%)*	*Negative (%)*	*Intensity of staining*
Control	55	45	++
Estradiol	73	27	+++
Estradiol plus R5020	44	56	++
R5020	35	65	+

[a]Cells were cultured for 8 days in the absence of steroids (control) or in the presence of estradiol (10^{-8} mol/L) or estradiol (10^{-8} mol/L) + R5020 (10^{-7} mol/L) alone.

(Reproduced with permission from ref. *34*).

Finally, epithelial cell expression of receptors other than those for steroids also varies throughout the cycle. For example, epidermal growth factor receptors are more highly expressed in the luteal phase compared with the follicular phase *(35)*, also suggesting a hormonal dependency of such receptors.

C-*MYC* PROTO-ONCOGENE EXPRESSION IN HBE CELLS

In breast cancer cell lines, the stimulatory effect of estradiol on cell growth can partly operate through the stimulation of proto-oncogene expression *(36)* and growth factor production. The proto-oncogene c-*myc* is involved in the stimulation of cell replication and can itself be stimulated by numerous mitogens including estradiol. Estradiol stimulation of c-*myc* was demonstrated in human breast cancer cell lines and also in noncancerous estradiol-dependent target tissues *(37)*. By contrast, progestins and triphenylethynelic antiestrogens inhibit c-*myc* expression *(38)*. We have demonstrated that E2 stimulates at both the molecular and the proteic level the expression of *c-myc* in HBE cells. Early stimulation of mRNA occurred 30 min after estradiol treatment followed by later stimulation after 2 h *(39)*. By immunocytochemistry, expression of the protein appears to be exclusively nuclear and heterogeneous, and the intensity of staining varies from cell to cell. In addition, c-*myc* expression is hormone modulated: the number of positive cells and the intensity of staining increase following estradiol treatment and decrease after addition of R5020 to estradiol *(40)*.

HUMAN STUDIES

Histologic Findings Associated with Endogenous Hormones

Histologic findings in vivo are important to discern changes in breast structure and function during the menstrual cycle that could predispose to malignant changes. Several groups have used the uptake of tritiated thymidine (^{3}HTdR) for calculating a thymidine labeling index as a measure of the proliferative activity of the normal breast tissue at different times of the human cycle in women undergoing breast surgery *(13,41–46)*.

In some studies *(13,43)* the mitotic activity of breast epithelial cells was reported to be higher during the follicular than during the luteal phase in normal cycling women, whereas other authors have shown a peak of mitotic activity of epithelial cells and DNA synthesis in the late luteal phase *(41,42,44–46)*. As this period of the menstrual cycle immediately follows the peaks of secretion of both progesterone and estrogen, these authors inferred that progesterone is involved in the promotion of breast epithelial cell mitoses, in contrast to the well-documented antiproliferative effect of progesterone on the endometrium *(8)*. However, this hypothesis remains to be confirmed as the exact timing of the biopsy within the menstrual cycle was sometimes questionable. In addition, several authors argue that breast cells would react to the cumulative effect of estrogens and progesterone secreted over several cycles rather than to the daily change in hormonal production *(47,48)*.

The recent development of monoclonal antibodies against specific cell proliferation marker antigens has also made possible a measurement of proliferation in cytologic breast cell samples. Three recent studies have shown the feasibility of mammary fine-needle aspiration biopsy in healthy women *(49–51)*. The study by Söderqvist et al. *(51)* analyzed proliferation of breast epithelial cells in healthy women during the menstrual cycle. Late luteal phase was associated with high mitotic activity of epithelial cells compared with early follicular phase. Furthermore, the putative specific role of progesterone, mainly based on a temporal relationship, could not be separated from a possible cumulative effect of estrogen. Hence, the selection of the different times for mammary needle aspiration appears to be determinant for interpreting data on breast epithelial cells in healthy women during the menstrual cycle.

Histological Findings with Exogenous Hormones

Interesting results on the interaction and effects of estradiol and progesterone on breast cell multiplication have recently been obtained in vivo *(52,53)*. Women undergoing surgery for benign breast disease were randomly treated with either estradiol or progesterone or a placebo, applied locally to the breast between day 11 and 13 of the follicular phase of the menstrual cycle prior to surgery. The number of mitoses in the epithelial cells of the normal part of the breast was counted. After estradiol treatment, both estradiol concentration in breast and the number of mitoses were high (0.83/1000 cells). After progesterone administration, progesterone concentration in breast tissue was high, but the number of mitoses was low (0.17/1000 cells). In the placebo group, the number of mitoses was low (0.5/1000 cells). The authors concluded that in vivo high intratissular concentrations of progesterone were able to decrease the mitotic activity of the normal lobular epithelial cells.

EPIDEMIOLOGIC DATA

Hormonal Risk Factors

Hormonal risk factors for breast cancer have been extensively studied in the past 20 years *(54,55)*. Nulliparity, early age at menarche, late age at first full-term pregnancy, and late age at menopause have been shown for many years to be associated with an increased risk of breast cancer. The results concerning the different characteristics of the menstrual cycle remain more controversial.

One finding reported quite consistently in recent studies is that a shorter menstrual cycle length over the age range 20–39 years is associated with an increased risk *(56–59)*. In a case-control study, we found that a previous history of cyclical mastalgia was associated with an increased risk of breast cancer *(60)*. Table 2 shows that cyclical mastalgia was associated with a twofold increase of relative risk, with a symptom-duration effect. In the same way, severe pain was found to be associated with a higher risk of breast cancer *(61)*. Olsson et al. reported that the number of menstrual cycles prior to the first full-term

Table 2
Association Between Duration of Cyclical Mastalgia (CM) and Risk of Breast Cancer[a]

	Cases, n *(%)*	*Controls,* n *(%)*	*Adjusted RR (95% CI)*
Cumulative duration of CM (months)			
<6	113 (54)	161 (77)	1.00
6–48	36 (17)	32 (15)	1.12 (0.61–2.05)
49–96	16 (8)	6 (3)	2.24 (0.77–6.52)
97+	45 (21)	11 (5)	5.54 (2.79–13.39)
p value[b]			<0.0001

*A*Abbreviations: RR, Relative risk of breast cancer adjusted on age, age at first full-term pregnancy, familial history of breast cancer, oral contraceptive use, history of benign breast disease and age at menarche; 95% CI, 95% confidence interval.

[b]p value for significant trend.

(From ref. *60*, with permission)

pregnancy may be particularly important. In 1980, Korenman *(62)* suggested that anovulatory menstrual cycles associated with estrogen unopposed by progesterone and with infertility increased the woman's risk of breast cancer.

These findings could be explain in two ways. For some authors *(3,62)*, these characteristics of the menstrual cycle associated with increased risk of breast cancer represent a situation of estrogen–progesterone imbalance leading to an "unopposed estrogen effect." Progesterone appeared to oppose the estrogen effects on the breast epithelial cells. Based on this rationale, some clinicians, at least in our country, propose progestin treatment for various benign breast diseases and menstrual disorders. Other authors consider that progesterone acts synergistically with estrogens *(4)*. Hence, the cumulative number of ovulatory menstrual cycles may represent an important etiologic factor, and some epidemiologic hormonal risk factors for breast cancer could be explained by this "estrogen augmented by progestogen" hypothesis.

Role of Exogenous Hormones on Breast Cancer Risk

Oral Contraception

The evaluation of carcinologic risks associated with various types of oral contraceptives remains unclear, because of the constant evolution of composition and dosages in estrogen and progestogen of pills. Since the introduction of oral contraceptives 30 years ago, numerous epidemiologic studies have analyzed the association between oral contraceptives and breast cancer risk *(63)*. The recent meta-analysis of the Collaborative Group on Hormonal Factors in Breast Cancer provides a large dataset *(64)*. Original data from 54 studies representing about 90% of the published epidemiologic studies were reanalyzed. The main finding was that a small increase in breast cancer risk was diagnosed in current users of combined oral contraceptives and in women who stopped use in the past 10 years. There was no evidence of an increase in risk more than 10 years after stopping use. In addition, the cancers diagnosed in women who had used oral contraceptives are less advanced clinically than the cancers diagnosed in women who had not used them.

No modification of breast cancer risk was associated with the use of progestin-only contraceptive pills or with any progestin amounts contained in combined estro-progestin pills.

Hormonal Replacement Therapy

Many epidemiologic studies have also been conducted to analyze the association between hormonal replacement therapy (HRT) and breast cancer risk. Several meta-analyses *(65–68)* have shown an increased risk *(30%)* in long-term users (5–10 years). This result essentially concerns estrogen-alone use. Few studies have focused on combined estro-progestin HRT. This relates to the recent coprescription of progestins with estrogens for menopausal therapy, especially in the United States, where most of the large epidemiologic studies were conducted. Table 3 shows the results of the main studies concerning combined HRT and breast cancer risk. The three most recent studies showed contradictory results. In the Nurses Health Cohort Study *(69)*, which involved 70,000 women followed for up to 16 years, the relative risk (RR) of breast cancer was significantly increased among women who were current users of estrogens (RR 1.32; 95% confidence limit [CI] 1.14–1.54) or of combined estrogens and progestins (RR 1.41; CI 1.15–1.74). No difference was observed between the two groups using either estrogens alone or combined HRT. The main finding was related to an earlier appearance of risk, after only 5 years of use of HRT. In the two population-based control studies published shortly after the Nurses Health Study, no increase in risk of any group of HRT users with long-term use was observed *(70,71)*. Stanford et al. *(71)* also reported a significant reduction in risk for long-term users of combined HRT.

These conflicting data have resulted in an active controversy as to whether progestins should be added to estrogens in HRT and especially whether hysterectomized women would need progestins *(47)*.

Progestogen Use

Except for medroxyprogesterone acetate used as a long-acting contraception and for progestin-only contraceptive pills, no study has directly addressed the potentially harmful or beneficial effect of progestin treatment on breast cancer risk. The term *progestogens* designates a large family of molecules characterized by their affinity for the progesterone receptors but with various binding capacities to androgen receptors and different metabolisms *(72,73)*. This implies that they should be considered distinct, yet related, therapeutic agents. Considering the widespread use of progestins in France, this was an important health issue. Women with benign breast disease were clearly a perfect target, considering their higher incidence of breast cancer. Indeed, any design including a minimum of events to be conclusive as well as a 10-year follow-up was not common at this time in this field. It was also clear that the ideal design would be a randomized trial. Therefore an analytical epidemiologic approach was chosen. We have conducted a cohort study of 1150 premenopausal French women who had benign breast disease, with a follow-up of 10 years *(74)*. Table 4 shows the main results. Neither overall progestogen use nor the duration of use was found to be significantly associated with breast cancer risk. When progestogens were classified into two categories according to their hormonal potency (19-nortestosterone derivatives vs. other progestogens), 19-nortestosterone derivative use was found to be significantly associated with a lower risk of breast cancer (RR 0.48; 95% CI 0.25–0.90). In addition, there was a linear trend in the decrease of the RR of breast cancer with duration of use. These results do not support the hypothesis that

Table 3
Relative Risk Estimates of Breast Cancer in Relation to Combined Hormone Replacement Therapy (HRT)

Author	*Country*	*Study design*	*Number of women*	*Relative risk (95% CI)*
Gambrell, 1983	USA	Cohort	48,669 person-years	0.3 (0,1–0.8)
Ewertz, 1988	Denmark	Case-control	834 cases 786 controls	1.4 (1.0–1.9)
Bergkvist, 1989	Sweden	Cohort	23,244	0.5 (0.2–1.8) duration <6 months 0.7 (0.3–1.3) duration 7–36 months 0.9 (0.3–2.6) duration 37–72 months 4.4 (0.9–22.4) duration >72 months
Kaufman, 1991	USA	Case-control	1,686 cases 2,077 controls	1.7 (0.9–3.6)
Palmer, 1991	Canada	Case-control	607 cases 1,214 controls	0.6 (0.2–1.9)
Nachtigall, 1992	USA	Random study	168	No breast cancer in HRT users
Yang, 1992	Canada	Case-control	452 cases 451 controls	1.2 (0.6–2.2)
Colditz et al., 1995 *(69)*	USA	Cohort	28,946 person-years	1.4 (1.1–1.7) current users
Stanford et al., 1995 *(71)*	USA	Case-control	526 cases 480 controls	0.4 (0.2–1.0) duration ≥8 years
Newcomb et al., 1995 *(70)*	USA	Case-control	3,130 cases 3,698 controls	1.0 (0.8–1.3)

Table 4
Relative Risk of Breast Cancer (RR)
Associated with the Cumulative Duration of Progestogen Use

Duration of progestogen use, months	*Group size*	*Number of breast cancer*	*RR*[a]	*95% CI (p trend)*[b]
All categories of progestogens				
0	384	20	1.00[c]	
1–36	435	15	0.82	0.42–1.63
37–72	124	4	0.52	0.17–1.54
73+	207	5	0.49	0.18–1.39 (0.11)
Ever use: yes	766	24	0.68	0.37–1.25
19-Nortestosterone derivatives				
0	551	29	1.00[c]	
1–36	363	10	0.57	0.28–1.18
37–72	101	3	0.43	0.13–1.45
73+	135	2	0.27	0.06–1.17 (0.02)
Ever use: yes	599	15	0.48	0.25–0.90
Other progestogens				
0	677	28	1.00[c]	
1–36	377	13	1.20	0.61–2.38
37–72	69	2	0.71	0.17–3.05
73+	27	1	0.93	0.12–7.04 (0.96)
Ever use: yes	473	16	1.14	0.60–2.15

[a]RR, relative risk calculated with the Cox model, adjusted on socioeconomic status, age at menarche, family history of breast cancer in first-degree relatives, type of benign breast disease, oral contraceptive use and change, in menopausal status during the follow-up period. Age and progestogen use are time-varying covariables.

[b]χ^2 for trend.

[c]Reference category.

(From ref. *74*, with permission)

progestogens might increase breast cancer risk. They suggest instead that high doses of 19-nortestosterone derivatives may have a beneficial effect on the risk of breast cancer in women with benign breast disease.

CARCINOGENESIS MODELING

Considering all these data on the effects of estrogen and progesterone on the mammary gland, speculations about their respective roles in the process of carcinogenesis may be attempted. The theoretical model of Moolgavkar and the experimental one of Russo are interesting from this perspective.

Moolgavkar Model

Moolgavkar's model for carcinogenesis *(75)* considers two steps in the evolution of normal cells to cancer cells. A normal cell has two possibilities: either it divides into new cells or it undergoes maturation, differentiation, and finally cell death. However, if the normal cell is exposed to an initiator of carcinogenesis, it can evolve into an "intermediate" (precancerous) cell.

"Intermediate" cells in turn can also undergo division or differentiation and cell death. In this model, if a second process of initiation occurs at this stage of intermediate cell, the cell definitively evolves into a cancerous cell. Cell division is a vulnerable phase as the cells are highly exposed to replication errors, oncogene activation, and intervention of exogenous carcinogens. It is speculated that estrogens, by stimulating cell multiplication, would increase the risk of replication errors, thus acting as carcinogenesis promoters, whereas progesterone and progestins, by orienting cells toward maturation, would exclude them from the pool of vulnerable dividing cells. In this model, under the previous speculations, any endogenous or exogenous situation of estrogen–progesterone imbalance favoring an "unopposed estrogen effect" should be avoided and/or corrected.

Russo Model

The model of Russo emphasizes the importance of differentiation of breast cells for mammary carcinogenesis. Experimental animal model studies provided evidence (1) that chemical carcinogens were causative agents of mammary cancer, (2) that the initiation of the disease required the interaction of the carcinogen with an undifferentiated and highly proliferating mammary gland, and (3) that first full-term pregnancy protected the mammary gland from chemically induced neoplastic transformation through the induction of differentiation *(76, 77)*. These findings indicate that the susceptibility of the breast to undergo malignant transformation is influenced by its stage of development and differentiation and its proliferative activity. Russo has performed a detailed classification of the lobular development that allowed estimation of the risk of malignant transformation according to lobular type. Hence a trend to a higher proliferative activity in lobules with a higher risk of malignant transformation was observed during the follicular phase of the menstrual cycle in comparison with the activity during the luteal phase. These results are consistent with the Laidlaw experiment *(16)*, which demonstrated that human breast tissue transplanted to nude mice receiving physiologic doses of estrogens displayed an increase in cell proliferation.

The protection afforded by early first full-term pregnancy in women could be explained by the higher degree of differentiation of the mammary gland when a carcinogenic agent might operate. These two findings (that cell proliferation is important for breast cancer initiation, whereas differentiation is a powerful inhibitor), should provide novel tools for developing rational strategies for breast cancer prevention.

SUMMARY

In most target cells of the female genital tract, adequate cell differentiation is obtained via the successive and synergistic actions of estradiol and progesterone. This is primarily because PR synthesis involves the prior action of estradiol via its receptor (ER). In normal breast, estradiol stimulates the growth of the ductal system, whereas lobular development depends on progesterone secretion. In other words estradiol plus progesterone, when secreted in an adequate balance, permit the complete and proper development of the mammary gland. On the other hand, progesterone may also have an antagonistic action against estradiol. The antiestrogen activity of progesterone is mediated through a decrease in the replenishment of ER along with the synthesis of 17β-hydroxysteroid dehydrogenase, which leads to accelerated metabolism of estradiol to estrone in the target organ itself. These biochemical events, well documented in the endometrium, have been shown in cultures of normal breast epithelial cells as well as in differentiated fibroadenomas with high cellular density. In addition, data from the literature show that estradiol added to human breast cells increases cell multiplication, possibly because of the synthesis of growth factors. Progesterone and progestins have opposite effects to estrogen. Data from our laboratory indicate that in normal cultured cells, estradiol and progesterone are likewise antagonistic with regard to cell multiplication. Based on these different data, it is inferred that in human beings, long periods of luteal phase defect leading to an unopposed estrogen effect might be a promoter agent involved in breast carcinogenesis.

REFERENCES

1. Kelsey JL, Horn-Ross PL (1993) Breast cancer: magnitude of the problem and descriptive epidemiology. Epidemiol Rev 15:7–16.
2. Feuer EJ, Wum LM, Boring CC, Flanders WD, Timmel MJ, Tong T (1993) The lifetime risk of developing breast cancer. J Natl Cancer Inst 85:892–897.
3. Mauvais-Jarvis P, Kuttenn F, Gompel A (1986) Antiestrogen action of progesterone in breast tissue. Breast Cancer Res Treat 8:179–187.
4. Key TJA, Pike MC (1988) The role of oestrogens and progestogens in the epidemiology and prevention of breast cancer. Eur J Cancer Clin Oncol 24:29–43.
5. Stanford JL, Thomas DB (1993) Exogenous progestins and breast cancer. Epidemiol Rev 15:98–107.
6. Wren BG, Eden JA (1996) Do progestogens reduce the risk of breast cancer? A review of the evidence. Menopause 1:4–12.
7. Bayard F, Damilano S, Robel P and Baulieu EE (1978) Cytoplasmic and nuclear estradiol and progesterone receptors in human endometrium. J Clin Endocrinol Metab 46:635–648.
8. Clarke CL, Sutherland RL (1990) Progestin regulation of cellular proliferation. Endocr Rev 2:266–301.
9. Eisen MJ (1932) The occurrence of benign and malignant mammary lesions in rats treated with crystalline estrogen. Cancer Res 2:632–644.
10. Lyons WR, McGinty DA (1941) Effects of estrone and progesterone on male rabbit mammary glands. 1. Variing doses of progesterone. Proc Soc Exp Biol Med 48:83–89.
11. Cowie AT, Folley ST, Malpress FH, Richardson KC (1952) Studies on the hormonal induction of mammary growth and lactation in the goat. J Endocrnol 8:64–88.
12. Asselin J, Kelly PA, Caron MG, Labrie F (1977) Control of hormone recpetor levels and growth of 7,12-dimethyl benz(a)anthracene induced mammary tumors by estrogens, progesterones and prolactin. Endocrinology 101:692–697.
13. Bassler R (1970) The morphology of hormone induced structural changes in female breast. Curr Top Pathol 53:1–89.
14. Asboe-Hansen G (1958) Hormonal effects on connective tissue. Physiot Rev 38:446–462.
15. McManus MJ, Welsch CW (1984) The effects of estrogen, progesterone, and human placental lactogen on DNA synthesis on human breast ductal epithelium ùaintained in athymic mice. Cancer 54:1920–1927.
16. Laidlaw IJ, Clarke RB, Howell A, Owen AW, Potten CS, Anderson E (1995) The proliferation of normal human breast tissue implanted into athymic nude mice is stimulated by estrogen but not progesterone. Endocrinology 136:164–171.
17. Longman SM, Buehring GC (1987) Oral contraceptives and breast cancer. *In vitro* effect of contraceptive steroids on human mammary cell growth. Cancer 59:281–287.
18. Segaloff A (1973) Inhibition by progesterone of radiation-estrogen-induced mammary cancer in rat. Cancer Res 33:1136–1137.
19. Grubbs CJ, Farnell DR, Hill DL, McDonough KC (1985) Chemoprevention of N, Nitroso-N-methyl urea induced mammary cancers by pretreatment with 17 β-estradiol and progesterone. J Nat Cancer Inst 74:927–931.
20. Russo J, Tay LK, Russo IH (1982) Differentiation of the mammary gland and susceptibility to carcinogenesis. Breast Cancer Res Treat 2:5–73.

21. Leavitt WW, Chen TJ, Do YS, Carklton BD, Allen TC (1978) Biology of progesterone receptors, In: *Receptors and Hormone Action II* (O'Malley BW, Birnbaumer L, eds.), New York Acad. Press, NY, pp. 157–188.
22. McGuire WL, Chamnes GC, Horwitz KB and Zava DT (1978) Hormones and their receptors in breast cancer In: *Receptors and Hormone Action II* (O'Malley BW, Birnbaumer L, eds.), Academic Press, New York, pp. 401–441.
23. Lubahn DB, Moyer JS, Golding TS, Couse JF, Korach KS, Smithies O (1993) Alteration of reproductive function but not prenatal sexual development after insertional disruption of the mouse estrogen receptor gene. Proc Natl Acad Sci USA 90:11162–11166.
24. Lydon JP, DeMayo FJ, Funk CR, Mani SK, Hughes AR, Montgomery CA Jr, et al. (1995) Mice lacking progesterone receptor exhibit pleiotropic reproductive abnormalities. Genes Dev 9:2266–2278.
25. Humphreys RC, Lydon JP, O'Malley BW, Rosen JM (1997) Mammary gland development is mediated by both stromal and epithelial progesterone receptors. Mol Endocrinol, 11:801–811.
26. Gompel A, Malet C, Spritzer P, Kuttenn F, Mauvais-Jarvis P (1986) Progestin effect on cell proliferation and 17β-hydroxysteroid dehydrogenase activity in normal human breast cells in culture. J Clin Endocrinol Metab 63:1174–1180.
27. Musgrove EA, Lee CS, Sutherland RL (1991) Progestins both stimulate and inhibit breast cancer cell cycle progresssion while increasing expression of transforming growth factor α, epidermal growth factor receptor, c-fos, and c-myc genes. Mol Cell Biol 11:5032–5043.
28. Prudhomme JF, Malet C, Gompel A, Lalardrie JP, Ochoa C, Boué A, et al. (1984) 17β-Hydroxysteroid dehydrogenase activity in human breast epithelial cell and fibroblast cultures. Endocrinology 114:1483–1489.
29. King RJB (1993) Estrogen and progestin effects in human breast carcinogenesis. Breast Cancer Res Treat 27:3–15.
30. Carpenter S, Georgiade G, McCarty KS Sr, McCarty KS Jr (1989) Immunohistochemical expression of estrogen receptor in normal breast tissue. Proc R Soc Edinb 95:59–66.
31. Anderson E, Clarke RB, Howell A (1997) Changes in the normal human breast throughout the menstrual cycle: relevance to breast carcinogenesis. Endocr Rel Cancer 4:23–33.
32. Sarf M, Gorski J (1971) Control of estrogen binding protein concentration under basal conditions and after estrogen administration. Biochemistry 10:2557–2562.
33. Kuttenn F, Fournier S, Durand JC, Mauvais-Jarvis P (1981) Estradiol and progesterone receptors in human breast firoadenomas. J Clin Endocrinol Metab 52:1225–1229.
34. Malet C, Gompel A, Yaneva H, Cren H, Fidji N, Mowszowicz I, et al. (1991) Estradiol and progesterone receptors in cultured normal human breast epithelial cells and fibroblasts—immunocytochemical studies. J Clin Endocrinol Metab 73:8–17.
35. Gompel A, Martin A, Simon P, Schoevaert D, Plu-Bureau G, Hugol D, et al. (1996) Epidermal growth factor receptor and c-erbB-2 expression in normal breast tissue during the menstrual cycle. Breast Cancer Res Treat 38:227–235.
36. Dubik D, Shiu RPC (1988) Transcriptional regulation of c-*myc* oncogene expression by estrogen in hormone responsive human breast cancer cells. J Biol Chem 253:12705–12708.
37. Weisz A, Bresciani F (1988) Estrogen induces expression of c-*fos* and c-*myc* protooncogenes in rat uterus. Mol Endocrinol 2:816–824.
38. Santos GF, Scott GK, Lee WMF, Liu E, Benz C (1988) Estrogen-induced post-transcriptional modulation of c-*myc* protooncogene expression in human breast cancer cells. J Biol Chem 263:9565–9568.
39. Leygue E, Gol-Winkler R, Gompel A, Louis-Sylvestre C, Soquet L, Staub S, et al. (1995) Estradiol stimulates c-*myc* proto-oncogene expression in normal human breast epithelial cells in culture. J Steroid Biochem Mol Biol 52:299–305.
40. Leygue E, Louis-Sylvestre C, Gol R, Malet C, Baudot N, Cumins C, et al. (1993) Estrogen regulation of c-*myc* in normal human breast epithelial (HBE) cells in culture. Presented in the *75th Annual Meeting of the American Endocrine Society,* Las Vegas, abstract #1914.
41. Meyer JS (1977) Cell proliferation in normal human breast ducts, fibroadenomas, and other ductal hyperplasias measured by nuclear labeling with tritriated thymidine. Effects of menstrual phase, age and oral contraception. Hum Pathol 8:67–81.
42. Masters JRW, Drife JO, Scarisbrick JJ (1977) Cyclic variation of DNA synthesis in human breast epithelium. J Natl Cancer Inst 58:163–165.

43. Vogel PM, Georgiade NG, Setter BF, Vogel S, McCarty K (1981) The correlation of histologic changes in the human breast with the menstrual cycle. Am J Pathol 104:23–34.
44. Ferguson DJP, Anderson TJ (1981) Morphological evaluation of cell turnover in relation to the menstrual cycle in the "resting" human breast. Br J Cancer 44:177–181.
45. Longacre TA, Bartow SA (1986) A correlative morphology study of human breast and endometrium in the menstrual cycle. Am J Surg Pathol 10:382–393.
46. Potten CS, Watson RJ, Williams GT, et al. (1988) The effect of age and menstrual cycle upon proliferative activity on the normal human breast. Br J Cancer 258:163–170.
47. Sitruk-Ware R (1992) Estrogens, progestins and breast cancer risk in postmenopausal women: state of the ongoing controversy in 1992. Maturitas 15:129–139.
48. Wren BG (1995) Hormonal replacement therapy and breast cancer. Eur Menopause J 2:13–19.
49. Dabrosin C, Ollinger K, Ungerstedt U, Hammar M (1997) Variability of glutathione levels in normal breast tissue and subcutaneous fat during the enstrual cycle: an in vivo study with microdialysis technique. J Clin Endocrinol Metab 82:1382–1384.
50. Miller NA, Thomas M, Martin LJ, et al. (1997) Feasibility of obtaining breast epithelial cells from healthy women for studies of cellular proliferation. Breast Cancer Res Treat 43:201–210.
51. Söderqvist G, Isaksson E, Von Schoulz B, Carlström K, Tani E, Skoog L (1997) Proliferation of breast epithelial cells in healthy women during the menstrual cycle. Am. J. Obst Gynecol. 176:123–128.
52. Barrat J, Lignieres B de, Marpeau L, Larue L, Fournier, S, Nahoul K, et al. (1990) Effet in vivo de l'administration locale de progesterone sur l'activité mitotique des galactophores humains. J Gynecol Obstet Biol Reprod 19:269–274.
53. Chang KJ, Lee TT, Linares-Cruz G, Fournier S, de Lignières B (1995) Influence of percutaneous administration of estradiol and progesterone on human breast epithelial cell in vivo. Fertil Steril 63:785–791.
54. Miller AB, Bulbrook, RD (1980) The epidemiology and etiology of breast cancer. N Engl J Med 303:1246–1248.
55. Kelsey JL, Gammon MD, John EM (1993) Reproductive factors and breast cancer. Epidemiol Rev 15:36–47.
56. Soini I (1977) Risk factors of breast cancer in Finland. Int J Epidemiol 6:365–373.
57. Olsson H, Landin-Olsson M, Gullberg B (1983) Retrospective assessment of menstrual cycle length in patients with breast cancer, in patients with benign breast disease, and in women without breast disease. J Natl Cancer Inst 70:17–20.
58. Yuan JM, Yu MC, Ross RK, Gao YT, Henderson BE (1988) Risk factors for breast cancer in Chinese women in shanghai. Cancer Res 48:1949–1953.
59. Whelan EA, Sandler DP, Root J, Smith UR, Weinberg CR (1992) Menstrual cycle patterns and risk of breast cancer. Am J Epidemiol 140:1081–1090.
60. Plu-Bureau G, Thalabard JC, Sitruk-Ware R, Asselain B, Mauvais-Jarvis P (1992) Cyclical mastalgia as a marker of breast cancer susceptibility: results of a case-control study among french women. Bri J Cancer 65:945–949
61. Goodwin PJ, Deboer G, Clark RM, Catton P, Redwood S, Hood N, et al. (1995) Cyclical mastopathy and premenopausal breast cancer risk: results of a case-control study. Breast Cancer Res Treat 33:63–73.
62. Korenman SG (1980) The endocrinology of breast cancer. Cancer 46:874–878.
63. Malone KE, Daling JR, Weiss NS (1993) Oral contraceptives in relation to breast cancer. Epidemiol Rev 15:80–97.
64. Collaborative Group on Hormonal Factors in Breast Cancer (1996) Breast cancer and hormonal contraceptives: further results. Contraception 3S:1–106.
65. Colditz GA, Egan KM, Stampfer MJ (1993) Hormone replacement therapy and risk of breast cancer: results from epidemiologic studies. Am J Obstet Gynecol 168:1473–1480.
66. Dupont WD, Page DL (1991) Menopausal estrogen replacement therapy and breast cancer. Arch Intern Med 151:67–72.
67. Sillero-Arenas M, Delgado-Rodriguez M, Rodigues-Canteras R, Bueno-Cavanillas A, Galvez-Vargas R (1992) Menopausal hormone replacement therapy and breast cancer: a meta-analysis. Obstet Gynecol 79:286–294.
68. Steinberg, K.K., Thacker SB, Smith SJ, Stroup DF, Zack MM, Flanders WD, et al. (1991) A meta-analysis of the effect of estrogen replacement therapy on the risk of breast cancer. JAMA 265:1985–1990.
69. Colditz GA, Hankinson SE, Hunter DJ, Willett WC, Manson JE, Stampfer MJ, et al. (1995) The use of estrogens and progestins and the risk of breast cancer in postmenopausal women. N Engl J Med 332:1589–1593.

70. Newcomb PA, Longnecker MP, Storer BE, Mittendorf R, Baron J, Clapp RW, et al. (1995) Long term hormone replacement therapy and risk of breast cancer in postmenopausal women. Am J Epidemiol 142:788–795.
71. Stanford JL, Weiss NS, Voigt LF, Daling JR, Habel LA, Rossing MA (1995) Combined estrogen and progestin hormone replacement therapy in relation to risk of breast cancer in middle-aged women. JAMA 274:137–142.
72. Mauvais-Jarvis P (1983) Progesterone and progestins: a general overview, In: *Progesterone and Progestins* (Bardin CW, Milgrom E, Mauvais-Jarvis P, eds.), Raven Press, New-York, pp. 1–16.
73. Horwitz KB, Wei LL, Sedlacek SM, D'Arville CN (1985) Progestin action and progesterone receptor structure in human breast cancer: a review. Recent Prog Horm Res 41:249–316.
74. Plu-Bureau G, Lê M, Sitruk-Ware R, Thalabard JC, Mauvais-Jarvis P (1994) Progestogen use and risk of breast cancer in a cohort study of premenopausal women with benign breast disease. Br J Cancer 70:270–277.
75. Moolgavkar SH, Day NE, Stevens RC (1980) Two stage model for carcinogenesis: epidemiology of breast cancer in females. J Natl Cancer Inst 65:559–569.
76. Russo J, Calaf G, Sohi N, Tahin Q, Zhang PL, Alvarado ME, et al. (1993) Critical steps in breast carcinogenesis. Ann NY Acad Sci 698:1–20
77. Russo J, Russo IH (1997) Role of differentiation in the pathogenesis and prevention of breast cancer. Endocr Rel Cancer 4:7–21.

3 Expression and Regulation of Insulin-like Growth Factors and Their Binding Proteins in the Normal Breast

Monica M. Richert, PhD
and Teresa L. Wood, PhD

STAGES OF MAMMARY GLAND DEVELOPMENT

Embryonically, the mammary gland first appears as an epithelial bud that penetrates the underlying mesenchyme. The mammary gland at birth consists of the epithelial parenchyma and the stroma, which includes connective tissue and the mammary fat pad. The epithelial parenchyma at this stage is rudimentary and consists of a small ductal tree. Each branch is composed of several layers of epithelial cells surrounding a central lumen. Beneath the epithelial cells, the myoepithelial cells form a discontinuous layer that rests on a basement membrane separating the parenchymal and the stromal compartments. Development of rodent and human mammary glands are parallel at most stages except for embryonic and prepubertal stages *(1,2)*. Human mammary glands in both males and females are more developed at birth than are rodent glands *(3)*. Human glands then regress during prepuberty and reinitiate growth at puberty. In rodents, the glands do not regress during prepuberty but maintain a small ductal tree, which, like the human gland, initiates rapid growth at the onset of puberty.

Most growth in the mammary gland occurs postnatally in two major phases: ductal growth that is initiated with puberty and alveolar differentiation that occurs during pregnancy. Ductal growth involves lengthening and branching of the parenchyma, which ultimately extends to the limits of the fat pad. Alveolar differentiation represents the terminal differentiation of the gland and involves the formation of the milk-secreting units.

Ductal and alveolar growth are controlled by specific combinations of the ovarian hormones, estrogen and progesterone, and the lactogenic hormones, including prolactin, growth hormone, and placental lactogen, produced by the pituitary and placenta. These hormones mediate mammary growth both indirectly through modulating other endocrine factors as well as directly through binding to their cognate receptors on glandular epithelial and stromal cells. In addition to direct actions of ovarian and lactogenic hormones,

From: *Contemporary Endocrinology: Endocrinology of Breast Cancer*
Edited by: A. Manni © Humana Press Inc., Totowa, NJ

local control of mammary growth and differentiation also is mediated by epithelial and stromal production of peptide growth factors. Major growth factor families implicated in normal mammary development include the epidermal growth factor family that consists of epidermal growth factor (EGF) and transforming growth factor-α (TGF-α), the transforming growth factor-β (TGF-β) family, the fibroblast growth factor (FGF) family, and the insulin-like growth factors (IGFs), IGF-I and IGF-II.

We review here postnatal stages of mammary development and discuss evidence that locally produced growth factors mediate growth and differentiation of mammary epithelium. While much of the data presented have been obtained from experiments in rodent mammary glands, we include correlative information on development of human glands where it is known. Finally, we present data that support a role for the IGFs and their primary modulators, the IGF binding proteins, in normal mammary development and discuss a possible model for their actions in the mammary gland.

Ductal Growth

The period of most rapid ductal growth occurs during puberty. Prior to puberty, the mammary epithelium consists of a small ductal tree that has initiated growth into one end of the mammary fat pad *(3)*. During pubertal and postpubertal growth, the ducts lengthen and branch to form secondary and tertiary ducts that ultimately extend to fill the mammary fat pad. In rodents, postpubertal ductal growth continues until the ducts reach the limits of the fat pad at 5–6 months of age. In humans, the mammary gland at puberty initially enlarges due to an increase in stromal and fatty tissue. Subsequently, the ductal structures elongate and branch similar to what is seen during puberty in rodents *(3,4)*. The primary difference between rodent and human glands during ductal growth is that, in humans, progressive ductal branching forms multiple individual functional units that contain both terminal end buds (TEBs) and alveolar buds. These immature structures are called type 1 terminal ductal lobular units (TDLUs) *(2)*.

Terminal End Buds

The main epithelial structure in both rodent and human mammary glands at the start of ductal growth is the TEB *(2,5,6)*. TEBs are bulbous structures located at the tips of the growing ducts, and they represent the sites of highest proliferation in the gland *(6,7)*. TEBs consist of four to six layers of epithelium with an outer layer of undifferentiated, pluripotent stem cells called cap cells, which sit on the basal lamina. Cap cells have the highest proliferative rate of any cell population in the mammary gland and give rise to the epithelial and myoepithelial cells of the ducts *(6,7)*. Cell division drops significantly in the trailing end bud cells as they differentiate into luminal, ductal, and myoepithelial cells. At the same time, branches form along the growing ducts. During postpubertal growth, TEBs as well as secondary and tertiary ductal branches begin to form alveolar buds that cleave to form rudimentary alveolar structures. In nonpregnant human glands, the type 1 TDLUs gradually progress to type 2 and type 3 TDLUs with the continued sprouting and division of alveolar buds into more differentiated lobule units *(2)*.

Hormonal Regulation of Ductal Growth

With the onset of puberty in both humans and rodents, ductal growth is cyclical in parallel with the estrus cycle. The highest proliferation rates occur during diestrus, and the lowest proliferation rates occur during estrus *(3)*. Proliferation in the TEBs is mediated primarily through the ovarian hormone estrogen *(3)*. Ovariectomy during pubertal growth results in regression of the ducts; TEB proliferation and ductal lengthening is reinitiated on treatment of these animals with estrogen *(6)*. Consistent with these studies, mice carrying a null mutation in the estrogen receptor gene demonstrate rudimentary ductal growth *(8)*. Evidence that the effect of estrogen is at least in part through local actions on the gland itself comes from two major sources: (1) the estrogen receptor is expressed in TEBs and ductal epithelium *(9)*, and (2) local implants of antiestrogens block ductal growth during puberty *(10)*.

The pituitary hormone most implicated in TEB proliferation is growth hormone (GH). In hypophysectomized and ovariectomized female rats, local treatment of glands with a combination of estrogen and GH induced normal TEB development *(11,12)*. In similar experiments, the combination of estrogen and prolactin was unable to promote normal TEB growth.

TEBs and Breast Tumors

Since extensive discussion of breast cancer is reviewed elsewhere in this volume, we will not cover it here except to point out the relationship between TEBs and development of breast tumors. Since the TEBs have the highest proliferative rates of any cell type in the mammary gland, they are also the most susceptible to transformation *(13)*. Moreover, TEB cells have the lowest percentage of cell death *(13)*. Therefore, any changes in the genome of these cells are more likely to be transmitted to daughter cells. When rat mammary glands are treated with chemical carcinogens, the DNA of TEB cells bind more carcinogen, produce more adducts, and are less efficient at removing them and repairing their DNA than are more differentiated cells with a slower cell cycle *(13)*. This lack of repair results in permanent changes to the genome during further growth and proliferation. Differentiation of TEBs to alveoli reduces the number of stem cells available for transformation and, therefore, reduces the risk of tumor development *(13)*.

Similarly, in the human breast, the type 1 TDLUs are the least differentiated structures with the highest proliferative capacity *(2,13)*. TEBs and type 1 TDLUs are equivalent in their carcinogenic potentials. Both are the sites of carcinogen binding to the DNA in vitro, and both express phenotypes of transformation after treatment with carcinogens *(2,13)*. Consistent with these data, the type 1 TDLUs are the sites of highest breast tumor origination in women. Since many of the GF signaling pathways implicated in breast cancer also have roles in normal mammary epithelial growth, these data provide an important additional basis for studying the role of locally produced factors in mediating TEB proliferation.

Alveolar Growth

As discussed above, the development of alveolar buds is initiated in the postpubertal gland with each menstrual cycle. These buds subdivide and form rudimentary alveolar structures in both rodents and humans as postpubertal growth continues. However, progression of these alveolar structures or alveolar units into fully differentiated milk-secreting units only occurs during pregnancy-induced growth of the mammary gland.

Lobuloalveolar Differentiation

The peak of mammary differentiation occurs during pregnancy and culminates with formation of alveoli and a fully lactating gland *(3,6)*. Initial pregnancy-induced mammary growth involves massive proliferation of ductal branches and formation of alveolar buds. During the second half of pregnancy, the alveolar buds progressively differentiate into individual alveoli that ultimately become lobules, the milk-secreting units of the lactating gland. This later stage of differentiation is commonly referred to as the lobuloalveolar phase of mammary growth. By the end of pregnancy, the alveoli completely fill the fat pad, at which time the gland is capable of milk production. Fully developed alveolar structures remain until the completion of lactation. At the end of lactation, the gland goes through a process of involution whereby the alveolar structures regress through a process of programmed cell death.

Hormonal Regulation of Alveolar Differentiation

The combination of estrogen, progesterone, and prolactin is sufficient to induce alveolar development in rodents that have been hypophysectomized, ovariectomized, and adrenalectomized *(3)*. Treatment of ovariectomized mice with estrogen in combination with progesterone, or with high levels of progesterone alone, induce alveolar development. Estrogen controls alveolar development indirectly by inducing synthesis and release of prolactin from the pituitary. In addition, estrogen has direct effects on alveolar growth by inducing transcription of the progesterone receptor (PR) gene *(14)*. The presence of PRs is essential for the process of alveolar development, as demonstrated in mice carrying a null mutation in the gene for the PR. Female PR-deficient mice show severely reduced alveolar development during pregnancy and are lactation deficient *(15,16)*. Similarly, mice carrying a gene deletion in the prolactin receptor have a phenotype similar to that seen in the PR null mutant; mice carrying either of these mutations demonstrate normal ductal growth but lack lobuloalveolar development *(15–17)*. Since all the lactogenic hormones (including prolactin, GH and the placental lactogens) can bind the prolactin receptor, it is unknown which of these hormones is directly responsible for alveolar development.

GROWTH FACTORS AND MAMMARY GLAND DEVELOPMENT

Normal mammary epithelial growth is dependent on the local induction of peptide growth factors. Among the growth factor families that have demonstrated roles in, or are highly implicated, in mammary growth and differentiation are the EGF, TGF-β, FGF, and IGF families.

EGF and TGF-α are positive effectors of TEB proliferation and ductal growth *(18–20)*. Both EGF and TGF-α are expressed in TEBs during ductal growth *(20,21)*. Similar to their role in ductal proliferation, EGF and TGF-α are positive effectors of alveolar growth *(22,23)*. However, TGF-α, but not EGF, is expressed in mammary epithelium during pregnancy-induced growth *(20,21)*. Both factors signal through the same receptor, which has been found at all stages of mammary growth *(20,21)*. A definitive role for this signaling pathway in mammary growth was demonstrated in the waved-2 mutant mouse. Waved-2 mice carry a point mutation in the kinase domain of the EGF receptor and have defects both in ductal growth and in development of secretory alveoli during pregnancy *(23)*.

In contrast to EGF and TGF-α, the TGF-β isoforms have consistent anti-proliferative actions both on mammary epithelial cells in culture and when added exogenously to mammary glands in vivo *(24–26)*. Endogenous expression of the TGF-β family members suggests that they may have similar roles during normal development. All TGF-β family members are present in the epithelium throughout pre- and postpubertal growth and during pregnancy *(26)*. The TGF-β1 protein has been localized in the extracellular matrix (ECM) during prepubertal growth, and levels of this factor are decreased in the region around the TEBs, suggesting that local depletion of this factor is necessary for ductal growth *(27)*. Finally, recently developed transgenic mice that overexpress TGF-β1 under the control of the whey acidic protein promoter fail to develop alveoli and lobules during pregnancy *(28)*.

Studies to date on the expression of the FGF growth factor family show complex temporal and spatial patterns of expression for the individual members of this family during mammary development *(29)*. FGF signaling clearly has a prominent role in alveolar growth since mice carrying the dominant-negative form of the FGFR2 receptor have significant deficits in lobuloalveolar development *(30,31)*.

Insulin-Like Growth Factors

It has long been known that superphysiologic concentrations of insulin (in the micromolar range) are required for maintenance and growth of mammary gland explants and mammary epithelial cells in culture *(32,33)*. Insulin at these concentrations stimulates growth by activating the IGF type I receptor (IGF-IR), a tyrosine kinase receptor structurally related to the insulin receptor *(34–39)*. The IGF-IR binds IGF-I and IGF-II with high affinity (dissociation constant K_d approx $1–2 \times 10^{-9}$) and insulin with 500–1000-fold lower affinity. Functional studies using both in vivo and in vitro approaches have demonstrated that IGF signaling through the IGF-IR accelerates cell cycle progression in fibroblasts *(37,40–42)*. Taken together, these data support a role for IGF signaling in mammary growth.

Additional support for an endogenous role for the IGFs in mammary growth comes from evidence that the mechanism by which GH induces mammary growth is through local induction of IGF-I. GH is the major inducer of circulating IGF-I and is one of the lactogenic hormones that mediates mammary growth. When given either systemically or locally to gonadectomized, hypophysectomized, and estrogen-treated male or female rats, GH induces ductal as well as alveolar growth *(11,12)*. IGF-I can substitute for GH in this paradigm, suggesting that this may be the mechanism by which GH induces mammary growth *(43)*. That this is due to IGF induction at the local level is suggested by studies showing that treatment of mammary tissue with GH induces mammary expression of IGF-I mRNA in a dose-dependent manner *(44)*.

The IGFs also may have important survival functions for mammary epithelial cells. Overexpression of IGF-I from a milk-protein promoter blocks involution through disrupting the normal process of cell death in the mammary epithelium *(45,46)*. These experiments support the hypothesis that reduction of the IGFs is important for normal involution.

Data on the expression of the IGFs during normal mammary development are limited. IGF-I mRNA has been found in extracts from rat and bovine mammary tissue *(47,48)* and in the stroma of normal human breast tissue *(49)*. We have shown high expression of IGFs, particularly that of IGF-II, in mammary epithelium during both ductal and alveolar growth in mice *(50)*. Similarly, we have shown high levels of IGF-IR in TEBs, ductal epithelium, and alveolar epithelium throughout postnatal mammary growth *(50)*. Data implicating IGF-II in normal mammary epithelial growth are of particular interest since overexpression of IGF-II (but not IGF-I) in the mammary gland of mice results in mammary tumors *(45,46,51)*. Moreover, in human breast tumors, expression of IGF-II is highly correlated with both malignancy and invasiveness *(52,53)*.

IGF Binding Proteins

The family of IGF binding proteins (IGFBPs) modulate IGF actions by a variety of mechanisms that include increasing IGF serum half-life, transporting the IGFs across capillary membranes, localizing the IGFs to specific tissues and cell types, and either blocking or enhancing IGF binding to cell surface receptors *(39,54–59)*. Whether the IGFBPs inhibit or enhance IGF action depends on alterations in their binding affinities for the IGFs. In serum or tissue fluids, the binding proteins have a higher affinity for the IGFs than that of the receptor *(39,55,57)*. By contrast, association of the IGFBP with the cell surface or ECM results in a drop in its affinity for the IGFs to a range similar to that of the receptor *(39,55,57)*. This then facilitates receptor binding and results in IGF-induced protein and DNA synthesis. These studies support a model whereby IGFs in solution preferentially partition to the IGFBPs and are unavailable for binding to the receptor. By contrast, IGFBPs anchored to the ECM or to the cell surface may localize and release the IGFs to the receptor, thereby enhancing IGF actions. At least four of the IGFBPs have the ability to bind to the cell surface or ECM. Included in this group are IGFBP-1 and -3, which bind to specific receptors on the cell surface, and IGFBP-2, -3, and -5, which associate with the ECM *(8,57,60–63)*.

Other mechanisms for regulating IGFBP affinity for the IGFs are through phosphorylation and proteolytic cleavage *(39,57,58)*. IGFBP-1 is phosphorylated on serine residues, which results in increased affinity for IGF-I and IGF-II. Dephosphorylation of IGFBP-1 reduces its affinity for the IGFs and potentiates IGF-mediated DNA synthesis *(58)*. Finally, several of the IGFBPs, including IGFBP-2, -3, -4, and -5, can be proteolytically cleaved, resulting in changes in their affinities for the IGFs *(39,57,58)*. Proteolysis of the IGFBPs usually reduces their affinities for the IGFs, often completely abolishing IGF binding *(58)*. Cleavage of IGFBP-4 reduces its inhibitory actions *(58)*. By contrast, proteolytic cleavage of IGFBP-5 abolishes its ability to localize IGF-I to fibroblast ECM and thus decreases IGF-I-mediated cell proliferation *(57,61,64,65)*. Such mechanisms have potential relevance to IGFBP regulation of IGF actions in the mammary gland since sequestration and release of growth factors from the ECM play a major role in regulating epithelial growth during mammary development.

To begin to ascertain whether the IGFBPs have an endogenous role in normal mammary development, we have used in situ hybridization histochemistry to determine the expression patterns of IGFBP mRNAs during ductal and alveolar growth in mice. Data on mRNA expression of IGFBP-1, -3, -4, and -6 are presented here.

Expression of IGFBP mRNAs During Ductal Growth

IGFBP mRNAs in TEBs. As described above, the TEB is the predominant structure during pubertal and postpubertal development of the mammary gland. We have detected mRNAs for IGFBPs-1–6 in TEBs during pubertal or postpubertal ductal growth. Expression patterns and levels for each IGFBP vary widely during these growth phases. IGFBP-3 mRNA is highly expressed in the TEBs but is limited to the outer layer of TEB cells (Fig. 1B). This hybridization pattern is what would be expected for expression in the highly proliferative cap cells of the TEBs. By contrast, BP-1, -4, and -6 mRNAs are expressed throughout the TEB (Fig. 1A,C,D). Of these, IGFBP-4 mRNAs are the most highly expressed. The relative expression of the mRNAs at all stages was determined by hybridizing adjacent sections with different IGFBP RNA probes of equivalent specific activity and then exposing them to autoradiographic emulsion for identical lengths of time.

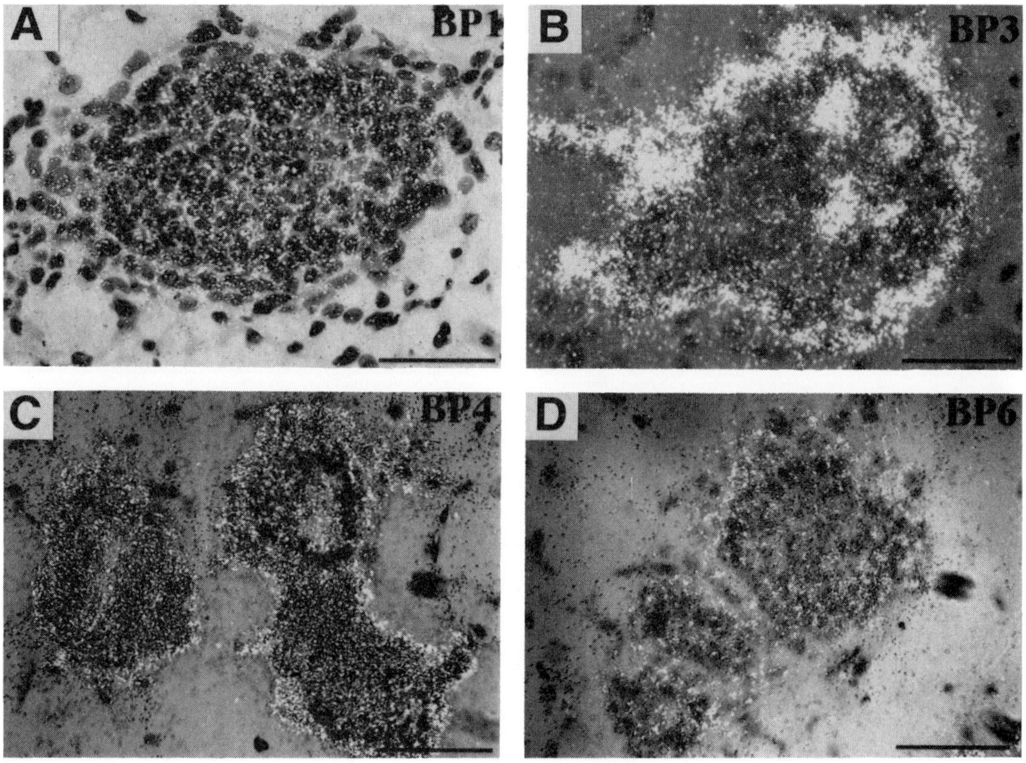

Fig. 1. In situ hybridization showing mRNA expression for IGFBP-1 **(A)**, IGFBP-3 **(B)**, IGFBP-4 **(C)**, and IGFBP-6 **(D)** in TEBs during ductal growth of mouse mammary glands taken from virgin female mice at either 5 weeks or 2–3 months of age. Fresh frozen sections of mammary glands were hybridized with ^{35}S-labeled antisense RNA probes according to standard procedures *(83)*. Sections were analyzed following 4–6 weeks of exposure to autoradiographic emulsion. Photomicrographs were taken using epifluorescence microscopy such that the exposed silver grains appear white against the hematoxylin-stained tissue sections. Scale bars = 50 µm.

IGFBP mRNAs in Ducts and Stroma. Similar to what was observed for the TEBs, IGFBP-1, -3, -4, and -6 mRNAs were all expressed in ductal epithelium during pubertal and postpubertal ductal growth (Fig. 2A-D). In addition, IGFBP-4 mRNA was expressed at high levels in the dense stroma surrounding the ducts (Fig. 2C). IGFBP-6 mRNAs showed a similar pattern to that for IGFBP-4, except its expression was lower in ductal epithelium and higher in selective cells throughout the stroma (Fig. 2D).

IGFBP mRNAs During Lobuloalveolar Differentiation

Expression patterns for most IGFBP mRNAs changed significantly during lobuloalveolar differentiation (compare Fig. 2 and 3). At mid- to late pregnancy stages, IGFBP-1 mRNA was no longer detectable in the mammary gland (Fig. 3A) at exposure times equivalent to those used to detect IGFBP-1 mRNAs during ductal growth (Figs. 1A and 2A). Similarly, IGFBP-4 and -6 mRNAs were no longer detectable in ductal epithelium and also were not seen in alveolar epithelium (Fig. 3C and 3D, respectively). However, the specific patterns of stromal expression observed for both IGFBP-4 and -6 were maintained during lobuloalveolar differentiation. IGFBP-3 mRNA expression was

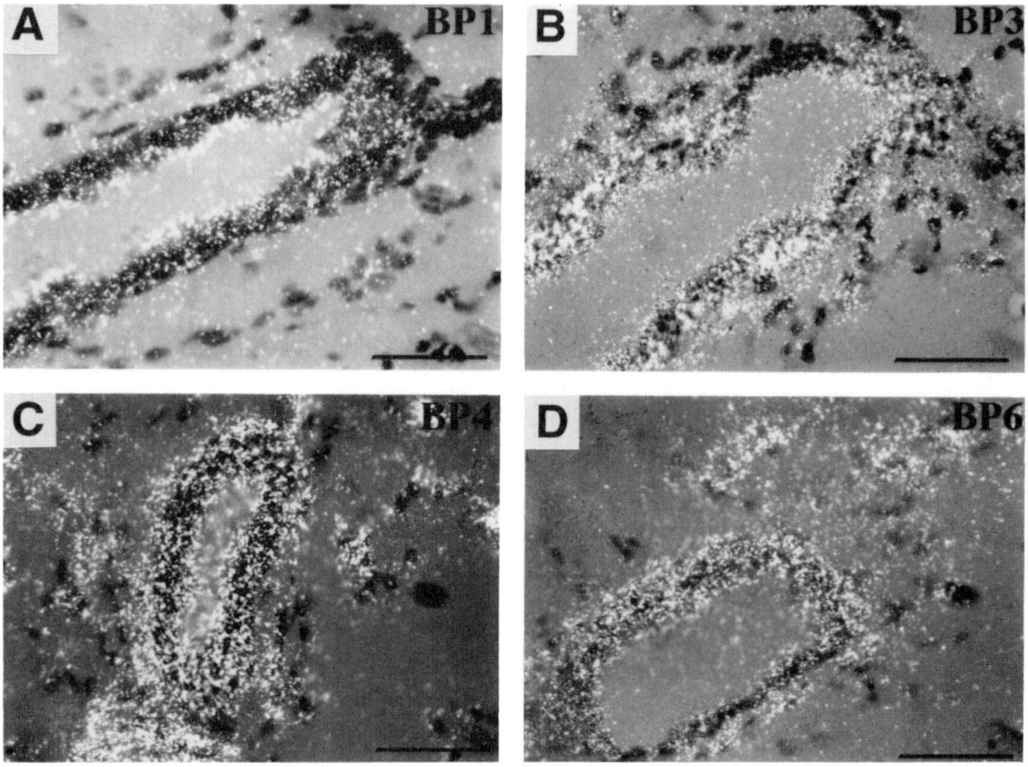

Fig. 2. In situ hybridization showing mRNA expression for IGFBP-1 **(A)**, IGFBP-3 **(B)**, IGFBP-4 **(C)**, and IGFBP-6 **(D)** during ductal growth of mouse mammary glands taken from virgin female mice at 2–3 months of age. Fresh frozen sections of mammary glands were hybridized with ^{35}S-labeled antisense RNA probes according to standard procedures *(83)*. Sections were analyzed following 4–6 weeks of exposure to autoradiographic emulsion. Photomicrographs were taken using epifluorescence microscopy such that the exposed silver grains appear white against the hematoxylin-stained tissue sections. Scale bars = 50 μm.

maintained in ductal epithelium and also was observed in alveolar epithelium during pregnancy-induced growth (Fig. 3B).

A MODEL FOR IGFBP ACTION DURING NORMAL MAMMARY GLAND DEVELOPMENT

IGFBPs as Modulators of Normal Mammary Growth

Our data demonstrate that multiple members of the IGFBP family are expressed during ductal and alveolar growth phases of mammary development. Moreover, mRNA expression of individual members of the IGFBP family is highly distinct and regulated during these postnatal growth phases. Based on these data and on previously published data on IGFBP actions in other systems, we propose several possible roles for the IGFBPs in modulating growth of the mammary gland, including (1) IGFBP enhancement of IGF-mediated mammary growth through ECM or cell surface binding, (2) IGFBP inhibition of IGF-mediated mammary growth, and (3) IGF-independent IGFBP actions.

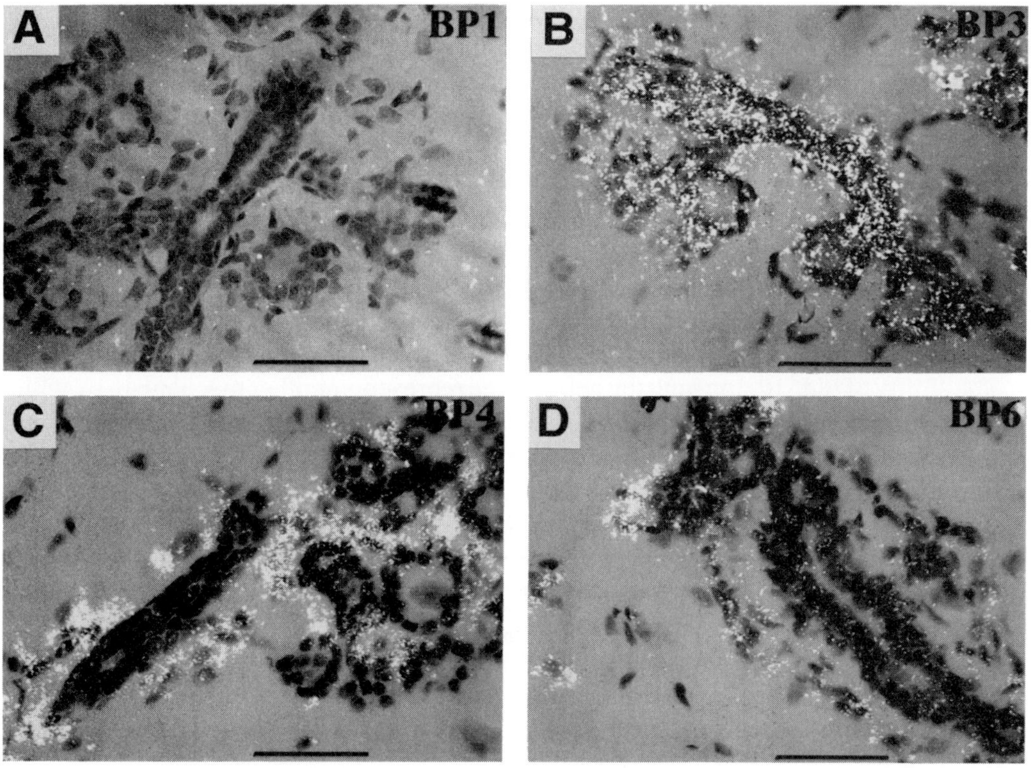

Fig. 3. In situ hybridization showing mRNA expression of IGFBP-1 **(A)**, IGFBP-3 **(B)**, IGFBP-4 **(C)**, and IGFBP-6 **(D)** in ducts, alveoli, and stroma during alveolar growth of mouse mammary glands taken from pregnant female mice on days 13–16 of pregnancy. Fresh frozen sections of mammary glands were hybridized with ^{35}S-labeled antisense RNA probes according to standard procedures *(83)*. Sections were analyzed following 4–6 weeks of exposure to autoradiographic emulsion. Photomicrographs were taken using epifluorescence microscopy such that the exposed silver grains appear white against the hematoxylin-stained tissue sections. Scale bars = 50 μm.

IGFBPs as Positive Modulators of IGF-Mediated Epithelial Growth

We propose a model for IGFBP action in promoting IGF-mediated epithelial proliferation in the mammary gland. This model is dependent on association of one or more of the IGFBPs to the ECM. When bound, these IGFBPs then localize the IGFs to the ECM and enhance IGF binding to epithelial IGF receptors. Leading candidates for these actions are IGFBPs-2, -3, and -5, all of which have demonstrated ability to bind to the ECM and are highly expressed in the mammary gland during ductal and alveolar growth.

Numerous lines of evidence support a critical role for the basement membrane in regulating epithelial proliferation and differentiation *(27,66,67)*. Abnormal breakdown of the ECM results in precocious growth of mammary epithelium *(67)*, suggesting that the ECM is a reservoir for growth-promoting agents. Components of the ECM vary with the stage of mammary development *(68,69)* and even locally along the ducts *(27)*. These data support a dynamic model of the ECM whereby ECM remodeling controls local proliferation and differentiation of developing mammary epithelium.

The ECM sequesters a number of growth factors including the FGFs and TGF-β *(3)*. Binding of the FGFs to the basement membrane extends their biologic potency by protecting them from degradation. This association is required for basic FGF activity and receptor interaction. By contrast, local depletion of TGF-β from the ECM surrounding TEBs appears to be critical for TEB and ductal growth *(27)*. These data support the hypothesis that alterations in the ECM promote TEB proliferation. It is potentially important that mRNAs for both IGF-I and -II, the IGF-IR, and the IGFBPs are expressed in the TEBs. Our model proposes that IGF-IGFBP association with the ECM allows release of IGFs to cell surface IGF receptors, thereby promoting epithelial proliferation. Thus, it will be of great interest to determine whether the IGFs and specific members of the IGFBPs are associated with the ECM around the TEBs and growing ducts.

The ability of IGFBP-1 to bind the cell surface represents another mechanism by which the IGFBPs may enhance mammary growth. IGFBP-1 binds the α5β1 integrin on cell surfaces through its carboxy-terminal Arg-Gly-Asp sequence *(39,70)*. IGFBP-1 binding to this integrin promotes cell migration through both IGF-dependent and IGF-independent mechanisms *(39,70–72)*. It is possible, then, that the expression of IGFBP-1 in TEBs and ductal epithelium specifically during ductal growth is important for extension of these structures through the stromal compartment.

IGFBPs as Inhibitors of IGF-Mediated Proliferation

Inhibitory actions of the IGFBPs on IGF-mediated cell proliferation are well demonstrated for a variety of cell types *(39,55–57)*. As discussed previously, IGFBP inhibitory effects are observed when the BP is in solution and not cell surface or ECM associated. Whereas most of the IGFBPs in solution can inhibit IGF-mediated cell proliferation, IGFBP-4 is the only member of the IGFBP family that appears to exclusively inhibit IGF actions. This binding protein has no demonstrated ability to bind either cell surfaces or the ECM and has consistent IGF-inhibitory actions on numerous cell types in vitro *(39,55–57,73)*. It is of potential interest that the mRNAs for IGFBP-4 are expressed at high levels in the dense stroma just outside the basement membrane throughout postnatal mammary development. This expression pattern suggests that IGFBP-4 may block IGF proliferative effects in the stroma and limit IGF actions to epithelial proliferation during mammary growth.

IGF-Independent IGFBP Actions

Several studies have suggested IGF-independent actions for IGFBP-3 *(74,75)*. These reports have potential significance for mammary development since IGFBP-3 (1) has antiproliferative effects on mammary epithelial cells *(74,76,77)* and (2) is regulated by members of the TGF-β family including TGF-β1 in breast cancer cells *(74–77)*. These results support the hypothesis that induction of BP-3 is one mechanism by which TGF-β inhibits growth of mammary epithelium. Whereas TGF-β induction of IGFBP-3 provides the possibility for IGF-dependent growth inhibition by IGFBP-3, the recent demonstration that IGFBP-3 binds to the type V TGF-β receptor on cell surfaces suggests a mechanism by which IGFBP-3 may directly inhibit proliferation of mammary cells *(78)*.

IGFBPs and Breast Cancer

Finally, in addition to potential roles for the IGFBPs in normal growth of the mammary gland, the IGFBPs also may have significant roles in proliferation of breast cancer cells.

Data supporting this hypothesis are presented in detail elsewhere in this volume. However, it is of interest to mention these data briefly here to stress the added importance of understanding the function of this family of proteins in mammary growth. Breast cancer cells in vitro and in vivo produce large amounts of IGF binding proteins *(79–81)*. Moreover, the IGFBP expression pattern in breast tumor cells is related to the estrogen responsiveness of the tumor or cell line *(79–81)*. For example, estrogen receptor positive cells produce IGFBPs-2,-4, and -5, and estrogen receptor negative cells secrete IGFBPs-1, -3, -4, and -6. Taken together with data supporting a role for the IGFs in breast cancer, it is likely that the IGFBPs are critical components of IGF-mediated breast tumor growth.

Second, IGFBPs have been proposed as therapeutics to block IGF-mediated growth of breast tumors *(82)*. It is then imperative to understand the individual functions of each IGFBP in growth of the mammary gland to determine which BP is most likely to inhibit rather than enhance IGF-mediated growth. Thus, understanding the mechanisms by which these factors mediate normal growth will provide important clues as to their function in abnormal growth of mammary tissue.

REFERENCES

1. Waugh D, van der Hoeven E (1962) Fine structure of the human adult female breast. Lab Invest 11:220–228.
2. Russo J, Gusterson B, Rogers A, Russo I, Wellings S, van Zweiten M (1990) Biology of Disease: Comparative study of human and rat mammary tumorigenesis. Lab Invest 62:244–278.
3. Imagawa W, Yang J, Guzman R, Nandi S (1994) Control of mammary gland development, In: *The Physiology of Reproduction*, 2nd Edition (Knobil E, Neill JD, eds.), Raven Press, New York, pp. 1033–1063.
4. Monaghan P, Perusinghe N, Cowen P, Gusterson B (1990) Peripubertal human breast development. Anat Rec 226:501–508.
5. Russo I, Medado J, Russo J (1989) Endocrine influences on the mammary gland, In: *Integument and Mammary Glands* (Jones T, Mohr U, Hunt R, eds.), Springer-Verlag, New York, pp. 252–266.
6. Russo IH, Russo J (1996) Mammary gland neoplasia in long-term rodent studies. Environmental Health Perspectives 104:938–967.
7. Russo J, Russo I (1991) Mammary tumorigenesis, In: *Modification of Tumor Development in Rodents*, vol. 33 in Progressive Experimental Tumor Research (Ito N, Sugano H, eds.), Karger, Basel, pp. 175–191.
8. Jones J, Gockerman A, Busby WJ, Camacho-Hubner C, Clemmons D (1993) Extracellular matrix contains insulin-like growth factor binding protein-5: potentiation of the effects of IGF-I. J Cell Biol 121:679–687.
9. Haslam S., Nummy K (1992) The ontogeny and cellular distribution of estrogen receptors in normal mouse mammary gland. J Steroid Biochem Mol Biol 42:589–595.
10. Silberstein G, Van Horn K, Shyamala G, Daniel C (1994) Essential role of endogenous estrogen in directly stimulating mammary growth demonstrated by implants containing pure antiestrogens. Endocrinology 134:84–90.
11. Kleinberg D, Ruan W, Catanese B, Newman C, Feldman F (1990) Non-lactogenic effects of growth hormone on growth and insulin-like growth factor-I messenger ribonucleic acid of rat mammary gland. Endocrinology 126:3274–3276.
12. Kleinberg D (1997) Early mammary development: Growth hormone and IGF-1. J Mam Gland Biol Neoplasia 2:49–57.
13. Russo I, Russo J (1996) Mammary gland neoplasia in long-term rodent studies. Environ Health Perspect 104:938–967.
14. Muldoon T (1987) Prolactin mediation of estrogen-induced changes in mammary tissue estrogen and progesterone receptors. Endocrinology 121:141–149.
15. Lydon J, DeMayo F, Funk C, Mani S, Hughes A, Montgomery J, et al. (1995) Mice lacking progesterone receptor exhibit pleiotropic reproductive abnormalities. Genes Dev 9:2266–2278.
16. Lydon JP, DeMayo FJ, Conneely OM, O'Malley BW (1996) Reproductive phenotpes of the progesterone receptor null mutant mouse. J Steroid Biochemi Mol Biol 56:67–77.
17. Ormandy CJ, Camus A, Barra J, Damotte D, Lucas B, Buteau H, et al. (1997) Null mutation of the prolactin receptor gene produces multiple reproductive defects in the mouse. Genes Dev 11:167–178.

18. Edery M, Pang K, Larson L, Colosi T, Nandi S (1985) Epidermal growth factor receptor levels in mouse mammary glands in various physiological states. Endocrinology 117:405–411.
19. Liscia D, Merlo G, Ciardiello F, Kim N, Smith G, Callahan R, Salomon D (1990) Transforming growth factor-α messenger RNA localization in the developing adult rat and human mammary gland by in situ hybridization. Dev Biol 140:123–131.
20. Snedeker S, Brown C, DiAugustine R (1991) Expression and functional properties of transforming growth factor α and epidermal growth factor during mouse mammary gland ductal morphogenesis. Dev Biol 88:276–280.
21. Coleman S, Silberstein G, Daniel C (1988) Ductal morphogenesis in the mouse mammary gland: evidence supporting a role for epidermal growth factor. Dev Biol 127:304–315.
22. Vonderhaar B (1987) Local effects of EGF, alpha-TGF, and EGF-like growth factor on lobuloalveolar development of the mouse mammary gland in vivo. J Cell Physiol 132:581–584.
23. Fowler K, Walker F, Alexander W, Hibbs M, Nice E, Bohmer R, et al. (1995) A mutation in the epidermal growth factor receptor in waved-2 mice has a profound effect on receptor biochemistry that results in impaired lactation. Proc Natl Acad Sci USA 92:1465–1469.
24. Silberstein G, Daniel C (1987) Reversible inhibition of mammary gland growth by transforming growth factor-β. Science 237:291–293.
25. Daniel C, Silberstein G, van Horn K, Strickland P, Robinson S (1989) TGF-β1-induced inhibition of mouse mammary ductal growth: developmental specificity and characterization. Dev Biol 135:20–30.
26. Robinson S, Silberstein G, Roberts A, Flanders K, Daniel C (1991) Regulated expression and growth inhibitory effects of transforming growth factor-β isoforms in mouse mammary gland development. Development 113:867–878.
27. Silberstein G, Flanders K, Roberts A, Daniel C (1992) Regulation of mammary morphogenesis: evidence for extracellular matrix-mediated inhibition of ductal budding by transforming growth factor-β1. Dev Biol 152:354–362.
28. Jhappan C, Geiser A, Kordon E, Bagheri D, Henninghausen L, Roberts A, et al. (1995) Targeting of a transforming growth factor β1 transgene to the pregnant mammary gland inhibits alveolar development and lactation. EMBO J 12:1835–1845.
29. Coleman-Krnacik S, Rosen J (1994) Differential temporal and spatial gene expression of fibroblast growth factor family members during mouse mammary gland development. Mol Endocrinol 8:218–229.
30. Jackson D, Bresnick J, Rosewell I, Crafton T, Poulson R, Stamp G, et al. (1997) Fibroblast growth factor signaling has a role in lobuloalveolar development of the mammary gland. J Cell Sci 110:1261–1268.
31. Jackson D, Bresnick J, and Dickson C (1997) A role for fibroblast growth factor signaling in the lobuloalveolar development of the mammary gland. J Mam Gland Biol Neoplasia 2:385–392.
32. Imagawa W, Spencer E, Larson L, Nandi S (1986) Somatomedin-C substitutes for insulin for the growth of mammary epithelial cells from normal virgin mice in serum-free collagen gel cell culture. Endocrinology 119:2695–2699.
33. Deeks S, Richards J, Nandi S (1988) Maintenance of normal rat mammary epithelial cells by insulin and insulin-like growth factor. Exp Cell Res 174:448–460.
34. Rechler MM, Nissley SP (1985) The nature and regulation of the receptors for insulin-like growth factors. Annu Rev Physiol 47:425–442.
35. Rechler MM, Nissley SP (1990) Insulin-like growth factors, In: *Peptide Growth Factors and Their Receptors I*, vol. 95 (Sporn MB, Roberts AB, eds.), Springer-Verlag, Heidelberg, pp. 263–267.
36. LeRoith D, Adamo M, Werner H, Roberts CT, Jr (1991) Insulin-like growth factors, their binding proteins and receptors as growth regulators in normal physiology and pathological states. Trends Endocrinol Metab 2:134–139.
37. Werner H, Woloschak M, Stannard B, Shen-Orr Z, Roberts CT, Jr, LeRoith D (1991) The insulin-like growth factor I receptor: molecular biology, heterogeneity and regulation, In: *Insulin-Like Growth Factors: Molecular and Cellular Aspects* (LeRoith D, ed.), CRC Press, Boca Raton, pp. 17–47.
38. Werner H, Roberts CT, Jr, LeRoith D (1994) The regulation of IGF-I receptor gene expression by positive and negative zinc-finger transcription factors. Adv Exp Biol Med 343:91–103.
39. Jones J, Clemmons D (1995) Insulin-like growth factors and their binding proteins: biological actions. Endocr Rev 16:3–34.
40. Baker J, Lie J-P, Robertson EJ, Efstratiadis A (1993) Role of insulin-like growth factors in embryonic and postnatal growth. Cell 75:73–82.
41. Liu J-P, Baker J, Perkins AS, Robertson EJ, Efstratiadis A (1993) Mice carrying null mutations of the genes encoding insulin-like growth factor I *(Igf-1)* and type 1 IGF receptor *(Igf1r)*. Cell 75:59–72.

42. Baserga R, Sell C, Porcu P, Rubini M (1994) The role of the IGF-I receptor in the growth and transformation of mammalian cells. Cell Prolif 27:63–71.
43. Ruan W, Newman C, Kleinberg D (1992) Intact and amino-terminally shortened forms of insulin-like growth factor I induce mammary gland differentiation and development. Proc Natl Acad Sci USA 89:10872–10876.
44. Ruan W, Catanese V, Wieczorek R, Feldman M, Kleinberg D (1995) Estradiol enhances the stimulatory effect of insulin-like growth factor (IGF-1) on mammary development and growth hormone-induced IGF-1 messenger ribonucleic acid. Endocrinology 136:1296–1302.
45. Neuenschwander S, Schwartz A, Wood T, Roberts J, Henninghausen L, LeRoith D (1996) Involution of the lactating mammary gland is inhibited by the IGF system in a transgenic mouse model. J Clin Invest 97:2225–2232.
46. Hadsell D, Greenberg N, Fligger J, Baumrucker C, and Rosen J (1996) Targeted expression of des(1-3) human insulin-like growth factor I in transgenic mice influences mammary gland development and IGF-binding protein expression. Endocrinology 137:321–330.
47. Murphy L, Bell G, Friesen H (1987) Tissue distribution of insulin-like growth factor I and II messenger ribonucleic acid in the adult rat. Endocrinology 120:1279–1282.
48. Hauser S, McGrath M, Collier R, Krivi C (1990) Cloning and in vivo expression of bovine growth hormone receptor mRNA. Mol Cell Endocrinol 72:187–200.
49. Yee D, Paik S, Lebavic G, Marcus R, Favoni R, Cullen K, et al. (1989) Analysis of IGF-I gene expression in malignancy—evidence for a paracrine role in human breast cancer. Mol Endocrinol 3:509–517.
50. Richert M, Wood T (1997) Expression and function of the IGFs in the development of the mouse mammary gland. Presented at *the Endocrine Society, 79th Annual Meeting,* Minneapolis, MN, p. 175.
51. Bates P, Fisher R, Ward A, Richardson L, Hill D, Graham C (1995) Mammary cancer in transgenic mice expression insulin-like growth factor II (IGF-II). Bri J Cancer 72:1189–1193.
52. Giani C, Cullen K, Campani D, Rasmussen A (1996) IGF-II mRNA and protein are expressed in the stroma of invasive breast cancers: an in situ hybridization and immunohistochemistry study. Breast Cancer Res Treat. 41:43–50.
53. Cullen K, Smith H, Hill S, Rosen N, and Lippman M (1991) Growth factor messenger RNA expression by human breast fibroblasts from benign and malignant lesions. Cancer Res 51:4978–4985.
54. McCusker RH, Clemmons DR (1992) The insulin-like growth factor binding proteins: structure and biological functions, In: *The Insulin-Like Growth Factors: Structure and Biological Functions* (Schofield PN, ed.), Oxford University Press, New York, pp. 110–150.
55. Clemmons DR, Jones JI, Busby WH, Wright G (1993) Role of insulin-like growth factor binding proteins in modifying IGF actions. Ann NY Acad Sci 692:10–21.
56. Clemmons DR (1993) IGF binding proteins and their functions. Mol Reprod Dev 35:368–375.
57. Clemmons D, Busby W, Arai T, Nam T, Clarke J, Jones J, et al. (1995) Role of insulin-like growth factor binding proteins in the control of IGF actions. Prog Growth Factor Res 6:357–366.
58. Clemmons DR (1994) Role of post translational modifications in modifying the biologic activity of insulin-like growth factor binding proteins. Adv Exp Biol Med 343:245–253.
59. Mohan S, Baylink D (1996) Editorial: insulin-like growth factor (IGF)-binding proteins in serum—do they have additional roles besides modulating the endocrine IGF actions? J Clin Endocrinol Metab 81:3817–3820.
60. Arai T, Parker A, Busby WJ, Clemmons D (1994) Heparin, heparan sulfate, and dermatan sulfate regulate formation of the insulin-like growth factor-I and insulin-like growth factor-binding protein complexes. J Biol Chem 269:20388–20393.
61. Hakeda Y, Kawaguchi H, Hurley M, Pilbeam C, Abreu C, Linkhart T, et al. (1996) Intact insulin-like growth factor binding protein-5 (IGFBP-5) associates with bone matrix and the soluble fragments of IGFBP-5 accumulated in culture medium of neonatal mouse calvariae by parathyroid hormone and prostaglandin E2–treatment. J Cell Physiol 166:370–379.
62. Arai T, Clarke J, Parker A, Busby WJ, Nam T, Clemmons D (1996) Substitution of specific amino acids in insulin-like growth factor (IGF) binding protein 5 alters heparin binding and its change in affinity for IGF-I in response to heparin. J Biol Chem 271:6099–6106.
63. Parker A, Clarke J, Busby WJ, Clemmons D (1996) Identification of the extracellular matrix binding sites for insulin-like growth factor-binding protein 5. J Biol Chem 271:13523–13529.
64. Arai T, Arai A, Busby WJ, Clemmons D (1994) Glycosaminoglycans inhibit degradation of insulin-like growth factor-binding protein-5. Endocrinology 135:2358–2363.
65. Nam T, Busby WJ, Clemmons D (1994) Human fibroblasts secrete a serine protease that cleaves insulin-like growth factor-binding protein-5. Endocrinology 135:1385–1391.

66. Lin C, Bissell M (1993) Multi-faceted regulation of cell differentiation by extracellular matrix. FASEB J 7:737–743.
67. Sympson C, Talhouk R, Alexander C, Chin J, Clift S, Bissell M, et al. (1994) Targeted expression of stromelysin-1 in mammary gland provides evidence for a role of proteinases in branching morphogenesis and the requirement for an intact basement membrane for tissue-specific gene expression. J Cell Biol 125:681–693.
68. Beck J, Lekutis C, Couchman J, Parry G (1993) Stage-specific remodeling of the mammary gland basement membrane during lactogenic development. Biochem Biophys Res Commun 190:616–623.
69. Keely P, Wu J, Santoro S (1995) The spatial and temporal expression of the $\alpha2\beta1$ integrin and its ligands, collagen I, collagen IV, and laminin, suggest important roles in mouse mammary morphogenesis. Differentiation 59:1–13.
70. Jones J, Gockerman A, Busby W, Jr, Wright G, Clemmons D (1993) Insulin-like growth factor binding protein 1 stimulates cell migration and binds to the $\alpha5\beta1$ integrin by means of its Arg-Gly-Asp sequence. Proc Natl Acad Sci USA 90:10553–10557.
71. Gockerman A, Prevette T, Jones J, Clemmons D (1995) Insulin-like growth factor (IGF)-binding proteins inhibit the smooth muscle cell migration responses to IGF-I and IGF-II. Endocrinology 136:4168–4173.
72. Jones J, Doerr M, Clemmons D (1995) Cell migration: interactions among integrins, IGFs and IGFBPs. Prog Growth Factor Res 6:319–327.
73. Mohan S, Nakao Y, Honda Y, Landale E, Leser U, Dony C, et al. (1995) Studies on the mechanisms by which insulin-like growth factor (IGF) binding protein-4 (IGFBP-4) and IGFBP-5 modulate IGF actions in bone cells. J Biol Chem 270:20424–20431.
74. Oh Y, Gucev Z, Ng L, Muller H, Rosenfeld R (1995) Antiproliferative actions of insulin-like growth factor binding protein (IGFBP)-3 in human breast cancer cells. Prog Growth Factor Res 6:503–512.
75. Rajah R, Valentinis B, Cohen P (1997) Insulin-like growth factor (IGF)-binding protein-3 induces apoptosis and mediates the effects of transforming growth factor-beta1 on programmed cell death through a p53- and IGF-independent mechanism. J Biol Chem 272:12181–12188.
76. Oh Y, Muller H, Ng L, Rosenfeld R (1995) Transforming growth factor-beta-induced cell growth inhibition in human breast cancer cells is mediated through insulin-like growth factor-binding protein-3 action. J Biol Chem 270:13589–13592.
77. Gucev Z, Oh Y, Kelley K, Rosenfeld R (1996) Insulin-like growth factor binding protein 3 mediates retinoic acid- and transforming growth factor beta2–induced growth inhibition in human breast cancer cells. Cancer Research 56:1545–1550.
78. Leal S, Liu Q, Huang S, Huang J (1997) The type V transforming growth factor beta receptor is the putative insulin-like growth factor-binding protein 3 receptor. J Biol Chem 272:20572–20576.
79. Figueroa J, Yee D (1992) The insulin-like growth factor binding proteins (IGFBPs) in human breast cancer. Breast Cancer Res Treat 22:81–90.
80. Manni A, Badger B, Wei L, Zaenglein A, Grove R, Khin S, et al. (1994) Hormonal regulation of insulin-like growth factor II and insulin-like growth factor binding protein expression by breast cancer cells in vivo: evidence for stromal epithelial interactions. Cancer Res 54:2934–2942.
81. McGuire S, Hilsenbeck S, Figueroa J, Jackson J, Yee D (1994) Detection of insulin-like growth factor binding proteins (IGFBPs) by ligand blotting in breast cancer tissues. Cancer Letters 77:25–32.
82. Yee D (1994) The insulin-like growth factor system as a target in breast cancer. Breast Cancer Res Treat 32:85–95.
83. Wood TL, O'Donnell SL, Levison SW (1995) Cytokines regulate IGF binding proteins in the CNS. Prog Growth Factor Res 6:181–187.

II

CARCINOGENESIS

4 Estrogens and Breast Cancer

An Epidemiologic Perspective

Heather Spencer Feigelson, PhD
and Brian E. Henderson, MD

The past 20 years of research have identified several risk and protective factors for breast cancer. All these factors can be understood as measures of the cumulative exposure of the breast to estrogen and, perhaps, progesterone. These ovarian hormones affect the rate of cell division and thus manifest their effect on the risk of breast cancer by causing proliferation of breast epithelial cells *(1)*. Proliferating cells are susceptible to genetic errors during DNA replication, which, if uncorrected, can ultimately lead to a malignant phenotype.

This chapter provides a brief overview of the primary risk factors for breast cancer and also reviews the evidence for the role of endogenous estrogens with their two most common sources, combined oral contraceptives (COCs) and hormone replacement therapy (HRT). Finally, the role of genetic susceptibility to breast cancer and the possible interaction between genetic alterations and estrogen exposure are presented.

BREAST CANCER RISK FACTORS

The known risk and protective factors for breast cancer are shown in Table 1. Early menarche and late menopause maximize the number of ovulatory cycles and therefore the cumulative estrogen "dose" to the breast epithelium. In general, about a 20% decrease in breast cancer risk results from each year menarche is delayed, and women who experience natural menopause before age 45 are estimated to have only half the breast cancer risk of those whose menopause occurs after age 55 *(2)*.

The primary source of estrogens in postmenopausal women is from the conversion of androstenedione to estrone in peripheral tissues, including adipose; thus, postmenopausal obesity increases the risk of breast cancer through increased production of estrogens. Obesity is also associated with decreased sex hormone binding globulin (SHBG) production and increased proportions of free- and albumin-bound estradiol, which are understood to be the biologically active estrogens *(3)*. Alcohol appears to increase plasma estrogen levels. Although alcohol consumption may confer a small increased risk for breast cancer, results across studies have been inconsistent. As summarized in a meta-analysis by Howe et al. *(4)*, women who consume three or more alcoholic drinks per day

From: *Contemporary Endocrinology: Endocrinology of Breast Cancer*
Edited by: A. Manni © Humana Press Inc., Totowa, NJ

Table 1
Risk Factors and Protective Factors for Breast Cancer

Risk factors (increased exposure to estrogen and progesterone)
Early menarche
Late menopause
Postmenopausal obesity
Hormone replacement therapy
Alcohol consumption
Protective factors (decreased exposure to estrogen and progesterone)
Early first full-term pregnancy
Lactation
Physical activity

have about a 50–70% increase in breast cancer risk compared with nondrinkers. For lower levels of consumption, the risks are correspondingly lower and confidence intervals generally include 1.0.

The protective effect of early age at first birth is complex. During the first trimester of pregnancy, the level of free estradiol rises rapidly. However, as the pregnancy continues, prolactin and free estradiol levels decrease, while SHBG levels increase, giving a net overall benefit with respect to the endogenous estrogen profile, which is associated with a permanent reduction in breast cancer risk *(3)*. Prolonged lactation and, more importantly, physical activity can reduce the number of ovulatory cycles. Bernstein et al. *(5)* found that the risk of breast cancer among women who exercised 4 or more hours per week during their reproductive years was nearly 60% lower than that of inactive women.

ENDOGENOUS ESTROGENS

Animal studies have repeatedly demonstrated that estrogens can induce and promote mammary tumors in rodents and that removing the ovaries or administering an antiestrogenic drug has the opposite effect *(6)*. One source of epidemiologic evidence of the role of endogenous estrogens in breast cancer etiology has come from studies of serum and urine hormone levels in populations at low and high risk. Shimizu et al. *(7)* reported higher levels of serum estrone and estradiol in postmenopausal white women in the United States compared with postmenopausal women living in rural Japan. Bernstein et al. *(8)* found higher serum estradiol levels in premenopausal cases compared with controls in two concurrent studies in Shanghai and the United States after carefully controlling for day of menstrual cycle. Furthermore, they showed that U.S. controls had higher estradiol concentrations than their Shanghai counterparts. Higher levels of estrone and estradiol were also found in postmenopausal cases of breast cancer compared with controls in Los Angeles *(9)*. Finally, numerous case-control and cohort studies have been conducted that compared serum hormone levels in breast cancer cases and healthy women. Key and Pike *(10)* summarized the results of early studies of serum hormones and breast cancer and concluded that postmenopausal breast cancer cases are exposed to more endogenous estrogen than controls. Recent studies have continued to support this conclusion and are discussed below. Table 2 summarizes the findings of six recent studies.

Lipworth et al. *(11)* conducted a population-based case-control study that included 122 pairs of postmenopausal women. In comparisons between the highest and lowest quartiles

Table 2

Summary of Recent Studies of Endogenous Hormones and Breast Cancer[a]

Study	*Type of study*	*Location*	*Menopausal Status*	*Cases/controls*	*Serum hormones*	*RR (95% CI)*
Lipworth et al. *(11)*	Population-based case-control (retrospective)	Sweden	Post	122/122	Estrone[b]	1.9 (0.7–5.2)
					Androstenedione	2.4 (0.9–6.6)
					Testosterone	0.5 (0.1–1.9)
					SHBG	0.3 (0.1–0.7)
Toniolo et al. *(12)*	Population-based case-control (prospective)	USA	Post	130/251	Total E2[b]	1.8 (0.8–3.8)
					Free E2	2.9 (1.3–6.6)
					% SHBG-bound E2	0.3 (0.1–0.7)
					% Albumin-bound E2	3.3 (1.4–7.4)
					Estrone	2.5 (0.8–7.8)
Berrino et al. *(13)*	Population-based case-control (prospective)	Italy	Post	24/88	Estradiol[c]	5.5 (0.8–37)
					Testosterone	7.0 (1.4–36)
					SHBG	0.3 (0.1–1.3)
					DHEAS	2.6 (0.6–11.1)
Thomas et al. *(14)*	Population-based case-control (prospective)	UK	Pre	62/182	Estradiol[d]	1.5 (0.9–2.6)
					Progesterone	0.8 (0.4–1.5)
					Testosterone	1.2 (0.6–2.4)
					SHBG	1.8 (0.8–4.1)
Thomas et al. *(15)*	Population-based case-control (prospective)	UK	Post	61/179	Estradiol[c]	5.0 (2.0–12.5)
					Testosterone	2.4 (1.0–5.7)
					SHBG	0.4 (0.2–0.9)
Dorgan et al. *(16)*	Population-based case-control (prospective)	USA	Post	71/133	Total E2[b]	2.7 (0.8–9.1)
					Free E2	5.2 (1.5–18.5)
					E1S/E1	0.3 (0.1–0.9)
					Testosterone	6.2 (2.0–19.0)
					SHBG	1.3 (0.5–3.9)

[a]Abbreviations: SHBG, sex hormone binding globulin; E2, estradiol; DHEAS, dehydroepiandrosterone sulfate.
[b]RR in this study correspond to comparisons between lowest and highest quartile.
[c]Comparisons between lowest and highest tertile.
[d]Per unit increase in log-transformed values

of serum hormone concentration, a positive association with breast cancer was found with estrone (odds ratio [OR] 1.20; 95% confidence interval (CI) 0.93–1.55) and androstenedione (OR 1.32; 95% CI 1.05–1.65), and inverse associations were found with SHBG (OR 0.71; 95% CI 0.48–1.04) and testosterone (OR 0.48; 95% CI 0.12–1.90) after mutual adjustment for hormonal variables and body mass index (BMI). Although neither of the adjusted associations of estrone or androstenedione are large, some of the effect of estrone would be underestimated when androstenedione is included in the model, since androstenedione is a precursor of estrone. The authors also found evidence of statistical interaction between BMI and SHBG. The OR for women with high SHBG and high BMI was 0.14 and the 95% CI 0.04–0.53 after adjusting for the other hormonal variables compared with women with low BMI and low SHBG. As the authors discuss, one explanation for this finding may be that reduced levels of SHBG imply higher estrogen bioavailability. Alternatively, low SHBG may reflect high circulating levels of insulin or insulin-like growth factor I (IGF-I), which are powerful negative regulators of SHBG synthesis in vitro *(11)*. One potential source of bias in this study is the possibility that the recent surgery among cases altered the serum steroid hormone levels. However, serum samples were all drawn at least 1 week postoperatively, which should be sufficient time for steroid levels to normalize. Such bias can be eliminated by using a prospective study design.

Toniolo et al. *(12)* found that free estradiol, albumin-bound estradiol, and estrone were all associated with increased risk of breast cancer after adjusting for BMI among 130 cases and 251 controls in a prospective study. Comparing the highest quartile with the lowest quartile, the adjusted RR for free (i.e., unbound) estradiol was 2.9 (95% CI 1.3–6.6), the adjusted RR for albumin-bound estradiol was 3.3 (95% CI 1.4–7.4), the adjusted RR for estrone was 2.5 (95% CI 0.8–7.8), and the adjusted RR for estrone comparing the third with the lowest quartile was 3.7 (95% CI 1.4–10.2). Levels of total estradiol and SHBG-bound estradiol were also elevated among cases but did not reach statistical significance.

Among 24 postmenopausal breast cancer cases and 88 matched control subjects from a prospective study, Berrino et al. *(13)* found higher serum levels of total estradiol, dehydroepiandrosterone sulfate (DHEAS), total testosterone, and free testosterone, and lower levels of SHBG among cases compared with controls. The age-adjusted RR of breast cancer comparing the highest serum tertile to the lowest tertile was 5.5 (95% CI 1.5–22.2) for total estradiol, 7.0 (95% CI 1.4–36.4) for total testosterone, 5.7 (95% CI 1.5–22.2) for free testosterone, 2.6 (95% CI 0.6–11.1) for DHEAS, and 0.3 (95% CI 0.1–1.3) for SHBG.

Thomas et al. examined serum hormone concentrations and breast cancer risk in two nested case-control studies among premenopausal *(14)* and postmenopausal *(15)* women on the island of Guernsey (UK).

Sixty-two premenopausal cases were matched to 182 cohort control subjects on day of menstrual cycle (that blood was collected), age, and year of blood collection. Although the results of this study did not reach statistical significance, cases had 12% higher mean estradiol than controls over the whole menstrual cycle, with a large difference at midcycle (75% higher, $p = 0.04$). The trends for estradiol and testosterone are consistent with those reported in other studies *(12,13)*. However, Thomas et al. *(14,15)* found higher SHBG among premenopausal cases compared with controls, a finding inconsistent with results of other studies and with the hypothesized relationship between SHBG and breast cancer.

Their second study *(15)* included 61 cases of postmenopausal cases matched on age, year of blood collection, and number of years since menopause with 179 control women from the cohort. Compared with controls, breast cancer cases had a 29% higher mean estradiol (E2) ($p = 0.004$), 22% higher testosterone ($p = 0.005$), and 12% lower SHBG ($p = 0.053$). Compared with those with serum E2 in the lowest tertile, women with E2 levels in the highest tertile were five times more likely to develop breast cancer (RR 5.03; 95% CI 2.0–12.5). Women in the highest tertile of serum testosterone were also at significantly increased risk compared to women with serum testosterone in the lowest tertile (RR 2.39; 95% CI 1.0–5.7), whereas the highest tertile of serum SHBG had a protective effect on risk of breast cancer (RR 0.37; 95% CI 0.15–0.89).

Finally, Dorgan, et al. *(16)* also found that postmenopausal women with elevated serum levels of E2 are at increased risk for developing breast cancer in a nested case-control study including 71 cases and 133 matched controls. The authors found an increased risk of breast cancer for both total E2 and for non-SHBG E2 (i.e., the biologically available fraction). Compared with the lowest quartile, women with non-SHBG E2 in the upper quartile were five times more likely to develop breast cancer (RR 5.2; 95% CI 1.5–18.5). Women in the highest quartile of serum testosterone, androstenedione, DHEAS, and SHBG were also at increased risk compared with women in the lowest quartile. Neither serum estrone (E1) nor estrone sulfate (E1S) were associated with the risk of developing breast cancer. However, the E1/E1S ratio, which in part may reflect the body's ability to inactivate E1, was strongly inversely associated with risk (RR 0.3; 95% CI 0.1–0.9 for the highest quartile compared with the lowest).

The findings of 29 epidemiologic studies of endogenous hormones and postmenopausal breast cancer, including the ones reviewed in detail here, have recently been summarized in a meta-analytic review *(17)*. Taken together, the six prospective studies published to date show that postmenopausal women who subsequently develop breast cancer have a 15% higher mean serum estradiol concentration than unaffected women ($p = 0.0003$). The more recent studies were more likely to show a positive association, perhaps because more stringent study conditions were imposed on the collection and laboratory analysis of the serum samples. Summary data from case-control studies showed a similar result; however, significant heterogeneity existed between studies. The summary estimates did not take into account the possible effects of time since menopause or body weight, both of which may confound the association between serum estrogen and breast cancer. However, the authors point out that the affect of body weight on breast cancer risk may be mediated through the association of weight with estradiol; thus, it would not be appropriate to adjust for body weight.

Taken together, the epidemiologic evidence strongly supports the theory that endogenous estrogens play a crucial role in breast carcinogenesis. This is in spite of the well-known problems that arise when attempting to measure steroid hormones accurately. Serum hormone measurements are subject to variation by many factors, for example, time of day, age, disease status, and laboratory imprecision. Further work is necessary to resolve the conflicting findings of the role of SHBG and breast cancer, and to confirm the association with testosterone and other androgens reported in these studies. There is a scientific basis for the association between risk of breast cancer and serum androgens, as androgens could provide a large pool of substrate for conversion to estrogen via the action of aromatase in breast tissue. As discussed later, underlying genetic differences in hormone metabolism among individuals may also introduce unmeasured confounding that may distort the results of studies of serum hormone levels.

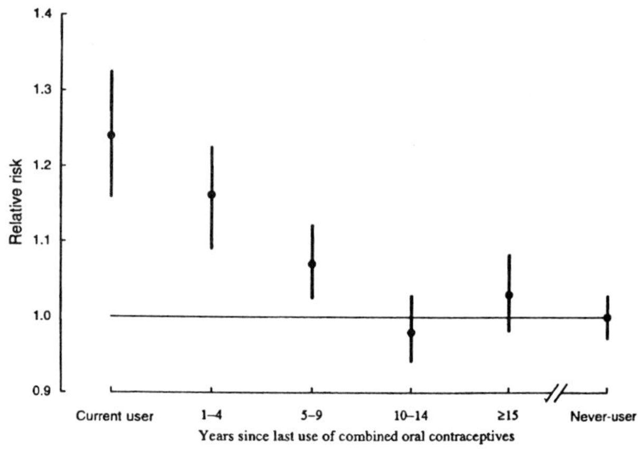

Fig. 1. Relative risk of breast cancer by time since last use of combined oral contraceptives. (From ref. *18*, with permission.)

ORAL CONTRACEPTIVES

COCs have been widely used since the early 1960s. By 1978, the World Health Organization estimated that more than 80 million women had been exposed to these drugs worldwide. A substantial body of literature now exists on the relation between COC use and risk of breast cancer; however, the conclusions have been mixed and controversial. A recent meta-analysis of 54 different studies that included a total of 53,297 women with breast cancer and 100,239 controls has provided many important answers about the risk of breast cancer among COC users *(18)*.

One important question has been whether the timing of COC use affects the risk of breast cancer. Many studies have suggested that COC use at an early age or before a first pregnancy increased the risk of breast cancer. Other studies have suggested that timc since first use, or time since last use, were important determinants of risk. Since these four indices are highly correlated, they are difficult to separate in a small study. This meta-analysis had sufficient power to examine adequately these four parameters independently and found that increased risk of breast cancer was associated with current (RR 1.24; $p < 0.00001$) and recent (RR 1.16; $p < 0.00001$) COC use. (Recent use was defined by use 1–4 years prior to diagnosis of breast cancer.) As demonstrated in Figure 1, this excess risk does not persist, and there is no evidence of an increased risk of breast cancer 10 or more years after cessation of COC use.

Few factors appeared to modify the risk associated with recent use of COCs, despite the large number of possibilities considered. The only factor identified that had much effect on risk that was associated with recent use was the age at first use. For recent users, the risks were greatest for those who began COC use before the age of 20 than for those who began at later ages, and tended to decline with increasing age at diagnoses. Neither total duration of COC use, nor duration of use prior to a first pregnancy, were associated with increased risk of breast cancer once recency of use was accounted for, and these relationships were consistent across all age groups. Possible confounders such as family history of breast cancer, ethnicity, menopausal status, age at menarche, and weight did not modify the magnitude of risk. However, family history data was not detailed and, as discussed later, certain subgroups of women may be at much higher risk based on individual genetic susceptibility.

Another significant finding of this study is that the cancers diagnosed in women who have ever used COCs are less likely to have spread beyond the breast than in women who have never used COCs (RR 0.88; $p = 0.002$). Furthermore, the magnitude of the relative deficit of more extensive disease did not vary significantly with time since last COC use, and the relative deficit is still evident 10 or more years after use (RR 0.85; $p = 0.001$). Thus, the excess risk in recent users was largely associated with tumors localized to the breast. It is not possible to infer from this study whether this finding is due to earlier diagnosis of cancer among ever-users (possibly resulting from increased medical surveillance), a biologic effect of COCs, or a combination of reasons.

Although the scope of this study is broad, there is still little information beyond 10 years after cessation of use. Moreover, most women who stopped use 10 or more years ago had used COCs for only short periods *(18)*. In the next decade, women who began use as teenagers will reach their late 40s and early 50s. At that time, it will be important to reexamine the effects of long-term and early use of COCs.

HORMONE REPLACEMENT THERAPY

The most commonly prescribed HRT for menopausal women in the United States includes conjugated equine estrogens (CEE), with a preferred dose of 0.625 mg/d for 25 days in a 28-d treatment cycle. This dose is lower than those commonly prescribed during the 1970s. Progestogens, usually 10 mg/d of medroxyprogesterone acetate, are sometimes added during days 14–25.

Most early studies of the possible effects of HRT on risk of breast cancer were uncontrolled follow-up studies. Early case-control studies that reported findings on menopausal estrogens and breast cancer were often limited by small numbers, insufficient data on dose and duration of use, and definite possibility of bias. Since the early 1980s, dozens of case-control studies using healthy population controls and large cohort studies have been published *(19)*. Overall, these studies found small to moderate increases in breast cancer risk after long-term use of estrogen replacement alone, although some variation existed across studies for ovarian status (intact versus removed) or antecedent surgical menopause, and some important sources of bias were not adequately addressed.

A recent meta-analysis including 52,505 women with breast cancer and 108,411 controls from 51 studies has clarified the relationship between HRT and breast cancer *(19)*. This study has also confirmed the important effects of age at menopause on breast cancer risk. Numerous sources of bias must be considered when evaluating any study of menopausal hormone use and breast cancer risk. Perhaps the most important confounder is the interaction between onset of menopause and onset of hormone use. Timing of menopause (early age of onset vs later age of onset) is associated with risk of breast cancer. Replacement therapy typically begins at the onset of menopausal symptoms and therefore masks the actual onset of menopause. Women who have early age at menopause have a reduced risk of breast cancer, but this may be confounded by replacement therapy at the onset of symptoms. Similarly, onset of menopause is masked in women who have a hysterectomy without bilateral oophorectomy. Furthermore, hysterectomized women may receive estrogen-only therapy while all other women are much more likely to receive progestin also.

This meta-analysis was of sufficient size to address these sources of bias by excluding from the analysis any woman having an unknown age at menopause. Thus, women who reported starting HRT use before their stated age at natural menopause and women who

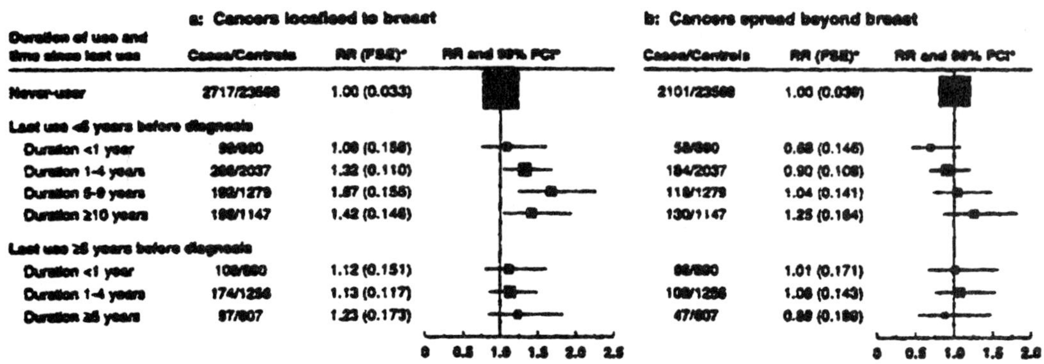

Fig. 2. Relative risk of breast cancer by duration and time since last use of hormone replacement therapy according to extent of tumor spread. (From ref. *19*, with permission.)

reported hysterectomy without bilateral oophorectomy before the natural menopause were excluded from the analysis. Altogether, this resulted in exclusion of about 18% of the study population.

In this large study, important aspects of menopause on breast cancer risk could be examined among never-users of HRT, and the findings confirmed long-standing hypotheses. The relation between age at menopause and breast cancer risk was similar for women with a natural menopause and those with a bilateral oophorectomy. As expected, women with an early menopause have a reduced risk of breast cancer. In postmenopausal women, the risk of breast cancer was related to BMI, increasing by 3.1% for each kg/m^2.

Among postmenopausal controls, ever-use of HRT was also related to BMI. Women with lower BMI were more likely to be current HRT users and to have used HRT for 5 years or longer. Based on these findings, the subsequent analyses were stratified by BMI, but not by type of menopause (natural vs surgical).

The main findings of the meta-analysis, displayed in Figure 2, show that for current or recent use of HRT, the risk for breast cancer increases in relation to increasing duration of use. For women whose last use of HRT was <5 years before diagnosis, there was strong evidence of increasing risk of breast cancer with increasing duration of use. Risk increased by 2.3% (i.e., RR 1.023; $p = 0.0002$) for each year of use. However, for women who stopped HRT use ≥5 years before diagnosis, there is no significant increase in the risk of breast cancer, either overall or in relation to duration of HRT use. After taking these timing factors into account, no other index of timing was important, including age at first use or time between menopause and first use. Furthermore, other potentially confounding factors, including family history, ethnicity, and education, did not modify the results. The only factor that seemed to modify the effect of HRT in current or recent users was BMI, with increased risk more pronounced in women with lower body weight. (A finding that is expected based on what we know about BMI and endogenous estrogens among postmenopausal women.)

Another important finding in this study, and similar to the findings for COC use, is that tumors among ever-users of HRT were less likely to have spread to axillary lymph nodes or to more distant sites compared with women who had never used HRT.

Users of HRT may have different opportunities for breast cancer diagnosis. For example, they may be screened for breast cancer before being prescribed HRT, and they may have more frequent mammographic or physician examinations than women who are not currently taking HRT. Other important differences between women who are prescribed HRT compared with never-users exist. Women with a family history of breast cancer are more likely to be never-users but are at increased risk of breast cancer, which may result in bias toward the null. Women who use HRT are more likely than never-users to be higher educated and of higher social class. Laya et al. *(20)* have provided direct evidence that current HRT use reduces the sensitivity and specificity of mammographic screening, most likely by increasing radiographic breast density. This differential misclassification could result in more breast cancer being missed on mammographic exam among HRT users, and thus an underestimation of the true risk of breast cancer associated with HRT use. However, because a similar finding was seen in the meta-analysis of COC use *(18)*, it is possible that these exogenous hormone preparations have a biologic effect on the breast that manifests in tumor characteristics; this should be examined in laboratory models.

Although the large size and comprehensive nature of this study has clarified many questions about the use of HRT and risk of breast cancer, some remain unanswered. As the authors point out, virtually no information about HRT and breast cancer risk beyond the age of 75 exists. Although this study found no marked variation in risk according to a broad classification of type or dose of HRT preparation used, the data were insufficient to permit reliable conclusions about different hormonal preparations on breast cancer risk. Key and Pike *(10)* have asserted that combined estrogen-progestogen therapy could be more carcinogenic than estrogen alone, and only about 12% of women in this meta-analysis would be expected to have used a combination estrogen-progestogen therapy. Finally, an important source of confounding that has not been addressed in any study to date is the possible role of underlying genetic susceptibility to breast cancer, which may affect the breast cancer risk associated with exposure to both endogenous and exogenous ovarian hormones.

GENETIC SUSCEPTIBILITY

Remarkable advances in molecular biology and careful study of cancer-prone families led to the identification of two breast cancer susceptibility genes, BRCA1 and BRCA2 (collectively referred to here as BRCA). Women who inherit a mutated copy of either gene have a high risk of developing breast cancer. Some estimates suggest that the risk is 87% by the age of 70 years *(21)*; however, this estimate is under heavy debate as more population-based studies emerge. The true lifetime risk may actually be much lower *(22)*, and it is well recognized that not all BRCA mutations will carry equal risk: some may be highly penetrant, while others may be silent.

One important determinant of penetrance may be the interaction of BRCA mutations with other known risk factors for breast cancer. We can hypothesize that both endogenous and exogenous hormonal factors may affect gene penetrance and expression. A recent study by Ursin et al. *(23)* begins to address this issue. In a population-based sample of 50 young Ashkenazi Jewish breast cancer patients, long-term OC use (over 4 years of use) was associated with an elevated risk of being classified as having a BRCA mutation (odds ratio [OR] 7.8; 95% CI 1.1–55.0). The results suggest that OC use may increase breast cancer risk substantially more in carriers of a mutated copy of BRCA. This study is the first to address the important issue of gene-environment interaction in carriers of mutant

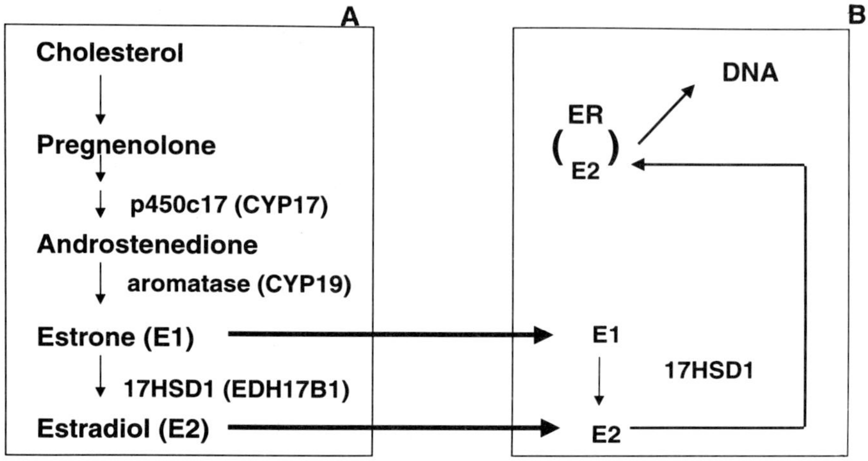

Fig. 3. Schematic presentation of estrogen metabolism in the ovaries and breast epithelium and four candidate genes that may play a role in breast cancer etiology. The genes of interest are the cytochrome P450c17α(CYP17) gene, the aromatase cytochrome P450 (CYP19) gene, the 17β-hydroxy steroid dehydrogenase 1 (HSD17B1) gene, and the estrogen receptor (ER) gene.

BRCA, and the results should be interpreted cautiously, given the small sample size of the study.

Although the impact of BRCA1 and BRCA2 is significant, probably no more than 5–10% of all breast cancers in the United States are attributable to these two loci *(24)*. Additional genes probably contribute to breast cancer risk. Much more common are multiple susceptibility genes, which have low absolute risk, but potentially high population-attributable risk. One such class of genes is that which codes for enzymes or receptors that control the metabolism and intracellular transport of estrogens.

We have used the paradigms that have been developed from studies of bladder cancer to propose a model for individual susceptibility to breast cancer *(25)*. We have assumed that within and between ethnic groups there exist genetic differences that affect steroid hormone metabolism and transport. Markers (i.e., genetic polymorphisms) of these differences are likely to provide a more precise measure of risk than circulating levels of steroid hormones. The polygenic model that we have developed for breast cancer assumes that there are functionally important polymorphisms in genes that encode enzymes involved in steroid hormone biosynthesis and metabolism that lead to differences in individual susceptibility to breast cancer and may interact with exogenous hormone exposures.

Figure 3 shows the schematic presentation of estrogen metabolism in the ovaries and breast epithelium and four candidate genes that may play a role in breast cancer etiology. The genes of interest are the cytochrome P450c17α (CYP17) gene, the aromatase P450 (CYP19) gene, the 17β -hydroxy steroid dehydrogenase 1 (HSD17B1) gene, and the estrogen receptor (ER) gene. CYP17 codes for the cytochrome P450c17α enzyme that mediates both steroid 17α-hydroxylase and 17-20-lyase activities and functions at key branch points in human steroidogenesis *(26)*. 17α -Hydroxylase activity converts steroids to precursors of the glucocorticoid cortisol, and 17-20-lyase activity yields precursors to estradiol and testosterone. Aromatase, the product of CYP19, catalyzes three consecutive hydroxylation reactions converting the C19 androgens to aromatic C18 estrogenic steroids *(27)*. The HSD17B1 gene codes for the enzyme 17 β-hydroxy steroid dehydrogenase type 1 (17HSD1), which catalyzes the final step of estradiol biosynthesis, namely, the interconversion of estrone into the more biologically active estrogen fraction, estradiol *(28)*. The primary role of steroid receptors, like ER, is to regulate the rate of transcription of certain genes by binding as a hormone-receptor complex to specific sequences of DNA called hormone response elements (HREs). Interaction between the receptor and HRE can result in either up- or downregulation of transcription, depending on binding and action of auxiliary factors specific to the target gene and the tissue. Polymorphisms in the ER gene may affect estrogen binding and subsequent transcription in target genes.

We have recently presented the first epidemiologic evidence to support this model *(29)*. The 5' untranslated region of CYP17 contains a single base pair polymorphism 34 bp upstream from the initiation of translation, and 27 bp downstream from the transcription start site *(30)*. This base pair change creates a recognition site for the *Msp*AI restriction enzyme and has been used to designate two alleles, A1 (the published sequence) and A2. We found a 2.5-fold increased risk of advanced breast cancer associated with the CYP17 A2 allele (95% CI 1.1–5.9). Furthermore, we showed that the A2 allele is associated with an earlier age at menarche among control subjects, and that there was an interaction between CYP17 genotype and age at menarche for risk of breast cancer.

One important question left unanswered in this first study was whether serum hormone levels differed by CYP17 genotype. Accordingly, we conducted a second study to examine the association between serum hormone levels and CYP17 genotype among a group of healthy, premenopausal, nulliparous women *(31)*. E2 measured on day 11 of the menstrual cycle was 11% and 57% higher ($p = 0.04$), respectively, among women hetero- or homozygous for the CYP17 A2 allele compared with A1/A1 women. Similarly, on cycle day 22, E2 was 7% and 28% higher ($p = 0.06$) and progesterone was 24% and 30% higher ($p = 0.04$). These data provide direct evidence of genetic control of serum hormone levels and help explain why measurement of postmenopausal hormone levels can be used to predict breast cancer risk.

Similar studies are under way for other relevant polymorphisms in the genes outlined in our model of genetic susceptibility to breast cancer.

PERSPECTIVES

It is widely accepted that cancer causation is the result of the combined influence of genetic susceptibility and environmental exposures (including endogenous hormone exposure). To understand and ultimately prevent breast cancer, we must understand both the genetic and environmental components.

The primary risk factors for breast cancer can be understood as regulators of the lifetime endogenous estrogen exposure on breast epithelium. Exogenous estrogens, namely COCs and HRT, probably make modest contributions to breast cancer risk. However, these risks must be weighed against the well-known benefits afforded by their use. In a recent report from the Nurses Health Study *(32)*, the authors found that current HRT users had a lower risk of death than women who had never used HRT. However, this apparent benefit decreased with long-term HRT use (10 or more years) because of an increase in mortality from breast cancer.

Metabolic genes and their role in carcinogenesis comprise a relatively new area of research with scant information at present. Individual differences in estrogen metabolism attributed to genetic polymorphisms and mutations should help us define women who may be at greater risk of breast cancer for certain exposures, such as exogenous estrogens, compared with other women who may be relatively genetically "insensitive" to the same exposure. Explicit epidemiologic studies of gene-cancer relationships need to be conducted to further our understanding of breast cancer etiology, control, and ultimately prevention. Although these types of investigations are still in their infancy, it is time to begin to capitalize on the rapid advancement of molecular biology techniques and integrate them into epidemiologic studies.

REFERENCES

1. Preston-Martin S, Pike MC, Ross RK, et al. (1990) Increased cell division as a cause of human cancer. Cancer Res 50:7415–221.
2. Henderson BE, Bernstein L (1996) Endogenous and exogenous hormonal factors. In: Diseases of the Breast (Harris JR, Morrow M, Lippman ME, Helman S, eds.), Lippincott-Raven, Philadelphia, pp. 185–200.
3. Bernstein L, Ross RK (1993) Endogenous hormones and breast cancer risk. Epidemiol Rev 15:48–65.
4. Howe G, Rohan T, et al. (1991) The association between alcohol and breast cancer risk: evidence from the combined analysis of six dietary case-control studies. Int J Cancer 47:707–710.
5. Bernstein L, Henderson BE, Hanisch R, et al. (1994) Physical exercise activity reduces the risk of breast cancer in young women. J Natl Cancer Inst 86:1403.
6. Dao TL (1991) The role of ovarian steroid hormones in mammary carcinogenesis, In: Hormones and Breast Cancer (Pike MC, Siiteri PK, Welsch CW, eds.), Banbury Report no. 8. Cold Spring Harbor Laboratory, Cold Spring Harbor, NY, pp. 281–295.
7. Shimizu H, Ross RK, Bernstein L, Pike MC, Henderson BE (1990) Serum oestrogen levels in postmenopausal women: comparison of American whites and Japanese in Japan. Br J Cancer 62:451–453.
8. Bernstein L, Yuan JM, Ross RK, et al. (1990) Serum hormone levels in pre-menopausal Chinese women in Shanghai and white women in Los Angeles: results from two breast cancer case-control studies. Cancer Causes Control 1:51–58.
9. Bernstein L, Ross RK, Pike MC, Brown JB, Henderson BE (1990) Hormone levels in older women: a study of post-menopausal breast cancer patients and healthy population controls. Br J Cancer 61:298–302.
10. Key TJA, Pike MC (1988) The role of oestrogens and progestogens in the epidemiology and prevention of breast cancer. Eur J Cancer Clin Oncol 24:29–43.
11. Lipworth L, Adami HO, Trichopoulos D, Carlstrom K, Mantzoros C (1996) Serum steroid hormone levels, sex hormone-binding globulin, and body mass index in the etiology of postmenopausal breast cancer. Epidemiology 7:96–100.
12. Toniolo PG, Levitz M, Zeleniuch-Jacquotte A, et al. (1995) A prospective study of endogenous estrogens and breast cancer in postmenopausal women. J Natl Cancer Inst 87:190–197.
13. Berrino F, Muti P, Micheli A, et al. (1996) Serum sex hormone levels after menopause and subsequent breast cancer. J Natl Cancer Inst 88:291–296.
14. Thomas HV, Key TJ, Allen DS, Moore JW, Dowsett M, Fentiman IS, et al. (1997) A prospective study of endogenous serum hormone concentrations and breast cancer risk in premenopausal women on the island of Guernsey. Br J Cancer 75:1075–1079.
15. Thomas HV, Key TJ, Allen DS, Moore JW, Dowsett M, Fentiman IS, et al. (1997) A prospective study of endogenous serum hormone concentrations and breast cancer risk in postmenopausal women on the island of Guernsey. Br J Cancer 76:401–405.
16. Dorgan JF, Longcope C, Stephenson HE, et al. (1996) Relation of prediagnostic serum estrogen and androgen levels to breast cancer risk. Cancer Epidemiol Biomarkers Prev 5:533–539.
17. Thomas HV, Reeves GK, Key TJA (1997) Endogenous estrogen and postmenopausal breast cancer: a quantitative review. Cancer Causes Control, 8(6):922–928.
18. Collaborative Group on Hormonal Factors in Breast Cancer (1996) Breast cancer and hormonal contraceptives: collaborative reanalysis of individual data on 53,297 women with breast cancer and 100,239 women without breast cancer from 54 epidemiological studies. Lancet. 347:1713–1727.

19. Collaborative Group on Hormonal Factors in Breast Cancer. Breast cancer and hormone replacement therapy: collaborative reanalysis of data from 51 epidemiological studies of 52,705 women with breast cancer and 108,411 women without breast cancer. Lancet 1997; 350:1047–1059.
20. Laya MB, Larson EB, Taplin SH, White E (1996) Effect of estrogen replacement therapy on the specificity and sensitivity of screening mammogrpahy. J Natl Cancer Inst 88:643–649.
21. Ford DF, Easton DF, Bishop DT, Narod SA, Goldgar DE (1994) Risks of cancer in BRCA1-mutation carriers. Lancet 343:692–695.
22. Healy B (1997) BRCA genes—bookmaking, fortunetelling, and medical care. N Engl J Med 336:1448–1449.
23. Ursin G, Henderson BE, Haile RW, Pike MC, Zhou N, Diep A, et al. (1997) Does oral contraceptive use increase the risk of breast cancer in women with BRCA1/BRCA2 mutations more than in other women? Cancer Res 57:3678–3681.
24. Castilla LH, Couch FJ, Erdos MR et al. (1994) Mutations in the BRCA1 gene in families with early-onset breast and ovarian cancer. Nature Genet 8:387–391.
25. Feigelson HS, Ross RK, Yu MC, Coetzee GA, Reichardt JKV, Henderson BE (1996) Genetic susceptibility to cancer from exogenous and endogenous exposures. J Cell Biochem 25S:15–22.
26. Brentano ST, Picado-Leonard J, Mellon SH, Moore CCD, Miller WI (1990) Tissue-specific cyclic adenosine 3',5'-monophosphate-induced, and phorbol ester-repressed transcription from the human P450c17 promoter in mouse cells. Mol Endocrinol 4:1972–1979.
27. Watanabe J, Harada N, Suemasu K, Hagashi Y, Gotoh O, Kawajiri K (1997) Arginine-cysteine polymorphism at codon 264 of the human CYP19 gene does not affect aromatase activity. Pharmacogenetics 7:419–424.
28. Poutanen M, Isomaa V, Lehto V-P, Vihko R (1992) Immunological analysis of 17β -hydroxysteroid dehydrogenase in benign and malignant human breast tissue. Int J Cancer 50:386–390.
29. Feigelson HS, Coetzee GA, Kolonel LN, Ross RK, Henderson BE (1997) A polymorphism in the CYP17 gene increases the risk of breast cancer. Cancer Res 57:1063–1065.
30. Carey AH, Waterworth D, Patel K, White D, Little J, Novelli P, et al. (1994) Polycystic ovaries and premature male pattern baldness are associated with one allele of the steroid metabolism gene CYP17. Hum Mol Genet 3:1873–1876.
31. Feigelson HS, Shames LS, Pike MC, Coetzee GA, Stanczyk FZ, Henderson BE (1998) CYP17 polymorphism is associated with serum estrogen and progesterone concentrations. Cancer Res, 58:585–587.
32. Grodstein F, Stampfer MJ, Colditz GA, et al. (1997) Postmenopausal hormone therapy and mortality. N Engl J Med 336:1769–1775.

5 Androgens, Estrogens, and Breast Cancer Risk

V.H.T. James, MD

INTRODUCTION

There is little controversy over the proposition that steroid hormones play a fundamental role in breast cancer. Ever since the work of Beatson *(1)* carried out at the end of the last century, it has been recognized that the ovarian hormones, notably estradiol, are fundamentally involved in the development of the disease. We also have an improving, if as yet imperfect, view of the mechanisms by which estrogens control tumor growth, and this basic knowledge has provided the rationale for estrogen ablation, which has long been the key therapeutic intervention in the treatment of the disease and is an option still to be bettered. Nevertheless, whereas therapy may be improving, it is far from perfect, and our understanding of the hormonal factors that may cause or predispose to breast cancer is poor. In particular, the precise role of androgen and estrogen metabolism is unclear, and in spite of a considerable volume of research, the question of whether abnormal steroid metabolism plays a part in determining cancer risk is still unresolved.

The hypothesis that exposure to estrogen is a risk factor for breast cancer receives support from epidemiologic studies *(2)*. These have suggested that women who experience a longer period of reproductive activity, i.e., an early menarche and a late menopause, are at greater risk of breast cancer. The observations that breast cancer is rare in men and that women castrated early in life are at lower risk also support the theory. Exposure to long-term estrogen for contraceptive reasons also appears to increase breast cancer risk, although only to a very small extent *(3)*. Thus there is some evidence that long-term overexposure to estrogen may unfavorably affect the risk of developing breast cancer. That being so, it follows that altered estrogen metabolism, leading to enhanced estrogen exposure, might be a general mechanism that could explain the relatively high incidence of the disease. However, the complexities of steroid metabolism and the fact that any such metabolic abberations are likely to be only very small, bearing in mind that it is lifetime exposure to such small changes that may be significant, has made the investigation of this proposition extremely difficult. Nevertheless, there have been sustained attempts to advance our knowledge of steroid metabolism in breast cancer and these have shed some light on the problem.

From: *Contemporary Endocrinology: Endocrinology of Breast Cancer*
Edited by: A. Manni © Humana Press Inc., Totowa, NJ

SOURCES OF ANDROGENS AND ESTROGENS

In the premenopausal woman, the adrenal cortex and the ovaries are the principal sources of steroid hormones. Estradiol is secreted directly by the ovary, and both the adrenal and the ovary produce androgens, notably androstenedione. The adrenal uniquely produces dehydroepiandrosterone, (DHA), and its sulphate (DHAS), and this latter steroid is quantitatively the major steroid hormone produced by the adrenal glands. During reproductive life, direct ovarian production of estradiol renders other sources relatively unimportant, but after the menopause, this picture changes, and the indirect production of estrogens assumes a far more important role. At this time, the conversion of androgens to estrogens in peripheral tissue, notably of androstenedione to estrone, takes over as the major estrogen source *(4,5)*. The key enzyme involved, aromatase, is widely distributed throughout body tissues. Adipose tissue is of particular importance because of its relatively large mass, and also neural tissues and bone. Further metabolism of estrone to estradiol requires the intervention of hydroxysteroid dehydrogenase (HSD), and both HSD and aromatase are present in normal and malignant breast tissue *(6,7)*. Thus, after the menopause the principal source of estrogens is peripheral production, and the details of the various steps involved are now reasonably well understood *(8,9)*.

Apart from the production of estrogen in peripheral body tissues, which contributes to the general body pool, there is also significant local accumulation or production of estrogen in both normal breast tissue and in some breast tumors *(6,7,10)*. Although the amounts are quantitively small, the fact that it is being produced directly within the breast implies that local concentration of estrogens may be relatively high; if exposure to estrogens is indeed a risk factor, then the possibility that abnormal production of estrogen is occurring either peripherally or locally may constitute a risk factor for the disease. This idea has attracted attempts to disclose altered steroid metabolism in women with breast cancer, which have involved urinary studies (mainly of androgen excretion), examination of blood levels of estrogen, and investigation of peripheral steroid metabolism and local production of estrogen in normal and malignant breast tissue. These aspects will be briefly surveyed in this chapter.

STUDIES OF ANDROGEN EXCRETION

Early attempts to establish an increase in estrogen production by women with breast cancer compared with normal women were based on measurements of urinary estrogen excretion, but the results were inconclusive, and given the analytical problems associated with these assays and the complexity of estrogen metabolism (which makes interpretation of the results difficult) this was unsurprising. What did appear to be promising was the unexpected observation that urinary excretion of other, adrenal steroid metabolites appeared to have some prognostic significance. Patients who had a relatively low excretion of androgen metabolites (17-oxosteroids) in relation to corticoid metabolites responded less favorably to endocrine ablation than did those with a higher ratio *(11)*.

Some support for the hypothesis that adrenal androgens are fundamentally involved in breast cancer was obtained from a major prospective trial in Guernsey in which urine samples were collected from a relatively static population of women; when breast cancer developed subsequently, the results were analyzed. They suggested that a low excretion of androgen metabolite was associated with a greater risk of developing cancer *(11)*. The results were not completely clear-cut, and the role that androgens play remained obscure.

Since the source of the major urinary androgens is DHA and its sulphate, it seems possible that this steroid is in some way involved. Changes in DHA secretion might be expected to be revealed by examination of blood levels, but this has not entirely clarified the situation. Although one careful study revealed no differences between controls and cancer patients *(12)*, another group has found that in a prospective study of premenopausal cancer patients, DHA levels in women who subsequently developed breast cancer were 10% lower than in controls, whereas in postmenopausal patients, DHA plasma levels were elevated and thus associated with increased risk *(13,14)*.

Although research into the biologic role of DHA has been pursued for many years, no clear function has yet emerged. It has been suggested that DHA may play some protective role against a variety of malignancies, and whereas this has been shown to be so in some animal studies *(15)*, it can also cause cancer in others *(16)*. More recently, interest has emerged in the possible immunologic effects of DHA. Administration of DHA can reduce elevated interleukin-6 (IL-6) levels in aging mice *(17)*, and since IL-6 is one of the factors that can stimulate aromatase activity, and thus estrogen production *(18)*, this might explain the role of DHA. Further work showed that the conversion of T-cells to Th2, the source of IL-6, is mediated by the ratio of cortisol to DHA; an increase in cortisol or a fall in DHA increases conversion to Th2 and production of IL-6 *(19)*.

These immunological effects of DHA led Bulbrook et al. *(11)* to consider that the low ratio of DHA to corticoid metabolites in the cancer cases may indicate that they are exposed to an immunosuppressive environment. Reed *(20)* suggests that the increased production of IL-6 increases the production of estrogen in the (presumably preclinical) breast tumor. This latter thesis that an altered ratio of cortisol to androgens may influence the activity of Th2 cells and thus cytokine production, which in turn can enhance estrogen production, is interesting. However, if valid, women in whom the ratio is altered by disease, or by therapy (e.g., patients with adrenal insufficiency receiving corticosteroid replacement therapy, or those receiving corticosteroids for asthma or rheumatoid arthritis), might also be expected to be at greater risk of breast cancer, but there does not appear to be any evidence that this is so. Furthermore in some patients with breast cancer, administration of glucocorticoids has proved effective in obtaining a remission. So, although a role for DHA as a protective agent against malignancies is attractive, further clinical evidence to support the idea has not been forthcoming so far.

ESTROGENS IN BLOOD

The thesis that continuing overexposure to estrogen may increase the risk of developing breast cancer is consistent with much of the evidence, but attempting to obtain proof that this may explain the high incidence of the disease is fraught with difficulty. Throughout reproductive life estrogen levels fluctuate constantly, not just through the month, but also through the day, and random blood or urine samples cannot reflect estrogen exposure in anything other than a very general way, and at a particular point in time. Although gross abnormalities may be revealed (e.g., patients with polycystic ovarian disease have elevated plasma levels of estrone compared with controls), any small changes would be masked by the larger fluctuations, and so probably rendered undetectable. The prospects are better in postmenopausal women, in whom the fluctuating ovarian production of estrogen is minimal and the estrogen produced derives from peripheral production from the precursors androstenedione, and to a smaller extent testosterone and DHA. However, in this situation, analytical problems become more important because of the lower concentrations of estrogens involved. Nevertheless, a number of investigators have studied postmenopausal women in an attempt to discover whether a difference exists between patients with cancer and controls. The problem with such a research program is obtaining proper controls, as well as excluding the possibility that any effect found is indeed causal and not an alteration in metabolism secondary to the development of cancer.

With the advent of methods for the analysis of estrogens in blood, renewed attempts were made to investigate the problem, and there have been several studies of plasma estrogen concentrations in women with breast cancer, seeking to find a difference between the cancer patients and normal women. In premenopausal women, no consistent differences in total plasma estrogen concentration has been found *(9,21)*. As pointed out above, there are considerable difficulties in selecting an appropriate and representative blood sample from a woman experiencing normal cycles, and a single blood sample represents only the situation at a single point in time. It is perhaps not too surprising that the results have not been conclusive.

In postmenopausal women there is better consensus, and several authors have reported results showing that the plasma levels of estrone and estradiol are slightly elevated compared with controls, although generally still within the normal range *(21)*. However, these studies have in general been retrospective, and so it is not clear whether the results may be due to the disease process, rather than reflecting a preexisting situation.

Data exist from prospective studies in which blood samples were taken prior to the onset of the disease and the samples from the cancer cases were analyzed at the time the cancer presented clinically together with those taken contemporaneously from controls. This experimental design eliminates to an extent the possibility that the presence of disease itself is a factor.

Two groups were unable to find any differences between cases and controls *(22,23)*. Three other groups did find a difference. Toniolo et al. *(24)* measured estrone and estradiol in 260 controls and 130 women who subsequently developed breast cancer. Compared with earlier studies, this is a substantial number of patients. Although the cases had hormone levels within the normal range, the women who subsequently developed breast cancer tended to show higher levels of estrone, total estradiol, and free estradiol, and a lower percentage of estradiol bound to sex hormone binding globulin than the women who did not develop cancer. In another study, Berrino et al. *(25)* studied a total of 24 cases and 88 controls and found that total testosterone, free testosterone, and estradiol were all significantly higher in the cases. More recently another investigation has provided additional supportive evidence. Thomas et al. *(26)* examined blood samples that had been taken from a large number of postmenopausal women in Guernsey several years prior to the onset of breast cancer. There were 61 patients, and 179 controls and the results showed that the women who developed breast cancer had a 29% higher mean plasma estradiol level than those who were still healthy. They also found an association between the development of breast cancer and plasma levels of testosterone. The mean concentration of sex hormone binding globulin was lower in the cases.

The results from these latter investigations are similar, and they suggest that some women who subsequently develop cancer are exposed to higher concentrations of estradiol than are women who do not. They are also consistent with data from other groups who have measured the concentration of free estradiol in plasma on the premise that it is this element that is biologically active *(27–30)* and have found that in the cancer patients the free fraction is increased. This fraction also correlates positively with the metabolic clearance of estradiol *(29)*, which is in agreement with the concept that it is free estradiol which is biologically important *(27)*.

The recent data are therefore consistent in showing that plasma estradiol is apparently a predictor for the development of breast cancer, but they do not reveal what role, if any, this increased estrogen exposure plays. Since tumor growth will undoubtedly have been initiated in these women many years earlier, the results of these studies may be indicating that the rate of tumor growth is increased by the higher levels of estrogen and that the women with higher estrogen concentrations are therefore showing clinical evidence of tumor growth at an earlier time.

The observation that plasma estrogen levels may be elevated in women who subsequently develop breast cancer raises the question of the source of the hormone and the reason for the increased production or exposure. Elevated plasma estrogen levels could be due to increased production, or altered clearance of estrogen, although there is no evidence for the latter. The possibility that increased estrogen production is occurring has attracted attention, and the principal enzyme system involved, aromatase, has been extensively studied. It has been known for some time that aromatase activity is increased in women who are obese *(31)* and that it is increased in relation to age *(5)*. Obese women are at higher risk of breast cancer, and risk is also age related *(2)*. However, when these factors are taken into account by using appropriate controls, there does not appear to be any general increase in peripheral conversion of androstenedione to estrone in women with breast cancer; if such a phenomenon exists, it must be very small, or may be only localized to target tissue.

Although it appears that the unbound fraction of plasma estradiol is increased in cancer patients, this finding has not attracted as much interest as might have been expected. It has been reported that plasma from breast cancer patients contains some material that interferes with the binding process *(27)*; this observation would appear to merit further study.

LOCAL ESTROGEN PRODUCTION

The possibility that local estrogen production in the breast or in breast tumors is an important factor has attracted considerable attention. Although a knowledge of circulating estrogen levels may give some indication of tissue exposure to estrogens, examination of tissue concentrations of steroids in women with breast cancer has shown that these are influenced by several factors and do not simply reflect blood estrogen levels *(32,33)*. Whereas in premenopausal women estradiol levels predominate over estrone, the reverse is true after the menopause because the major source of estrogen in these women is peripheral conversion of androstenedione to estrone. Examination of breast tumor tissue in postmenopausal patients shows that, in contrast to peripheral blood, the concentration of estradiol exceeds that of estrone *(33,34)*, implying that there is either selective uptake of estradiol or that biosynthesis or conversion of estrone to estradiol is occurring locally in the tumor. It has been known for some time that breast tumors and breast tissue contain aromatase, dehydrogenase, and sulphatase, i.e., all the enzymes necessary for local steroid biosynthesis. In addition, by infusing the appropriate radiolabeled steroids, it is possible to distinguish the source of the estrogen present. Using this technique, it was found that in some breast tumors the predominant source is by accumulation, whereas in others it is from uptake of precursor and subsequent biosynthesis *(35)*. Thus, some breast tumors have the capability to biosynthesize significant quantities of estrogen, which because of its local production may be present at relatively high concentration. For an estrogen-dependent tumor, this clearly offers an important biologic advantage. It has also been shown that the breast tissue surrounding the tumor has higher steroid enzyme activity than does tissue remote from the tumor *(6)*. Furthermore, the aromatase activity in the quadrant of the breast that contains the tumor is usually higher than that found in the other quadrants *(36)*. These observations are consistent with the supposition that some breast tumors secrete substances that can enhance the activity of steroid biosynthetic enzymes and thus increase local production of estrogen. Although they have not yet been fully identified, it appears that certain cytokines (especially IL-6 and tumor necrosis factor-α) and an albumin-like protein are significant agents *(37)*.

Quantitatively, the amounts of estrogen produced or sequestered in a breast tumor are relatively small, but it should be remembered that analytical studies of these tissues with current techniques require disruption of the tissue and extraction prior to analysis. It is not yet possible to examine local production or accumulation at the cellular level and so we do not know anything about the local estrogen concentrations to which the individual cells are exposed; it is possible that local steroid concentrations in the breast may be very high.

The possibility that clinically premalignant breast tissue may express aberrant steroid metabolic processes, which in turn favor the development of breast tumors, is an attractive thesis, but one that is difficult to study for obvious reasons. However, studies of patients with cystic disease of the breast may be of some relevance, since some data suggest that as a group, patients with some types of cystic disease may be at higher risk of developing breast cancer than are women without breast disease. Examination of breast cyst fluid has demonstrated that this contains remarkably high concentrations of some steroids and especially of DHA *(38)*. Classifying cysts by electrolyte content allows separation into high- and low-risk categories—types I and II respectively *(39)*. The cyst fluid from type I contains the highest concentrations of DHA *(38)*. Other studies have shown that this steroid is concentrated by an unknown mechanism against the plasma gradient. In addition to cyst fluid, nipple aspirate also contains DHA in large amounts *(40)*. Thus it appears that breast tissue is exposed to DHA, which may be present in abnormally high concentrations in patients with breast cysts. These observations have again brought DHA into focus as a possibly important factor in human breast cancer. What role this steroid androgen plays and whether an abnormal concentration in breast tissue is important in relation to cancer risk are still undetermined.

The biologic role of DHA is unknown, in spite of claims that it may influence a variety of metabolic processes *(41)*. Thus it has been shown that DHA in animal models may protect against cancer or may predispose to it. It can also act as an antiobesity agent and has been claimed to influence the aging process favorably. Such a variety of actions suggest that it may act at a central point in metabolism; it has been proposed that it inhibits the activity of glucose-6-phosphatase *(42,43)*. Alternatively, it may be the metabolic products of DHA that are the significant factors. Conversion of DHA to estrogens is not a major metabolic pathway, but an important metabolite is 5-androstenediol. This unusual steroid has both androgenic and estrogenic activity *(44)*, and it is possible that this might be an important aspect of the biology of DHA. We are nevertheless left with an enigma yet to be solved over the role that DHA plays in breast cancer, and indeed in human metabolism generally.

CONCLUSIONS

In spite of many years of patient and careful research, the significance of altered androgen and estrogen metabolism in human breast cancer is still far from clear. It seems that there is now some agreement that some women who eventually develop breast cancer do have slightly elevated estrogen levels and estrogen exposure compared with women who do not. We do not know what the relevance of this observation is, but these changes may have some importance in deciding the rate of progression of the disease. The results suggest that there is some increase in estrogen production in breast cancer patients, but no clear evidence for altered peripheral conversion has been found. Several reports suggest that altered steroid metabolism in breast tissue, and in breast tumors particularly, may have a role in influencing tumor growth. The adrenal and ovarian androgen androstenedione has a clear function as a precursor of estrone, but the major adrenal steroid DHA and its sulfate continue to pose unanswered questions about the part they may play, if any, in the disease process. If one exists, it must be rather early in the disease history. There are still numerous unanswered questions in this field, but they are well worth answering since they could provide us with additional and much needed information that might help with both the prevention and treatment of breast cancer.

REFERENCES

1. Beatson GT (1896) On the treatment of inoperable cases of carcinoma of the mamma: suggestions for a new method of treatment with illustrative cases. Lancet 2:104–107.
2. Kelsey JL (1979) A review of the epidemiology of human breast cancer. Epidemiol Rev 1:74–49.
3. Kelsey JL, Berkovitz GS (1988) Breast cancer epidemiology. Cancer Res 48:5615–5623.
4. Siiteri and MacDonald PC (1973) Role of extraglandular estrogen in human endocrinology, in Handbook of Physiology vol. 2, Part 1 (Greep RO, Astwood EB, eds.), pp. 615–629.
5. Hemsell DL, Grodin J, Breuner PF, Siiteri PK, MacDonald PC (1974) Plasma precursors of estrogen. II. Correlation of the extent of conversion of plasma androstenedione to estrone with age. J Clin Endocrinol Metab 38:376–379.
6. Bonney RC, Reed MJ, Davidson K, Beranek PA, James VHT (1983) The relationship between 17β-hydroxysteroid dehydrogenase activity and oestrogen concentrations in human breast tumours and in normal breast tissue. Clin Endocrinol (Oxf) 19:727–739.
7. James VHT, McNeill JM, Lai LC, Newton CJM, Ghichik MW, Reed MJ (1987) Aromatase activity in normal breast and breast tumour tissue: in vivo and in vitro studies. Steroids 50:523–535.
8. Simpson ER, Zhao Y, Buhin SE, Mendelson CR, Agarwal VR (1997) Mesenchymal-epithelial interactions and breast cancer. Endocr Rel Cancer 4:407–422.
9. Pasqualini JR, Chetrite G (1996) Activity, regulation and expression of sulphatase, sulphotransferase, and 17β-hydroxysteroid dehydrogenase in breast cancer, In: Hormone Dependent Cancer (Pasqualini JR, Katzenellenbogen BS, eds.), Marcel Dekker, New York.
10. Miller WR (1997) Uptake and synthesis of steroid hormones by the breast. Endocr Rel Cancer 4:307–312.
11. Bulbrook RD, Thomas BS, Wang DY (1997) A retrospective view of androgen and corticoid metabolites in the aetiology and clinical course of breast cancer. Endocr Rel Cancer 4:285–288.
12. Jones DL, James VHT (1987) Determination of dehydroepiandrosterone and dehydroepiandrosterone sulphate in blood and tissues; studies of normal women and women with breast or endometrial cancer. J Steroid Biochem 26:151–159.
13. Helzlsouer KJ, Gordon GB, Alberg AJ, Bush TL, Comstock GW (1992) Relationship of prediagnostic serum levels of dehydroepiandrosterone and dehydroepiandrosterone sulphate to the risk of developing premenopausal breast cancer. Cancer Res 52:1–4.
14. Gordon GB, Bush TL, Helzsouer KJ, Miller SR, Comstock GW (1990) Relationship of serum levels of dehydroepiandrosterone and dehydroepiandrosterone sulphate to the risk of developing breast cancer. Cancer Res 50:3859–3862.
15. Schwartz AG (1979) Inhibition of spontaneous breast cancer in female C3H (Avy/a) mice by long term treatment with dehydroepiandrosterone. Cancer Res 39:1129–1132.

16. Beamer WG, Schultz KL ,Tennent BJ (1988) Induction of ovarian granulosa cell tumours in SWXJ-9 mice with dehydroepiandrosterone. Cancer Res 48:2788–2792.
17. Daynes RA, Araneo BA, Ershler WB, Maloney C, Li G-Z, Ryu S-Y (1993) Altered regulation of IL-6 production with normal aging. J Immunol 150:5219–5230.
18. Reed MJ, Purohit A (1997) Breast cancer and the role of cytokines in regulating estrogen synthesis: an emerging hypothesis. Endocr Rev, 18:701–715.
19. Rook GAW, Hernandez-Pando R, Lightman SL (1994) Hormones, peripherally activated prohormones and regulation of the Th1/Th2 balance. Immunol Today 15:301–303.
20. Reed MJ (1995) The discriminant function test: a marker of Th1/Th2 cell cytokine secretion and breast tumour oestrogen synthesis. Mol Med Today 1:98–103.
21. Key TJ, Pike MC (1988) The role of oestrogens and progestogens in the epidemiology and prevention of breast cancer. Eur J Cancer Clin Oncol 24:29–43.
22. Wysowski DK, Comstock GW, Helsing KJ, Lau HL (1987) Sex hormone levels in serum in relation to the development of breast cancer. Am J Epidemiol 125:791–799.
23. Garland CF, Friedlander NJ, Barrett-Conner E, Khaw KT (19XX) Sex hormones and postmenopausal breast cancer: a prospective study in an adult community. Am J Epidemiol 135:1220–1230.
24. Toniolo PG, Levitz M, Zeleniuch-Jacquette A, Banerjee S, Koenig KL, Shore RE, et al. (1995) A prospective study of endogenous estrogens and breast cancer in postmenopausal women. J Natl Cancer Inst 87:190–197.
25. Berrino F, Muti P, Micheli A, Bolelli G, Krogh V, Sciajno R, et al. (1996) Serum sex hormone levels after menopause and subsequent breast cancer. J Natl Cancer Inst 88:291–296.
26. Thomas HV, Key TJ, Allen DS, Moore JW, Dowsett M, Fentiman IS, et al. (1997) A prospective study of endogenous serum hormone concentrations and breast cancer risk in postmenopausal women on the island of Guernsey. Br J Cancer, 75:1075–1079.
27. Siiteri PK (1981) Extraglandular oestrogen formation and serum binding of oestradiol: relationship to cancer. J Endocrinol 89:119.
28. Reed MJ, Cheng RW, Noel CT, Dudley HAF, James VHT (1983) Plasma levels of estrone, estrone sulphate and estradiol and the percentage of unbound estradiol in postmenopausal women with and without breast disease. Cancer Res 43:3940–3943.
29. Reed MJ, Beranek P, Cheng RW, Ghilchik M, James VHT (1985) The distribution of estradiol in plasma from postmenopausal women with and without breast cancer. Int J Cancer 35:457–460.
30. Moore JW, Clark GM, Hoare SA, Millis RR, Hayward JL, Quinlan MK, et al. (1986) Binding of oestradiol to blood proteins and aetiology of breast cancer. Int J Cancer 38:625–630.
31. Erdman CD, MacDonald PC (1978) Effect of obesity on conversion of plasma androstenedione to oestrone in ovulatory and anovulatory young women. Am J Obstet Gynec 130:456 461.
32. McNeill JM, Reed MR, Beranek PA, Bonney RC, Robinson DJ, James VHT (1986) A comparison of the in vivo uptake and metabolism of 3H estradiol by normal breast and breast tumour tissue in post-menopausal women. Int J Cancer 38:193–196.
33. James VHT, Reed MJ, Adams EF, Ghilchik M, Lai LC, Coldham NG, et al. (1989) Oestrogen uptake and metabolism in vivo Proc Roy Soc Edinburgh 97B:185–193.
34. Van Landeghem AAJ, Portman J, Nabuurs M, Thijssen JHH (1985) Endogenous concentrations and subcellar distribution of estrogens in normal and malignant breast tissue. Cancer Res 45:2900–2906.
35. Reed MJ, Owen AM, Lai LC, Coldham NG, Ghilchik MW, Shaik NA, et al. (1989) In situ oestrone synthesis in normal breast and breast tumour tissue: effect of treatment with 4-hydroxy androstenedione Int J Cancer 44:233–237.
36. O'Neill JS, Elto RA, Miller WR (1988) Aromatase activity in adipose tissue from breast quadrants: a link with tumour site Br. Med. J. 296:742–743.
37. Purohit A, Wang DY, Ghilchik MW, Reed MJ (1999) J Endocrinol 150:565–571.
39. Bradlow HL, Schwartz MK Fleisher M, Nisselbaum J, Boyar R, O'Connor J, et al. (1979) Accumulation of hormones in breast cyst fluid 1979 J Clin Endocr Metab 49:778–782.
39. Dixon JM, Lumsden AB, Miller WR (1985) The relationship of cyst type to risk factors for breast cancer in patient with breast cystic disease Eur J Cancer Clin Oncol 21:1047–1050.
40. Miller WSR, Hanenuik V, Forrest APM (1981) Factors affecting dehydroepiandrosterone sulphate levels in human breast secretions Breast Cancer Res Treat 1:267–272.
41. Herbert J (1995) The age of dehydroepiandrosterone Lancet 345:1193–1194.
42. Marks PA, Banks JA (1960) Inhibition of mammalian glucose-6-phosphate dehydrogenase by steroids Proc Natl Acad Sci USA 46:447.

43. Gordon GB, Newitt JA, Shantz LM, Weng DE, Talalay P (1986) Inhibition of the conversion of 3T3 fibroblast clones to adipocytes by dehydroepiandrosterone and related anticarcinogenic steroids Cancer Res 46:3389–3395.
44. Adams JB, Garcia M, Rochfort H (1981) Estrogenic effects of physiological concentrations of 5-androstene-3β, 17β-diol and its metabolism in MCF7 human breast cancer cells. Cancer Res 41:4720–4726.

6 Local Estrogen Production

Is Aromatase An Oncogene?

Rajeshwar Rao Tekmal, PHD
and Richard J. Santen, MD

INTRODUCTION

Breast cancer is one of the most prevalent types of cancer observed in women. Approximately one in eight women will develop breast cancer during her lifetime. The etiology of breast cancer is thought to involve a complex interplay of genetic (hereditary and somatic), hormonal (endogenous and exogenous), and environmental factors that influence the physiologic status of the host. Epidemiologic studies indicate that early menarche, decreased parity, late age at first birth, obesity and excess weight gain, and late age at menopause can increase a women's risk of developing breast cancer *(1–3)*. These findings implicate the involvement of steroid hormones, especially estrogen, in the development of breast cancer.

The mitogenic and proliferative effects of estrogens have long been recognized and are known to correlate with breast tissue estrogen and progesterone receptors in tumor tissue *(4)*. Interestingly, the proportion of patients with hormone-sensitive tumors is higher among postmenopausal patients than premenopausal patients. In addition, the sources of sex steroids differ between pre- and postmenopausal women. Estrogens can be synthesized by the ovary or by extraglandular tissues and then delivered via the endocrine route to breast tissue. The synthesis of estrogens is catalyzed by an enzyme complex known as aromatase, whose activity results in aromatization of the A ring of androgens, to form the phenolic ring characteristic of estrogens. While many of the enzymes involved in steroid biosynthesis are ubiquitous, the aromatase enzyme is expressed in very few cell types and acts as the rate-limiting step in estrogen biosynthesis *(5–8)*.

In premenopausal women, estrogen is produced via aromatase in the ovary. This hormone is then secreted into blood, where it is delivered via an endocrine mechanism to several target tissues. After the menopause, the ovary ceases to synthesize estrogen and extraglandular sites become important. Adipose tissue is probably the main site of peripheral estrogen synthesis. Local production in the target tissue itself, particularly in the breast, can occur as well. The role of local estrogen synthesis via aromatase in breast tissue could be important for initiation of breast cancer as well as for its promotion *(5–8)*. The capacity of certain breast carcinomas to synthesize estrogens as a result of

From: *Contemporary Endocrinology: Endocrinology of Breast Cancer*
Edited by: A. Manni © Humana Press Inc., Totowa, NJ

intratumoral aromatase has been established for almost 20 years *(9)*. The potential clinical importance of this intracrine growth support has led to widespread clinical and laboratory investigations. Whereas estrogen synthesis in adipose tissue in postmenopausal women is a major source of estrogen, local formation in the breast tumor itself could be more important for mediating tumor estradiol levels.

Estrogen is known to be a promoter of breast cancer growth. Because of this, aromatase inhibitors have been used to treat women with hormone-dependent breast cancer *(7)*. Evidence also suggests that estrogen might initiate breast cancer. This process would be more likely to occur in tissues that synthesize estradiol locally and produce high local concentrations of estrogen. This chapter will focus on the possibility that estrogens might initiate as well as promote breast cancer and that these processes occur in breast tissues that overexpress the aromatase enzyme.

CLINICAL OBSERVATIONS: THE ROLE OF AROMATASE IN BREAST TUMORS

Estrogen Levels in Breast Tissue

Estrogens are the most important hormones involved in supporting the growth of hormone-dependent breast cancers *(10,11)*. The biosynthesis of estrogens is catalyzed by an enzyme called aromatase, a cytochrome P450 enzyme localized in the endoplasmic reticulum. Breast tumors from postmenopausal women maintain a high estrogen content, even though the plasma levels of estradiol fall to low levels following menopause *(12,13)*. In postmenopausal women, estrogens are no longer synthesized by the ovaries but exclusively by peripheral tissues. Adipose tissue is the main source of circulating estrogens. As a result of the functional cessation of the ovaries, plasma estrogen levels decrease dramatically in postmenopausal women and remain unchanged or increase slightly by the time of breast carcinoma development *(14–21)*. By contrast, concentrations of estradiol in breast tumors from postmenopausal patients remain as high as in premenopausal patients' plasma *(12,22–25)*. In addition, tumor levels are higher than estrogen concentrations in normal breast tissue. Van landeghem et al. reported that the concentrations of estradiol in malignant tissue in pre- and postmenopausal patients were similar despite the large differences in the peripheral plasma levels. The calculated ratio of tissue to plasma estradiol is 1:1 for premenopausal and 10–50:1 for postmenopausal patients. Maintenance of high tumor estrogen concentrations reflects the in situ estradiol production from plasma estrogen precursors. One pathway for in situ synthesis involves the conversion of androstenedione to estrone/estradiol catalyzed by aromatase *(25)*.

Aromatase Activity and its Prognostic Significance

Sixty to 70% of breast carcinomas contain measurable quantities of aromatase when assessed by biochemical methods that quantify the activity of enzyme *(9,26,27)*. A number of studies (but not all) have also shown a significant correlation between aromatase activity and clinical response to endocrine therapy with aromatase inhibitors *(6,7,28–30)*. Studies from the Dowsett group have shown aromatase activity in breast carcinomas in the range of 5–80 pmole/g protein/h, which is equivalent to 0.02–0.09% conversion of androstenedione to estrone *(8)*. Opinions differ as to whether this activity is sufficient to produce mitogenic concentrations of estradiol locally *(31,32)*. Other previous studies also measured tissue/plasma gradients for androstenedione, using either an isotope infusion technique *(33)* or a radioimmunologic method *(23)*. In both investigations, significant tumor/plasma gradients were detected for androstenedione with concentrations in tumors being almost eightfold higher than in plasma. Thus the amount of estrogen derived from androstenedione is likely to be higher than originally estimated *(31)*. Some recent studies of Pasqualini et al. *(34)* have also clearly shown that in situ concentrations of the estrogens in breast tumors of postmenopausal patients are significantly higher than those found in plasma.

A study using a double isotope infusion technique was performed by Reed et al. *(33)* to determine the relative contribution of local aromatization to estrogen levels in normal breast and breast tumor tissue. Seven postmenopausal patients with advanced breast tumor were infused with ^{3}[H]androstenedione and ^{14}[C]estrone for 12 h before operation. At surgery, normal breast and breast tumor biopsy samples were obtained and ^{3}[H]androstenedione, ^{3}[H]estrone, and ^{14}[C]estrone were measured. In two-thirds of samples examined, in situ synthesis of ^{3}[H]estrone from ^{3}[H]androstenedione accounted for the major fraction (84.4 ± 9%) of the ^{3}[H]estrone detected in both tumors and surrounding normal tissue *(33)*. In a recent study Lu et al. *(35)* showed a positive correlation between aromatase activity level in the tumor and expression of proliferating cell nuclear antigen, a marker for cell proliferation. They also showed that DNA synthesis was stimulated by estradiol and testosterone, an aromatase substrate, in the specimens with high levels of aromatase activity *(35)*. These studies are suggestive of the functional importance of in situ aromatization in breast cancer.

LOCAL AROMATASE ACTIVITY IN BREAST TISSUES

Aromatase Activity in Malignant Breast Tissues

Based on a number of early reports that human breast carcinoma tissues could convert androgens to estrogens *(36–38)*, numerous studies have been done to identify the aromatase enzyme protein in malignant breast tissues and to reveal the biologic significance of intratumoral aromatase. Brodie's group *(35)* performed a study to determine the location of aromatase enzyme in human breast cancers using both immunocytochemistry and in situ hybridization. Of the 19 tumors investigated, 10 (52.6%) showed significant immunoreactivity to antiaromatase antibody in the cytoplasm of tumor epithelial cells and in surrounding stromal cells. The aromatase mRNA detected by in situ hybridization was also located in tumor epithelial cells and stromal cells, and the pattern of expression was the same as with immunocytochemistry *(35)*. Berstein et al. *(39)* conducted an immunocytochemical study on 23 breast cancer samples and obtained a similar result, i.e., aromatase was found in different cell types, but the most intensive staining was found in malignant cells. Several other groups have reported that aromatase, as detected by specific antibody *(40,41)*, and aromatase messenger RNA *(42,43)* were mainly distributed in stromal cells around carcinomatous glands. Using competitive polymerase chain reaction (PCR) to quantitate aromatase mRNA in breast adipose tissues obtained from the four breast quadrants, Bulun et al. *(44,45)* found that the highest aromatase transcript levels colocalized to the quadrants bearing tumors. Taken together, these studies clearly demonstrate aromatase immunochemical localization and its mRNA in breast tumor tissue and the importance of in situ aromatase activity. However, no consensus has yet been reached regarding the relative importance of stromal vs tumor epithelial sources of aromatase.

Aromatase Activity in Benign Breast Tissues

A number of investigators concurrently examined aromatase in normal breast tissue and the surrounding breast cancer using radiometric aromatase enzyme assays. Each of these studies demonstrated that aromatase was present in normal breast tissues *(22–24)* and made a major contribution to the tissue estrogen levels *(33)*. In additional studies, Santner et al. *(43)* measured aromatase activities in primary culture of breast stromal cells prepared from both benign and cancerous breast tissues. They found aromatase activity in both malignant and benign breast tissue stromal cells. The enzyme activities were inducible nearly 10,000-fold by dexamethasone, cyclic adenosine monophosphate (cAMP) and phorbol ester, the factors known to upregulate aromatase activity in normal adipose fibroblasts. The aromatase present in the benign component of breasts containing tumors could be the result of factors secreted by the tumor. Because of this possibility, it is critically important to demonstrate aromatase in benign breast tissue obtained from women without breast cancer. Bulun et al. *(46)* accomplished this by quantitating adipose fibroblast aromatase transcript levels in tumor-free breasts of women undergoing reduction mammoplasty. Using an elegant competitive PCR assay, they detected aromatase message in all benign breast tissues studied. Of great interest was the fact that 67% of the highest fibroblast-to-adipocyte ratios and 64% of the highest aromatase transcript levels were detected in the upper outer quadrant of the breast, the region in which breast tumors occur in 71% of cases *(46)*.

Several observations suggest that aromatase may be overexpressed in benign breast tissues under certain circumstances. Published studies have shown increased aromatase activities in skin fibroblasts in patients with familial or nonfamilial gynecomastia *(47,48)*. More direct evidence derives from a striking example that occurs under physiologic circumstances. Mammary tissue from goats markedly increase breast tissue aromatase activity during late pregnancy. The majority of estradiol formed by the goat during this period originates from breast tissue *(49)*. These data, taken together with observations made in malignant breast tissue, suggest that aromatase is not only present in normal breast tissue but can be induced under certain physiologic circumstances to make exceedingly large amounts of estrogen.

IS AROMATASE AN ONCOGENE?

Breast Cancer Cells Overexpressing Aromatase Activity: A Model for Aromatase Role in Tumorigenesis

Studies employing the well-characterized breast cancer cell line (MCF-7) examined the biologic role of aromatase in vitro and provided a means to examine in vivo events. Hormone-responsive tumors can be formed in athymic nude mice with these cells. Tumor growth is negligible without estradiol supplementation even in intact females, suggesting the critical need for estrogen made by the tumor cells. Recent studies of Santner et al. *(50)* provide further direct biologic evidence for the importance of aromatase in breast carcinoma. These studies show that the growth of wild-type MCF-7 cells does not increase when cells are provided solely with androstenedione. These cells express low levels of aromatase. By contrast, aromatase-transfected MCF-7 cells respond to androstenedione with increased proliferation due to changes in the levels of aromatase. Furthermore, this proliferative effect can be blocked by an aromatase inhibitor. Studies of Yue et al. *(51)*

have also shown that local estrogen production in vivo from tumors formed from MCF-7 cells transfected with aromatase cDNA was sufficient to stimulate tumor growth without exogenous or ovarian estrogen. The tumor growth in these animals was nearly completely abrogated when the animals were given an aromatase inhibitor. These studies clearly indicate that increased aromatase activity is needed for in situ estrogen production, which contributes to enhanced tumor growth *(51,52)*. Using aromatase overexpressing MCF-7 breast tumors in ovariectomized mice, Santen's group *(53)* has clearly demonstrated that increased tumor aromatase activity contributes to increased levels of estrogens in breast tumor tissue. The autocrine/paracrine effects of aromatase provide higher estrogen and tumor growth than endocrine-mediated actions. Furthermore, recent studies from our group *(54)* have shown that overexpression of aromatase in tissue can increase local estradiol production to a biologically greater extent than plasma uptake. Taken together, these studies clearly demonstrate the importance of in situ estrogen production in mammary tumor proliferation.

Preneoplastic HAN Model

Gray et al. *(55)* and others *(56)* have studied precancerous, hyperplastic alveolar nodules (D2, C4, and C5 HAN) that were induced by either mammotrophic hormones or 7,12-dimethylbenz (a)-anthracene (DMBA) in BALB/c mice. They demonstrated that these lesions also contain one or more newly integrated MMTV proviral DNA copies. Recently we cloned *int*-5 (formerly called *int*-H) from mouse precancerous D2 HAN genomic DNA and its normal allele from BALB/c genome *(57)*. The localization of *int*-5 on chromosome 9 unequivocally distinguishes this gene from any other *int* genes. The expression of *int*-5 in D2 tumors is 5–10-fold greater than in normal mammary gland, indicating that *int*-5 is overexpressed in mammary tumor. Recently we have shown that the cellular gene at the MMTV integration site in the *int*-5 locus is identical to the gene encoding aromatase (CYP19), a member of the cytochrome P450 gene superfamily *(58)*. MMTV is integrated within the 3' untranslated region of the aromatase gene, and this integration is responsible for the overexpression of this gene (hereafter the *int*-5 locus is referred to as *int-5/aromatase*).

Using a cell line derived from the D2 tumor, we have demonstrated the effect of the aromatase substrate, androstenedione, on the proliferation of tumor cells. Proliferative effects of androstenedione were blocked by an aromatase inhibitor, providing evidence for the role of *int-5/aromatase* in this process. Furthermore, the androstenedione-mediated proliferation was inhibited by addition of the antiestrogen ICI 164,384, suggesting that the estrogen formed from the conversion of androstenedione by *int-5/aromatase* acts like a mitogen to stimulate the growth of D2 tumor cells.

These results raised the hypothesis that overexpression of aromatase may not only stimulate tumor growth but may also be responsible for mammary tumorigenesis. Our results provided the first demonstration of integration of MMTV in a cellular gene that plays a role in hormone-dependent breast cancer *(58–60)*. To determine whether production of estrogen by the mammary tumor cells could stimulate in vivo tumor growth in the absence of ovarian estrogen, D2 mammary tumor cells were inoculated into ovariectomized (OVX) mice. The growth of these tumors was rapid, with palpable tumors appearing in <10 days. In 5 weeks D2 mammary tumors reached a mean weight of 855 ± 39 mg with minimal variation in size and growth rate in different OVX mice. When OVX mice with D2 mammary tumors supplemented with androstenedione were treated with the aromatase inhibitor (CGS 16949A), tumor growth was significantly inhibited. These results indicate that the overexpressed *int-5/aromatase* provides a mechanism for an endogenous, nonovarian source of estrogen synthesis. The amount of estrogen formed stimulates tumor growth; this growth can be inhibited by aromatase inhibitors *(60)*.

Overexpression of Aromatase in Breast Tissue: In Vivo Transgenic Model

Since aromatase was first detected in breast tumors, the problem of assessing its functional significance has attracted considerable attention and controversy. A number of recent studies provide evidence to support a biologic role for tumor aromatase. Aromatase activity is higher in tumor-bearing quadrants than in normal quadrants. Tumor concentrations of androstenedione are known to be higher than plasma levels and contribute to significant in situ tumor estrogen synthesis. Increased aromatase protein expression by immunohistochemical localization in tumors compared with normal areas of the breast is detected. Breast tumor-specific transcriptional regulation of aromatase gene occurs. In addition, breast tumor aromatase activity can be correlated with markers of cell proliferation such as PCNA *(35)*. All these studies provide evidence that locally overexpressed aromatase has a direct biologic role in the growth of breast tumors *(6,7,28,35,46,51,61)*.

An intriguing hypothesis is that local estrogen is directly involved in the initiation of either preneoplastic or neoplastic (or both) changes in mammary epithelium. To address this question directly, we have generated an *int-5/aromatase* transgenic mice model and shown for the first time that the transgenic virgin and postlactational females that overexpress *int-5/aromatase* develop various preneoplastic histopathologic changes *(62)*. These transgenic animals respond to carcinogens such as DMBA with nearly uniform development of neoplasms compared with no neoplastic changes in nontransgenic wild-type animals similarly exposed to DMBA *(63)*.

The expression of *int-5/aromatase* mRNA is about 8–10-fold higher in transgenic mice mammary tissue compared with nontransgenic mice mammary tissue. To determine if the overexpression of *int-5/aromatase* contributes to increased mammary tissue estrogen levels, we determined the tissue estrogen levels from both nontransgenic and transgenic females of 10 weeks. Our data show that estrogen levels are about fivefold higher in transgenic mice mammary tissue than the same tissue in nontransgenic mice. This observation suggests that overexpression of *int-5/aromatase* contributes to increased mammary tissue estrogen levels. Estrogen and progesterone receptor levels are also higher in transgenic mice mammary tissue compared with nontransgenic mice mammary tissue. These results indicate that overexpression of *int-5/aromatase* contributes to increased mammary tissue estrogen levels, which induces its own receptor as well as the progesterone receptor.

Mammary Glands from MMTV-*int-5/aromatase* Transgenic Females Exhibit Various Preneoplastic/neoplastic Abnormalities

Virgin Females. Mammary glands from 7–8 week-old nontransgenic virgin females consisted of extensive ducts, with a few alveoli growing from terminal branches at the end buds of the ducts. In transgenic virgin females we observed both increased and the enlarged ductal growth, compared to nontransgenic litter mates. Of these ducts several had hyperplastic and dysplastic lesions and fibroadenomas (Fig. 1). This suggests that early estrogenic activity as a result of *aromatase* overexpression is sufficient for hyperplastic changes to occur in mammary epithelial cells of transgenic mice.

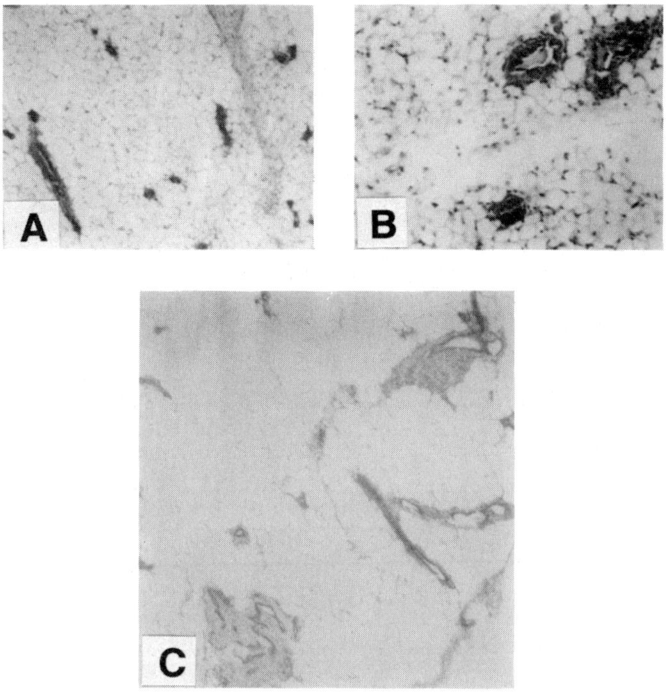

Fig. 1. Morphological appearance of nontransgenic and transgenic mammary glands from 8-wk-old virgin females: (A,B) Histological sections of mammary glands from nontransgenic virgin females. Note the presence of normal ductal and glandular growth. (C) Histological section (representative of mammary gland from *aromatase* transgenic virgin female mice. Note the presence of enlarged ducts with hyperplastic and dysplastic changes along with fibroadenoma like lesion.

Postlactational Females. Mammary glands from postlactational nontransgenic females consisted of extensive ducts with the presence of minimal lobular alveolar growth. By contrast, mammary glands of transgenic females showed significant alveolar hyperplasia throughout all the mammary glands. In the transgenic mice there were abundant alveolar glands and numerous terminal ducts compared with nontransgenic animals, which had retained only simple ductal development after involution.

Histologic examination of mammary glands of transgenic female mice that had gone through one pregnancy, 3 weeks of lactation, and 8 weeks of involution showed a range of histologic abnormalities including formation of HAN, atypical ductal and glandular hyperplasia, ductal and lobular dysplasia, and hyperplastic lesions with excessive fibrous tissue around them, similar to fibroadenomas. In addition, mammary glands in transgenic mice exhibited an increased occurrence of multinucleated cells, and some nuclei were enlarged (karyomegaly), with a hyperchromatic appearance. In general the involuted mammary glands of transgenic mice contained a pattern of postpregnancy involution different from that of the control. There is a significant increase in periductal, peri-, and intralobular fibrosis. Interestingly, these changes are similar to what is observed in the breast tissue from women with a history of breast cancer (Fig. 2).

Persistence of ductal hyperplasia and dysplasia was evident even after several months of involution in mammary glands from transgenic females. In many postlactational

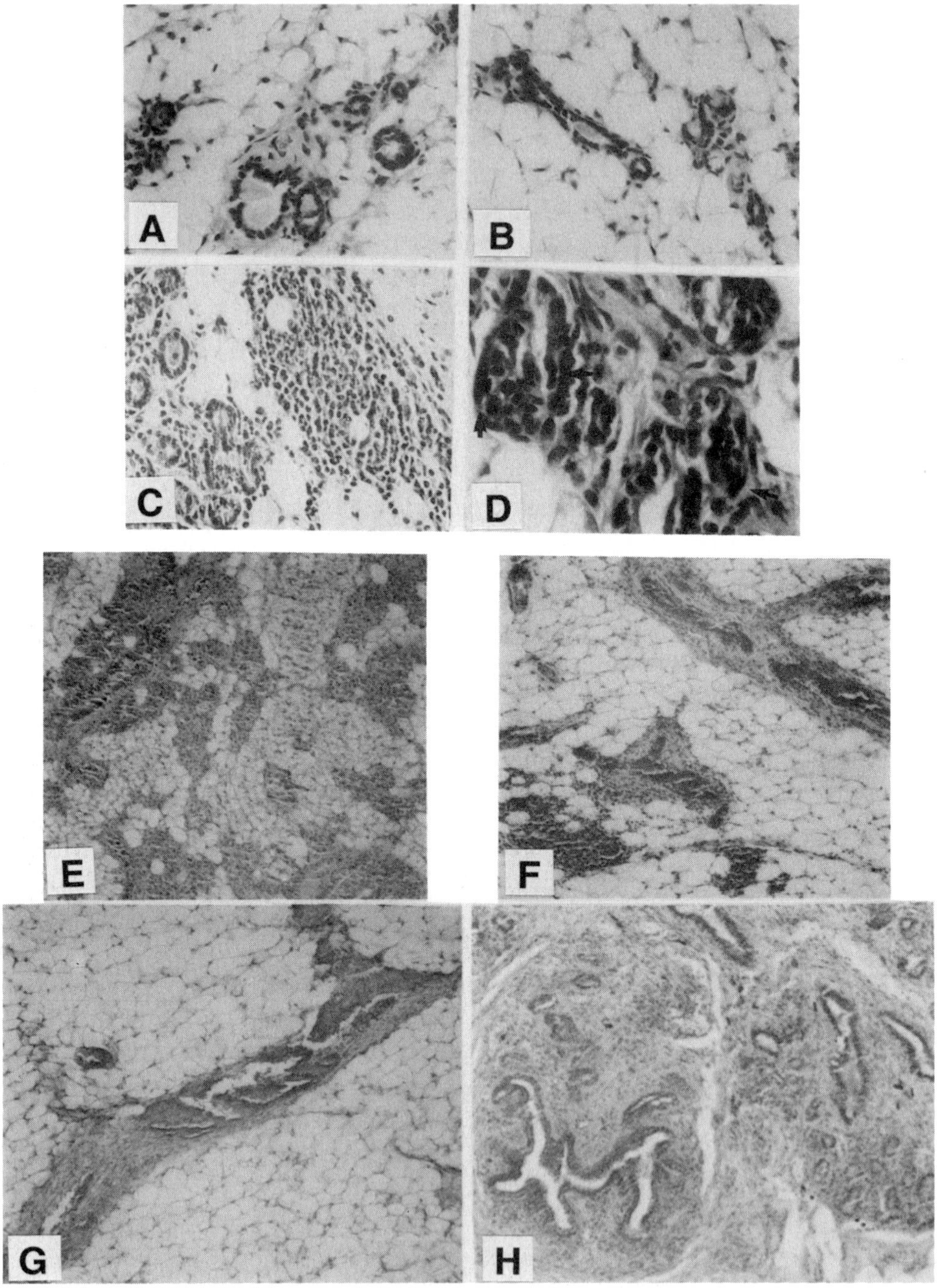

Fig. 2. Morphological appearance of nontransgenic and transgenic mammary glands from postlactational females. (A,B) Histological appearance of involuting mammary gland (4 wk after weaning) from nontransgenic female. Note the presence of only rudimentary ductal and glandular growth. (C–H) Histological sections of involuting mammary glands from transgenic female mice. Note the persistence of dysplastic ducts (C) and hyperplasia with multinucleated and hyperchromatic nuclei (D). Persistence of hyperplasia and dysplasia was evident even after 6 mo after involution (E–G). Some females develop neoplastic changes similar to ductal carcinoma *in situ* during involution (H).

females, the progression of hyperplastic and dysplastic changes to more prominent preneoplastic/neoplastic changes was very significant with the age. However, we have not observed any frankly invasive tumors. Our unpublished data show that preneoplastic and neoplastic changes persist even in the absence of ovarian estrogen in ovariectomized virgin and postlactational females. These results clearly demonstrate that increased mammary estrogen alone without the influence of circulating ovarian estrogen is sufficient to induce and maintain various preneoplastic/neoplastic changes.

Development of preneoplastic/neoplastic lesions to complete, invasive tumors is rare in this model. Nonetheless these data indicate the possibility that continued mammary estrogenic activity may be involved in the progression of preneoplastic changes to neoplastic changes and provide evidence that mammary estrogen is involved in the initiation and progression of breast cancer.

Overexpression of *int-5/aromatase* in Male Mammary Glands Leads to Increased Epithelial Growth and Hyperplasia

Our studies (unpublished) show that overexpression of *int-5/aromatase* in male transgenic mice results in increased epithelial glandular growth as early as 10 weeks of age. Histologic examination of these glands shows clear evidence of hyperplastic and dysplastic changes that are similar to gynecomastia (a benign condition). These results clearly demonstrate that increased mammary estrogen alone without the influence of circulating gonadal estrogen is sufficient to induce various proliferative changes and support the prior hypothesis that increased aromatase may contribute to gynecomastia *(48)*

CARCINOGENIC ROLE OF BREAST TISSUE ESTROGEN

Two general but not exclusive possibilities have been proposed to explain how estrogens exert carcinogenic effects: (1) receptor-mediated, epigenetic, facilitative effects; and (2) direct genotoxic actions. Via the first mechanism, estradiol at physiologic concentrations binds to the estrogen receptor and enhances the mitotic rate. Via the second mechanism, estradiol is metabolically transformed to catechol estrogens and quinones, which directly or indirectly may cause DNA damage and resultant mutations. While the genotoxic mechanism could take place at concentrations similar to those required for receptor binding, proportional increases in estradiol levels would be expected to enhance these effects correspondingly.

Additivity or synergy between mechanisms could also occur. DNA damage would not necessarily be harmful in nonproliferative or slowly proliferating cells, in which the adducts formed can be effectively removed by DNA repair machinery. By contrast, in rapidly growing cells, inadequate repairing of damaged DNA might occur, which would result in a statistically significant increase in the number of genetic mutations. These interactions, whether additive or synergistic, might then be responsible for increasing the carcinogenic effect of estrogens.

The use of estrogens has increasingly been associated with human cancer. For example, the administration of diethylstilbestrol, the synthetic estrogen, to pregnant women is associated with an increased risk of mammary cancer in these women and of vaginal adenocarcinomas in their daughters *(64,65)*. Use of steroidal estrogens has been implicated in the rising incidence of endometrial adenocarcinoma. Estrogens have also been reported to induce tumors in laboratory animals, i.e., kidney tumors in hamsters, uterine tumors in mice, Leydig cell tumors in mice, and pituitary tumors in rats *(66)*. Among those, estrogen-induced renal carcinoma in Syrian hamsters is a well-characterized animal model, which provides insight into the potential mechanisms of carcinogenic action of estrogens.

High-dose external estrogenic exposure has long been associated with experimental mammary cancer. Several studies have reported that administration of natural estrogens in large doses for long periods induced hyperplasia and multiple benign and malignant neoplasms in the mammary gland and other organs *(66–72)*. Estrogens also significantly enhance or promote the carcinogenic effects of other chemical carcinogens, such as DMBA, and consequently they enhance mammary tumors in mice and rats (initiated by DMBA). Estrogens may also directly act to damage cells.

Steroidal estrogens are thought to act as carcinogens by alternate metabolic transformations. Estradiol and the oral contraceptive ethinyl estradiol may be metabolized to reactive hydroxylated intermediates (2OH and 16αOH). These compounds are thought to be genotoxic through reactive semiquinone formation. Both DNA and proteins may be substrates of such damage. Interestingly, both types of reactive intermediates bind the estrogen receptor, and the 16αOH form of estradiol appears to form a covalent adduct with the estrogen receptor *(73–76)*. Recent studies have shown that 16α-hydroxylation of estradiol is increased in women who have a high inherited risk of developing breast cancer or who have developed breast cancer, and oncogenes and tumor-associated viruses affect the extent of 2- and 16α-hydroxylation in a pro-risk direction *(73–76)*. Estrogens can also be metabolized to 4-hydroxy-estrogens *(77)*. In rodent models, 4-hydroxyestradiol formation has been found to be predominant in estradiol-induced tumors, whereas in these rodents' livers, in which tumors are not induced, 2-hydroxylation of estradiol predominates.

For estrogen metabolites to be carcinogenic factors in breast tissue, it is important to know whether the metabolic machinery exists for catalyzing the necessary steps. Studies from the Cavalieri group *(78,79)* postulate that oxidation of catechol estrogens (CE) to catechol estrogen quinones results in formation of quinone compounds that covalently bind to DNA to form depurinating adducts, i.e., adducts that are lost from DNA by cleavage of the bond between the deoxyribose and the purine base. On repurination of DNA, point mutations occur at sites of depurinated DNA. The resultant point mutations in critical genes could initiate tumors. Thus, the genotoxic effects of specific metabolites of estrogen can be at the origin of many human cancers, including breast cancer. CE production has been reported to occur in human breast cancer tissues *(80)* and in MCF-7 breast cancer cells *(81)*. Spink et al. *(82)* demonstrated that the formation of 4-hydroxy estradiol in MCF-7 cells is catalyzed by cytochrome P450 IBl, which is inducible by 2,3,7,8-tetrachlorodibenzo-p-dioxin (TCDD), a common environmental pollutant. Liehr and Ricci *(77)* found that in microsomes prepared from normal human mammary tissue, the rate of 2-hydroxylation of estradiol did not differ markedly from that of 4-hydroxylation. However, in microsomes of mammary fibroadenomas and of adenocarcinomas, rates of formation of 4-OHE2 exceeded those of 2-OHE2 formation by almost fourfold *(77)*. Generally two CEs are mainly inactivated by *O*-methylation catalyzed by catechol-*o*-methyltransferases. If conjugation is insufficient, the CE may be oxidized to quinones. These quinones (specially CE-2,3) can react with DNA to form stable adducts that remain in DNA unless repaired *(83)*. The CE-3,4 quinones, if not inactivated, react with DNA to form depurinating adducts, more specifically two rotational conformers bound to the N-7 of guanine (4-OHE$_{1or2}$-1(αβ)-N7Gua) *(84)*. These data suggest that 4-hydroxyestradiol-mediated DNA damage may be involved in tumor initiation or malignant transformation of benign breast disease.

An additional carcinogenic mechanism has also been suggested to result from the metabolism of estradiol to 4-hydroxy estradiol to 3,4 quinone and back to 4-hydroxy estradiol *(78)*. This metabolic pathway generates oxygen free radicals and functions as a redox cycle. The free radicals released could indirectly activate polycyclic aromatic hydrocarbons such as DMBA to produce compounds capable of binding to guanine bases and inducing depurination. For example, N-7 guanine-DMBA adducts form. Through this mechanism, estrogen metabolism could result in increased carcinogenicity of DMBA. Increased production of estrogen in tissue, as mediated by aromatase overexpression, would then act synergistically with DMBA to produce neoplasms. This is an intriguing hypothesis to explain our observations of increased neoplastic changes in transgenic animals receiving DMBA.

REFERENCES

1. Harris JR, Lippman ME, Veronesi U, Willett W (1992) Breast cancer. N Engl J Med 327:319328; 390–398; 473–480.
2. Lambe M, Hsieh CC, Chan HW, Ekbom A, Trichopoulos D, Adami HO (1996) Parity, age at first and last birth, and risk of breast cancer: a population-based study in Sweden. Breast Cancer Res Treat 38:305–311.
3. van den Brandt PA, Dirx MJ, Ronckers CM, van den Hoogen P, Goldbohm RA (1997) Height, weight, weight change, and postmenopausal breast cancer risk: The Netherlands Cohort Study. Cancer Causes Control 8:39–47.
4. McGuire WL (1980) An update on estrogen and progesterone receptors in prognosis for primary and advanced breast cancer. In: Hormones and Cancer (Iacobelli S, et al., eds.), Raven Press, New York, pp. 337–344.
5. Siiteri PK (1982) Review of studies on estrogen biosynthesis in the human. Cancer Res 42:3269s–3275s.
6. Reed MJ (1994) The role of aromatase in breast tumors. Breast Cancer Res Treat 30:7–17.
7. Brodie AMX, Santen RJ (1994) Aromatase and its inhibitors in breast cancer—overview and perspective. Breast Cancer Res Treat 30:1–6.
8. Dowsett M, Detre S, Rowlands M, Grimshaw R (1996) Oestrogen formation in breast clinical and biological importance. J Endocrinol 150:S59–S63.
9. Miller WR, CYNeill J (1976) Oestradiol synthesis from C19 steroids by human breast cancers. Brit J Cancer 33:116–118.
10. Clarke R, Dickson RB, Lippman ME (1992) Hormonal arspects of breast cancer. Growth factors, drugs and stromal interactions. Crit Rev Oncol Hematol 12:1–23.
11. Lippman ME, Dickson RB (1989) Mechanisms of growth control in normal and malignant breast epithelium. Recent Prog Horm Res 45:383–440.
12. van Landeghem AAJ, Poortman J, Nabuurs M, Thijssen JHH (1985) Endogenous concentration and subcellular distribution of estrogens in normal and malignant human breast tissue. Cancer Res 45:2900–2906.
13. Fishman J, Nisselbaum JS, Menedez-Botet CJ, Schwartz MK (1977) Estrone and estradiol content in human breast tumors: relationship to estradiol receptors. J Steroid Biochem 8:893–896.
14. Wysowski DK, Comstock GW, Helsing KJ, Lau HL (1987) Sex hormone levels in serum in relation to the development of breast cancer. Am J Epidemiol 125:791–799.
15. Moore JW, Clark GM, Bulbrook RD, Hayward JL, Murai JT, Hammond GL, et al. (1982) Serum concentrations of total and non-protein-bound oestradiol in patients with breast cancer and in normal controls. Int J Cancer 29:17–21.
16. Teruel M, Bolufer P, Rodriguez A, Antonio P, Salabert MT (1989) Plasma sex steroids and SHBG in patients with breast cancer and their relation to tumor oestrogen-dependency. Exp Clin Endocrinol 93:37–44.
17. Bernstein L, Ross RK, Pike MC, Brown JB, Henderson BE (1990) Hormone levels in older women: a study of post-menopausal breast cancer patients and healthy population controls. Br J Cancer 61:298–302.
18. Toniolo PG, Levitz M, Zeleniuch-Jacquotte A, Banerjjee S, Koenig KL, Shore RE, et al. (1995) A prospective study of endogenous estrogens and breast cancer in postmenopausal women. J Natl Cancer Inst 87:190–197.
19. Petrakis NL, Wrensch MR., Emster VL, Miike T, Murai J, Simberg N (1987) Influence of pregnancy and lactation on serum and breast fluid estrogen levels: implications for breast cancer risk. Int J Cancer 40:587–591.

20. Emster VL, Wrensch MR, Petrakis NL, King EB, Miike T, Murai J, et al. (1987) Benign and malignant breast disease: initial study results of serum and breast fluid analyses of endogenous estrogens. J Natl Cancer Inst 79:949–960.
21. Garland CF, Friedlander NJ, Barrett-Connor E, Khaw KT (1992) Sex hormones and postmenopausal breast cancer: a prospective study in an adult community. Am J Epidemiol 135:1220–1230.
22. Bonney RC, Reed MJ, Davidson K, Beranek PA, James VHT (1983) The relationship between 17β-hydroxysteroid dehydrogenase activity and estrogen concentration in human breast tumors and in normal breast tissue. Clin Endocrinol 19:727–739.
23. Vermeulen A, Deslypere JP, Paridaens R, Leclercq G, Roy F, Heuson JC (1986) Aromatase, 17β-hydroxysteroid dehydrogenase and intra-tissular sex hormone concentrations in cancerous and normal glandular breast tissue in postmenopausal women. Eur J Cancer Oncol 22:515–525, 1986.
24. Mehta RR, Valcourt L, Graves J, Green R, Das Gupta TK (1987) Subcellular concentration of estrone, estradiol, androstenedione and 17β-hydroxysteroid dehydrogenase (17-β-OH-SDH) activity in malignant and non-malignant human breast tissues. Int J Cancer 40:305–308.
25. Santen RJ, Leszczynski D, Mallet N, Feil PD, Wright C, Manni A, et al. (1986) Enzymatic control of estrogen production in human breast cancer: relative significance of aromatase versus sulfatase pathways, In: Endocrinology of the Breast Basic and Clinical Aspects (Angel A, Bradlow HL, Dogliotti L, eds.), New York Academy of Science, pp. 126–137.
26. Lipton A, Santner SJ, Santen RJ, Harvey HA, Deil PD, White-Hershey D, et al. (1987) Aromatase activity in primary and metastatic human breast cancer. Cancer 59:779–783.
27. Silva MC, Rowlands MG, Dowsett M, Gusterson B, M[cKinna JA, Fryatt I, et al. (1989) Intratumoral aromatase as prognostic factor in human breast carcinoma. Cancer Res 49: 2588–2591.
28. Evans TRJ, Rowlands MG, Silva MC, Law M, Coombes RC (1993) Prognostic significance of aromatase and estrone sulfatase enzymes in human breast cancer. J Steroid Biochem Mol Biol 44:583–587.
29. Lipton A, Santen RJ, Santner SJ, Harvey HA, Sanders SI, Matthews YL (1992) Prognostic value of breast cancer aromatase. Cancer 70:1951–1955.
30. Bezwoda WR, Manson N, Dansey R (1987) Correlation of breast tumor aromatase activity and response to aromatase inhibition with aminoglutethimide. Oncology 44:345–349.
31. Bradlow HL (1982) A reassessment of the role of breast tumor aromatization. Cancer Res 42:3382S–3386S.
32. Miller WR, Anderson TJ, Jack WJL (1990) Relationship between tumor aromatase activity, tumor characteristics and response to therapy. J Steroid Biochem Mol Biol 37:1055–1059.
33. Reed MJ, Owen AM, Lai LC, Coldham NG, Ghilchik MW, Shaikh NA, et al. (1989) *In situ* oestrogen synthesis in normal breast and breast tumor tissues: effect of treatment with 4-hydroxyandrostenedione. Int J Cancer 44:233–237.
34. Pasqualini JR, Chetrite G, Blacker C, Feinstein M-C, Delalonde L, Talbi M, et al. (1996) Concentrations of estrone, estradiol, and estrone sulfate and evaluation of sulfatase and aromatase activities in pre- and postmenopausal breast cancer patients. J Clin Endocrinol Metab 81:1460–1464.
35. Lu Q, Nakamura J, Savinov A, Yue W, Weisz J, Dabbs DJ, et al. (1996) Expression of aromatase protein and messenger ribonucleic acid in tumor epithelial cells and evidence of functional significance of locally produced estrogen in human breast cancers. Endocrinology 137:3061–3068.
36. Abul-Hajj YJ (1975) Metabolism of dehydroepiandrosterone by hormone dependent and hormone independent human breast carcinoma. Steroids 26:488–500.
37. Adams JB, Li K (1975) Biosynthesis of 17β-estradiol in human breast carcinoma tissue and a novel method for its characterization. Br J Cancer 31:429–433.
38. Miller WR, Forrest APM (1974) Oestradiol synthesis by human breast carcinoma. Lancet 2:866- 868.
39. Berstein LM, Larionov AA, Kyshtoobaeva ASh, Pozharisski KM, Semiglazov VF, Ivanova OA (1996) Aromatase in breast cancer tissue—localization and relationship with reproductive status of patients. J Cancer Res Clin Oncol 122:495–498.
40. Santen RJ, Martel J, Hoagland M, Naftolin F, Roa L, Harada N, et al. (1994) Stromal spindle cells contain aromatase in human breast tumors. J Clin Endocrinol Metab 79:627–632.
41. Sasano H, Frost AR, Saitoh R, Harada N, Poutanen M, Vihko R, et al. (1996) Aromatase and 17β-hydroxysteroid dehydrogenase type 1 in human breast carcinoma. J Clin Endocrinol Metab E'1:4042–4046.
42. Price T, Aitken J, Head J, Mahendroo MS, Means GO, Simpson ER (1992) Determination of aromatase cytochrome P450 messenger RNA in hurman breast tissues by competitive polymerase chain reaction amplification. J Clin Endocrinol Metab 74:1247–1252.
43. Santner SJ, Pauley RL, Tait L, Kaseta J, Santen RJ (1997) Aromatase activity and expression in breast cancer and benign breast tissue stromal cells. J Clin Endocrinol Metab 82:200–208.

44. Bulun SE, Price TM, Aitken J, Mahendroo MS, Simpson ER (1993) A link between breast cancer and local estrogen biosynthesis suggested by quantification of breast adipose tissue aromatase cytochrome P450 transcripts using competitive polymerase chain reaction after reverse transcription. J Clin Endocrinol Metab 77:1622–1628.
45. Bulun SE, Simpson ER (1994) Regulation of aromatase expression in human tissues. Breast Cancer Res Treat 30:19–29.
46. Bulun SE, Sharda G, Rink J, Sharma S, Simpson ER (1996) Distribution of aromatase P450 transcripts and adipose fibroblasts in the human breast. J Clin Endocrinol Metab 81:1273–1277.
47. Berkovitz GD, Guerami A, Brown TR, MacDonald PC, Migeon CJ (1985) Familial gynecomastia with increased extra glandular aromatization of plasma C-19-steroids. J Clin Invest 75:1763–1769.
48. Bulard J, Mowszowicz I, Schaison G (1987) Increased aromatase activity in pubic skin fibroblasts from patients with isolated gynecomastia. J Clin Endocrinol Metab 64:618–623.
49. Peaker M, Taylor E (1990) Oestrogen biosynthesis by the goat mammary gland: transient aromatase activity during late pregnancy. J Endocrinol 125: R1–R3.
50. Santner SJ, Chen S, Zhou D, Korsunsky Z, Martel J, Sa;nten RJ (1993) Effect of androstenedione on growth of untransfected and aromatase-transfected MCF-7 cells in culture. J Steroid Biochem Mol Biol 44: 611–616.
51. Yue W, Zhou D, Chen S, Brodie A (1994) A new nude mouse model for postmenopausal breast cancer using MCF-7 cells transfected with the human aromatase gene. Cancer Res 54:5092.
52. Yue W, Wang J, Savinov S, Brodie A (1995) The effects of aromatase inhibitors on growth of mammary tumors in a nude mouse model. Cancer Res 55:3073–3077.
53. Yue W, Wang JP, Hamilton C, Demers L, Santen RJ (1996) Estrogen produced *in situ* by breast tumors increases estradiol level and tumor growth rate more than blood borne estradiol, In: Proceedings of the IVth Aromatase Conference, abstract B3, p. 26.
54. Masamura S, Santner SJ, Gimotty P, George J, Santen RJ (1997) Mechanism of maintenance of high breast tumor estradiol concentrations in the absence of ovarian function: role of very high affinity tissue uptake. Breast Cancer Res Treat 42:215–226.
55. Gray DA, McGrath CM, Jones RF, Morris VL (1986) A common mouse mammary tumor virus integration site in chemically induced precancerous mammary hyperplasias. Virology 30:360–368.
56. Ashley RL, Cardiff RD, Fanning TG (1980) Reevaluation of the effect of mouse mammary tumor virus infection on the BALB/c mouse hyperplastic outgrowth. J Natl Cancer Inst 65:977–986.
57. Morris VL, Rao TR, Kozak CA, Gray DA, Lee Chan, ECM, Cornell TJ, et al. (1991) Characterization of *int-5*, a locus associated with early events in mammary carcinogenesis. Oncogene Res 6:53–63.
58. Durgam VR, Tekmal RR (1994) The nature and expression of *int-5*, a novel MMTV integration locus gene in carcinogen-induced mammary tumors;. Cancer Lett 87:179–186.
59. Tekmal RR, Durgam VR (1995) The overexpression of *int-5/aromatase,* a novel MMTV integration locus gene, is responsible for D2 mammary tumor cell proliferation. Cancer Lett 88:147–155.
60. Tekrnal, RR, Durgam, VR (1997) A novel in vitro and in vivo breast cancer model for testing inhibitors of estrogen biosynthesis and action using D2 tumor cells with an activated *int-5/aromatase* gene. Cancer Lett. 118:21–28.
61. Harda N, Utsumi T, Takagi Y (1993) Tissue-specific expression of the human aromatase P-450 gene by alternative use of multiple exons 1 and promoters, and switching of tissue-specific exons in carcinogenesis. Proc Natl Acad Sci USA 90:11312–11316.
62. Tekmal RR, Ramachandra N, Gubba S, Durgam, VRi, Mantione J, Toda K, et al. (1996) Overexpression of *int-5/aromatase* in mammary glands of transgenic mice results in the induction of hyperplasia and nuclear abnormalities. Cancer Res 56:3180–3185.
63. Keshava N, Fang C, Bhalla KN, Tekmal RR (1997) Environmental mutagen (DMBA) acts synergistically in *int-5/aromatase* transgenic mice that have increased mammary estrogen activity. Muta Res 379:S151.
64. Greenberg ER, Barnes AB, Resseguie Z, Barrett JA, Burnide S, Lanza LL, et al. (1984) Breast cancer in mothers given diethylstilbestrol in pregnancy. N Engl J Med 311:1393–1398.
65. Herbst AL, Ulfelder H, Poskanzer DC (1971) Adenocarcinoma of the vagina: association of maternal stilbestrol therapy with tumor appearance in young women. New Engl J Med 284:878–881.
66. Lupulescu A (1983) Hormones and Carcinogenesis, Praeger Scientific, New York, pp. 89–144.
67. Warner MR (1976) Effect of various doses of estrogen to BALB/c Crgl neonatal female mice on mammary growth and branching at 5 weeks of age. Cell Tissue Kinet 9:429–438.
68. Jones LA, Bern HA (1979) Cervicovaginal and mammary gland abnormalities in BALB/c Crgl mice treated neonatally with progesterone and estrogen, alone or in combination. Cancer Res 39:2560–2567.

69. Warner MR, Yu L, Rosen JM (1980) Long term effects of perinatal injection of estrogen and progesterone on the morphological and biochemical development of the mammary gland. Endocrinology 106:823–832.
70. Tomooka Y, Bern HA (1982) Growth of mouse mammary glands after neonatal sex hormone treatment. J Natl Cancer Res Inst 69:1347–1352.
71. Sattin RW, Rubin GL, Wingo PA, Webster LA, Ory HW (1988) The Cancer and Steroid Hormone Study of the Centers for Disease Control and the National Institute of Child Health and Human Development. N Engl J Med 315:405–411.
72. Furth J (1982) Hormones as etiological agents in neoplasia, In: Cancer, vol I (F Becker, ed.), Plenum Press, New York, pp. 89–134
73. Fishman J (1983) Aromatic hydroxylation of estrogens. Annu Rev Physiol 45:61–72.
74. Bradlow HL, Hershcopf RJ, Marucci CP (1986) 16α-Hydroxylation of estradiol in women with breast cancer. Ann NY Acad Sci 464:138–151.
75. Fishman J, Osborne MP, Telang NT (1995) The role of estrogen in mammary carcinogenesis. Ann NY Acad Sci 768:91–100.
76. Bradlow HL, Sepkovic DW, Telang NT, Osborne MP (1995) Indole-3-carbinol: a novel approach to breast cancer prevention. Ann NY Acad Sci 768:180–200.
77. Liehr JG, Ricci MJ (1996) 4-Hydroxylation of estrogens as marker of human mammary tumors. Proc Natl Acad Sci USA 93:3294–3296.
78. Cavalieri E, Rogan E (1997) Mechanisms of tumor initiation by polycyclic aromatic hydrocarbons in mammals, In: The Handbook of Environmental Chemistry, vol. 3. PAHs and Related Compunds (Nelson A, ed.), Pergamon Press, New York.
79. Rogan E, Stack D, Cerny R, Edney J, Johannson S, Higginbotham S, et al. (1997) GC/MS analysis of catechol estrogen metabolites in breast tissue samples, In: Proceedings of the Department of Defense Breast Cancer Research Program Meeting, 3:743.
80. Levin M, Weisz J, Bui QD, Santen RJ (1987) Peroxidatic catechol estrogen production by human breast tissue *in vitro*. J Steroid Biochem 28:513–520.
81. Spink DC, Lincoln DW, Dickerman HW, Gierdly JF (1990) 2,3,7,8-Tetrachloro-dibenzo p-dioxine causes an extensive alteration of 17β-estradiol metabolism in MCF-7 breast tumor cells. Proc Natl Acad Sci USA 87:6917–6921.
82. Spink DC, Hayes CL, Young NR, Christou M, Sutter TR, Jefcoate CR, et al. (1994) The effects of 2,3,7,8-tetrachlorodibenzodioxin on estrogen metabolism in MCF-7 breast cancer cells: evidence for induction of a novel 17β-estradiol 4-hydroxylase. J Steroid Biochem Mol Biol 51:251–258.
83. Dwivedy I, Devanesan P, Cremonesi P, Rogan E, Cavalieri E (1992) Synthesis and characterization of estrogen 2,3- and 3,4 quinonens. Comparison of DNA adducts formed by the quinones versus horseradish peroxidase-activated catechol estrogens. Chem Res Toxicol 5:828–833.
84. Stack DE, Byun J, Gross ML, Rogan KG, Cavelieri E (1996) Molecular characteristics of catachol estrogen quinones in reactions with deoxyribonucleosides. Chem Res Toxicol 9:851–859.

7 Oncogenes and Mammary Carcinogenesis

Maria Luisa Veronese, MD,
Florencia Bullrich, PhD,
and Carlo M. Croce, MD

INTRODUCTION

Breast cancer is the most common malignancy among women in the United States, accounting for nearly 32% of all cancers and for nearly 20% of all cancer deaths in women *(1)*. Breast cancer is a multifactorial disease, and several factors are thought to influence the risk of breast cancer development, including geography, radiation exposure, and reproductive and family history. A family history of breast cancer constitutes the major risk factor, although familial breast cancer accounts for only 5% of all cases *(1)*. Although breast cancer deaths declined by 5% between 1989 and 1992 *(2)*, the incidence of breast cancer is expected to increase by 2–3% annually *(1)*, and efforts to decrease mortality significantly, including new therapeutic approaches and early diagnosis, have been relatively unsuccessful. One of the critical factors in determining the therapeutic approach to breast cancer, along with the presence or absence of lymph node metastasis, is the estrogen and progesterone receptor (ER and PR) status of the tumor. Indeed, ER- and/or PR-positive tumors have been found to be more likely to respond to endocrine therapy and are associated with a better prognosis *(1)*. An understanding of the genetic changes involved in breast cancer and of its biologic behavior, including possible interactions between hormones and oncogenes or tumor suppressor genes, will undoubtedly aid in the design of new therapies as well as in prevention and diagnosis of this disease.

It is thought that breast cancer, like other cancers, results from the sequential accumulation of specific genetic changes. These changes involve deactivating mutations in tumor suppressor genes such as *p53* and activating alterations in oncogenes such as *C-MYC*. Certain tumors such as retinoblastoma, Wilms' tumor, and tumors associated with neurofibromatosis and Li-Fraumeni syndrome are known to result from inherited mutations. Li-Fraumeni syndrome results from the transmission of a mutated *p53* gene and is associated with an increased risk of developing cancer including breast cancer *(3)*. Inherited predisposition to breast cancer found in breast and ovarian cancer families is also associated with transmission of mutations in the *BRCA1* or *BRCA2* genes located on chromosomes 17q21 and 13q12-13, respectively *(4,5)*. However, neither *BRCA1* nor

From: *Contemporary Endocrinology: Endocrinology of Breast Cancer*
Edited by: A. Manni © Humana Press Inc., Totowa, NJ

BRCA2 are mutated in sporadic tumors, indicating that additional genes must be involved in the initiation and progression of breast cancer.

Indeed, numerous loci containing putative tumor suppressor genes involved in breast cancer have been identified through loss of heterozygosity studies, including loci on chromosomes 1, 3, 11, 13, 16, and 17 *(3)*. DNA amplification resulting in activation of oncogenes occurs in 15–20% of cases and is the most frequently observed cytogenetic abnormality in breast cancer *(6)*. These oncogenes include genes encoding growth factor receptors, transcription factors, and regulators of apoptosis. This chapter examines the role of oncogenes in breast carcinogenesis and their possible use as prognostic factors. First, the classes of oncogenes and their function will be described, and second, the oncogenes, that have been shown to play an important role in breast cancer will be presented.

ONCOGENES

Oncogenes were first identified in animal retroviruses as the genes necessary for tumor induction by the virus *(7,8)*. These genes were later found to be mutated copies of normal host genes (proto-oncogenes) *(9)*. To date almost 100 oncogenes have been discovered by various methods, but only a small subset seems to play an important role in human cancer *(10)*. In human cells proto-oncogenes can induce tumorigenicity through activation by amplification, mutation, or chromosomal translocation. Functional studies have indicated two general mechanisms by which proto-oncogene activation can result in cellular transformation. Oncogenes can promote cell growth by accelerating the frequency of cell division and/or inhibit cell death by increasing the cell's life span. Functionally, proto-oncogenes can be upstream or downstream regulators of cell division and/ or cell death. Indeed, proteins activated in human malignancy include growth factors, their cell surface receptors and cytoplasmic signal transducers, nuclear transcription factors, and proteins involved in cell cycle control and apoptosis regulation. Members of each of these functional subsets are directly or indirectly implicated in breast cancer initiation and/or progression and lead to tumorigenesis by contributing to the induction of one or more of the transforming pathways described below.

Classes of Oncogenes

Growth Factors

Growth factors function as extracellular signals to induce cell proliferation through their interaction with a specific receptor on the target cell. Examples of this group include platelet derived growth factor (*PDGF*), epidermal growth factor (*EGF*), nerve growth factor (*NGF*), and fibroblast growth factor (*FGF*) *(11)*. The *PDGF* gene was recently found rearranged in soft tissue tumors through the t(17;22) translocation, which results in constitutive activation of the PDGF molecule and therefore, presumably, of PDGF-regulated cell growth pathways *(12)*. Molecules like EGF activate pathways regulating cell growth through a family of cell surface receptors (such as epidermal growth factor receptor [EGFR]) known to play an important role in breast cancer pathogenesis (see below). Therefore, these growth factors can be directly or indirectly involved in mammary gland tumorigenesis *(3,13)*.

Growth Factor Receptors

Growth factor receptors are integral membrane proteins with intrinsic tyrosine kinase activity. Binding of a growth factor to the receptor stimulates the tyrosine kinase activity of the receptor and results in the phosphorylation of cytoplasmic proteins with the consequent activation of cellular pathways regulating cell growth and differentiation. Examples are *ERBB/EGFR*, *ERBB-2*/neu/HER2, PDGFR, *KIT, MET, RET,* and *TRK (14)*. The *PDGFR* gene, located on chromosome 5, is involved in leukemogenesis through the t(5;12) translocation, which fuses its tyrosine kinase domain with the *TEL* gene on chromosome 12, thought to encode a DNA binding protein *(15)*. As mentioned above, growth factor receptors are commonly amplified in breast cancer and are thought to play an important role in mammary gland tumorigenesis. Overexpression of members of the *EGFR* family occurs in 20–40% of breast tumors and is thought to contribute to breast carcinogenesis through induction of mitogenic pathways activated by the receptor's tyrosine kinase.

Signal Transducers

Signal transducers are proteins involved in the transmission of signals from the cell surface to the nucleus. They include non-receptor protein kinases and quanosine triphosphate (GTP) binding proteins. The prototype non-receptor kinase involved in human tumors is ABL, which is constitutively activated in the *BCR/ABL* fusion protein resulting from the t(9;22) translocation characteristic of chronic myelogenous leukemia (CML) *(16)*. Another important class of oncogenic signal transducers is found in the RAS family of GTP binding proteins. RAS proteins activate downstream signal transducers such as MAP kinase in a cascade that leads to gene expression and cell division. Constitutive activation of these proteins results in cellular transformation through increased proliferation and occurs through both mutation and amplification in numerous human tumors, including breast cancer *(17–19)*.

Transcription Factors

Transcription factors are nuclear proteins involved in the regulation of gene expression. Transcription factors are often deregulated by amplification or by translocation. Aberrant and/or ectopic transcription factor activity results from overexpression or from the formation of chimeric proteins with one gene contributing to the DNA binding domain and the other contributing to transactivation domain *(20)*. Transformation is thought to occur through loss of control over gene expression and a resulting increase in cellular proliferation. The prototype transcription factor involved in tumorigenesis is C-MYC, a member of the bHLH group of DNA binding proteins *(21)*. *MYC* can be activated through chromosomal translocations that result in its overexpression, such as in the t(8;14) of Burkitt's lymphomas *(22)*, or through amplification such as occurs in solid tumors including breast cancer *(3,6,17)*.

Cell Cycle Proteins

Cell cycle proteins involved in human tumors include positive and negative cell cycle regulators, which are involved in numerous human tumors. Indeed, deregulation of cell cycle progression represents one of the major strategies for cellular transformation by both oncogene and tumor suppressor genes. Negative cell cycle regulators include tumor suppressors such as p53 and p16 that are inactivated by deletion or mutation *(23–25)*, whereas positive cell cycle regulators like *BCL-1*/PRAD1/CyclinD1 are activated by translocations or amplification *(3,26–28)*. For both negative and positive cell cycle regulators, transformation is thought to be due primarily to an increase in cellular proliferation.

Regulation of Programmed Cell Death or Apoptosis

Apoptosis is an important target for cellular transformation and represents the major mechanism of cell killing by antineoplastic drugs. Apoptosis plays crucial roles in organ development, in the regulation of cell number, and as a mechanism to eliminate unwanted or damaged cells such as self-reactive lymphocytes, cells infected by pathogens, and tumor cells *(29–31)*. Both oncogenes and tumor suppressor genes have been implicated in the control of cell death, and transformation by regulators of apoptosis is thought to result from increased cell survival. In addition to its role as a negative cell cycle regulator, the *p53* tumor suppressor gene is thought to be primarily responsible for the induction of cell death following DNA damage *(23,32)*. The *BCL-2* proto-oncogene, which was identified through its involvement in chromosomal translocations in B-cell malignancies *(33)* and was later found to be overexpressed in many other lymphoid and solid tumors *(34)*, is a potent inhibitor of apoptosis *(35)*.

MECHANISMS OF ONCOGENE ACTIVATION

3.1. Chromosomal Translocations

Chromosomal translocations are most common in hematologic malignancies and result in transcriptional activation of proto-oncogenes or in the formation of fusion proteins with transforming activity. In B-cell lymphomas the t(8;14)(q24;q32), t(11;14)(q13;q32), and t(14;18)(q32;q21) translocations result in the transcriptional activation, respectively, of *C-MYC* on chromosome 8q24, *BCL1*/CCND1/PRAD1 on chromosome 11q13, and *BCL2* on chromosome 18q21. Upregulation of *C-MYC*, *BCL1*, or *BCL2* expression occurs when these rearrangements place the proto-oncogene under the influence of regulatory sequences of constitutively expressed immunoglobulin genes on chromosome 14q32 *(22,26)*. Fusion proteins resulting from chromosomal translocations are involved in both hematopoietic and solid tumors. The t(9;22)(q34;q11) translocation of CML mentioned above results in the fusion of the *ABL* gene on chromosome 9q34 with the *BCR* gene on chromosome 22q11 *(16)*. Oncogenic transformation by *BCR/ABL* depends on constitutive activation of the ABL kinase *(36)*. In addition, membrane-bound proteins such as RET and PDGFR are involved in the formation of chimeric proteins with aberrant activity in hematopoietic and solid tumors *(15,37)*.

Mutations

Mutations, in the form of base substitutions, deletions, and insertions, usually in critical regulatory regions of the protein, can also result in constitutive activation of proto-oncogene function such as the one described above for *C-ABL*. This is exemplified by the ras family of GTPases, involved in tyrosine kinase growth factor receptor signal transduction *(38)*. Mutations resulting in permanently active enzymes have been described in a high percentage of colon cancers *(18,19,39)* and other tumors including a small percentage of breast cancers *(40)*.

DNA Amplification

DNA amplification, because it results in an increase in gene copy number, can result in proto-oncogene activation through overexpression *(41)*. DNA amplification, in the form of double minute chromosomes (DMINs), was first observed in cultured cells after selection for drug resistance *(42)*. In human tumors, the first report of gene amplification described *C-MYC* amplification in the HL-60 cell line and in primary leukemic cells derived from the patient. *C-MYC* was found to lie either within DMINs or within homogenous staining regions *(43,44)*. Since then proto-oncogene amplification has been described in numerous malignancies *(17,41)* and is now known to occur in a significant number of breast, ovarian, and lung tumors *(3,6,13,45)*. Amplified DNA fragments can be very large (more than 1 mega base) and the amplification unit (amplicon) often includes more than one gene. The process leading to gene amplification is thought to represent a particular form of DNA instability involving disproportionate DNA replication *(41)*. Several reports suggest a correlation between inactivation of a putative tumor suppressor gene on the short arm of chromosome 1 (perhaps regulating DNA stability) and *N-MYC* and *C-MYC* amplification *(46–48)*, suggesting that DNA amplification may be controlled by distinct recessive loci.

ONCOGENES AND BREAST CANCER

ERBB-2

The *EGFR*, *ERBB-2/HER-2/neu*, *ERBB-3/HER-3*, and *ERBB-4/HER4* genes are involved in mammary tumorigenesis through amplification and overexpression *(3,6)*. The *ERBB-2/HER-2/neu* gene was first identified in rat neuroblastomas as a gene with transforming activity *(49–51)*. The human homolog was independently cloned and named *HER-2* and *cC-ERBB-2 (52,53)*. The protein product of this gene, now interchangably called ERBB-2, HER-2, or neu, is a member of the EGF receptor family. Members of this group belong to the tyrosine kinase receptor superfamily and include the EGFR itself as well as erbB-2/HER-2/neu, erbB-3/HER-3, and erbB-4/HER4 *(54,55)*. Signaling through the EGFR family, as through other protein kinase receptors, is initiated after ligand binding. Ligand binding leads to receptor dimerization, autophosphorylation, transphosphorylation, and finally activation of the receptor dimer as a kinase for cytoplasmic substrates *(55)*. Activated receptor complexes bind and phosphorylate src homology domain (SH2) containing proteins such as Grb2. Grb-2 associates with the Sos protein through its SH3 domains to form the Grb2/Sos complex, which recruits and activates ras proteins to the cellular membrane, thus directing a series of phosphorylation steps leading to gene expression, DNA synthesis, and cellular proliferation *(56,57)* (Fig. 1). Because of their role as inducers of cellular proliferation, tyrosine kinase receptors represent important targets for involvement in tumorigenesis and are indeed often activated through mutation, translocation, or amplification in human tumors. A ligand termed heregulin (HRG) or neu differentiation factor (NDF) was discovered and shown to induce tyrosine phosphorylation of erbB-2 *(58–60)*. Later studies indicate that ligand binding and signaling through the EGFR family involve the formation of heterodimers such as erbB-2/erbB-3 or erbB-2/erbB-4 and that these heterodimers all show affinity for the HRG/NDF ligand *(61–63)*. It has been proposed that heterodimerization in response to ligand binding regulates EGFR family activity by directing the selection of particular cytoplasmic targets by different receptor complexes *(63)*. In breast cancer, amplification of individual members of the EGFR family may favor the formation of certain heterodimers versus others, activating signal transduction pathways that are particularly effective in achieving transformation of breast epithelium.

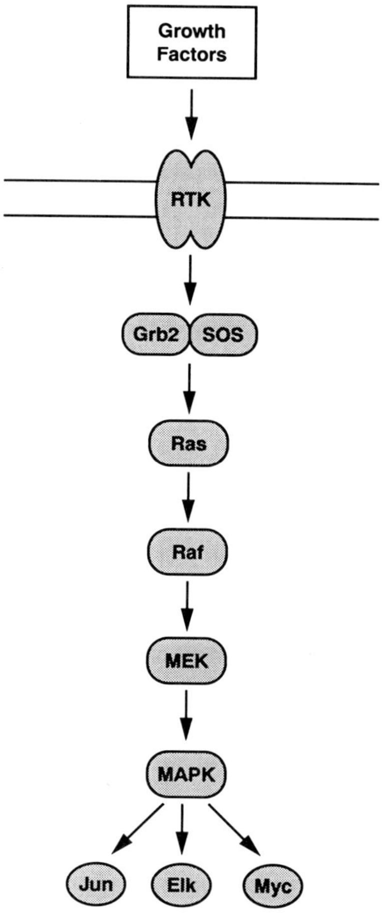

Fig. 1. Signal transduction through receptor tyrosine kinases (RTK). Ligand-mediated activation of the kinase activity of the membrane-associated RTK leads to ras activation, which in turn leads to induction of a cascade of serine/threonine kinases resulting in increased transcription of genes such as *JUN, ELK,* and *MYC.* (Adapted from ref. 40, with permission.)

In breast cancer, signal transduction pathways regulated by the EGFR family are activated through *ERBB-2/HER-2/neu* amplification in approximately 20% of all tumors *(3,64).* In addition, in agreement with the hypothesis that *ERBB-2/HER-2/neu* overexpression contributes to transformation through induction of cell proliferation, *ERBB-2/HER-2/neu* amplification was found to be inversely related to ER and PR status *(64)* and positively correlated with high mitotic index, topoisomerase II expression, and poor prognosis *(6,65).*

The proposed mechanism involving receptor heterodimerization in EGFR family signaling and the identification of the HRG/NDF ligand indicate that studies of receptor coexpression and ligand mediated activation of specific heterodimers receptor formed in breast cancer cells should provide important clues to the role of the EGFR family in breast carcinogenesis.

RAS

The *RAS* genes, *H-RAS*, *K-RAS*, and *N-RAS*, encode guanine nucleotide binding proteins which play a critical role in signal transduction with receptor tyrosine kinases by controlling cellular growth and differentiation *(38)*. Ras proteins are plasma membrane associated and cycle between an active GTP-bound form and an inactive GDP-bound form *(66)*. Ras function is positively regulated by proteins such as Sos, which, as mentioned above, is involved in signaling through the EGFR family *(56,57,67)*. Negative regulation of ras, on the other hand, is achieved by stimulating its intrinsic GTPase activity, by shifting the balance toward an increase in the GDP-bound form of ras *(68)*. Multiple mitogenic pathways can be activated by ras including the RAF, PI3K, and MEKK pathways (Fig. 1). Activation of upstream serine/threonine kinases involves displacement of the kinase to the cell membrane and results in activation of a cascade involving downstream kinases such as JNK, MAP, and Rho. These then translocate to the nucleus, where they activate transcription factors such ELK, JUN, MYC, and AP1 *(67)*.

Ras family genes are frequently mutated in human tumors *(69)*, particularly in colon and pancreatic carcinomas *(19,70)*. Mutant ras proteins have a decreased GTPase activity and are insensitive to regulatory stimuli *(68,71)*, leading to transformation through constitutive activation of the ras signaling pathway (Fig. 1). *RAS* is mutated in less than 5% and overexpressed in 20–60% of breast cancers *(40,72–74)*. Although ras overexpression seems not to be associated with tumor sensitivity to hormonal treatment or overall survival *(75)*, the limited number of studies performed so far suggest that ras overexpression in breast tumors could be associated with disease progression and more malignant phenotypes *(74)*.

MYC

The *C-MYC* proto-oncogene on chromosome 8q24 was found to be rearranged and activated as a result of the t(8;14)(q24;q32) translocation characteristic of Burkitt's lymphomas *(76,77)*. The myc protein is a transcription factor and contains an amino terminal transactivation domain and a basic helix-loop-helix leucine zipper (bHLHLZ) motif involved in dimerization and sequence-specific DNA binding *(21)*. Like other members of the bHLHLZ family, myc is active as a transcription factor only when complexed with max, another bHLHLZ transcription factor *(78,79)*. The myc /max heterodimer was shown to bind specifically to the CACGTG target sequence on DNA *(21,80)*. This sequence has been found in the promoters of several genes that control for cell death, proliferation, and differentiation including the *p53* promoter genes *(81)*. The expression of *C-MYC* itself is tightly regulated in normal cells, and *C-MYC* mRNA is only synthesized in response to mitogenic stimuli. Aberrant or increased expression of *C-MYC* is thought to contribute to tumorigenesis through loss of control of the expression of growth-regulating genes by myc/max heterodimers *(82–84)*.

Myc has been reported to be amplified and overexpressed in up to 20% of breast cancers *(64,74)* and is likely to play an important role in the pathogenesis of breast cancer. *MYC* amplification in breast tumors is more common in PR-negative cases *(64)* and is associated with high mitotic index *(85)*, high histologic grade *(86,87)*, advanced patient age *(85,88)*, and tumor aggressiveness. Subsequent studies have evaluated the prognostic significance of coexpression of several oncogenes and of *p53*. Coexpression of *C-MYC*, *Ha-RAS*, and *C-FOS* was found to be a strong indicator of recurrence and shortened survival *(74)*, whereas coamplification of *BCL1* and *C-MYC* and of *BCL1* and *c-ERBB-2* was associated with high histologic grade *(85)*. As mentioned above, the amplification of myc family genes in neuroblastomas and breast cancers is associated with loss of heterozygosity on the short arm of chromosome 1, suggesting that a putative tumor

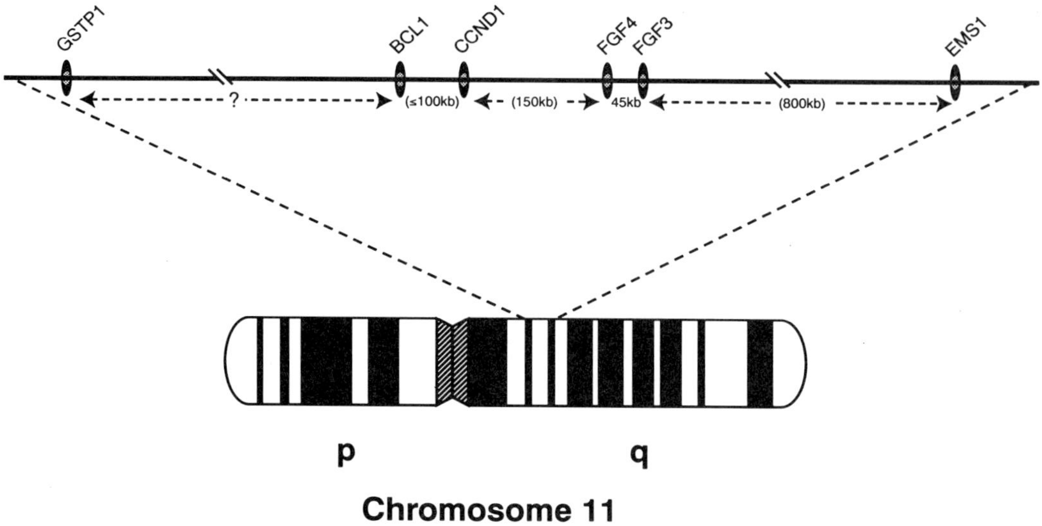

Fig. 2. 11q13 amplicon in breast cancer. (From ref. 3, with permission.)

suppressor on 1p controls myc amplification in several human tumors *(46–48)*. The association of *C-MYC* amplification with high cell kinetics and poor prognosis is in accordance with its role as a regulator of cell cycle progression, as well as with its known involvement in a high-grade malignancy such as Burkitt's lymphoma. In follicular lymphomas with a t(14;18) translocation involving the *BCL2* gene, the acquisition of a t(8;14) translocation results in development of a more aggressive disease *(89)*, indicating that *C-MYC* activation can also play an important role in tumor progression.

11q13 Amplication

Band q13 on chromosome 11 is amplified in 15–20% of breast cancers *(3,6)*. Since the initial reports, the number of candidate genes has fluctuated with new gene discoveries, functional experiments, and better physical characterization of the amplified 11q13 region. Indeed, as mentioned previously, amplified DNA segments can be quite large and include more than one gene. Furthermore, detailed physical mapping within the region indicates that there may be more than one independent amplicon at 11q13 and therefore more than one target gene *(90)*. Nevertheless, a region that appears amplified in the majority of tumors with 11q13 amplification has been defined (Fig. 2). The first candidate genes within this region to be proposed as targets were two FGF genes, *FGF3* and *FGF4* *(3)*. Although MMTV insertional activation of *FGF3* and *FGF4* is associated with mouse breast carcinogenesis *(91)*, neither gene has been found overexpressed in human mammary tumors, suggesting that they do not represent the target of 11q13 amplification. Two other genes within the region, the *EMS1* gene, encoding a protein of unknown function *(92)*, and *CCND1/PRAD1/BCL1* gene, encoding cyclin D1 *(28)*, are overexpressed in almost all tumors with 11q13 amplification and represent the strongest candidates for involvement in breast tumorigenesis. The *BCL1* locus was initially discovered by cloning of the t(11;14) translocation characteristic of mantle cell lymphomas *(93)*. The gene rearranged by this translocation was found to code for Cyclin D1/CCND1 and to be involved in translocations in parathyroid tumors *(27,28)*. Cyclin D1 plays a crucial role in cell

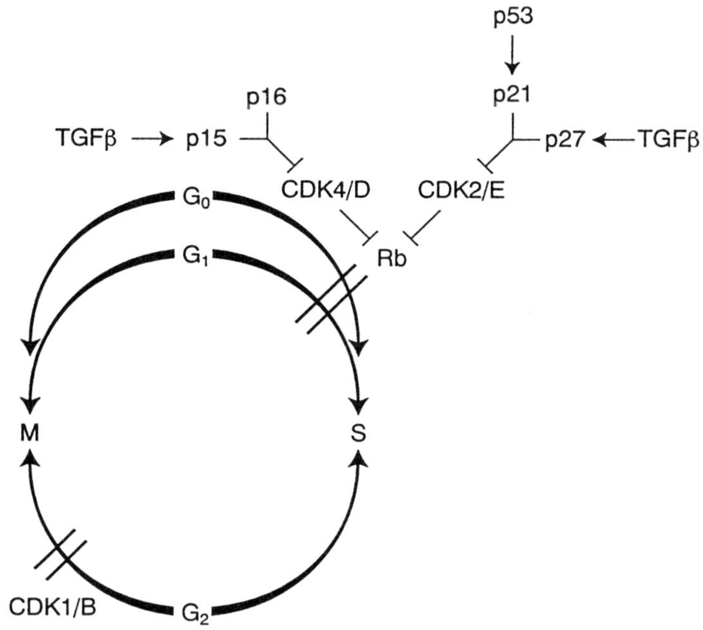

Fig. 3. The cell cycle and a simplified view of the molecular pathways of its control. The double bars represent "checkpoints" where progression through the cycle may be arrested. No attempt has been made to distinguish G_0 arrest from G_1 arrest. Arrows represent activation; blunt-ended bars represent inhibition. Kinases and phosphatases that regulate the cyclin-dependent kinases (CDKs) are not shown. p15, p16, p21, p27, CDK inhibitors; p53, tumor suppressor; Rb, retinoblastoma gene product; TGF-β, transforming growth factor-β. (From ref. 94, with permission.)

cycle control, and, as mentioned above, loss of fidelity in the regulation of cell division is one of the major mechanisms of cellular transformation. Several genes, including *Cyclin D1,* with a direct involvement in cell cycle control, are altered in human tumors. This cell cycle control is achieved through the coordinated activation and deactivation of cyclin-dependent kinases (CDKs). The association of cyclins with their corresponding cdks is necessary for CDK activation and phosphorylation of downstream proteins such as the retinoblastoma protein (Rb). Cyclin/CDK complexes are then inactivated by proteins named CDK inhibitors such as p16 *(94,95)*. Cyclin D1 activates cell cycle kinases CDK4 and CDK6, which form the complexes Cyclin D1/CDK4 or Cyclin D1/CDK6 that can be inactivated by p16 *(94)* (Fig. 3). This pathway for Rb phosphorylation thus contains three genes involved in human cancer: *CCND1, CDK4,* which is amplified in sarcomas *(96)*, and *p16,* which is mutated in both hematopoietic and solid tumors *(24,25)*. The findings that transgenic mice overexpressing CCND1 exhibit a high incidence of mammary tumors *(97)* and that Cyclin D1 can transform cells *(98)*, as well as its known role as a positive regulator of cell cycle progression, indicate that CCND1 is likely to play an important role in mammary tumor initiation and/or progression. Growth factors such as EGF and basic fibroblast growth factor (bFGF), as well as steroid hormones including estrogen and progesterone, are known to induce proliferation of breast cells. The observed stimulatory effect on cell division is partly due to the induction of expression of genes such as *C-MYC* and *Cyclin D1 (99,100)*. Therefore, amplification of *C-MYC* and/or *CyclinD1/BCL1/PRAD1* and the resulting overexpression of these genes represents a means for cancer cells to achieve growth factor independence and to escape normal control of proliferation. Interestingly, an inverse relationship between ER positivity and 11q13 amplification has been reported *(64)*. More than half of ER- or PR-positive tumors (which constitute approximately 50% of all tumors) respond to hormonal therapy. It is possible that Cyclin D1/*BCL1*/PRAD1 amplification contributes to hormonal therapy resistance of ER- or PR-positive unresponsive tumors. In addition, 11q13 amplification has been associated with more advanced disease (tumors with lymph node metastasis), shorter relapse-free survival, and increased mortality, suggesting that 11q13 amplification may mark a group of higher risk patients *(3)*.

BCL2

Control of a cell's life span is necessary for normal development and, in adult life, for the maintenance of tissue homeostasis. This control is achieved through an active form of programmed cell death named apoptosis and characterized by chromatin condensation, blebbing of the plasma membrane, presence of apoptotic bodies, and fragmentation of genomic DNA *(101)*. Several genes that regulate apoptosis are involved in the pathogenesis of human tumors, most notably *p53, C-MYC,* and *BCL2*. The *BCL2* gene, the most widely studied inhibitor of cellular death, was discovered as the target of chromosomal rearrangements resulting from the t(14;18) translocation in follicular lymphomas *(33)*. The *BCL2* gene, which is overexpressed in follicular lymphomas as a result of the translocation *(102)*, codes for a membrane-associated protein that has been found to promote cell survival *(35)* and to inhibit apoptosis induced by a variety of stimuli including glucocorticoids, anticancer drugs, growth factor withdrawal, and radiation *(103)*. In addition, *BCL2* has recently been proposed to play a role in G2-M checkpoint *(104)*. Several mammalian homologs of *BCL2* have been isolated with either apoptotic *(105)* or antiapoptotic functions *(106,107)*. In particular, heterodimerization of bcl2 with the proapoptotic protein bax inhibits the antiapoptotic effect of bcl-2 *(108)*. It is thought that the ratio of bcl-2 to bax is a crucial determinant in the control of apoptosis *(34)*; therefore, *BCL2* overexpression such as that observed in follicular lymphomas *(102)* contributes to tumorigenesis by disrupting the bcl2/bax balance and increasing cell survival. In normal mammary epithelium *BCL2* mRNA levels have been shown to vary with the menstrual cycle *(109)*, suggesting that *BCL2* expression may be under hormonal control. In addition, in the MCF-7 ER-positive breast cancer cell line, removal of estrogen from the growth medium was shown to result in loss of *BCL2* mRNA, whereas the levels of bax protein were not affected by estrogen exposure *(110)*. In breast tumors a strong association between good prognostic indicators such as estrogen and progesterone receptor positivity and *BCL2* expression has been reported by several investigators *(111–113)*. Loss of *BCL2* expression is associated with poor prognostic indicators such as high mitotic index, *EGFR* and *C-ERBB-2/neu* amplification, and mutant *p53* positivity *(111,114,115)*. Conversely, a strong association between bcl2 negativity/bax positivity and negative histopathologic features has been documented *(116)*. It is possible that high bcl2/low bax expression, by increasing cell survival in low-grade slowly dividing tumors, may favor the accumulation of genetic changes and the subsequent progression to a more aggressive phenotype. Particularly interesting is the observation that both wild-type and mutant *p53* can downregulate *BCL2* expression *(117)*. In fact, levels of mutant *p53* in human breast tumors are inversely related to levels of *BCL2* protein *(109)*.

BCL2 has been shown to protect cells from death induced by several anticancer drugs including cyclophosphamide, etoposide, and cysplatin *(34)*. The mechanism for *BCL2*-induced drug resistance in ER-positive breast carcinomas may involve estrogen-mediated pathways for control of *BCL2* expression. Indeed, the sensitivity of the ER-positive breast cancer cell line MCF-7 to Adriamycin was markedly increased when cells were grown in the absence of estrogen or in the presence of estrogen and antiestrogen and correlated with low levels of *BCL2* expression *(110)*. Recently, the *BCL2* protein was shown to be inactivated by phosphorylation induced by drugs that interfere with microtubule polymerization or depolymerization but not by drugs that induce DNA damage *(104,118,119)*. bcl2 phosphorylation and cell death were shown to occur in response to taxol, taxotere, vincristine, and vinblastine, suggesting that induction of bcl2 phosphorylation by these drugs represents an important therapeutic target and can be used to overcome bcl2-mediated cell death protection.

SUMMARY AND CONCLUSIONS

The development of breast cancer requires the progressive accumulation of specific genetic changes. Although the precise sequence in which these alterations occur, leading, for example, from atypical hyperplasia to invasive carcinoma, cannot be established at this time, several genes including the *p53* tumor suppressor gene, as well as the *BCL1, C-MYC, ERBB-2,* and *BCL2* oncogenes described in this chapter, are known to play important roles in breast cancer progression. *BCL1*, *C-MYC*, and *ERBB-2* are activated through amplification, resulting in their overexpression, and are thought to contribute to breast tumorigenesis by increasing the rate of cell division. *BCL2* expression is thought to play a role in breast carcinogenesis by increasing the cell's life span and may be implicated in drug resistance by inhibiting cell death caused by anticancer drugs. The discovery that oncogene and tumor suppressor gene alterations form the genetic basis of neoplasia, and that specific genetic alterations are important determinants of proliferative rate and metastatic potential, suggested that these genetic changes could be used as prognostic factors. Today, lymph node metastasis, tumor size, tumor grade, and hormone receptor status constitute the major factors in determining prognosis and treatment approaches to breast cancer. An understanding of the functions of oncogenes and their interactions as well as their roles in the particular environment of the mammary gland will provide important clues to the biochemical mechanisms leading to breast cancer initiation and/or progression. Molecular diagnostic approaches should prove particularly useful in identifying patients with histologically undetectable metastasis, as well as in the detection of early hematogenous spread and minimal residual disease. Additional investigations are necessary to obtain a better definition of prognostic subtypes and their association with particular genetic abnormalities. Furthermore, an understanding of oncogene function can provide the basis for new therapeutic approaches and may lead to more effective treatment of this disease.

ACKNOWLEDGMENTS

We thank Juan Palazzo (Department of Pathology, Jefferson Medical College, Philadelphia, PA) and Teresa Druck (Kimmel Cancer Institute, Jefferson Medical College, Philadelphia, PA) for their helpful comments on the manuscript.

REFERENCES

1. Tavassoli FA (1992) *Pathology of the Breast,* Elsevier Science Publishing, New York.
2. Abeloff MD (1995) Breast. Curr Opin Oncol 7:489–494.
3. Bieche I, Lidereau R (1995) Genetic alterations in breast cancer. Genes Chromosomes Cancer 14:227–251.
4. Miki Y, Swensen J, Shattuck-Eidens D, Futreal PA, Harshman K, Tavitigian S, et al. (1994) A strong candidate for the breast and ovarian cancer susceptibility gene BRCA1. Science 266:66–71.
5. Tavtigian SV, Simard J, Rommens J, Couch F, Shattuck-Eidens D, Neuhaunsen S, et al. (1996) The complete BRCA2 gene and mutations in chromosome 13q-linked kindreds. Nature Genet 12:333–337.
6. Devilee P, Schuuring E, van de Vijver MJ, Cornelisse CJ (1994) Recent developments in the molecular genetic understanding of breast cancer. Crit Rev Oncog 5:247–270.
7. Weiss R, Teich N, Varmus H, Coffin J (1982) *RNA Tumor Viruses: Molecular Biology of tumor viruses, 2nd ed.,* Cold Spring Harbor Laboratory Cold Spring Harbor NY.
8. Weiss R, Teich N, Varmus H, Coffin J (1985) *RNA Tumor Viruses: Molecular Biology of tumor viruses, Supplement to 2nd ed.,* Cold Spring Harbor Laboratory Cold Spring Harbor NY.
9. Bishop JM (1983) Cellular oncogenes and retroviruses. Annu Rev Biochem 52:301–354.
10. Levine AJ (1995) The genetic origins of neoplasia. JAMA 273:592.
11. Cross M, Dexter TM (1991) Growth factors in development, transformation, and tumorigenesis. Cell 64:271–280.
12. Simon MP, Pedeutour F, Sirvent N, Grosgeorge J, Minoletti F, Coindre JM, et al. (1997) Deregulation of the platelet-derived growth factor B-chain gene via fusion with collagen gene COL1A1 in dermatofibrosarcoma protuberans and giant-cell fibroblastoma. Nature Genet 15:95–98.
13. Hoskins K, Weber BL (1995) Recent advances in breast cancer biology. Curr Opin. Oncol 7:495–500.
14. Yarden Y, Ullrich A (1988) Growth factors and receptor tyrosine kinases. Annu Rev Biochem 57:443–478.
15. Golub TR, Barker G, Lovett M, Gilliland DG (1994) Fusion of PDGF receptor β to a novel *ets*-like gene, *tel,* in chronic myalomonocytic leukemia with t(5;12) chromosomal translocation. Cell 77:307–316.
16. Shtivelman E, Lifshitz B, Gale RP, Canaani E (1985) Fused transcript for abl and bcr genes in chronic myelogenous leukemia. Nature 315:550–554.
17. Bishop J Ms (1986) *Amplification of Proto-Oncogenes in Tumorigenesis.* (Oldstone ALN, ed.), Springer-Verlag New York, pp. 71–78
18. Bos JL, Fearon ER, Hamilton SR, Verlaan-de-Vries M, Van Boom JH, Van der Eb AJ, Vogelstein B (1987) Prevalence of *ras* mutations in human colorectal cancers. Nature 327:293–297.
19. Forrester K, Almonguera C, Han K, Grizzle WE, Perucho M (1987) Detection of high incidence of *K-ras* oncogenes during colon tumorigenesis. Nature 327:298–303.
20. Rabbitts TH (1994) Chromosomal translocations in human cancer. Nature 372:143–149.
21. Amati B, Land H (1994) Myc-Max-Mad: a transcription factor network controlling cell cycle progression, differentiation and death. Curr Opin Genet Devel 4:102–108.
22. Croce CM, Nowell PC (1985) Molecular basis of human B-cell neoplasia. Blood 65:1–7.
23. Hollstein M, Sidransky D, Vogelstein B, Harris C (1991) p53 mutations in human cancers. Science 253:49–53.
24. Ohta M, Nagai H, Shimizu M, Rasio D, Berd D, Mastrangelo M, et al. (1994) Rarity of Somatic and germline mutations of the cyclin-dependent kinase 4 inhibitor gene CDK4I, in melanoma. Cancer Res 54:5269–5272.
25. Rasool O, Heyman M, Borgonovo L, Liu Y, Grander D, Soderhall S, et al. (1995) p15/ink4B and p16/ink4 gene inactivation in acute lymphocytic leukemia. Blood 85:3431–3436.
26. Showe L, Croce C (1987) The role of chromosomal translocations in B- and T-cell neoplasia. Annu Rev Immunol 5:253–277.
27. Rosenberg CL, Kim HG, Shows TB, Kronenberg HM, et al. (1991) Rearrangement and overexpression of D11S287E, a candidate oncogene on chromosome 11q23 in benign parathyroid tumors. Oncogene 6:449–453.
28. Motokura T, Bloom T, Kim HG, Juppner H, Ruderman JV, Kronenberg HM, Arnold A (1991) A novel cyclin encoded by a bcl-1 linked oncogene. Nature 350:512–515.
29. Nagata S, Golstein P (1995) The Fas death factor. Science 267, 1449–1456.
30. Steller H (1995) Mechanisms and genes of cellular suicide. Science 267:1445–1449.
31. Whyte M, Evan G (1995) The last cut is the deepest. Nature 376:17–18.
32. Lowe SW, Schmitt EM, Smith SW, Osborne BA, Jacks T (1993) p53 is required for radiation-induced apoptosis in mouse thymocytes. Nature 362, 847–849.

33. Tsujimoto Y, Finger LR, Yunis J, Nowell PC, Croce CM (1984) Cloning of the chromosome breakpoint of neoplastic B cells with the t(14;18) chromossome translocation. Science 226:1097–1099.
34. Reed JC (1995) Regulation of apoptosis by bcl-2 family proteins and its role in cancer and chemoresistance. Curr Opin Oncol 7:541–546.
35. Vaux DL (1988) Bcl-2 gene promotes hematopoietic cell survival and cooperates with c-myc to immortalize pre-B cells. Nature. 335, 440–442.
36. Konopka JB, Watanabe SM, Witte ON (1984) An alteration of the human c-abl protein in K562 leukemia cells unmasks associated tyrosine kinase activity. Cell 37:1035–1042.
37. Pierotti MA, Santoro M, Jenkins RB, Sozzi G, Bongarzone I, Grieco M, et al. (1992) Characterization of an inversion on the long arm of chromosome 10 juxtaposing D10S170 and RET and creating the oncogenic sequence RET/PTC. Proc Natl Acad Sci USA 85:1616–1620.
38. Lowy DR, Willumsen M (1993) Function and regulation of ras. Annu Rev Biochem 62:851–891.
39. Barbacid M (1987) Ras genes. Annu Rev.Biochem 56:779–827.
40. Clark GJ, Der CJ (1995) Aberrant function of the ras signal transduction pathway in human breast cancer. Breast Cancer Res Treat 35:133–134.
41. Alitalo K, Schwab M (1986) Oncogene amplification in tumor cells. Adv Cancer Res 47:235–281.
42. Alt FW, Kellems RE, Bertino JR, Schimke RT (1978) Selective multiplication of dihydrofolate reductase genes in methotrexate-resistant variants of cultured murine cells. J Biol Chem 253:1357–1370.
43. Schimke R, ed. (1982) *Gene Amplification.* Cold Spring Harbor Laboratory, Cold Spring Harbor New York.
44. Alitalo K, Schwab M, Lin CC, Varmus HE, Bishop JM (1983) Homogeneously staining chromosomal regions contain amplified copies of an abundantly expressed cellular oncogene (c-myc) in malignant neuroendocrine cells from a human colon carcinoma. Proc Natl Acad Sci USA 80:1707–1711.
45. Nau MN, Brooks BJ, Battey J, Sausville E, Gazdar AF, Kirsch IR, et al. (1985) L-myc, a new myc-related gene amplified and expressed in human small cell lung cancer. Nature 318:69–73.
46. Fong CT, Dracopoli NC, Write PS, Merril PT, Griffith RC, Housman DE, et al. (1989) Loss of heterozygosity for the short arm of chromosome 1 in human neuroblastomas: correlation with n-myc amplification. Proc Natl Acad Sci USA 86:3753–3757.
47. Caron H, van Sluis P, van Hoeve M, de Kraker J, Bras J, Slater R, et al. (1993) Allelic loss of chromosome 1p36 in neuroblastoma is of preferential maternal origin and correlates with n-myc amplification. Nature Genet 4:187–190.
48. Bieche I, Champeme MH, Lidereau R (1994) A tumor suppressor gene on chromosome 1p32–pter controls the amplification of myc family genes in breast cancer. Cancer Res 54:474–476.
49. Shih C, Padhy LC, Murray M, Weinberg RA (1981) Transforming genes of carcinomas and neuroblastomas introduced into mouse fibroblasts. Nature 290:261–264.
50. Padhy LC, Shih C, Cowing D, Finkelstein R, Weinberg RA (1982) Identification of a phosphoprotein specifically induced by the transforming DNA of rat neuroblastomas. Cell 28:865–871.
51. Schechter AL, Hung MC, Vaidyanathan L, Weinberg RA, Yang-Feng TL, Francke U, et al. (1985) The neu gene: an erbB-homologous gene distinct from and unlinked to the gene encoding the EGF receptor. Science 229:976–978.
52. Coussens L, Yang-Feng TL, Liao YC, Chen E, Gray A, McGrath J, et al. (1985) Tyrosine kinase receptor with extensive homology with EGF receptor shares chromosomal location with neu oncogene. Science 230:1132–1139.
53. Semba K, Kamata N, Toyoshima K, Yamamoto T (1985) A v-erb related protooncogene, c-erbB2, is distinct from c-erbB1/epidermal growth factor receptor gene and is amplified in a human salivary gland adenocarcinoma. Proc Natl Acad Sci USA 82:6497–6501.
54. Ullrich A, Schlessinger J (1990) Signal transduction by receptors with tyrosine kinase activity. Cell 61:203–212.
55. van der Geer P, Hunter T, Lindberg RA (1994) Receptor protein-tyrosine kinases and their signal transduction pathways. Annu Rev Cell Biol 10:251–337.
56. Schlessinger J (1994) SH2/SH3 signaling proteins. Curr Opin Oncol 4:25–30.
57. Chrysogelos S, Dickson RB (1994) EGF receptor expression, regulation, and function in breast cancer. Breast Cancer Res Treat 29:29–40.
58. Peles E, Bacus SS, Koski RA, Lu HS, Wen D, Ogden SG, et al. (1992) Isolation of the neu/HER-2 stimulatory ligand: a 44 kd glycoprotein that induces differentiation of mammary tumor cells. Cell 69:205–216.
59. Wen D, Peles E, Cupples R, Suggs SV, Bacus SS, Luo Y, et al. (1992) Neu differentiation factor: a transmembrane glycoprotein containing an EGF domain and an immunoglobulin homology unit. Cell 69:559–572.

60. Holmes WE, Sliwkowski MX, Akita RW, Henzel WJ, Lee J, Park JW, Yansura D, Abadi N, Raab H, Lewis GD, et al. (1992) Identification of heregulin, a specific activator of p185erbB2. Science 256:1205–1210.
61. Plowman GD, Green JM, Culouscou JM, Carlton GW, Rothwell VM, Buckley S (1993) Heregulin induces tyrosine phosphorilation of HER4/p180erbB4. Nature 366:473–475.
62. Sliwkowski MX, Schaefer G, Akita RW, Lofgren JA, Fitzpatrick VD, Nuijens A, et al. (1994) Coexpression of erbB2 and erbB3 proteins reconstitutes a high affinity receptor for heregulin. J Biol Chem 269:14661–14665.
63. Carraway KL, Cantley LC (1994) A neu acquaintance for erbB3 and erbB4: a role for receptor heterodimerization in growth signaling. Cell 78:5–8.
64. Berns EMJJ, Klijn JGM, van Staveren IL, Portengen H, Noordegraaf E, Foekens JA (1992) Prevalence of amplification of the oncogenes c-myc, her2/neu, and int2 in one thousand human breast tumors: correlation with steroid receptors. Eur J Cancer 28:697–700.
65. Jarvinen AH, Kononen J, Pelto-Huikko M, Isola J (1996) Expression of topoisomerase IIa is associated with rapid cell proliferation, aneuploidy, and c-erbB2 overexpression in breast cancer. Am J Pathol 148:2073–2082.
66. Vojtek AB, Hollenberg SM, Cooper JA (1993) Mammalian Ras interacts directly with the serine/threonine kinase raf. Cell 74:205–214.
67. Quilliam LA, Khosravi-Far R, Huff SY, Der CJ (1995) Guanine nucleotide exchange factors: activators of the Ras superfamily of proteins. BioEssays 17:395–404.
68. Trahey M, McCormick F (1987) A cytoplasmic protein stimulates normal p21 ras GTPase, but does not affect oncogenic mutants. Science 238:542–545.
69. Rodenhuis S (1992) ras and human tumors. Semin Cancer Biol 3:241–247.
70. Almoguera C, Shibata D, Forrester K, Martin J, Arnheim N, Perucho M (1988) Most human carcinomas of the exocrine pancreas contain mutant K-ras genes. Cell 53:549–554.
71. Gibbs BG, Sigal IS, Poe M, Scolnick EM (1984) Intrinsic GTPase activity distinguishes normal and oncogenic ras p21 molecules. Proc Natl Acad Sci USA 81:5704–5708.
72. Thor A, Ohuchi N, Hand PH, Callahan R, Weeks MO, Theillet C, et al. (1986) ras gene alterations and enhanced levels of ras p21 expression in a spectrum of benign and malignant human mammary tissues. Lab Invest 55:603–615.
73. Spandidos DA, Yiagnisis M, Papadimitriou K, Field JK (1989) Ras, c-myc, and c-erb-2 oncoproteins in human breast cancer. Anticancer Res 9:1385–1394.
74. Bland KI, Konstadoulakis MM, Vezeridis MP, Wanebo HJ (1995) Oncogene protein co-expression. Value of Ha-ras, c-myc, c-fos, and p53 as prognostic discriminants for breast carcinoma. Ann Surg 221:706–720.
75. Archer SG, Eliopoulos A, Spandidos D, Barnes D, Ellis IO, Blamey RW, et al. (1995) Expression of ras p21, p53, and c-erbB-2 in advanced breast cancer and response to first line hormonal therapy. Adv. Breast Cancer. 1260–1266.
76. Croce CM, Thierfelder W, Erikson J, Nishikura K, Finan J, Lenoir GM, et al. (1983) Transcriptional activation of an unrearranged and untranslocated c-myc oncogene by translocation of a cλ locus in Burkitt lymphoma cells. Proc Natl Acad Sci USA 80:6922–6926.
77. Erikson J, Nishikura K, ar-Rushdi A, Finan J, Emanuel B, Lenoir G, et al. (1983) Translocation of an immunoglobulin κ locus to a region 3' of an unrearranged c-myc oncogene enhances c-myc transcription. Proc Natl Acad Sci USA 80:7581–7585.
78. Blackwood EM, Eisenman RN (1991) Max: a helix-loop-helix zipper protein that forms a sequence-specific DNA-binding complex with myc. Science 251:1211–1217.
79. Prendergast GC, Lawe D, Ziff EB (1991) Association of Myn, the murine homolog of Max, with c-Myc stimulates methylation-sensitive DNA binding and Ras cotransformation. Cell 65:395–407.
80. Blackwell TK, Kretzner EM, Blackwood EM, Eisenman RN, Weintraub H (1990) Sequence-specific DNA binding by the c-myc protein. Science 250:1149–1151.
81. Reisman D, Elkind NB, Roy B, Beamon J, Rotter V (1993) c-myc transactivates the p53 promoter through a required down-stream CACGTG motif. Cell Growth Differ 4:57–65.
82. Marcu KB, Bossone SA, Patel AJ (1992) Myc function and regulation. Annu Rev Biochem 61:809–860.
83. Amati B, Brooks MW, Levy N, Littlewood TD, Evan GI, Land H (1993) Oncogenic activity of the c-myc protein requires dimerization with max. Cell 72:233–245.
84. Vastrik I, Makela TP, Koskinen PJ, Klefstrom J, Alitalo K (1994) Myc protein: partners and antagonists. Crit Rev Oncog 5:59–68.

85. Contegiacomo A, Pizzi C, De Marchis L, Alimandi M, Delrio P, Di Palma E, et al. (1995) High cell kinetics is associated with amplification of the int-2, bcl-1, myc and erbB-2 proto-oncogenes and loss of heterozygosity at the DF3 locus in primary breast cancers. Int. J Cancer 61:1–6.
86. Varley JM, Swallow JE, Brammar WJ, Whittaker JL, Walker RA (1987) Alterations to either c-erbB-2 (neu) or c-myc proto-oncogenes in breast carcinomas correlate with poor short-term prognosis. Oncogene 1:423.
87. Tavassoli M, Quirke P, Farzaneh F, Lock NJ, Mayne LV, Kirkham N (1989) c-erbB-2/c-erbA coamplification indicative of lymph node metastasis, and c-myc amplification of high tumor grade, in human breast carcinoma. Br. J Cancer 60:505–.
88. Escot C, Theillet C, Lidereau R, Spyratos F, Champeme MH, Gest J, et al. (1986) Genetic alterations of the c-myc protooncogene (MYC) in human primary breast carcinomas. Proc Natl Acad Sci USA 83:4834.
89. Gauwerky CE, Haluska FG, Tsujimoto Y, Nowell PC, Croce CM (1988) Evolution of B-cell malignancy: pre-B-cell leukemia resulting from MYC activation in a B cell neoplasm with a rearranged BCL2 gene. Proc Natl Acad Sci USA 85:8548–8552.
90. Kerlseder J, Zeillinger R, Schneeberger C, Czerwenka K, Speiser P, Kubista E, et al. (1994) Patterns of DNA amplification at band q13 of chromosome 11 in human breast cancer. Genes Chromosom Cancer 9:42–48.
91. Shackleford GM, MacArthur CA, Kwan HC, Varmus HE (1993) Mouse mammary tumor virus infection accelerates mammary carcinogenesis in wnt1 transgenic mice by insertional activation of int2/FGF3 and Hst/FGF4. Proc Natl Acad Sci USA 90:740–744.
92. Schuuring E, Verhoeven E, Mooi WL, Michalides R (1992) Identification and cloning of two overexpressed genes U21B31/PRAD1 and EMS1, within the amplified chromosome 11q13 region in human carcinomas. Oncogene 7:355–361.
93. Tsujimoto Y, Yunis J, Onorato-Showe L, Erikson J, Nowell PC, Croce CM (1984) Molecular cloning of the chromosomal breakpoint of B-cell lymphomas and leukemias with the t(11;14) translocation. Science 224:1403–1406.
94. Kamb A (1995) Cell-cycle regulators and cancer. Trends Genet 11:136–140.
95. Motokura T, Arnold A (1993) Cyclin D, oncogenesis. Curr Opin Genes Dev 3:5–10.
96. Khatib ZA, Matsushime H, Valentine M, Shapiro DN, Sherr CJ, Look AT (1993) Coamplification of the CDK4 gene with MDM2 and GLI in human sarcomas. Cancer Res. 53, 5535–5541.
97. Wang TC, Cardiff RD, Zukerberg L, Lees E, Arnold A, Schmidt EV (1994) Mammary hyperplasia and carcinoma in MMTV-cyclin D1 transgenic mice. Nature 369:669–671.
98. Hinds PH, Dowdy SF, Eaton EN, Arnold A, Weinberg RA (1994) Function of a human cyclin gene as an oncogene. Proc Natl Acad Sci USA 91:709–713.
99. Musgrove EA, Sutherland RL (1994) Cell cycle control by steroid hormones. Cancer Biol 5:381–389.
100. Sutherland RL, Hamilton JA, Sweeney KJE, Watts CKW, Musgrove EA (1995) Expression and regulation of cyclin genes in breast cancer. Acta Oncol 5:651–656.
101. Wyllie AH (1987) Apoptosis: cell death in tissue regulation. J Pathol 153:313–316.
102. Tsujimoto Y, Cossman J, Jaffe E, Croce CM (1985) Involvement of the bcl-2 gene in human follicular lymphoma. Science 228:140–144.
103. Nunez G, London L, Hockenbery D, Alexander M, McKearn JP, Korsmeyer SJ (1990) Deregulated bcl-2 gene expression selectively prolongs survival of growth factor-deprived hemopoietic cell lines. J Immunol 144:3602–3610.
104. Haldar S, Basu A, Croce CM (1997) Bcl2 is the guardian of microtubule integrity. Cancer Res 57:229–233.
105. Boise LH, Gonzalez-Garcia M, Postema CF, Ding L, Lindstein T, Turka LA, et al. (1993) Bcl-X, a bcl-2 related gene that functions as a dominant regulator of apoptotic cell death. Cell 76:597–608.
106. Oltvai ZN, Milliman CL, Korsmeyer S (1993) Bcl-2 heterodimerizes with a conserved homolog Bax, that accelerates programmed cell death. Cell 74:609–619.
107. Chittenden T, Harrington EA, O'Connor R, Flemington C, Lutz RJ, Evan GI, et al. (1995) Induction of apoptosis by the bcl-2 related gene that functions as a dominant regulator of apoptotic cell death. Nature 374:733–736.
108. Sato T, Hanada M, Bodnig S, Irie S, Iwana N, Boise LH, et al. (1994) Interactions among members of the bcl-2 protein family analyzed with a yeast two-hybrid system. Proc Natl Acad. Sci USA 91:9238–9242.
109. Lu QL, Abel P, Foster CS, Lalani EN (1996) bcl-2: role in epithelial differentiation and oncogenesis. Hum Pathol 27:102–110.

110. Teixeira C, Reed JC, Pratt MAC (1995) Estrogen promotes chemotherapeutic drug resistance by a mechanism involving bcl-2 proto-oncogene expression in human breast cancer cells. Cancer Res 55:3902–3907.
111. Leek RD, Kaklamanis L, Pezzella F, Gatter KC, Harris AL (1994) bcl-2 in normal human breast and carcinoma, association with oestrogen receptor-positive, epidermal growth factor receptor-negative tumors and in situ cancer. Br J Cancer 69:135–139.
112. Hellemans PA, van Dam PA, Weyler J, van Oosterom AT, Buytaert P, Van Mark E (1995) Prognostic value of bcl-2 expression in invasive breast cancer. Br J Cancer 72:354–360.
113. van Slooten HJ, Clahsen PC, van Dierendonck JH, Duval C, Pallud C, Mandard AM, et al. (1996) Expression of bcl-2 in node-negative breast cancer is associated with various prognostic factors, but does not predict response to one course of perioperative chemotherapy. Br J Cancer 74:78–85.
114. Joensuu H, Pylkkanen L, Toikkanen S (1994) Bcl-2 protein expression and long-term survival in breast cancer. Am. J Pathol. 145, 1191–1198.
115. Silvestrini R, Veneroni S, Daidone MG, Benini E, Boracchi P, Mezzetti M, et al. (1994) The bcl-2 protein: a prognostic indicator strongly related to p53 protein in lymph node-negative breast cancer patients. J Natl Cancer Ins 86:499–504.
116. Binder C, Marx D, Binder L, Schauer A, Hiddemann W (1996) Expression of Bax in relation to Bcl-2 and other predictive parameters in breast cancer. Ann Oncol 7:129–133.
117. Haldar S, Negrini M, Monne M, Sabbioni S, Croce CM (1994) Down-regulation of bcl-2 by p53 in breast cancer cells. Cancer Res 54:2095–2097.
118. Haldar S, Jena N, Croce CM (1995) Inactivation of bcl-2 by phosphorylation. Proc Natl Acad Sci USA 92:4507–4511.
119. Haldar S, Chintapalli J, Croce CM (1996) Taxol induces bcl-2 phosphorylation and death of prostate cancer cells. Cancer Res 56:1253–1255.

8 Categorization of Breast Cyst Fluid and Breast Cancer Risk

Luigi Dogliotti, MD, PHD
and Pasquale Caraci, MD

INTRODUCTION

Gross cystic disease of the breast (GCD) is a well-defined clinical and pathologic entity, commonly occurring in the premenopausal decade. Its prevalence was estimated to be about 7% in western countries *(1)*. Although the cyst itself is not considered a premalignant lesion, several studies with long-term follow-up indicate that bearers have a two- to fourfold increased risk of developing cancer, in the same or in the contralateral breast *(1–7)*. Studies on the composition of the aspirated fluid (breast cyst fluid [BCF]) have demonstrated that this "biochemical space" has a peculiar composition with unusual profiles of many constituents, including ions, steroid and peptide hormones, growth factors, enzymes, immunoglobulins, cytokines, and other proteins *(8–11)*. Furthermore, certain constituents show not only an enormous range of cyst fluid levels, but also a distribution of values consistent with the existence of distinct subpopulations. In particular, two major subgroups of cysts have been identified on the basis of the electrolyte composition and more specifically on the K^+/Na^+ ratio *(12–14)*. Cationic categorization of cysts has gained wide acceptance as an useful tool to evaluate individual patients in relation to the natural history of cystic disease and could be of significance in predicting the breast cancer risk *(6–9,14)*.

BIOCHEMICAL AND PATHOPHYSIOLOGIC BASES OF BREAST CYST FLUID CATIONIC CATEGORIZATION

Since the early observations *(15)*, Na^+ and K^+ concentrations of different cyst fluids have been found to vary widely, ranging from those characteristic of the extracellular fluids (high Na^+, low K^+) to levels approximating those found in the intracellular compartment (low Na^+, high K^+). It was then observed that the intracystic levels of these ions were inversely correlated and that the bimodal distribution of values for both K^+ and Na^+ (or K^+/Na^+ ratio) was in agreement with the existence of more than one population of cyst fluids *(12–14)*. Two major subsets and a third minor one were proposed: *type I*, with high K^+ and low Na^+; *type II*, with low K^+ and high Na^+; and *type III*, a minor subset with intermediate values *(13,14,16)*. Particularly interesting was the early observation of a

From: *Contemporary Endocrinology: Endocrinology of Breast Cancer*
Edited by: A. Manni © Humana Press Inc., Totowa, NJ

Table 1
Nonsteroidal Compounds Assayable at Significantly Higher Concentrations in Type I and Type II Cysts[a]

Higher in type I cysts	Higher in type II cysts
H^+	Cl^-
EGF	Albumin
IGF-II	CEA
Gastrin-releasing peptide	Thrombospondin
Cathepsin-D	β-Thromboglobulin
IgA-11S	IgA-7S
Relaxin	IgG
α-Fetoprotein	SHBG
γ-GT	CBG
α-Amylase	LDH
Triiodothyronine	TGF-β2

[a]Abbreviaitons: EGF, epidermal growth factor; IGF, insulin-like growth factor; γ-GT, γ-glutamil-transpeptidase; CEA, carcinoembryonic antigen; SHBG, sex hormone binding globulin; CBG, corticosteroid-binding globulin; LDH, lactate dehydrogenase; TGF, transforming growth factor.

highly significant positive correlation between K^+ (or K^+/Na^+ ratio) and dehydroepyandrosterone sulfate (DHEAS), which was shown to be accumulated in BCF, in concentrations up to 100-fold higher than in plasma *(13,14,16)*. It was also suggested that the measurement of Cl^- alone could be used to separate fluids in two main subsets, considering that the intracystic levels of Cl^- were positively correlated to Na^+ and negatively correlated to K^+ *(17)*.

Analysis of protein content has validated electrolyte categorization of cysts. Type I cysts display a polymorphic protein profile, clearly distinct from that of the serum; remarkably, they are rich in intracellular enzymes *(9)*, and contain the 11S secretory form of IgA and low levels of albumin *(18,19)*. Type II cysts show a protein profile more similar to that of human serum: they have higher levels of albumin and the 7S monomeric form of IgA *(9,18)*.

Based on electrolyte and protein composition, Molina et al. *(20)* distinguished two fluid forms: *nontransudative (intracellular) cyst fluids* (high K^+, low Na^+), accounted for by specific secretory breast activity or passive cell sloughing into the fluid; and *transudative cyst fluids* (low K^+, high Na^+), in which serum and interstitial fluids have a more direct influence on the cyst fluid composition, possibly as a consequence of an open cell-cell junction in the lining epithelium, in a manner similar to certain conditions of milk secretion *(21)*. It was suggested, moreover, that digoxin-like substances, present in higher concentrations in type I fluids, may play a role in determining the electrolyte profile by regulating the Na^+/K^+ ATPase activity *(22)*.

In recent years, comparative studies on the biochemical composition of BCF, as a function of cyst type, have confirmed that this categorization is meaningful, as the major subsets differ markedly in the levels of many components, including steroid hormones, growth factors, immunoglobulins, enzymes, and other specific and nonspecific proteins *(8–10,13,14,18–20,23–35)*. Tables 1 and 2 list a number of compounds that can be assayed at significantly different concentrations in opposing cationic subsets. It is worth

Table 2
Nonconjugated and Conjugated Steroids Assayable at Significantly Different Concentrations in Type I and Type II Cysts

Higher in type I cysts
Testosterone
Dihydrotestosterone
Androsterone
Androstane-3α, 17β-diol
Androst-5-ene-3β,17β-diol
Dehydroepiandrosterone sulfate (DHEAS)
Androsterone glucuronide
Androstan-3α, 17β-diolglucuronide
Estrone-3-sulfate
Estriol-3-sulfate
Estradiol
Higher in type II cysts
Progesterone
Pregnenolone

noting that type I fluids show remarkably high levels of androgen *(13,14,16)* and estrogen sulfates *(26–28)* and display an important androgenic milieu *(29,30)*. Furthermore, mitogenic peptides such as epidermal growth factor *(23–25)*, insulin-like growth factor II *(25)*, gastrin-releasing peptide *(31)*, and cathepsin-D *(32)* have also been found at higher concentrations in type I cysts, whereas transforming growth factor-β, which is claimed to have an inhibitory effect on growth of tumor cells of epithelial origin, is preferably accumulated in type II cysts *(35)*. These findings lend support to the view that the surrounding breast tissue is different for the opposite subsets of cysts. Accordingly, for certain women bearing breast cysts, BCF may be a "magnifying glass" for a hormonal and proliferative environment permissive to subsequent cancer growth.

Another distinctive feature of type I fluids is that they have a closer resemblance to nipple aspirates, having similar concentrations of DHEAS *(36)* and the 11S secretory form of IgA *(9,18)*. These observations also support the view that type I fluids reflect the secretory activity of the mammary cells.

RELATIONSHIP TO PATHOLOGY

In a classical study, Dixon et al. *(37)* correlated cyst type with the morphology of the lining epithelium: type I cysts were found to be specifically associated with apocrine metaplastic cells *(apocrine type)*, and type II cysts were lined by flattened cells with minimal apocrine changes *(flattened type)*. This dichotomy, however, has been subsequently questioned *(38)*.

In a computer-aided cytomorphometric study, we found that type I fluids were more frequently apocrine cell rich *(84%)* than type II fluids *(54%)*, suggesting a higher frequency of exfoliated apocrine cells in type I cysts *(39)*. The issue has been reexamined by Leis *(7)* in an extensive review on the significance of apocrine cells and their identification by cyst fluid analysis. Using a different cutoff value for segregating two cyst subsets by fluid analysis (Na^+/K^+ ratio = 3) and histologic examination of surgically excised cysts, he found that the electrolyte classification corresponded accurately to histologic features of the cells lining the cyst wall, in that BCFs with a low Na^+/K^+ ratio were aspirated exclusively from cysts of the *apocrine type*, and BCFs with a high Na^+/K^+ ratio were aspirated exclusively from cysts of the so-called *attenuated type*.

It is held that BCF cytology virtually never shows morphologic signs of preneoplastic or neoplastic significance. However, particular attention has to be paid to the surrounding and/or contralateral breast tissue of patients bearing breast macrocysts, since proliferative premalignant lesions can frequently be observed *(40)*. Interestingly, in a retrospective histopathologic study *(41)*, foci of apocrine metaplasia and epithelial hyperplasia of any degree, with or without atypia, were all seen more frequently in patients with type I or histologically apocrine cysts. In his review, Leis *(7)* reported on a histologic study of slides from 116 gross cysts that had been excised with a surrounding section of breast tissue. Epithelial hyperplasia with marked atypia was found in the adjacent breast tissue in about 15% of the 71 apocrine cysts but in none of the 45 attenuated cysts.

CATIONIC CATEGORIZATION AND RISK OF BREAST CANCER

It is matter of debate whether cationic typing of BCF may be predictive of breast cancer risk in individual patients. As previously stressed, it has been reported that patients with type I apocrine cysts were significantly more likely to have in situ carcinoma or foci of epithelial hyperplasia with or without atypia and apocrine metaplasia in their breasts than matched controls *(7,40)*. These findings rouse interest when considering that proliferative lesions such as atypical hyperplasia are admittedly reliable markers of increased breast cancer risk among women undergoing biopsy *(42)*. Moreover, apocrine changes in the breast are reportedly a more common finding in populations at high risk of breast carcinoma than in populations at low risk *(43)*.

Preliminary observations of Bradlow et al. *(9)* and Bundred and Mansel *(6)* suggested that women who have had one or more type I aspirated cysts are at increased risk of breast cancer. Other authors, however, have questioned whether the cationic categorization of cysts could give valuable information concerning breast cancer risk *(44,45)*. Nevertheless, one should consider with caution the claim of Ebbs and Bates *(44)* that cyst type does not predict breast cancer risk since their report is possibly invalidated by including patients who had their cancer previously diagnosed or diagnosed within a year of the initial cyst aspiration.

To evaluate the relationship between the risk of subsequent breast cancer and the biochemical characteristics of BCF in women affected by GCD, a prospective cohort study was undertaken in 1983 at the Cancer Prevention Center of Ravenna, Romagna, Italy. The results of this study were recently published *(46)*. In brief, between February 1983 and February 1993, 1323 consecutive women aged 30–69 years, with no previous or concomitant malignancy at any site including breast, underwent aspiration of one or more breast cyst >1 mL. Of these women, 229 were excluded from the study because they did not meet the eligibility criteria and a further 292 because their BCF was not assayed for cationic content. Thus 802 women were enrolled in the study and had BCF assayed for biochemical composition. The follow-up program has included physical examination and ultrasound scan every year and mammography every other year. The proportion of women lost to follow-up has been very low (<1%).

In regard to BCF, the electrolyte composition showed a bimodal distribution; the scatter plot of log K^+ vs log Na^+ suggested that fluids could be separated into three

Table 3
Incidence of Breast Cancer Among 802 Women with Gross Cystic Disease by Type of Breast Cyst Aspirated and Compared with Incidence Among General Female Population Covered by the Romagna Cancer Registry

	Type I (n = *417*)	*Type II* (n = *325*)	*Mixed* (n = *60*)	*Total* (n = *802*)
No. of cases of invasive cancer	12	2	1	15
Person-year of observation	2658.5	2054.9	389.2	5111.6
Expected no. of cases[a]	4.58	3.59	0.69	8.86
Age standardized ratio	2.62	0.56	1.44	1.69
(95% CI)	(1.40–4.40)	(0.09–1.72)	(0.08–6.33)	(0.97–2.70)

[a]Based on the age-specific incidence rates reported by the Romagna Cancer Registry

Table 4
Relative Risk of Invasive Breast Cancer Among 802 Women with Gross Cystic Disease by Cationic Type of Breast Cysts Aspirated at Enrollment

			Relative risk (95% CI)	
Type of cyst	*No. of subjects*	*No. of cancers*	*Univariate analysis*	*Multivariate analysis*
Type II	325	2	1.0	1.0
Type I	417	12	4.62 (1.26–29.7)	4.24 (1.12–27.5)
Mixed	60	1	2.57 (0.12 to 26.9)	1.98 (0.07 to 34.4)

subgroups: *type I cysts*, with $K^+/Na^+ >1.5$; *type II cysts*, with $K^+/Na^+ <0.25$; and *type III cysts*, with K^+/Na^+ 0.25–1.5.

By December 1994, 17 breast cancers had been diagnosed in the cohort, 15 cases of invasive breast cancer (14 epithelial cancers and 1 malignant phylloides tumor) and 2 cases of ductal carcinoma in situ. Fourteen of the cases, including the two cases of ductal carcinoma in situ, occurred in the women with type I cysts, two occurred in those with type II cysts, and one in those with mixed cysts. The incidence of invasive breast cancer in the whole cohort was higher than that expected from the rates reported by the Romagna Cancer Registry (age standardized incidence ratio 1.69; 95% confidence interval [CI] 0.97–2.70) *(47)*, as reported in Table 3. The increased risk was concentrated in the group of women with type I cysts: 12 cases observed vs 4.58 expected (age standardized incidence ratio 2.62; 95% CI 1.40–4.40); no excess was seen among the women with type II and mixed cysts. Table 4 shows the results of direct comparison among the three groups of women: the risk of invasive breast cancer among women with type I cysts was significantly higher than women with type II cysts, in both univariate (relative risk 4.62; 95% CI 1.26–29.7) and multivariate analysis (relative risk 4.24; 95% CI 1.12–27.5). The association was stronger when the two cases of ductal carcinoma in situ were included in the analyses (relative risks 5.41 [95% CI 1.51–34.4] and 5.06 [95% CI 1.33–32.5]), respectively. The relative risk of breast cancer remained virtually unchanged after adjusting for several known risk factors for breast cancer.

CONCLUSIONS

It has been stated that mammary cysts are complex endocrine entities capable of accumulating, metabolizing, and probably synthesizing certain hormones *(8)*. Biochemical, histopathologic and clinical findings indicate that the electrolyte composition is useful in classifying cyst fluids *(8,9,12–14,20)*. Patients bearing type I cysts have a higher risk of relapse *(7,48,49)* and present more frequently with multiple and bilateral cysts *(7,14,48–50)*.

Unfortunately, there has been insufficient agreement on the precise criteria to be used for defining the different subsets. Evidence indicates the existence of two fundamental cyst types, even if a third intermediate subset is sometimes defined in order to overcome the difficulty, on a mathematical basis, of identifying a single cation cutoff value *(51)*. We consider it appropriate, for practical and clinical purpose, to use a cutoff value of K^+/Na^+ ratio >1.5 to identify type I cysts: in the Italian cohort *(46,49)*, these patients have demonstrated a behavior relatively homogeneous with regard to the clinical course, showing a higher risk of relapse and presenting more often with multiple cysts.

Regarding breast cancer risk among women with gross cystic disease, the Italian study, the largest cohort study performed to date, shows that the overall relative risk (1.69) is lower than expected in comparison with previous studies *(1–4,6,7)*, paralleling data from Ciatto et al. *(5)* in the Florence study.

On the other hand, this study clearly shows that the increased risk of breast cancer is limited to a subgroup of women with gross cystic disease. Such women can be easily identified on the basis of a high K^+/Na^+ ratio in the cyst fluid. The clinical implications of this finding are noteworthy in the light of the simplicity, availability, and low cost of electrolyte measurement. However, the size and duration of the increased risk among women with type I cysts are still to be assessed and need to further explored by longer follow-up.

REFERENCES

1. Haagensen CD, Bodian C, Haagensen DE (1981) Breast Carcinoma: Risk and Detection, WB Saunders, Philadelphia.
2. Harrington E, Lesnick G (1981) The association between gross cysts of the breast and breast cancer. Breast 7:13–17.
3. Jones BM, Bradbeer JW (1980) The presentation and progress of macroscopic breast cysts. Br J Surg 67:669–671.
4. Roberts MM, Jones V, Elton RA, Fortt RW, Williams S, Gravelle IH (1984) Risk of breast cancer in women with history of benign disease of the breast. BMJ 288:275–278.
5. Ciatto S, Biggeri A, Del Turco MR, Bartoli D, Iossa A (1990) Risk of breast cancer subsequent to proven gross cystic disease, Eur. J Cancer., 26:555–557.
6. Bundred NJ, Mansel RE (1989) Clinical factors influencing the risk of breast cancer in women with gross cysts. Br J Clin Pract 43(suppl 68):103–105.
7. Leis HP Jr (1993) Gross breast cysts: significance of apocrine type, identification by cyst fluid analysis, and management. Breast Dis 6:185–194.
8. Dogliotti L, Orlandi F, Caraci P, Puligheddu B, Torta M, Angeli A (1990) Biochemistry of breast cyst fluid: an approach to understanding intercellular communication in the terminal duct lobular units. Ann NY Acad Sci 586:17–28.
9. Bradlow HL, Fleisher M, Schwartz MK, Nisselbaum J, Breed CN (1985) Classification of patients with gross cystic breast disease according to the biochemical composition of breast cyst fluid, In: *Fibrocystic Breast Disease*, (Dogliotti L, Mansel RE, eds.), Editio Cantor, Aulendorf, pp. 9–20.
10. Miller WR (1989) The biochemistry of cyst fluids. Br J Clin Pract 43(suppl 68):94–99.
11. Enriori CL, Novelli JE, Cremona MC, Hirsig RJP, Enriori PJ (1992) Biochemical study of cyst fluid in human breast cystic disease: a review. Breast Cancer Res Treat 24:1–9.

12. Bradlow HL, Skidmore FD, Schwartz MK, Fleisher M (1981) Cation levels in human breast cyst fluid. Clin Oncol 7:338–390.
13. Miller WR, Dixon JM, Scott WN, Forrest APM (1983) Classification of human breast cysts according to electrolyte and androgen conjugate composition. Clin Oncol 9:227–232.
14. Dogliotti L, Orlandi F, Torta M, Buzzi G, Naldoni C, Mazzotti A, et al. (1986) Cations and dehydroepyandrosterone-sulfate in cyst fluid of pre- and menopausal patients with gross cystic disease of breast. Evidence for the existence of subpopulations of cysts. Eur J Cancer Clin Oncol 22:1301–1307.
15. Fleisher M, Robbins GG, Breed CN, Fracchia AA, Urban JA, Schwartz MK (1974) Biochemistry of breast cyst fluid. Mem Sloan Kettering Cancer Center Clin Bull 3:94–97.
16. Bradlow HL, Skidmore FD, Schwartz MK, Fleisher M, Schwartz D (1983). Cations in breast cyst fluid, In: *Endocrinology of Cystic Breast Disease* (Angeli A, Bradlow HL, Dogliotti L, eds.), Raven Press, New York, pp. 197–201.
17. Fleisher M, Bradlow HL, Schwartz MK, Schwartz D, Breed CN (1984). Anion gap in human breast cyst fluid (HBCF): a possible high risk indicator for breast cancer. Clin Chem 30:940.
18. Yap PL, Miller WR, Roberts MM, Creel RJ, Freedeman B, Mirtle CL, et al. (1984) Protein concentrations in fluid from gross cystic disease of the breast. Clin Oncol 10:35–43.
19. Rosner W, Khan MS, Breed CN, Fleisher M, Bradlow HL (1985) Plasma steroid-binding proteins in the cysts of gross cystic disease of the breast. J Clin Endocrinol Metab 61:200–203.
20. Molina R, Filella X, Herranz M, Pratz M, Velazco A, Zanon G, et al. (1990) Biochemistry of cyst fluid in fibrocystic disease of the breast. Approach to classification and understanding of the mechanism formation. Ann NY Acad Sci 586:29–42.
21. Neville MC (1990) The physiological basis of milk secretion. Ann NY Acad Sci 586:1–11.
22. Chasalow FI, Bradlow HL (1990). Digoxin-like materials in human breast cyst fluid. Ann NY Acad Sci 586:107–116.
23. Boccardo F, Valenti G, Zanardi S, Cerruti G, Fassio T, Bruzzi P, et al. (1988) Epidermal growth factor in breast cyst fluid: relationship with intracystic cation and androgen conjugate content. Cancer Res 45:5860–5863.
24. Lai LC, Ghilchik MW, Shaikh NA, Reed MJ, James VHT (1989). Relationship between epidermal growth factor and dehydroepiandrosterone and its sulfate in breast cyst fluid. Br J Cancer 60:320–323.
25. Ness JC, Sedghinasab M, Moe RE, Tapper D (1993). Identification of multiple proliferative growth factors in breast cyst fluid. Am J Surg 166:237–243.
26. Raju U, Banerjee S, Levitz M, Breed CN, Bradlow HL, Fleisher M, Skidmore FD (1985) Correlation of concentrations of estriol-3-sulfate with those of potassium and sodium in human breast cyst fluid. Steroids. 45:341–346.
27. Orlandi F, Caraci P, Puligheddu B, Torta M, Dogliotti L, Angeli A (1990). Estrone-3-sulfate in human breast cyst fluid. Ann NY Acad Sci 586: 464–466.
28. Hawkins RA, Thomson ML, Killen E (1985) Oestrone sulphate, adipose tissue and breast cancer. Breast Cancer Res Treat 6:75–87.
29. Belanger A, Caron S, Labrie F, Naldoni C, Dogliotti L, Angeli A (1990) Levels of eighteen non-conjugated and conjugated steroids in human breast cyst fluid: relationships with cyst type. Eur J Cancer 26:277–281.
30. Secreto G, Recchione C, Ballerini P, Callegari L, Cavalleri A, Attili A, et al. (1991) Accumulation of active androgens in breast cyst fluids. Eur J Cancer 27:44–47.
31. Lai LC, Ghatei MA, Takahashi K, Patel KV, Schrey MP, Ghilchick MV, et al. (1990) Mitogenic peptide in breast cyst fluid: relationship with intracystic electrolyte ratios. Int J Cancer 46:1014–1016.
32. Scambia G, Beneditti Panici P, Ferrandina G, Battaglia F Rossi S, Bellantone R, et al. (1991) Cathepsin D and epidermal growth factor in human breast cyst fluid. Br J Cancer 64:965–967.
33. Miller WR, Dawes J (1985) Platelet associated proteins in human breast cyst fluids. Clin Chem Acta 152:37–42.
34. Dixon JM, Miller WR, Scott WN (1984) pH of human breast cyst fluid. Clin Oncol 10:721–724.
35. Lai LC, Siraj AK, Erbas H, Lennard TWJ (1995) Relationship between basic fibroblastic growth factor and transforming growth factor beta 2 in breast cyst fluid. Br J Surg 75:702–704.
36. Dixon JM (1989). Pathogenesis of cystic disease of the breast. Br J Clin Pract 43(suppl 68):90–93.
37. Dixon JM, Miller WR, Scott WN, Forrest APM (1983). The morphological basis of human breast cyst populations. Br J Surg 70:604–606.
38. Page DL, Dupont WD (1986) Are the breast cysts a premalignant marker? J Cancer Clin Oncol 22:635.

39. Beccati D, Grilli N, Schincaglia P, Naldoni C, Tavolazzi L, Ranaldi R, et al. (1988) Apocrine cells in human breast cyst fluid and their relationship to cyst type: a morphometric study. Eur J Cancer Clin Oncol 24:597–602.
40. Kern WH, Brooks RN (1969) Atypical epithelial hyperplasia associated with breast cancer and fibrocystic disease, Cancer 24:668–675.
41. Dixon JM, Lumsdeh AB, Miller WR (1985) The relationship of cyst type to risk factors for breast cancer and the subsequent development of breast cancer in patients with breast cystic disease. Eur J Cancer Clin Oncol 21:1047–1050.
42. Dupont WD, Parl FF, Hartmann WH, Brinton LA, Winfield AC, Worrell JA, et al. (1993) Breast cancer risk associated with proliferative breast disease and atypical hyperplasia. Cancer 71:1258–1265.
43. Schuerch C, Rosen PP, Hirota T, Itabashi M, Yamamoto H, Kinnie DW, et al. (1982) A pathologic study of benign breast disease in Tokyo and New York. Cancer 50:1899–1903.
44. Ebbs SR, Bates T (1988) Cyst type does not predict the natural history of cyst disease or breast cancer risk. Br J Surg 75:702–704.
45. Miller WR, Scott WN, Harris WH, Wang D (1992). Using biological measurements, can patients with benign breast disease who are at high risk for breast cancer be identified? Cancer Detect Prev 16:99–106.
46. Bruzzi P, Dogliotti L, Naldoni C, Bucchi L, Costantini M, Cicognani A, et al. (1997) Cohort study of association of risk of breast cancer with cyst type in women with gross cystic disease of the breast. BMJ 314:925–928.
47. Amadori D, Falcini F, Buzzi GF, Gambi A, Vignutelli P, Callea A (1992) *Registro Tumori della Romagna (1986–1988),* Istituto Oncologico Romagnolo, Forlì, Italy.
48. Bundred NJ, Walker RA, Jenkins A, Shaw D, Hall AV, Winder AF (1992) Biochemical analysis of breast cyst fluid predicts the natural history of breast cysts. Breast Dis 5:21–27.
49. Naldoni C, Costantini M, Dogliotti L, Bruzzi P, Bucchi L, Buzzi G, et al. (1992) Association of cyst type with risk factors for breast cancer and relapse rate in women with gross cystic disease of the breast. Cancer Res 52:1791–1795.
50. Dixon JM, Scott, WN, Miller WR (1985) Natural history of cystic disease: the importance of cyst type. Br J Surg 72:190–192.
51. Angeli A, Bradlow HL, Bodian CA, Chasalow FI, Dogliotti L, and Haagensen DE Jr (1990). Criteria for classifying breast cyst fluids. Ann NY Acad Sci 586:49–52.

III

Tumor Progression

9 The Role of Tumor Suppressor Genes in Breast Cancer Progression

Robert Callahan, PhD

INTRODUCTION

Breast cancer is the most frequent malignancy affecting women today. The etiology of this disease is influenced by a variety of factors such as menstrual and reproductive history, family history, long-term treatment with estrogen, diet, and previous atypical benign breast disease *(1–3)*. It seems probable that these factors provide a selective environment for the clonal outgrowth of mammary epithelial cells that contain somatic mutations. Some of these mutations could uncouple normal mammary gland development or contribute to the development of neoplasia. Alternatively, they could provide atypical nonmalignant as well as malignant cells with a selective growth advantage, the means to metastasize to distant organ sites, or evasion of host immunosurveillance. Because of the heterogeneity and multiplicity of factors necessary for the development of most epithelial tumors, the current view is that multiple somatic mutations act in concert to produce an invasive carcinoma with the ability to metastasize to distant organ sites. The identification of these mutations has been a major focus of molecular biologic studies of breast cancer for over a decade (reviewed in refs. *4* and *5)*. A driving force in this effort has been the hope that mutation of specific genes or groups of genes could be used as prognostic indicators in the management of the disease and/or targets for therapeutic intervention. This chapter focuses on recent work on the identification and characterization of tumor suppressor genes in hereditary and sporadic breast cancer.

The term *tumor suppressor genes* was originally coined to describe a class of genes that normally act to restrict neoplastic growth. Studies of hereditary retinoblastoma and the *RB1* gene established this disease as an early paradigm for the genetics of hereditary cancers *(6)*. In his "two-hit" hypothesis, Knudson *(6,7)* proposed that in hereditary retinoblastoma a recessive mutated allele of *RB1* was inherited from a parent and tumorigenesis initiated with the somatic mutation of the other allele in susceptible precursor cells. Nonhereditary retinoblastomas represent clonal outgrowth of a precursor cell that has sustained two somatic mutations of *RB1*. Confirmation that *RB1* is a tumor suppressor gene came from the demonstration that reintroduction of the wild-type *RB1* gene into retinoblastoma tumor cell lines suppressed neoplastic transformation *(8)*.

From: *Contemporary Endocrinology: Endocrinology of Breast Cancer*
Edited by: A. Manni © Humana Press Inc., Totowa, NJ

BREAST CANCER SUSCEPTIBILITY GENES

Approximately 5–10% of breast cancers have a familial component to the disease. Genome linkage analysis of families having a high incidence of breast cancer with highly polymorphic genetic markers has led to the identification over the past 7 years of perhaps four or five susceptibility genes (reviewed in ref. *9*).

BRCA1

BRCA1 is located on chromosome 17q21 *(10)* and is composed of 22 coding exons, which span over 100,000 kb of DNA and are expressed as 5592-bp RNA species *(11)*. Approximately 45% of families with pure site-specific breast cancer have linkage to *BRCA1 (12)*. The cumulative risk among gene carriers is 51% at age 50 years and 85% at age 70 years. The estimated gene frequency for *BRCA1* is 0.0006 *(13)*. The presence of two or more cases of early-onset breast cancer and two or more cases of ovarian cancer is associated with a 92% probability of being linked to *BRCA1 (14)*. Among 254 carriers of *BRCA1* mutations, 132 distinct mutations have been identified *(15)*. The most common mutations are 185delAG *(12%)* and 5382insC *(10%)*. As a consequence of the "founder effect," the 185delAG mutation may account for 16% of all breast cancer and 39% of all ovarian cancers diagnosed in Ashkenazi women before the age of 50 years *(16,17)*. The current Ashkenazi Jewish population is descended from a limited group of founders from Central and Eastern Europe *(18)*.

Studies of the temporal and spatial pattern of *BRCA1* RNA expression during normal mouse embryogenesis, in adult tissues, in the mammary gland during postnatal development, and in mammary glands of animals whose ovarian hormones were experimentally altered represented a first step in developing a foundation for understanding how the absence or mutation of the gene promotes carcinogenesis *(19,20)*. *BRCA1* RNA could first be detected in the otic vesicle of embryonic day 9.5 (E9.5) embryos. By E10.5 *BRCA1* RNA expression was detected in the neuroectoderm, followed by keratinocytes and whisker pad primordia at E11–12.5. At E14–17 *BRCA1* expression could be detected in the epithelial cells of the developing kidney. A survey of adult tissues revealed significant steady-state levels of *BRCA1* RNA in the thymus and testis. Lower levels of *BRCA1* RNA were detected in mammary gland, ovary, uterus spleen, lymph node, spleen, stomach, small intestine, and lung. No or barely detectable levels of *BRCA1* expression were found in the kidney, heart, brain, and skeletal muscle.

BRCA1 RNA expression in the mammary gland is restricted to ductal and alveolar epithelial cells, with the highest levels localized over the terminal end buds *(19,20)*. Terminal end buds contain rapidly proliferating cells that are undergoing differentiation. During pregnancy *BRCA1* RNA expression increased 10-fold by day 10 and remained high through day 17, but was diminished during lactation. The increased levels of *BRCA1* RNA during pregnancy raised the possibility that expression of the gene is modulated by ovarian hormones. *BRCA1* RNA levels in the mammary glands of ovarectomized mice are slightly lower than in mammary tissue from intact females. Treatment of the ovarectomized females with either 17β-estradiol or progesterone alone had no effect on *BRCA1* RNA levels, but treatment with both hormones together increased the steady-state levels of *BRCA1* RNA four- to fivefold. In related experiments it was found that steroid hormone depletion of estrogen receptor-positive human breast tumor cell lines followed by addition of either β-estradiol or progesterone was sufficient to induce *BRCA1*

RNA expression *(21)* whereas inhibition of *BRCA1* RNA expression was associated with growth acceleration of both normal and malignant mammary epithelial cells *(22)* and murine NIH3T3 cells *(23)*. These results are consistent with the conclusion that *BRCA1* is a hormone-induced growth regulator.

To investigate in vivo the role *BRCA1* plays during development and to create a mouse model for breast and ovarian carcinogenesis, four strains of mice have been created in which *BRCA1* has been disrupted by targeted mutagenesis *(24–27)*. Each of these mouse strains contain a small deletion (intron 10, 5' end of exon11, 5' end of exon 11, exons 5–6, and exon 2, respectively) in *BRCA1*. In each strain heterozygous animals appeared normal and healthy and are fertile, whereas nullizygous (*BRCA1-/-*) embryos die early during development. In three of the strains *(25–27)* embryos fail to develop much beyond E7.5 days of gestation. They display distinguishable embryonic and extraembryonic structures but fail to differentiate and form egg cylinders and thus are unable to form primitive streaks and undergo gastrulation. By contrast, the mutant mice reported by Gowen et al. *(24)* survive until midgestation and die in utero between days 10 and 13 of development. The basis for this difference is unclear, but it could be related to differences in the genetic background of this strain compared with the other three mouse strains or, as discussed below, it could be a function of this particular mutation.

The defect in *BRCA1* nullizygous embryos does not appear to affect apoptosis but does affect cell growth as defined by 5-bromo-2'-deoxyuridine incorporation, indicating that the proliferative capabilities of the mutant embryos are compromised. Moreover, the steady-state levels of the cell cycle inhibitor p21 are dramatically increased in the E4 day mutant embryo *(25)*. Expression of p21 is normally upregulated by the *p53* gene as a part of the G_1-phase cell cycle arrest, which is induced in response to DNA damage *(28,29)*. Genetic evidence for a link between *BRCA1* function in the developing embryo and *p53* was provide by morphologic examination of *BRCA1/p53* double nullizygotes *(27)*. It was found that the BRCA1 phenotype was less severe on the *p53-/-* genetic background. Thus, loss of *BRCA1* function during embryonic development appears to activate a growth arrest pathway.

There are two points of concern about these mouse models for studies of the role that *BRCA1* plays in development and tumorigenesis. Recently Boyd et al. *(30)* identified a 32-year-old patient who was homozygous for a *BRCA1* mutation that would be expected to express a protein of 900 amino acids. It may be significant that the longest BRCA1 protein that would be expected in the *BRCA1* nullizygous mouse strains is 300 residues *(26)*. Another potentially related concern is that heterozygous BRCA1 mutant mouse strains do not appear to develop mammary tumors by 15 months of age. This may mean that *BRCA1* germline mutations in mice are not predisposing to tumor development or that tumor development in these mouse strains has a much longer latency.

BRCA1 encodes a protein composed of 1863 amino acid residues *(11)*. Searches of the protein sequence for regions of functional similarity to other proteins suggested that the first 180 residues have significant homology with zinc finger domains (C3HC4) found in numerous nucleic acid binding proteins and that the remainder of the protein represents an "acidic blob" domain with transactivational activity *(11)*. One study showed that fusing the C-terminal portion of BRCA1 (residues 1528–1863) in frame to GAL4 DNA binding domain was capable of activating the transcription of a reporter gene in either yeast or mammalian cells *(31)*. This was further refined to residues 1760–1863 as the minimal transactivation domain *(32)*. In addition, two putative nuclear localization signal

(NLS) sequences have been identified (residues 501–507 and 607–614) *(33,34)*, which would be consistent with BRCA1 being a nuclear protein. These results provide further evidence that the consequences of germline *BRCA1* mutations differ in hereditary breast and ovarian cancers and that one of the functions of BRCA1 may be the regulation of transcription. However, Jensen et al. *(35)* have reported a "granin" consensus sequence at human BRCA1 residues 1214–1223. Granins are acidic proteins localized in secretory vesicles of the cell, which raises the possibility that BRCA1 is a secreted protein. The significance of granin consensus sequence has been recently challenged *(36)*.

A major stumbling block toward developing an understanding of BRCA1 's role in the normal regulation of mammary growth, differentiation, and carcinogenesis is the conflicting results that have been obtained on the subcellular localization and size of the protein using polyclonal antibodies raised against peptides corresponding to different portions of the protein. Chen et al. *(37–39)*, using polyclonal antibodies prepared against either sequences encoded by the 5' or 3' end of exon 11 and a commercial antibody preparation against a peptide near the C-terminus of the protein, presented evidence that in normal cells the 220-kDa BRCA1 protein is located in the nucleus, but in breast and ovarian cancer cell lines the protein is located in the cytoplasm. In a second independent study, Scully et al. *(40)*, using a polyclonal serum against a peptide near the C-terminus of BRCA1 and monoclonal antibodies against defined regions of BRCA1, identified a 220-kDa protein localized in the nucleus in both normal and malignant tumor cell lines. Similar results were obtained by Zhang et al. *(41)* with a polyclonal antisera raised against a peptide comprised of BRCA1 residues 903–919. Jensen et al *(35)* using the C-terminal 19 residue of BRCA1, raised a polyclonal antiserum that detects a 190-kDa protein that localizes to the secretory vesicles and is secreted by human mammary epithelial cells. Part of the confusion resulting from these studies may reflect crossreactivity of certain antisera with epidermal growth factor receptor or the related c-erbB2 protein *(42)*. Another possibility is the expression of splice variants of *BRCA1* in normal and tumor cell lines, which lack the sequences encoded by *BRCA1* exon 11 *(33,42)*. This exon encodes the NLS sequences. It has been shown that the protein encoded by splice variants lacking this sequence are located in the cytoplasm and therefore could have been confused with the wild-type protein in studies in which the antibody was not specific for exon 11b *(34)*. In addition, Wilson et al. *(34)* point out that most of the tumors studied so far contain both nuclear and cytoplasmic staining, indicating that the malignant process is not simply a matter of relocating the BRCA1 protein to the cytoplasm.

Most *BRCA1* mutations produce truncated proteins varying in length from 5 to 99% of the complete protein. Preliminary attempts to link specific genotypes with phenotypes suggests that in 60 high-risk families there is a correlation between *BRCA1* mutations located in the 3' third of the gene and a significantly lower risk of ovarian cancer *(43)*. This observation was confirmed in an independent analysis of 166 patients inheriting a *BRCA1* mutation *(44)*. In addition, transfection experiments have been carried out demonstrating that whereas wild-type *BRCA1* inhibits the growth of both breast and ovarian tumor cell lines, a C-terminal truncation mutant (1835Stop) inhibits the growth of only the ovarian carcinoma cell line *(44)*. This points to the possibility that the mechanism of tumor suppression by *BRCA1* differs in breast and ovarian cancers.

Insights into the normal function of BRCA1 have come from studies on the proteins with which BRCA1 interacts. In two reports *(38,40)* BRCA1 immunostaining is characterized by a "nuclear dot" pattern that appears in the S phase of the cell cycle. A homolog of bacterial REC A, hRAD51, is also detected as nuclear dots during the S phase of the cell cycle *(45)*. This protein is a member of a family of proteins known to be involved in DNA strand-exchange functions associated with normal recombination *(46)*. Scully et al. *(47)* have shown that the two proteins colocalize in vivo and coimmunoprecipitate. BRCA1 amino acid residues 758–1064 are required for binding to RAD51 in vitro *(47)*. Their results suggest a functional interaction between BRCA1 and RAD51 in meiotic and mitotic cell cycles and imply that BRCA1 is involved in the control of recombination and genome integrity.

In a separate study Scully et al. *(48)* demonstrated that BRCA1 copurifies through several chromatographic steps with the RNA polymerase II holoenzyme. In addition, immunopurification of BRCA1 also copurifies transcriptionally active RNA polymerase II and transcription factors TFIIF, TFIIe, and TFIIH. The interaction of BRCA1 with RNA polymerase II holoenzyme seems to be dependent on sequences near the C-terminus, since a BRCA1 protein lacking the last 11 residues binds significantly less efficiently to the RNA polymerase II holoenzyme than the wild-type protein. It seems probable that one function of BRCA1 is to affect the expression of one or more genes at the level of transcription. This may also relate to the association between position of germline mutations and the relative frequency of breast and ovarian cancers. However, how the association between BRCA1 and RNA polymerase II functionally relates to the interaction between BRCA1 and RAD51 remains a challenge for the future *(48)*.

BRCA2

BRCA2 was found to be linked to chromosome 13q12-q13 in 15 families at high risk for breast cancer in which *BRCA1* had been excluded *(49–51)*. The risk for ovarian cancer seems to be lower in these families than in those carrying a *BRCA1* mutation, but male breast cancer may be a significant component of this syndrome *(52)*. *BRCA2* is composed of 27 exons that encode a 11,385-bp RNA species; it spans 70 kb of genomic DNA *(49,51)*. All the mutations found in *BRCA2* cause premature termination of the encoded protein and are distributed evenly throughout the gene. Like *BRCA1*, the frequency of particular mutations appears to be abnormally high in certain populations as a consequence of the founder effect. For instance, 6 of 80 (8%) Ashkenazi Jewish women diagnosed with breast cancer prior to 40 years of age carry the 6174delT mutation *(53)*. Similarly, 27% of Icelandic women developing breast cancer between the ages of 30 and 39 years carried the 999del5 mutation *(54)*.

To develop an understanding of the role *BRCA2* plays in hereditary breast cancer, several studies have been undertaken to describe the expression pattern of *BRCA2* during normal embryonic development and in adult tissues. In cultured mammary epithelial cells, *BRCA2* is expressed in a cell cycle-dependent manner, peaking at the G_1/S boundary, and is upregulated in differentiating mammary epithelial cells in response to glucocorticoids *(55,56)*. Expression of *BRCA2* RNA is coordinate with *BRCA1* RNA, which suggests that these genes are induced by and may function in overlapping regulatory pathways involved in the control of cell proliferation and differentiation. Analysis of multiple fetal and adult tissues has shown that the pattern of *BRCA2* RNA expression is virtually indistinguishable from that of *BRCA1*. However, during pregnancy, upregulation of RNA expression by ovarian hormones is significantly greater for *BRCA1* than for *BRCA2 (57)*. This raises the possibility that gender-specific differences in phenotype associated with germline mutations in *BRCA2* compared with *BRCA1* may be related to the differential regulation of these genes by sex hormones.

Since the amino acid sequence of BRCA2 initially provided few structural clues to the function of the protein, three groups *(27,58,59)* have independently created strains of mice in which *BRCA2* has been inactivated (*BRCA2*$^{ex10-11}$, *BRCA2*^{ex11}, and *BRCA2*^{ex11}, respectively) in the germline. In each case nullizygous fetuses die before 9.5 days of development. Apoptosis is normal in these fetuses, but cellular proliferation is impaired. Moreover, the steady-state levels of the cyclin-dependent kinase inhibitor p21 is increased. Thus, the phenotype of the *BRCA2* mutants is similar to some of the *BRCA1* mutants *(25–27)*, but less severe. In addition, like *BRCA1/p53* double nullizygotes, *BRCA2/p53* double nullizygotes at day 10.5 of development were either indistinguishable from wild-type or were more developed than the most advanced *BRCA2* single mutants and exhibited exencephaly *(27)*. The similarity in phenotype of *BRCA1* and *BRCA2* mutants suggests that these genes have either cooperative roles or convergent functions during embryogenesis. In terms of development, the combined effect of *BRCA1* and *BRCA2* mutations in two recovered double nullizygous decidua fell within the range of phenotypes observed in *BRCA1* null mutants *(27)*.

A few clues to the function of BRCA2 during development have begun to emerge that again seem to parallel BRCA1. Milner et al. *(60)* found that the sequences encoded by exon 3 of BRCA2 are similar to the activation domain of c-JUN. They showed that BRCA2 residues 23–105 (exon3) have the potential to activate transcription in yeast when linked to the lexA DNA binding domain. The activation potential of the exon 3-encoded sequences is under negative control by flanking inhibitory sequences on either side of exon 3. The similarity between BRCA2 exon 3 and c-JUN also overlaps the δ-domain of the latter protein, which contains the binding site for the JUN N-terminal kinase (JNK). This suggests that BRCA2 activity may be regulated by signal transduction pathways that culminate in the stimulation of JNK-like kinases.

In another striking parallel with BRCA1, BRCA2 has been shown to interact physically with RAD51 in the yeast two-hybrid system *(59,61)*. This strongly suggests that BRCA1, BRCA2, and RAD51 act in concert during the normal response to DNA damage. Moreover, both *BRCA2 (59)* and *RAD51 (62)* mutant embryos have an increased sensitivity to radiation, directly implicating them as playing a role in DNA damage control.

BRCA3?

A study of eight breast cancer families with no linkage to either *BRCA1* or *BRCA2* has provided preliminary evidence for linkage with markers on chromosome 8p12-22 *(63)*. Recently, another analysis of two additional breast cancer families also found linkage on 8p12-p22 *(64)*. By incorporating loss of heterozygosity (LOH) data from tumors of affected family members, a maximum cumulative 3-point lod score of 3.30 at $q = 0.00$ was obtained in this study with D8S137 and D8S131. Four germline mutations of a gene *(WRN)* encoding a helicase have been identified in Werner's syndrome patients and are located very near D8S137 and D8S131 *(65)*. Werner's syndrome is characterized by premature aging and an increased incidence of cancer, including breast cancer. It remains to be determined whether *WRN* or a closely linked gene corresponds to *BRCA3*.

*Li-Fraumeni Syndrome (*TP53*)*

The Li-Fraumeni syndrome *(66)* is a rare inherited disease in which carriers contain a germline mutation in the *TP53* gene located on chromosome 17p13.1 *(67)*. This disease is defined by a sarcoma in the index case at <45 years of age, associated with breast cancer, primary brain tumor, leukemia, or adrenocortical tumor in a first-degree relative at <45 years of age, or a sarcoma at any age. It is estimated that at least 50% of the carriers will develop breast cancer by the age of 50 *(68)*; however, this syndrome accounts for only <1% of all diagnosed breast cancers *(69,70)*. The *TP53* gene is composed of 11 exons that span 16–20 kb of genomic DNA and encode a 2.2–2.5-kb RNA species and a 53-kDa protein (reviewed in ref. *71*). The 23 germline mutations that have been identified, most of which correspond to missense mutations, appear to be evenly distributed within the evolutionarily conserved exons 4–9 *(71)*. The *TP53* tumor suppressor gene mediates cell cycle perturbations in response to DNA damage and plays a role in cell death, genetic stability, and cancer susceptibility. Due to restrictions in the size of this chapter an adequate assessment of the current level of understanding of *TP53* function is not possible. Instead, the reader's attention is directed to two recent reviews on the subject *(72,73)*.

*Cowden's disease (*PTEN*)*

Cowden's disease is characterized by the formation of multiple benign tumors (hamartomas), as well as an increased susceptibility to malignant breast and thyroid tumors *(74–76)*. It has been estimated that 30% of the women affected by this hereditary disease have developed breast cancer *(74–76)*. The gene for Cowden's disease is located on chromosome 10q22-q23 *(77)*. Germline mutations of this gene have been found in four of five carriers of this very rare (probably less than 200 cases) disease *(78)*. The target gene encodes a protein having a tyrosine phosphatase domain and a large region of homology to chicken tensin. Hence, the gene has been named *PTEN* (*p*hospatase and *ten*sin homologue located on chromosome *ten*). Mutations of *PTEN* have also been found in glioblastomas and prostate tumors *(79,80)*. The demonstration that introduction of wild-type chromosome 10 suppresses the tumorigenicity of glioblastoma cells in mice is consistent with *PTEN* encoding a tumor suppressor gene *(81)*.

*Ataxia Telangiectasia (*ATM*)*

Ataxia telangiectasia (AT) is another rare autosomal recessive disorder characterized by cerebellar degeneration, immunodeficiency, chromosomal instability and cancer predisposition, radiation sensitivity, and cell cycle abnormalities *(82)*. Easton's *(83)* review of four independent studies estimated that the relative risk of breast cancer in AT heterozygotes is 3.9. An estimated 1% of the general population could be heterozygous for AT. This could translate into as much as 8% of breast cancer in patients younger than 40 years of age and 2% of patients from 40 to 60 years of age. Thus germline mutations could account for more breast cancers than *BRCA1* and *BRCA2* combined.

The affected gene *(ATM)* spans 150 kb of genomic DNA on chromosome 11q22-q23 and is expressed as a 13-kb RNA species *(84)*. The 9.168-kb open reading frame encodes a 350-kDa protein *(85,86)* and is present in the nucleus and cytoplasmic vesicles *(87)*. The C-terminal end of the protein contains a domain that is similar to several yeast and mammalian phosphatidylinositol-3' *(PI-3)* kinases *(88)*. These enzymes are involved in mitogenic signal transduction, meiotic recombination, and cell cycle control. Correction of the AT phenotype was achieved by introducing full-length *ATM* cDNA in an expression vector into AT cell lines expressing only truncated ATM protein *(85)*. The transfected cells had enhanced survival in response to radiation exposure, decreased radiation-induced chromosomal aberrations, reduced radioresistant DNA synthesis, partially corrected defective cell cycle checkpoints, and induction of stress-activated protein kinase.

ATM and *TP53* are both believed to mediate DNA damage-induced cell cycle checkpoints, apoptosis, genetic stability, and cancer susceptibility (see review in ref. *73*). In fact, using the yeast two-hybrid system, Watters et al. *(87)* demonstrated that the ATM protein binds to TP53 and that this association is defective in AT cells. Three laboratories have developed strains of mice that are null for *ATM*, which recapitulate the AT phenotype in humans *(89–91)*. Recent studies have focused on these mouse strains in conjunction with the *TP53* null mouse strains and double knockout mouse strains to dissect the role these two genes play in the signaling pathways involved in the phenotypes caused by their individual and collective loss of function. In one study it was found that *ATM* and *TP53* do not seem to interact in response to acute radiation toxicity, but do cooperate in apoptosis and tumor suppression *(92)*. These authors have also found that the abnormalities exhibited in radiation-induced G_1/S cell cycle checkpoint correspond to two separate pathways of interaction between *ATM* and *TP53*. One of these is linear, involving G_1/S cell cycle control; the another involves aspects of growth regulation. It may be pertinent with regard to the latter pathway that in AT cells or in thymocytes or fibroblasts from *ATM*-null mice, ionizing radiation-induced activation of the nuclear c-ABL tyrosine kinase does not occur *(93)*. This deficiency is corrected by the ectopic expression of functional ATM, suggesting that c-ABL is a downstream target for phosphorylation and activation by ATM.

LOSS OF HETEROZYGOSITY IN NONHEREDITARY PRIMARY HUMAN BREAST TUMORS

A preview of the complexity of somatic alterations that occur during sporadic (nonfamilial) human breast tumor progression was provided by earlier cytogenetic analysis of primary human breast tumor cells in culture *(94)*. The alterations include aneuploidy (either gain or loss of entire chromosomes) and rearrangements affecting chromosomes 1q (translocations), 6q (deletions and translocations), 7p (translocations, pericentric inversions, and isochromosomes), and 11q (translocations). LOH represents another common genetic alteration in primary human breast tumors and occurs as a consequence of either interstitial deletions, chromosome loss, or aberrant mitotic recombinational events. It is thought that LOH reveals within the affected region of the genome the presence of a recessive mutation in the remaining allele of a tumor suppressor gene(s) *(7)*. LOH represents the most frequent type of genetic alteration found in primary human breast carcinomas *(4,5)*. At the present time, 12 chromosome arms have been found to be frequently affected by LOH in primary breast tumors, including chromosomes 1p, 1q, 3p, 6q, 7q, 11p, 8p, 13q, 16 q, 17p, 17q, and 18q (reviewed in refs. *4* and *5*). Moreover, it is not uncommon for multiple regions within these chromosome arms to be independently affected by LOH.

Most of the studies aimed at defining regions of the genome affected by LOH have focused on invasive ductal carcinomas. Aldaz et al. *(95)* have extended this approach to include preinvasive ductal carcinoma (DCIS) and lobular carcinomas. Their findings suggest that allelic imbalances observed on chromosomes 7p, 7q, 13q, 16q, 17p, and 17q represent early abnormalities since they occur in approximately 30% of the DCIS samples. More recently chromosome 9p has also been found to be frequently affected by LOH in

DCIS *(96)*. LOH on chromosome 8p was found in 36% of the cases compared with 14% of invasive ductal carcinomas. Moreover, microsatellite instability was observed in 40% of lobular carcinomas compared with 13% of ductal carcinomas. This suggests that invasive lobular carcinomas may arise by a different mechanism of carcinogenesis than that of ductal breast carcinomas.

The identification of the target genes affected by LOH has represented a major goal in experimental breast cancer research. The apparent complexity of genetic alterations found in primary human breast tumors and the possibility that some them are a consequence of tumor progression rather than a cause has made this a daunting challenge. Analysis of the hereditary cancer susceptibility genes *BRCA1* (17q21), *BRCA2* (13q12-q13), *RB1* (13q14), and *TP53* (17p13.1) in nonfamilial or sporadic breast carcinomas has shown that only *TP53* frequently (25–45%) contains inactivating mutations *(97–100)*. Mature studies of the *PTEN* (Cowden's disease) or *ATM* (Ataxia telangiectasia) genes in nonhereditary breast cancer have not been reported.

Two general strategies are currently being pursued to identify putative tumor suppressor genes that are inactivated by mutation in primary human breast carcinomas. One of these approaches employs regional mapping of the chromosomes affected by LOH in primary human breast carcinomas to identify the smallest affected genomic region that is physically defined by yeast artificial chromosome or P1 phage clones of genomic DNA. Although at the present time this approach has not led to the identification of a target gene for LOH in sporadic human breast carcinomas, it seems high likely that as the Human Genome Project progresses these genes will be identified. In related studies, Negrini et al. *(101)* identified the *FHIT* (fragile histidine triad) gene on chromosome 3p14.2, which is frequently affected by LOH primary human breast carcinomas (reviewed in ref. *4*). The gene was originally identified as a target for internal homozygous deletions in a variety of tumor cell lines *(102–104)*. Its physiological function is not known, but 20% of breast tumor cell lines and primary breast tumors exhibit altered RNA transcripts. Another approach has been microcell-mediated chromosome transfer (MMCT) that identifies particular genomic DNA fragments which contribute to phenotypic changes in the growth of recipient breast carcinoma tissue culture cell lines. Using this approach it has been shown that chromosome 6q harbors two regions corresponding to 6q14-q15 and the distal end of 6q, which inhibit the tumorigenicity of the MDA-MB-231 breast tumor cell line in BALB/c-nu/nu mice *(105)*. These two regions of chromosome 6q are frequently affected by LOH in primary human breast tumors *(106,107)*. Similarly, it has been shown that chromosome 17q24-q25 contains sequences that have tumor suppressor activity *(108)*. This region of chromosome 17q is also known to be affected by LOH in primary human breast carcinomas *(109–113)*. To date the candidate tumor suppressor genes in each case have not been identified.

COMMON THEMES, UNANSWERED QUESTIONS, AND FUTURE DIRECTIONS

During the past 10 years the major advance in breast cancer research has been the identification of most, if not all, of the hereditary breast cancer susceptibility genes. Clearly, understanding their role in developmental biology, in general, and the mammary gland, in particular, will continue to constitute a major area of research interest. The theme that links *BRCA1* and *BRCA2* together is their apparent involvement in DNA damage response pathways. This is supported by the demonstrated physical interaction between *RAD51* and *BRCA1* or *BRCA2* and the similarity of phenotypes of developing mouse embryos that are nullizygous for one of these three genes. Similarly, the *TP53* and *ATM* genes are also known to play important roles in DNA damage response pathways. It seems likely that at least one consequence of the loss of function of any one of these genes during tumorigenesis is an increased mutation rate and a subsequent higher probability of the cellular outgrowths acquiring neoplastic or metastatic growth properties. If this senario is true, the basis of the tissue specificity of tumorigenesis in *BRCA1* and *BRCA2* carriers as well as the absence of their involvement in sporadic breast cancer remains a challenge for future studies. During the past decade a great deal of energy has been expended in attempting to define the regions of the genome affected by LOH in primary human breast tumors. Although to date the identities of the target genes for LOH are largely unknown, it seems likely that as the Human Genome Project continues to mature these barriers too will fall.

REFERENCES

1. Gompel G, van Kerkem C (1983) The breast, In: Principles of Surgical Pathology (Silverberg, S, ed.), Wiley Medical, New York, pp. 245–255.
2. Harris JR, Hellman S, Canellos GP, Fisher B (1982) Cancer of the breast, In: Cancer Principles and Practice of Oncology (DeVita VT, Rosenberg SA, eds.), JB Lippincott, Philadelphia, pp. 1119–1178.
3. Lynch HT, Albano WA, Danes S, Layton MA, Kimberling WJ, Lynch JF, et al. (1984) Genetic predisposition to breast cancer. Cancer 53:612–622.
4. Bieche I, Lidereau R (1995) Genetic alterations in breast cancer. Genes Chromosom Cancer 14:227–251.
5. Brenner AJ, Aldaz CM (1997) The genetics of sporadic breast cancer, In: Etiology of Breast and Gynecological Cancers, Wiley-Liss, New York, pp. 63–82.
6. Knudson AG (1985) Hereditary cancer, oncogenes, and antioncogenes. Cancer Res 45:1437–1441.
7. Knudson AG (1989) Hereditary cancers: clue to mechanisms of carcinogenesis. Br J Cancer 59:661–666.
8. Lee W-H, Shew J-Y, Hong F, Sery T, Donoso LA, Young LJ, Bet al. (1987) The retinoblastoma susceptibility gene encodes a nuclear phosphoprotein associated with DNA binding activity. Nature 329:642–645.
9. Greene MH (1997) Genetics of Breast Cancer. Mayo Clin Proc 72:54–65.
10. Hall JM, Lee MK, Newman B, Horrow JE, Anderson LA, Huey B et al. (1990) Linkage of early-onset familial breast cancer to chromosome 17q21. Science 250:1684–1689.
11. Miki Y, Swensen J, Shattuck-Eidens D, Futreal PA, Harshman K, Tavtigian S, et al. (1994) A strong candidate for the breast and ovarian cancer susceptibity gene BRCA1. Science 266:66–71.
12. Ford D, Easton DF (1995) The genetics of breast and ovarian cancer. Br J Cancer 72:805–812.
13. Easton D, Ford D, Peto J (1993) Inherited susceptibility to breast cancer. Cancer Surv 18:95–113.
14. Narod SA, Feunteun J, Lynch HT, Watson P, Conway T, Lynch J et al. (1995) An evaluation of the genetic heterogeneity in 145 breast-ovarian cancer families. Am J Hum Genet 56:254–264.
15. Couch FJ, Weber B (1996) Mutations and polymorphisms in the familial early-onset breast cancer (BRCA1) gene. Hum Mutat 8:8–18.
16. Tonin P, Serova O, Lenoir G, Lynch H, Durocher F, Simard J, et al. (1995) BRCA1 mutations in Ashkenazi Jewish woman (Letter). Am J Genet 57:189.
17. Struewing JP, Brody LC, Erdos MR, Kase RG, Giambaressi TR, Smith SA, et al. (1995) Detection of eight BRCA1 mutations in 10 breast/ovarian cancer families, including 1 family with male breast cancer. Am J Hum Genet 57:1–7.
18. Risch N, de Leon D, Kramer P, Almasy L, Singer B, et al. (1995) Genetic analysis of idiopathic torsion dystonia in Ashkenazi Jews and their recent descent from a small founder population. Nature Genet 9:152–159.
19. Marquis ST, Rajan JV, Wynshaw-Boris A, Xu J, Yin G-Y, Abel KJ, et al. (1995) The developmental pattern of BRCA1 expression implies a role in differentiation of the breast and other tissues. Nature Genet. 11:17–26.

20. Lane TF, Deng C, Elson A, Lyu MS, Kozak CA, Leder P (1995) Expression of Brca1 is associated with terminal differentiation of ectodermally and mesodermally derived tissues in mice. Genes & Devel. 9:2712–2722.
21. Gudas JM, Nguyen H, Li T, Cowan KH (1995) Hormone-dependent regulation of BRCA1 in human breast cancer cells. Cancer Res. 55:4561–4565.
22. Thompson ME, Jensen RA, Obermiller PS, Page DL, Holt JT (1995) Decreased expression of BRCA1 accelerates growth and is often present during sporadic breast cancer progression. Nature Genet 9:444–450.
23. Rao VN, Shao N, Ahmad M, Reddy ESP (1996) Antisense RNA to the putitive tumor suppressor gene BRCA1 transforms mouse fibroblasts. Oncogene 12:523–528.
24. Gowen LC, Johnson BL, Latour AM, Sulik KK, Koller BH (1996) BRCA1 deficiency results in early embryonic leathality characterized by neuroepithelial abnormalities. Nature Genet 12:191–194.
25. Hakem R, de la Pompa J, Sirard C, Mo R, Woo M, Hakem A, Wakeham A, et al. (1996) The tumor suppressor gene BRCA1 is required for embryonic cellular proliferation in the mouse. Cell 85:1009–1023.
26. Liu C-Y, Fleken-Nikitin A, Li S, Zeng Y, Lee W-H (1996) Inactivation of the mouse Brca1 gene leads to failure in the morphogenesis of the egg cylinder in early postimplantation development. Genes Dev 10:1835–1843.
27. Ludwig T, Chapman DL, Papaioannou VE, Efstratiadis A (1997) Targeted mutations of breast cancer susceptibility gene homologs in mice: lethal phenotypes of Brca1, Brca2, Brca1/Brca2, Brca1/p53, and Brca2/p53 nullizygous embryos. Genes Dev 11:1226–1241.
28. Deng C, Zhang P, Harper JW, Elledge SJ, Leder P (1995) Mice lacking p21CIP1/WAF1 undergo normal development, but are defective in G1 checkpoint control. Cell 82:675–684.
29. Brugarolas J, Chandrasekaran C, Gordon JI, Beach D, Jacks T, Hannon GJ (1995) Radiation-induced cell cycle arrest compromised by p21 deficiency. Nature 377:552–557.
30. Boyd M, Harris F, McFariane R, Davidson HR, Black DM (1995) A human BRCA1 gene knockout. Nature 375:541–542.
31. Chapman MS, Verma IM (1996) Transcriptional activation by BRCA1. Nature 382:678–679.
32. Monteiro AN A, August A, Hanafusa H (1996) Evidence for a transcription activation function of BRCA1 C-terminal region. Proc Natl Acad Sci USA 93:1395–13599.
33. Thakur S, Zhang HB, Peng Y, Le H, Carroll B, Ward T, et al. (1997) Localization of BRCA1 and a splice variant identifies the nuclear localization signal. Mol Cell Biol 17:444–452.
34. Wilson CA, Payton MN, Elliot GS, Buaas FW, Cajulis EE, et al. (1997) Differential subcellular localization, expression and biological toxicity of BRCA1 and the splice variant BRCA1-d11b. Oncogene 14:1–16.
35. Jensen RA, Thompson ME, Jetton TL, Szabo CI, van der Meer R, Helou B, et al. (1996) BRCA1 is secreted and exhibits properties of a granin. Nature Genet 12:303–308.
36. Bradley A, Sharan SK (1996) BRCA1 protein products and secreted tumour suppressors [Letter]. Nature Genet 13:268–269.
37. Chen YC, Chen P-L, Riley DJ, Lee W-H, Allred DC, Osborne CK (1996) Location of BRCA1 in human breast and ovarian cells (Technical Comments). Science 272:125–126.
38. Chen Y, Farmer AA, Chen C-F, Jones DC, Chen P-L, Lee, W.-H. (1996) BRCA1 is 220-kDa nuclear phophoprotein that is expressed and phophorylated in a cell cycle-dependent manner. Cancer Res 56:3168–3172.
39. Chen YC, Chen C-F, Riley DJ, Allred DC, Chen P-L, Von Hoff D, et al. (1995) Aberrant subcellular locatization of BRCA1 in breast cancer. Science 270:789–792.
40. Scully R, Ganesan S, Brown M, De Caprio JA, Cannistra SA, Feunteun J, et al. (1996) Location of BRCA1 in human breast and ovarian cells [Technical Comments]. Science 272:123–125.
41. Zhang H-T, Zhang X, Zhao H-Z, Kajino Y, Weber BL, Davis JG, et al. (1997) Relationship of p215BRCA1 to tyrosine kinase signaling pathways and the cell cycle in normal and transformed cells. Oncogene 14:2863–2869.
42. Wilson CA, Payton MN, Pekar SK, Zhang K, Pacifici RE, Gudas JL, et al. (1996) BRCA1 protein products: Antibody specificity [Correspondence]. Nature Genet 13:264–265.
43. Gayther SA, Warren W, Maziyer S, Russell PA, Harrington PA, Chiano M, et al. (1995) Germline mutations of the BRCA1 gene in breast and ovarian cancer families provide evidence for a genotype-phenotype correlation. Nature Genet 11:428–433.
44. Holt JT, Thompson ME, Szabo C, Robinson-Benion C, Arteaga CL, King M-C, et al. (1996) Growth retardation and tumour inhibition by BRCA1. Nature Genet 12:298–302.
45. Tashiro S, Kotomura N, Shinohara A, Tanaka K, Ueda K, Kamada N (1996) S phase specific formation of the human Rad51 protein nuclear foci in lymphocytes. Oncogene 12:2165–2170.

46. Baumann P, Beson FE, West SC (1996) Human Rad51 protein promotes ATP-dependent homologous pairing and strand transfer reactions in vitro. Cell 87:757–766.
47. Scully R, Chen J, Plug A, Xiao Y, Weaver D, Feunteun J, et al. (1997) Association of BRCA1 with Rad51 in mitotic and meiotic cells. Cell 88:265–275.
48. Scully R, Anderson SF, Chao DM, Wei W, Ye L, Young RA, et al. (1997) BRCA1 is a component of the RNA polymerase II holoenzyme. Proc Natl Acad Sci USA 94:5605–5610.
49. Tavtigian SV, Simard J, Rommens J, Couch F, Shattuck-Eidens D, Neuhausen S, et al. (1996) The complete BRCA2 gene and mutations in chromosome 13q-linked kindreds. Nature Genet 12:333–337.
50. Wooster R, Neuhausen SL, Mangion J, Quirk Y, Ford D, Collins N, et al. (1994) Localization of breast cancer suceptibility gene, BRCA2, to chromosome 13q12-13. Science 265:2088–2090.
51. Wooster R, Bignell G, Lancaster J, Swift S, Seal S, Mangion J, et al. (1995) Identification of the breast cancer susceptibility gene BRCA2. Nature 378:789–791.
52. Thorlacius S, Tryggvadottir L, Olafsdottir GH, Jonasson JG, Ogmundsdottir HM, Tulinius H, et al. (1995) Linkage to BRCA2 region in hereditary male breast cancer. Lancet 346:544–5.
53. Neuhausen S, Gilewski T, Norton L, Tran T, McGuire P, Swensen J, et al. (1996) Recurrent BRCA2 6174delT mutations in Ashkenazi Jewish women affected by breast cancer. Nature Genet 13:126–128.
54. Thorlacius S, Olafsdottir G, Tryggvadottir L, Neuhausen S, Tavtigian SV, Tulinius H, et al. (1996) A single BRCA2 mutation in male and female breast cancer families from Iceland with varied cancer phenotypes. Nature Genet 13:117–119.
55. Wang SC, Lin SH, Su LK, Hung MC (1997) Changes in BRCA2 expression during progression of the cell cycle. Biochem Biophys Res Commun 234:247–251.
56. Rajan JV, Wang M, Marquis ST, Chodosh LA (1996) Brca2 is coordinately regulated with Brca1 during proliferation and differentiation in mammary epithelial cells. Proc Natl Acad Sci USA 93:13078–13083.
57. Rajan JV, Marquis ST, Gardner HP, Chodosh LA (1997) Developmental expression of Brca2 colocalizes with Brca1 and is associated with proliferation and differentiation in multiple tissues. Dev Biol 184:385–401.
58. Suzuki A, de la Pompa JL, Hakem R, Elia A, Yoshida R, Mo R, et al. (1997) Brca2 is required for embryonic cellular proliferation in the mouse. Genes Dev 11:1242–1252.
59. Sharan SK, Morimatsu M, Albrecht U, Lim DS, Regel E, Dinh C, et al. (1997) Embryonic lethality and radiation hypersensitivity mediated by Rad51 in mice lacking Brca2. Nature 386:804–810.
60. Milner J, Ponder B, Hughes-Davies L, Seltmann M, Kouzarides T (1997) Transcriptional activation functions in BRCA2. Nature 386:772–773.
61. Mizuta R, LaSalle JM, Cheng HL, Shinohara A, Ogawa H, Copeland N, et al. (1997) RAB22 and RAB163/mouse BRCA2: proteins that specifically interact with the RAD51 protein. Proc Natl Acad Sci USA 94:6927–6932.
62. Lim DS, Hasty P (1996) A mutation in mouse rad51 results in an early embryonic lethal that is suppressed by a mutation in p53. Mol Cell Biol 16:7133–7143.
63. Kerangueven F, Essioux L, Dib A, Noguchi T, Allione F, Geneix J, et al. (1995) Loss of heterozygosity and linkage analysis in breast carcinoma: indication for a putative third susceptibility gene on the short arm of chromosome 8. Oncogene 10:1023–1026.
64. Seitz S, Rohde K, Bende E, Nothnagel A, Kolble K, et al. (1997) Strong indication for a breast cancer susceptibility gene on chromosome 8p12-p22: linkage analysis in German breast cancer families. Oncogene 14:741–743.
65. Yu CE, Oshima J, Fu YH, Wijsman EM, Hisama F, Alisch R, et al. (1996) Positional cloning of the Werner's syndrome gene. Science 272:193–194.
66. Li FP, Fraumeni JF J (1969) Soft-tissue sarcomas, breast cancer, and other neoplams: a familial syndrome? Ann Intern Med 71:747–752.
67. Malkin D, Li FP, Strong LC, Fraumeni JF, Nelson CE, Kim DH, et al. (1990) Germ line p53 mutations in a familial syndrome of breast cancer, sarcomas, and other neoplasms. Science 250:1233–1238.
68. Li FP, Fraumeni JFJ, Mulvihill JJ, Blattner WA, Dreyfus MG, Tucker MA, et al. (1988) A cancer family syndrome in twenty-four kindreds. Cancer Res 48:5358–5362.
69. Borresen AL, Andersen TI, Garber J, Barbier-Piraux N, Thorlacius S, Eyfjord J, et al. (1992) Screening for germ line TP53 mutations in breast cancer patients. Cancer Res 52:3234–3236.
70. Sidransky D, Tokino T, Helzlsouer K, Zehnbauer B, Rausch G, Shelton B, et al. (1992) Inherited p53 gene mutations in breast cancer. Cancer Res 52:2984–2986.
71. Eeles RA (1995) Germline mutations in the TP53 gene. Cancer Surv 25:101–124.
72. Levine AJ (1997) p53, the cellular gatekeeper for growth and division. Cell 88:323–331.

73. Morgan SE, Kastan MB (1997) p53 and ATM: cell cycle, cell death, and cancer. Adv. Cancer Res 71:1–25.
74. Brownstein MH, Wolf M, Bikowski JB (1978) Cowden disease: a cutaneous marker of breast cancer. Cancer 41:2393–2398.
75. Marra G, Armelao F, Vecchio FM, Percesepe A, Anti M (1994) Cowden's disease with extensive gastrointestinal polyposis. J Clin Gastroenterol 18:42–47.
76. Starink TM, van der Veen JP, Arwert F, de Waal LP, de Lange GG, Gille JJ, et al. (1986) The Cowden syndrome: a clinical and genetic study in 21 patients. Clin Genet 29:222–233.
77. Nelen MR, Padberg GW, Peeters EA, Lin AY, van den Helm B, Frants RR, et al. (1996) Localization of the gene for Cowden disease to chromosome10q22–23. Nature Genet 13:114–116.
78. Liaw D, Marsh DJ, Li J, Dahia PL, Wang SI, Zheng Z, et al. (1997) Germline mutations of the PTEN gene in Cowden disease, an inherited breast and thyroid cancer syndrome. Nature Genet. 16:64–67.
79. Li J, Yen C, Liaw D, Podsypanina K, Bose S, Wang SI, et al. (1997) PTEN, a putative protein tyrosine phosphatase gene mutated in human brain, breast, and prostate cancer. Science 275:1943–1947.
80. Steck PA, Pershouse MA, Jasser SA, Yung WK, Lin H, Ligon AH, et al. (1997) Identification of a candidate tumour suppressor gene, MMAC1, at chromosome 10q23.3 that is mutated in multiple advanced cancers. Nature Genet 15:356–362.
81. Hsu SC, Volpert OV, Steck PA, Mikkelsen T, Polverini PJ, Rao S, et al. (1996) Inhibition of angiogenesis in human glioblastomas by chromosome10 induction of thrombospondin-1. Cancer Res 56:5684–5691.
82. McKinnon PJ (1987) Ataxia-telangiectasia: an inherited disorder of ionizing radiation sensitivity in man. Progress in the elucidation of the underlying biochemical defect. Hum Genet 75:197–208.
83. Easton DF (1994) Cancer risks in A-T heterozygotes. Int J Radiat Biol 66(Suppl 6:):S177–S182.
84. Uziel T, Savitsky K, Platzer M, Ziv Y, Helbitz T, Nehls M, et al. (1996) Genomic Organization of the ATM gene. Genomics 33:317–320.
85. Zhang N, Chen P, Khanna KK, Scott S, Gatei M, Kozlov S, et al. (1997) Isolation of full-length ATM cDNA and correction of the ataxia-telangiectasia cellular phenotype. Proc Natl Acad Sci USA 94:8021–8026.
86. Greenwell PW, Kronmal SL, Porter SE, Gassenhuber J, Obermaier B, Petes TD (1995) TEL1, a gene involved in controlling telomere length in *S. cerevisiae,* is homologous to the human ataxia telangiectasia gene. Cell 82:823–829.
87. Watters D, Khanna KK, Beamish H, Birrell G, Spring K, Kedar P, Gatei M, et al. (1997) Cellular localisation of the ataxia-telangiectasia (ATM) gene product and discrimination between mutated and normal forms. Oncogene 14:1911–1921.
88. Savitsky K, Bar-Shira A, Gilad S, Rotman G, Ziv Y, Vanagaite L, Tagle DA, et al. (1995) A single ataxia telangiectasia gene with a product similar to PI-3 kinase. Science 268:1749–1753.
89. Elson A, Wang Y, Daugherty CJ, Morton CC, Zhou F, Campos-Torres J, et al. (1996) Pleiotropic defects in ataxia-telangiectasia protein-deficient mice. Proc Natl Acad Sci USA 93:13084–13089.
90. Barlow C, Hirotsune S, Paylor R, Liyanage M, Eckhaus M, Collins F, et al. (1996) Atm-deficient mice: a paradigm of ataxia telangiectasia. Cell 86:159–171.
91. Xu Y, Baltimore D (1996) Dual roles of ATM in the cellular response to radiation and in cell growth control. Genes Dev 10:2401–2410.
92. Westphal CH, Schmaltz C, Rowan S, Elson A, Fisher DE, Leder P (1997) Genetic interactions between atm and p53 influence cellular proliferation and irradiation-induced cell cycle checkpoints. Cancer Res 57:1664–1667.
93. Baskaran R, Wood LD, Whitaker LL, Canman CE, Morgan SE, Xu Y, et al. (1997) Ataxia telangiectasia mutant protein activates c-Abl tyrosine kinase in response to ionizing radiation. Nature 387:516–519.
94. Trent JM (1985) Cytogenetic and molecular biologic alterations in human breast cancer: a review. Breast Cancer Res Treat 5:221–229.
95. Aldaz CM, Chen T, Sahin A, Cunningham J, Bondy M (1995) Comparative allelotype of in situ and invasive human breast cancer: high frequency of microsatellite instability in lobular breast carcinomas. Cancer Res 55:3976–3981.
96. Fujii H, Marsh C, Cairns P, Sidransky D, Gabrielson E (1996) Genetic divergence in the clonal evolution of breast cancer. Cancer Res 56:1493–1497.
97. Osborne RJ, Merlo GR, Mitudomi T, Venesio T, Liscia DS, Cappa APM, et al. (1991) Mutations in the p53 gene in primary human breast cancer. Cancer Res 51:6194–6198.
98. Borg A, Zhang Q-X, Alm P, Olsson H, Sellberg G (1992) The retinoblastoma gene in breast cancer: allele loss is not correlated with loss of gene protein expression. Cancer Res 52:2991–2994.

99. Futreal PA, Liu Q, Shattuck-Eidens D, Cochran C, Harshman K, Tavtigian S, et al. (1994) BRCA1 mutations in primary breast and ovarian carcinomas. Science 266:120–122.
100. Lancaster J, Wooster R, Mangion J, Phelan CM, Cochran. C, Gumbs C, et al. (1996) BRCA2 mutations in primary breast and ovarian cancers. Nature Genet 13:238–240.
101. Negrini M, Monaco C, Vorechovsky I,Ohta M, Druck T, Baffa R, Huebner K, et al. (1996) The FHIT gene at 3p14.2 is abnormal in breast carcinomas. Cancer Res 56:3173–3179.
102. Kastury K, Baffa R, Druck T, Ohta M, Cotticelli MG, Inoue H, et al. (1996) Potential gastrointestinal tumor suppressor locus at the 3p14.2 FRA3B site identified by homozygous deletions in tumor cell lines. Cancer Res 56:978–983.
103. Lisitsyn N, Lisitsina NM, Dalbagni G, Barker P, Sanchez CA, Gnarra J, et al. (1995) Comparative genomic analysis of tumors: detection of DNA losses and amplification. Proc Natl Acad Sci USA 92:946–951.
104. Ohta M, Inoue H, Cotticelli MG, Kastury K, Baffa R, Palazzo J, et al. (1996) The FHIT gene, spanning the chromosome 3p14.2 fragile site and renal carcinoma-associated t(3;8) breakpoint, is abnormal in digestive tract cancers. Cell 84:587–597.
105. Negrini M, Sabbioni S, Possati L, Rattan S, Corallini A, Barbanti-Brodano G, et al. (1994) Suppression of tumorigenicty of breast cancer cells by microcell-mediated chromosome transfer: studies on chromosomes 6 and 11. Cancer Res 54:1331–1336.
106. Orphanos V, McGowan G, Hey Y, Boyle JM, Santibanezkoref M (1995) Proximal 6q, a region showing allele loss in primary breast cancer. Br J Cancer 71:290–293.
107. Sheng ZM, Marchetti A, Buttitta F, Champeme M-H, Campani D, Bistocchi M, et al. (1996) Multiple regions of chromosome 6q affected by loss of heterozygosity in primary human breast carcinomas. Br J Cancer 73:144–147.
108. Plummer SJ, Adams L, Simmons JA, Casey G (1997) Localization of a growth suppressor activity in MCF7 breast cancer cells to chromosome 17q24–q25. Oncogene 14:2339–2345.
109. Nagai MA, Yamamoto L, Salaorni S, Pacheco MM, Brentani MM, et al. (1994) Detailed deletion mapping of chromosome segment 17q12–21 in sporadic breast tumours. Genes Chromosome Cancer 11:58–62.
110. Kirchweger R, Zeillinger R, Schneeberger C, Speiser P, Louason G, Theillet C (1994) Patterns of allele losses suggest the existence of five distinct regions of LOH on chromosome 17 in breast cancer. Int J Cancer 56:193–199.
111. Devilee P, Cornelisse CJ (1994) Somatic genetic changes in human breast cancer. Biochim Biophys Acta 119:8:113–130.
112. Cropp CS, Champeme M-H, Lidereau R, Callahan R (1993) Identification of three regions on chromosome 17q in primary human breast carcinomas which are frequently deleted. Cancer Res 53:5617–5619.
113. Cropp CS, Nevanlinna HA, Pyrhonen S, Stenman U-H, Salmikangas P, Albertsen H, et al. (1994) Evidence for involvement of BRCA1 in sporadic breast carcinomas. Cancer Res 54:2548–2551.

10 Oncogene Activation and Breast Cancer Progression

Richard J. Pietras, PhD, MD
and Mark D. Pegram, MD

GENE ALTERATIONS IN HUMAN BREAST CANCER

Gene alterations play an important role in the origin and pathogenesis of human breast cancer. Three broad categories of gene changes that appear to contribute to tumor progression include tumor suppressor genes, repair-mutator genes, and oncogenes *(1)*. Inherited defects in some somatic genes appear to be responsible for development of hereditary and familial breast cancer, estimated at 1% and 5%, respectively, of all breast cancer cases. Identified alterations include mutations in tumor suppressor genes such as *p53* in Li-Fraumeni syndrome *(2,3)*. Mutations in the *BRCA1* gene at chromosome 17q21 have been documented in familial breast cancer *(4)*. A separate locus on chromosome 13q13, the *BRCA2* gene, was also associated with familial breast cancer *(5,6)*. Recent studies suggest that *BRCA1* may represent a repair-mutator gene, a gene responsible for maintaining the fidelity of DNA duplication *(7)*. The failure of gene surveillance can result in further alterations in gene function and thereby increase the mutation rate of other genes. Presumably, tumor suppressor genes and oncogenes would be prominent targets of faulty repair-mutator genes *(1,7)*.

Oncogenes are genes directly responsible for cancer progression and often present as altered versions of proto-oncogenes, which are normally involved in the control of cell growth and differentiation *(1,3)*. In the breast cancer cell, qualitative or quantitative differences are found between the proto-oncogene and its corresponding oncogene. The proto-oncogene can become an oncogene when a mutation in the coding region constituitively activates the biologic activity of the protein product without affecting the total amount of the product. Alternatively, a proto-oncogene can become an oncogene when excess product occurs from amplification (multiple copies) of the gene or from mutation, rearrangement, insertion, or deletion of the regulatory region of gene *(8)*. The oncogenes are, in turn, involved in the regulation of a complex series of cyclin-dependent kinases and other cell cycle modulators that determine progression through the cell division cycle *(3)*. Other categories of genes and their products that affect tumor progression include hormonal influences and angiogenic factors, topics that are detailed in other chapters of this volume.

From: *Contemporary Endocrinology: Endocrinology of Breast Cancer*
Edited by: A. Manni © Humana Press Inc., Totowa, NJ

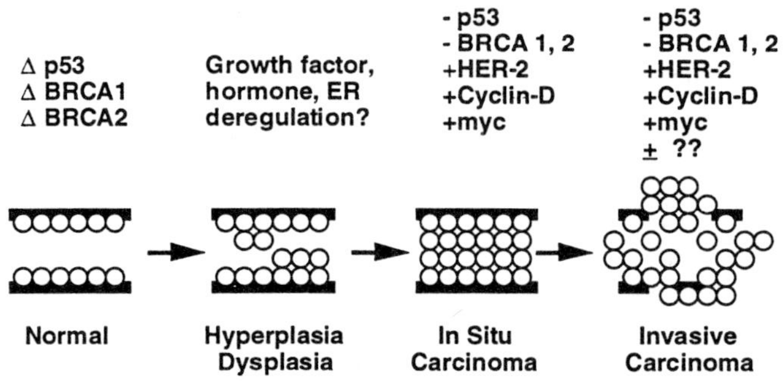

Fig. 1. Hypothetical scheme for malignant progression of human breast cancer. Some genes may be inherited in an altered (Δ*p53*), deleted (–*p53*), or amplified (+*HER-2*) form during the course of breast cancer development and progression. Amplification of the *HER-2/neu* gene is not found in normal breast tissue or hyperplasia/dysplasia (nonmalignant tissue) but is found in ductal in situ carcinoma and in invasive ductal carcinoma of the breast. In the early stages of tumorigenesis, *cyclin D* gene expression appears to be prevalent in noncomedo ductal carcinoma *in situ (96)*, whereas overexpression of the *HER-2/neu* gene tends to predominate in comedo-type ductal carcinoma in situ *(16)*. In more advanced breast malignancies, coamplification of c-*myc* and *HER-2/neu* genes appears to occur infrequently in most studies, suggesting that activation of these oncogenes may represent independent avenues in breast cancer development. See text and independent reviews *(134–136)* for additional details on other potential gene alterations in breast cancer progression. (Adapted from refs. *134–136*, with permission.)

MOLECULAR GENETICS OF BREAST CANCER PROGRESSION

Breast cancer progression is hypothesized to occur by an accumulated series of genetic and phenotypic changes in pathways regulating cell growth (Fig. 1). Intraductal carcinoma or ductal carcinoma *in situ* is the earliest histologic pattern considered a breast cancer. Cells within these malignant ducts have the cytologic features of more advanced malignancy but grow within the confines of an intact basement membrane without microscopic evidence of invasion (Fig. 1). Ductal carcinoma *in situ* appears capable of progression to invasive cancer. Inherited or somatic genetic changes in oncogenes, tumor suppressor genes, DNA repair machinery, and cell cycle checkpoints lead to *in situ* carcinoma and subsequently to invasion and metastasis. Familial disease may bypass one or more steps in this postulated cascade. With classic cytogenetic methods and studies of loss of heterozygosity (LOH), gene regions identified as commonly rearranged, amplified, or otherwise altered have been commonly detected at chromosomes 1, 3, 6, 7, 8, 9, 11, 13, 15, 16, 17, 18, and 20 *(3,6)*. Application of comparative genomic hybridization has also implicated chromosomes 10, 12, and 22 in the malignant process. As in most human cancers, the most common genetic abnormality in breast cancer is loss of specific chromosome arms. LOH analysis of polymorphic DNA markers points to chromosomes and subregions of chromosome arms likely to harbor tumor suppressor genes. LOH generally allows expression of a recessive mutant in an allele of a tumor suppressor gene by removal of a dominant normal allele, as in the case of *p53* expression *(1–3)*.

The second most common type of cytogenetic alteration in breast cancer appears to be gene amplification *(3,8)*. Karyotype analysis and chromosome *in situ* hybridization approaches such as comparative genomic hybridization or microfluorescent *in situ* hybridization (FISH) point to amplified chromosomal loci likely to harbor oncogenes. The initial step in gene amplification may involve the formation of extrachromosomal, self-

Fig. 2. Metaphase spread of chromosomal material from a breast cancer cell line that shows amplification of the *HER-2/neu* gene. The fluorescence in situ hybridization (FISH) method was used to evaluate SKBR3 cells that have overexpression of the *HER-2/neu* gene at the upper limit of that usually observed in clinical specimens. Punctate fluorescence is due to labeled probe specific for the *HER-2/neu* gene *(16)*. (Courtesy of Dr. G. Pauletti, UCLA School of Medicine, Los Angeles CA.)

replicating units termed double-minute chromosomes. These elements then become permanently incorporated into chromosomal regions and are termed homogeneous staining regions (Fig. 2). An amplified genetic unit (amplicon) is initially much larger than the actual size of the principal gene of biologic importance. Irrelevant or silent genes may also be coamplified with one or more expressed genes on an amplicon *(3,8)*.

ONCOGENE AMPLIFICATION IN BREAST CANCER PROGRESSION

The best established examples of amplified and functional genes for breast tumorigenesis (dominant oncogenes) include the growth factor receptor gene *c-neu/HER-2 (c-erb B2)* and the nuclear transcription factor c-*myc* (Table 1). However, the genetic diversity of breast cancer is reflected in the various oncogenes implicated in breast cancer progression *(3)*. Gene amplification occurs at the following loci: *HER-2/neu* (chromosome 17q12, 20–30% of tumors) and c-*myc* (8p24, 20% of tumors). Genes encoding cell cycle kinase regulatory proteins, such as cyclin D1 (*PRAD1/CYD1* [chromosome 11q13]), are also commonly amplified in about 15% of human breast cancers and are considered oncogenes (Table 2). Other candidate oncogenes showing amplification at specific loci include the fibroblast growth factor receptor oncogene *FLG* at chromosome 8p12 (10–15% of tumors) and *BEK* at chromosome 10q26 (10–15% of tumors), the insulin-like growth factor receptor oncogene *IGFR* at chromosome 15q24-25 (2% of tumors), and unidentified

Table 1
Proto-oncogene Abnormalities and Clinical Correlates in Human Breast Cancer[a]

Proto-oncogene	*Product*	*Abnormality*	*Clinical correlate*
HER-2/neu	185-kDa membrane growth factor receptor	Gene amplification/ overexpression; increased product	Poor prognosis; poor response to therapy
HER-1/EGFR	170-kDa membrane growth factor receptor	Gene overexpression	Poor prognosis?; predicts response to therapy
c-*myc*	67-kDa nuclear transcription factor	Gene amplification/ overexpression	Predicts early relapse, poor prognosis
c-*ras*	21-kDa G-binding membrane protein	Amplification; point mutation; rearrangement	Does not correlate with overall survival
cyclin D1/PRAD1	Regulator of G_1-S transition	Gene overexpression	Correlates with estrogen receptor

[a]Data derived from prior investigations on *HER-2 (3,6,8,14,15)*, *EGFR (43–48)*, c-*myc (52,69–74)*, c-*ras (77–81)*, and *cyclin D1 (93–96)*.

Table 2
Candidate Proto-oncogenes and Clinical Correlates in Human Breast Cancer[a]

Candidate gene	*Product*	*Abnormality*	*Clinical correlate*
AIB1	Steroid receptor coactivator	Gene amplification/ overexpression	?
int-2	27-kDa protein	Gene amplification	?
FLG, BEK	Fibroblast growth factor receptors	Gene amplification	?
IGFR	Insulin-like growth factor receptor	Gene amplification	?
Ornithine decarboxylase	Enzyme in polyamine biosynthesis	Gene overexpression	?
Cathepsin D	Proteinase	?	Poor prognosis?
MMTVenv-like gene	Undefined	?	?

[a]Data derived from prior investigations on *AIB1 (9)*, int-2 *(3,136,137)*, *FLG, BEK, IGFR (3,136,137)*, ornithine decarboxylase *(110,118)*, cathepsin D *(105–108)*, and *MMTV env*-like genes *(124–132)*.

genes at chromosomes 13q31, 17q22-24, and 20q11-13.2 (Table 2) *(3)*. AIB1, a steroid receptor coactivator amplified in approximately 10% of human breast cancers, was recently identified at chromosome 20q12. Altered expression of this protein may contribute to development of steroid-dependent cancers *(9)*.

With the exception of c-*myc* and *PRAD1/CYD1,* gene amplification in breast cancer commonly involves one of several growth factor receptors. Growth factor receptor pathways play a critical role in human breast cancer progression *(10)*. In particular, members of the epidermal growth factor receptor (EGFR) family of growth factor receptors (EGFR, HER-2/*neu*/erb B2, HER-3/erbB3, HER-4/erb B4) appear to play a critical role in breast cancer progression. Receptors for HER-2, HER-4, and EGFR

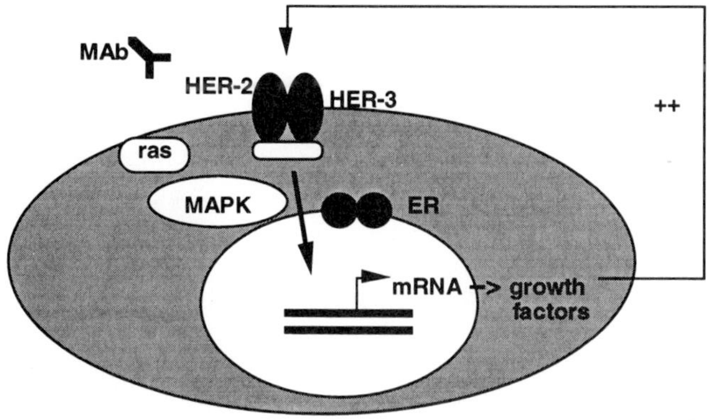

Fig. 3. Simplified model for growth factor receptor regulation of the growth of human breast cancer cells. The natural secretory products of mammary cells are abundant sources of growth factors that may contribute to breast carcinogenesis *(3)*. HER-2/*neu* receptor is a transmembrane tyrosine kinase that forms a heterodimer with HER-3 and other EGF receptor-related proteins for binding growth factors such as heregulin *(8,10,11)*. The HER-2/*neu* receptor signaling pathway is modulated by adaptor proteins, the mitogen-activated protein kinase (MAPK) pathway, and the ras signaling pathway to promote changes in nuclear transcription. Downstream elements such as phospholipase Cγ, PI-3-kinase, GTPase activating protein, and adaptor proteins such as SHC are part of the HER-2 receptor signaling machinery but are not shown here (see Fig. 5) *(10)*. In contrast to HER-2/*neu*, the tyrosine kinase catalytic site of HER-3 has absent or reduced kinase activity *(36)* and has sites that may afford specificity for activation of PI3 kinase *(37)*. Cross-communication between HER-2/*neu* signaling and estrogen receptor (ER) signaling also occurs in breast cancer *(29)*.

have up to 80% sequence homology, predominantly in the tyrosine kinase domain, and encode transmembrane glycoproteins with tyrosine kinase activity that appears essential for the signaling function of these molecules (Fig. 3). These receptors transmit growth and differentiation signals to the intracellular machinery (*ras*/MAP kinase cascades) in response to specific ligands such as heregulins or EGF. By contrast, the HER-3 receptor has substitutions in several important amino acids in its tyrosine kinase domain and may have reduced or absent enzymatic activity *(10)*. However, the HER2/*neu* receptor can form functional receptor heterodimers with HER-3 and with each of the other EGFR family members *(10,11)*.

Although several members of the EGFR family appear to be overexpressed in breast cancer *(6,10,11)*, amplification and overexpression of the *HER-2* gene has been studied most extensively. The gene known as *neu, erb B2,* or *HER-2* was first identified as a dominant transforming gene activated in chemically induced rat neuroectodermal tumors *(12)*. Although the original oncogenic alleles of *neu* were found to have a single point mutation in the transmembrane domain of the product *(13)*, the receptor is activated in human breast cancer only through amplification and overexpression of the wild-type gene. Reports by Slamon and colleagues *(14,15)* presented ideal studies of the changes in HER-2/*neu* oncogene expression in breast cancer specimens. The investigators used Southern, Northern, and Western blots and immunohistochemistry for HER-2/*neu* detection in 187 breast tumor specimens to analyze the amount of HER-2/*neu* expression at gene, RNA transcript, and protein levels. The latter work and ensuing studies established that 20–30% of breast tumors have amplification of the HER-2/*neu* gene and overexpress the encoded protein, a 185-kDa transmembrane tyrosine kinase receptor for growth

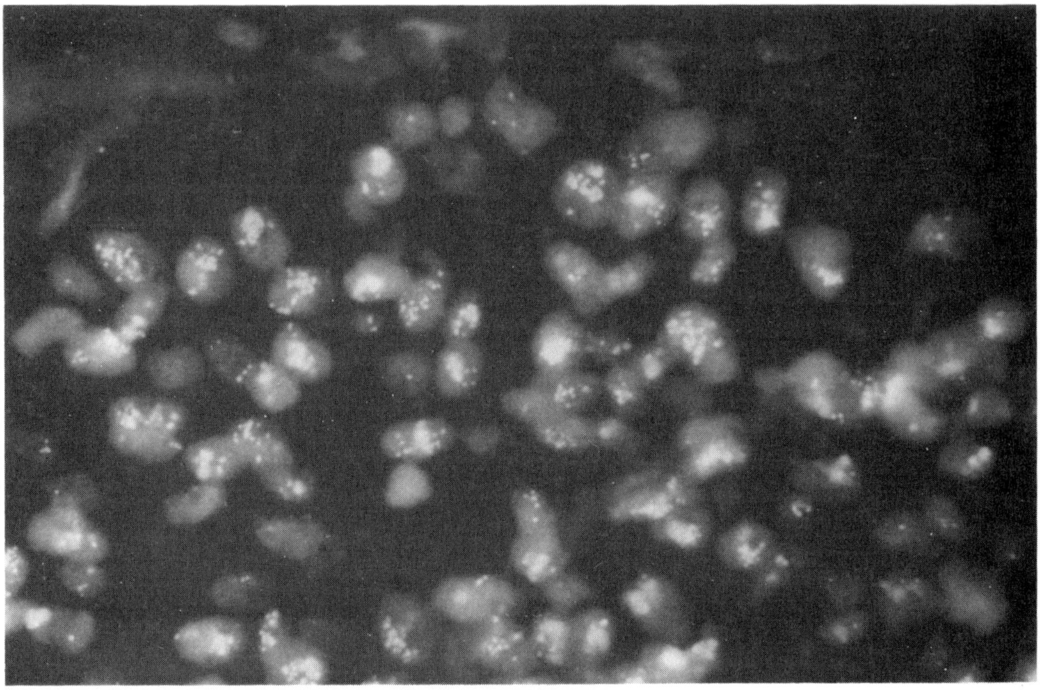

Fig, 4. Representative photomicrograph of breast tumor tissue after fluorescence in situ hybridization (FISH) using a labeled probe specific for the *HER-2/neu* gene *(16)*. Example shows amplification of the *HER-2/neu* gene as observed in a primary breast cancer specimen. (Courtesy of Dr. G. Pauletti, UCLA School of Medicine, Los Angeles, CA.)

factors *(3,10,11,14,15)*. The temporal occurrence of *HER-2* gene amplification in breast tumor progression has also been studied in several recent investigations. In one notable work, amplification of *HER-2/neu* was assessed by FISH in a range of proliferative and malignant ductal lesions of the breast, allowing for interphase analysis of gene copy number on a cell by cell basis (Fig. 4) *(16)*. Using the latter approach, *HER-2/neu* amplification was found to be restricted to ductal carcinoma *in situ*, predominantly in the comedo type, and to invasive carcinoma and was not detected in nonmalignant intraductal proliferations such as ductal hyperplasia and atypical ductal hyperplasia. Amplification was almost exclusively restricted to *in situ* and invasive carcinomas of high histologic grade *(16)*. The work suggests that *HER-2/neu* gene amplification is an early event in the development of high-grade ductal malignancies, but that oncogene alterations are not evident in early hyperproliferative or premalignant atypical ductal lesions *(16–18)*. Independent work shows that expression of HER-2/*neu* is maintained during progression from intraductal to invasive phases of growth in the same tumor tissue *(19–21)*. Overexpression of HER-2/*neu* is also maintained in metastatic lesions, suggesting a continuing function for HER-2/*neu (19)*. However, HER-2/*neu* overexpression probably represents only one histomorphologic pathway of breast tumorigenesis. A significant subset of breast carcinomas probably do not develop from HER-2/*neu* overexpression, and independent and/or complementary molecular events are required to explain these alternate pathways to malignancy (Table 1) *(2)*. As noted above, the development of cancer is a process that involves not only the activation

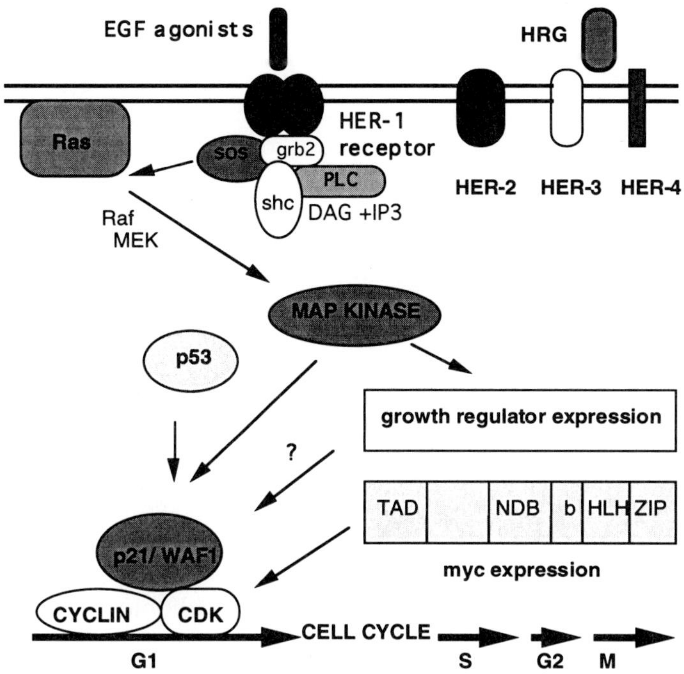

Fig. 5. Hypothetical scheme for interaction of a growth factor receptor pathway with that of other tumor suppressor and proto-oncogene products in the regulation of cell growth. The cell cycle is controlled by an ordered series of cyclins, cyclin-dependent kinases (CDKs) and their inhibitors, such as p21/WAF1, which is modulated, in turn, by p53 gene products *(1,41,42,138)*. Growth factor receptors (HER-1, HER-2, HER-3, HER-4) and their respective ligands (EGF ligands: HER-1; heregulin ligand family: HER-3, HER-4), ras signaling pathways (ras, REF, MEK, MAP kinase), and c-*myc* gene products are also postulated to influence these regulatory events. Functional domains of c-*myc* are indicated, including the transcriptional activation domain (TAD), nonspecific DNA-binding domain (NDB), basic specific DNA-binding domain (b), helix-loop-helix, and leucine zipper oligomerization domains (HLH-ZIP) *(136)*. See text for details.

of oncogenes but also the dysregulation of tumor suppressor and repair-mutator gene function *(1–3,17)* (Fig. 5).

CLINICAL IMPLICATIONS OF *HER-2/neu* GENE OVEREXPRESSION IN BREAST CANCER

HER-2/*neu* overexpression is associated with poor prognosis in patients with node-positive and node-negative breast cancers *(3,8,14,15,21)*. In addition, overexpression of the HER-2 receptor is associated with a poor clinical response to certain chemotherapeutic *(22–24)* and antihormonal drugs *(25–29)*. There is currently ongoing debate about the efficacy of standard chemotherapy in breast cancer patients whose tumors have high levels of HER-2 receptor *(3,30)*, but several studies suggest that patients whose tumors overexpress HER-2 respond worse to antihormone treatment *(31)*. Further well-designed clinical trials should help to clarify these important problems.

Since activation of the HER-2/*neu* signal transduction pathway correlates with the ability of HER-2/*neu* to transform breast epithelial cells, the occurrence of the HER-2/*neu* gene in human breast cancers has significant therapeutic implications *(8,10)*. Monoclonal antibodies directed to the extracellular domain of the HER-2/*neu* receptor reduce the proliferation of breast cancer cells that overexpress HER-2 receptors, thus providing a rationale for the therapeutic targeting of this growth pathway. In addition, monoclonal antibodies to the HER-2/neu receptor have been found to sensitize breast cancer cells to chemotherapeutic agents that elicit damage to cellular DNA *(32,33)*. A recombinant humanized monoclonal antibody to the HER-2 receptor is currently in phase III clinical trials alone and in combination with chemotherapeutic drugs *(34)*. Depending on the latter results, treatment with HER-2-specific monoclonal antibodies alone or in combination with other agents may prove to be an important new therapy for breast cancer.

THE ROLE OF THE EPIDERMAL GROWTH FACTOR RECEPTOR IN BREAST CANCER

The EGFR is a 170-kDa transmembrane receptor with tyrosine kinase activity *(35)*. EGFR shares considerable sequence homology with other members of the type I receptor tyrosine kinase family, HER-2/*neu*, HER-3, and HER-4 (Fig. 5) *(35–37)*. The structural motifs in this family include four conserved domains: two cysteine-rich extracellular domains, which are critical for ligand binding, a hydrophobic transmembrane domain, and a cytoplasmic kinase domain. In addition to the kinase activity of the cytoplasmic portion of EGFR, the phosphorylated form of EGFR has high-affinity recognition sites for Grb-2 (growth factor receptor bound-2), SHC, and SH2 (src homology type-2) domain-containing proteins (such as those found in phospholipase C-γ) *(38,39)*. As an adaptor protein forming a complex between activated tyrosine kinases and *ras*, Grb-2 serves a crucial link between EGFR and SOS, a *ras* guanosine triphosphate/guanosine diphosphate (GTP/GDP) exchange protein *(40,41)*. Formation of the EGFR/Grb-2/SOS complex serves to catalyze the *ras*-activated exchange of GTP for GDP. In a simplified model of receptor tyrosine kinase signal transduction (Fig. 5), activated *ras* stimulates *raf* kinase, which, in turn, phosphorylates MEK (a MAP-kinase kinase) and MAP kinases, leading to regulation of the function of nuclear transcription factors that direct mitogenesis or differentiation. The complexity of EGFR signaling is amplified by the several ligands that bind to EGFR, including EGF, transforming growth factor-α (TGF-α), amphiregulin, and cripto-1, and by the capability of EGFR to transactivate other type I tyrosine kinases including HER-2/*neu* and HER-3 receptors (Fig. 5) *(42)*.

The gene encoding EGFR, *c-erb-B,* is localized to chromosome 7 and is homologous to the *v-erb-B* oncogene. Although transfection of EGFR alone is insufficient for transformation of mammalian cells, cotransfection of EGFR with one of its activating ligands, such as EGF or TGF-α, does result in transformation, thus establishing EGFR as a proto-oncogene. A role for EGFR in the pathogenesis of breast cancer is suggested by the fact that the receptor and some of its ligands are overexpressed in a significant fraction of breast cancers compared with expression levels seen in normal breast tissues *(43,44)*. In contrast to the *c-erb B-2* gene, the *c-erb B* proto-oncogene is generally not amplified in breast cancers, with overexpression due to an increase in production of the protein product. The clinical importance of EGFR overexpression was first suggested by Sainsbury et al., who reported that EGFR is an independent predictor of early relapse and death in patients with breast cancer *(45)*. However, several following reports have offered widely conflicting results on the prognostic significance of EGFR expression in breast cancer.

Comprehensive reviews of the latter cohorts *(46,47)* conclude that (1) based on results from 40 studies comprising 5232 patients, EGFR overexpression is found in about 45% of all breast cancers (range 14–91%); (2) EGFR overexpression is often associated with shortened relapse-free, but not overall, survival by univariate analysis; (3) the prognostic significance of EGFR overexpression is lost on application of multivariate analyses that control for other prognostic variables such as *c-erb B-2* overexpression; (4) there is a lack of statistical association between EGFR and tumor size, lymph node status, tumor cell differentiation/grade, or menopausal status; (5) overexpression of both EGFR and HER-2/*neu* portends a particularly poor prognosis; and (6) there is a highly significant inverse correlation between EGFR expression and steroid (estrogen and progesterone) receptor expression *(47)*. Furthermore, there appears to be an inverse association between EGFR overexpression and the response to antiestrogen therapy in breast cancer *(48)*. These combined data suggest that, whereas EGFR expression may not be a useful prognostic factor in breast cancer, it may be a useful predictive factor for response to hormonal therapy. Support for this hypothesis is provided by laboratory experiments showing that transfection of EGFR into hormone-dependent breast cells results in hormone independence, loss of estrogen receptor (ER) and progesterone receptor (PgR) expression, and acquired resistance to tamoxifen *(49,50)*. Indeed, emerging data also suggest a potential role for EGFR in resistance to chemotherapy. Doxorubicin-resistant MCF-7 cells have increased expression of EGFR, and transfection of EGFR into breast cells confers resistance to certain chemotherapeutic drugs *(51)*. A main difficulty in the use of EGFR as a predictive marker in breast cancer is the lack of standardization in the measures of EGFR protein in tumor samples. Popular methods include immunohistochemical and radioligand binding assays. Unfortunately, antibodies, labeling approaches, and cutoff values to discriminate positive from negative results differ significantly in each study. Until uniform standards are established, the precise role of EGFR expression in breast cancer progression will remain uncertain. It is likely that tumor expression of EGFR ligands and other type I receptors transactivated by EGFR contributes to the clinical significance of EGFR expression and should be evaluated in parallel in future studies. The potential role of EGFR in tumor initiation or transition from preinvasive to invasive malignancy also remains to be assessed.

THE ROLE OF c-*myc* IN BREAST CANCER

The cellular homologue of v-*myc*, c-*myc,* is a 439-amino acid nuclear phosphoprotein that functions as a transcription factor. It is often overexpressed in breast cancer with amplification of the c-*myc* gene on chromosome 8q24 *(52)*. The structure of c-*myc* includes an amino-terminal transcription activation domain, a basic DNA binding domain, a helix-loop-helix motif, and a leucine-zipper motif (Fig. 5). The latter two motifs are responsible for the formation of both homo- and heterodimers. Heterodimeric complexes between *myc* and an 18-kDa helix-loop-helix protein, *max*, bind specifically to E-box DNA sequences (CACGTG), resulting in transcription activation. By contrast, *max* homodimers inhibit transactivation, and *max* complexed with another helix-loop-helix protein, *mad*, also inhibits transcription in conjunction with the corepressor protein, Sin3. *myc* expression is induced by a variety of growth factors, including EGF, TGF-α, insulin-like growth factor-I (IGF-I), and heregulin, and by steroid hormones such as estradiol and progesterone *(53–56)*. A specific estrogen-responsive region of the c-*myc* gene has been found *(57)*, and constitutive upregulation of c-*myc* expression is noted in ER-negative breast cells *(58)*. Inhibition of estrogen-induced expression of c-*myc* protein by an antisense oligonucleotide results in arrest of estrogen-stimulated cell proliferation *(59)*. c-*myc* expression is attenuated by antiestrogens in ER-expressing breast cell lines *(57)*, and also by TGF-β or oncostatin M, factors that inhibit the growth of mammary epithelial cells in vitro *(60,61)*. This regulation of c-*myc* expression by estrogen and by mitogenic growth factors that are known to be expressed in breast tissues suggests a role for dysregulation of c-*myc* in the malignant transformation of breast epithelia.

The transformation of normal epithelial cells by c-*myc* requires cooperation with other oncogenes or peptide growth factors. For example, human mammary A1N4 cells transfected with c-*myc* could only form colonies under anchorage-independent conditions with the addition of exogenous EGF, TGF-α, or basic fibroblast growth factor (bFGF) *(62)*. This suggests that c-*myc* overexpression alone is not sufficient for tumorigenesis. In support of this hypothesis, transgenic mice produced by microinjection with a mouse mammary tumor virus long terminal repeat (MMTV-LTR) c-*myc* construct into pronuclei of fertilized eggs results in mice that develop mammary tumors but only after a long latency period and/or multiple pregnancies. Such latency periods suggest that other genetic alterations must take place in addition to c-*myc* overexpression to result in malignant degeneration of breast epithelia *(63–65)*. The fact that double transgenic strains in which c-*myc* is co-overexpressed with v-Ha-*ras*, c-*neu*, or TGF-α results in a shorter latency to onset of breast tumors also supports this view *(66–68)*.

A summary of 30 studies published between 1986 and 1996 on the incidence and prognostic significance of c-*myc* gene amplification in breast cancer was recently reported by Watson et al. *(69)*. In this analysis, encompassing over 5,000 breast tumors, the amplification rate was about 15% (range 1%–33%). Wide variability in the results is probably due to technical differences in patient selection, cutoff points for gene amplification, contamination of tumor cell populations by stromal cells (in studies using Southern blot techniques), and the use of different control genes. Nonetheless, the incidence of c-*myc* amplification in these studies is near the approximate 20% incidence of c-*myc* amplification found in breast carcinoma cell lines *(70)*. Genetic rearrangements of c-*myc* are found infrequently in breast cancer *(71)*. Despite considerable variability in correlations between c-*myc* amplification and other established prognostic factors in breast cancer, there is a relatively consistent association detected with pathologic grade *(69)*. In addition, other reports have demonstrated an association between c-*myc* amplification and shortened relapse-free or overall survival, lymph node status, DNA ploidy, steroid hormone receptor status, cathepsin D expression, and inflammatory breast cancer *(52)*. With the exception of one study *(72)*, coamplification of c-*myc* and *c-erb B-2* appears to be a very infrequent occurrence. In one provocative report, a significant association between c-*myc* amplification and LOH on chromosome 1p was noted, suggesting the possibility of a tumor suppressor gene at this locus that, when lost, may facilitate c-*myc* amplification *(73)*. Overexpression of c-*myc* in the absence of gene amplification also occurs in breast cancer and, although there is general agreement in these studies that c-*myc* expression is increased in breast tumor cells relative to adjacent normal cells, it remains unclear what impact this event may have on prognosis. There is recent evidence that N-*myc* protein is also overexpressed in breast carcinomas in the absence of gene amplification, and this finding may correlate with tumor stage, grade, and clinical outcome *(74)*.

ras SIGNAL TRANSDUCTION PATHWAY IN BREAST CANCER

The three human *ras* proto-oncogenes encode four homologous 21-kDa proteins: H-*ras*, K-*ras* 4A, K-*ras* 4B, and N-*ras* *(75–78)*. As shown in Fig. 5, *ras* plays a key role as an intermediate for signal transduction initiated by ligand binding of receptor tyrosine kinases. Activated *ras* targets mitogen-activated serine/threonine protein kinases (MAP kinases) via *raf* and *MEK*. MAP kinases, in turn, translocate to the nucleus, where they regulate the activity of nuclear transcription factors. *ras* localization to the cell membrane is critical for its function, and *ras* undergoes a series of posttranslational modifications resulting in a mature form of the protein that is membrane associated. *ras* is initially prenylated, undergoes proteolytic cleavage of three C-terminal amino acid residues, and then undergoes methylation of the C-terminal carboxyl group of the prenylated cysteine residue exposed by proteolysis. Finally, *ras* proteins may be further modified by palmitoylation to stabilize membrane association *(75)*. The activity of mature *ras* proteins is regulated by binding of guanine nucleotides, such that GTP-bound *ras* is activated and GDP-bound *ras* is inactive *(76)*. Coordination of the phosphorylation of *ras*-bound guanine nucleotides is accomplished by guanine nucleotide exchange factors, such as SOS, and GTP-ase activating proteins (GAPs). Oncogenic activation of *ras* by point mutations in critical regions that govern *ras*-GDP/GTP cycling render *ras*-GTP resistant to GAP. *ras* is constitutively activated by such mutations. Although carcinogen-induced mammary cancers in rats frequently exhibit *ras* mutations, point mutations of *ras* are found in <5% of sporadic human breast carcinomas *(77)*. This low incidence of *ras* mutations does not exclude the possibility that alterations in the activity of normal *ras* proteins might be intimately involved in the pathogenesis of breast cancer. Indeed, several lines of evidence point to a role for *ras* activation in the emergence of breast malignancy.

First, overexpression of normal H-*ras* protein has been reported in human breast tumors *(78, 79)*. Transfection of activated *ras* into MCF-7 breast carcinoma cells also increases tumorigenicity *(80)*, and oncogenic *ras* transfection into normal breast epithelial cells (MCF-10A) results in cellular transformation *(81)*. Transgenic mice with mutant *ras* expression directed to breast tissue develop mammary tumors, and there is cooperation with other oncogenes such as c-*myc* in double transgeneic mice that develop mammary tumors at an even faster rate *(68)*. H-*ras* rare alleles, consisting of a variable number of tandem repeats of a 28-bp region capable of binding NF-κB transcription regulatory proteins, may also be associated with an increased risk of breast cancer *(82)*. Recently, data from Migliaccio et al. showed that estradiol can activate the p21*ras*-MAP kinase pathway in MCF-7 breast cells, possibly via activation of c-*src* protein *(83)*. Such data implicate *ras* as a possible intermediate for estrogen in breast cells. Our understanding of the role of *ras* proteins in initiation or progression of breast cancer is hampered by the fact that there is no reliable method available for measurement of *ras* activity in premalignant or malignant breast tissues. Several investigators have examined *ras* expression levels in malignant breast tissues and find that increased expression levels are detectable in 55–71% of cases. However, expression of *ras* does not appear to correlate with other clinicopathologic variables or with patient outcome *(84)*. It is possible that studies of new chemical agents that target and disrupt *ras* will help to elucidate further the role of *ras* signal transduction in breast neoplasia *(85)*.

AMPLIFICATION OF CHROMOSOME 11q13 AND EVIDENCE FOR CYCLIN D1 AND int-2/FGF-3 AMPLIFICATION IN BREAST CANCER

The earliest studies of the chromosome 11q13 region in breast cancer were driven by the observation that its mouse homolog is a frequent site for integration by MMTV. The observation that this region is sometimes amplified in breast cancers prompted a search for proto-oncogenes in this region. The MMTV integration site, designated int-2, involved a segment of DNA harboring two closely linked polypeptide growth factors, FGF-3 and FGF-4, which have oncogenic potential and may afford a selective growth advantage for cells with 11q13 amplification. However, neither of these genes are expressed in normal mammary epithelia; and, in human tumors with 11q13 amplification, there is no concordant increase in FGF-3 or FGF-4 transcripts. Thus, it appears that the latter genes may be silent passengers in this specific amplicon rather than genes with significant amplification/overexpression leading to an aberrant increase in protein activity as seen with other amplified oncogenes such as *c-erbB-2*. These findings prompted further inspection of the 11q13 amplicon to identify new candidate oncogenes.

Other lines of evidence pointed to this region as harboring an oncogene because the segment is the target of the t (11;14)(q13,q32) translocation in mantle cell lymphoma; and, in parathyroid adenomas, an inversion of part of chromosome 11 fuses the 11q13 region to the parathyroid hormone gene on 11p15 *(86,87)*. Ultimately, *cyclin D1* was recognized as the leading candidate gene operative on the 11q13 amplicon *(88)*. *cyclin D1* was isolated by differential screening of cDNAs from 11q13 amplified vs nonamplified libraries. *cyclin D1* expression was induced by various growth factors, and immunostaining localized cyclin D1 protein to the cell nucleus *(88)*. It was recognized that the yeast homolog of cyclin D1 was able to rescue the G_1-S transition in yeast cells that were deficient in G_1 cyclins, and sequence analysis revealed homology of the human product to other cyclin proteins. Coimmunoprecipitation experiments demonstrated association of cyclin D1 with cyclin-dependent kinases, resulting in a complex that is able to phosphorylate and inactive p105 Rb and p107 Rb-related proteins *(88)*. Furthermore, it is noteworthy that cyclin D1-/- knockout mice demonstrate absence of lobuloalveolar structures in breast tissues during terminal differentiation *(89)*. In a transgenic mouse model, under the control of the MMTV promoter, *cyclin D1* overexpression in mammary tissues results in hyperplasia and neoplasia *(90)*. However, when cyclin D1 driven by the immunoglobulin enhancer, transgenic mice do not develop overt lymphomas unless they are crossed with other oncogenes such as *myc* or *ras (91)*, suggesting that factors other than *cyclin D1* overexpression alone are required for the transition from benign to malignant growth. This hypothesis is supported by transfection studies in mammalian cells, which demonstrate a lack of transformation and an overall decrease in cell viability following cyclin D1 transfection, despite a decrease in the G_1-S transit time *(92)*.

In human breast cancer, amplification of 11q13 has been well studied (reviewed in ref. *93*). It is amplified in approximately 5–23% of breast tumors, with most studies detecting amplification rates of 15–20%. Amplification of this region is consistently accompanied by overexpression of *cyclin D1*, but emerging evidence suggests that the protein product is much more frequently overexpressed than would be predicted based on the observed amplification rate in breast cancer. Thus, other mechanisms of *cyclin D1* dysregulation may be operative in this malignancy *(94,95)*. In terms of the prognostic significance of *cyclin D1* amplification, several observations are noteworthy. There is clear evidence that *cyclin D1* overexpression is positively correlated with expression of the estrogen receptor *(94–96)*. In some, but not all studies, amplification was associated with lymph node involvement and/or adverse prognosis. In a recent comprehensive study of cyclin gene amplification and overexpression in breast cancer involving a series of 1171 breast tumors, *cyclin D1* amplification was prevalent in non-comedo-type ductal carcinoma *in situ*, suggesting that this amplification event may occur relatively early in the neoplastic process *(96)*. Higher rates of amplification in lobular as opposed to ductal breast carcinomas were also found. Furthermore, *cyclin D1* was frequently overexpressed in the absence of gene amplification, and no amplification of cyclins *A, D2, D3,* and *E* was found in human breast cancers *(96)*. Additional studies have evaluated protein expression of cyclin D1 in breast carcinomas, and, in contrast to work showing an adverse prognosis associated with 11q13 amplification, cyclin D1 protein overexpression paradoxically identifies a patient subset with a more favorable prognosis. The latter finding may be influenced by the fact that many of these cases are ER positive, and, thus, expression of *cyclin D1* may be due to induction by estrogens in malignant breast tissue *(95)*. Some data on the expression of cyclin E protein also suggests a possible role for this protein in tumorigenesis. Porter et al. *(97)* reported that high cyclin E levels portend a poor prognosis, even in node-negative breast cancer patients. However, in the latter analysis, the investigators did not control for ER expression. Using a more comprehensive, multivariate statistical model to control for ER expression, Nielsen et al. found that the prognostic value of cyclin E overexpression correlated strongly with an inverse correlation between ER expression and cyclin E levels *(98)*.

OTHER CANDIDATE ONCOGENES IN BREAST CANCER PATHOBIOLOGY

Cathepsin D

Many enzymes capable of degrading extracellular matrix, such as matrix metalloproteinases, cathepsins, and plasminogen activators, have been implicated in tumor progression and metastasis *(99–101)*. Cathepsin D is a lysosomal acid protease whose production in breast cancer cells is stimulated by estrogen *(102)*. Following translation, pro-cathepsin D is proteolytically cleaved to an active form *(103)*. The ability of the active species of cathepsin D to degrade extracellular matrix and to activate other proteolytic enzymes suggests a potential role for this protein in breast cancer invasion and metastasis *(99,103)*. Overexpression of cathepsin D in transformed cells enhances their malignant phenotype and metastatic potency. Furthermore, cathepsin D has mitogenic activity, and it may act in an autocrine or paracrine fashion to promote tumor cell proliferation *(103,104)*. Although initial clinical studies suggested that cathepsin D may provide significant prognostic information in patients with breast cancer, subsequent investigations have been conflicting *(105)*. Whether or not cathepsin D expression has prognostic or predictive value in breast cancer remains highly controversial. Despite a plethora of published work, data to date are too contradictory to draw meaningful conclusions. Differences in published studies are due to an unparalleled variety of assays, reagents, approaches, and arbitrary clinical cutoff values. Recent evidence from immunohistochemical studies suggests the further problem that an abundance of the cathepsin D found in tumor specimens may reside in the stromal cell compartment rather than in tumor cells. Some of the latter studies suggest that expression of cathepsin D by host fibroblasts and macrophages has prognostic significance in breast cancer and that such expression may represent the host response to tissue damage caused by advancing malignant cells *(106)*. Evidence from large cohorts of breast cancer patients suggests that determination of total cathepsin D in cytosol extracts from whole tumor specimens (tumor plus stroma) has no prognostic utility *(105,107,108)*. It is likely that only use of *in situ* hybridization methods or *in situ* immunohistochemical localization with monoclonal antibodies to cathepsin D or pro-cathepsin D will help to resolve the controversy on the prognostic utility of cathepsin D. Finally, evaluation of the role of related cathepsins in breast cancer may prove worthwhile *(109)*.

Ornithine Decarboxylase

Ornithine decarboxylase (ODC) is the first enzyme involved in the polyamine biosynthetic pathway. The polyamines, putrescine, spermidine, and spermine, are present in all cells, and levels are tightly regulated by (1) ornithine decarboxylase *(110)*, (2) S-adenosylmethionine decarboxylase, a rate-limiting enzyme in spermidine and spermine biosynthesis in some cell types *(111)*, and (3) by enzymatic degradation of polyamines or excretion via transport proteins *(112)*. Treatment of estrogen-responsive MCF-7 breast cancer cells with estradiol results in induction of ornithine decarboxylase gene expression *(110)*. This induction can be augmented by the addition of IGF-I and insulin. Polyamines may then exert growth regulatory effects by facilitating the interaction of the estrogen receptor complex with DNA and by regulating the expression of estrogen-inducible genes *(113,114)*. Growth-stimulatory effects of estradiol can be inhibited by DL-α-difluoro-methylornithine, an irreversible inhibitor of ODC *(115)*. Similarly, growth-inhibitory effects of tamoxifen can be reversed by the addition of polyamines, and tamoxifen has been shown to decrease ODC expression and activity *(116)*. Cell transformation by carcinogens, viruses, or oncogenes is often accompanied by constitutive activation of ODC *(117)*. In breast cancer specimens, malignant tumor cell populations have higher levels of polyamines than surrounding normal tissues *(118)*. Recent studies indicate that the ODC gene is a transcriptional target for c-*myc* and c-*fos* *(119,120)*. A role for ODC in tumorigenesis is supported by the transformation of NIH/3T3 fibroblasts on transfection with ODC cDNA *(121)*. Additional studies link increased polyamine biosynthesis with an aggressive breast cancer phenotype *(122)*. Despite these findings, ODC overexpression in transgenic mice was not found to induce murine tumors *(123)*. Although enzyme activity increased in almost all tissues, polyamine pools increased only in brain and testis, underscoring the complex regulation of polyamine pools by mechanisms independent of ODC expression *(123)*. Whether or not ODC has significant independent prognostic significance in breast cancer remains to be proven. However, targeting polyamine biosynthesis as a therapeutic strategy for breast cancer may prove useful *(110)*.

Detection of MMTV-Like Sequences in Breast Cancer

Studies of animal oncogenic retroviruses have been fundamental to the discovery of human cellular proto-oncogenes *(3,6,11)*. As noted above, MMTV is an agent associated with a high incidence of breast cancer in mice. It acts as an insertional mutagen and, on insertion into chromosomal DNA, activates genes not expressed in normal mammary tissue. Although efforts to demonstrate the presence of viruses in human breast cancer have often yielded contradictory results, several lines of evidence suggest a potential association between MMTV-like virus and human breast cancer. MMTV*env*-related antigenic reactivity has been detected in breast tumor tissue sections as well as in human milk, breast tumor cells in culture, and patient serum *(124–126)*. Sequence homology to MMTV has been noted in human DNA under low stringency conditions, and RNA related to MMTV has been detected in human breast cancer cells *(127,128)*. In addition, breast cancer patients show viral-specific T-cell responses to MMTV *(129)*, and viral particles have been detected in human breast cancer cell lines and in monocytes from affected patients *(130,131)*.

Using polymerase chain reaction (PCR) technology, Pogo and Holland identified a 660-bp sequence of the *MMTVenv* gene in 39% of 335 breast cancer samples *(132)*. By contrast, this PCR product was only detected in 1.6% of 121 normal breast tissue specimens from reduction mammoplasty. The product could not be amplified from lymphocytes from breast cancer patients or from other human cancers or cell lines. Sequencing of this PCR product revealed 95–99% homology to the *MMTVenv* gene but not to other known human endogenous retroviruses. Using reverse transcription PCR analysis, 65% of these cases had evidence for transcription of these sequences. These investigators were also able to identify a 630-bp segment with high homology to the MMTV-LTR. This segment contained both a glucocorticoid-responsive element and MMTV superantigen domains *(132)*. Taken together, these data suggest the possibility of an MMTV-like virus associated with a significant fraction of human breast cancers. The notion that viruses may play a role in the pathogenesis of human malignancies was recently promoted by the discovery of a member of the herpesvirus family associated with progression of Kaposi's sarcoma and multiple myeloma *(133)*. Elucidation of a possible viral etiology for breast cancer could have profound implications for breast cancer screening, prevention, and therapy.

CONCLUSIONS

Of the more than 100,000 genes contained in the genome of the human breast cancer cell, only a few have been proved to be altered in malignant progression. *HER-2/neu,* c-*myc,* and *cyclin D1* are among the oncogenes overexpressed and are probably involved in the pathogenesis of human breast cancer. With information from studies of clinical cancer specimens, some distinct patterns of gene alteration are beginning to emerge. The results of several investigations suggest that the pathway to cancerous growth will likely involve cooperative interactions and networking connections among oncogenes, tumor suppressor genes, and repair-mutator genes (Fig. 5). The products of oncogenes and their cross-communication with growth factor and hormone signaling pathways also appear to play a major role in breast cancer progression. The challenge for the future is to identify the specific sequence and pattern of gene activation in breast cancer and to intensify our search for other crucial molecular defects leading to unregulated cell growth. Furthermore, we must clarify the role of heritable gene alterations in this process. Hopefully, advances in this work will help us to devise novel therapeutics based on the unique biology of these cancers.

ACKNOWLEDGMENTS

We are very grateful to Dr. Dennis Slamon for advice and encouragement and to Dr. Giovanni Pauletti for providing data from fluorescence in situ hybridization experiments. This work was supported by grants from the USPHS (R29 CA 60835; RO1 AG14785), the US Army Breast Cancer Research Program (DAMD17-94-J-4370), and the California Breast Cancer Research Program (1RB-0297).

REFERENCES

1. Levine AJ (1995) The genetic origins of neoplasia. JAMA 273:592–593.
2. Li FP, Fraumeni JF Jr (1969) Soft tissue sarcomas, breast cancer and other neoplasms: a familial syndrome? Ann Intern Med 71:747–752.
3. Dickson RB, Lippman ME (1997) Cancer of the breast, In: Cancer: Principles & Practice of Oncology, 5th ed. (DeVita VT Jr, Hellman S, Rosenberg SA, eds.), Lippincott-Raven, Philadelphia, pp. 1541–1557.
4. Miki Y, Swansen J, Shattuck-Eidens D, Futreal PA, Harshman K, Tavtigian S, et al. (1994) A strong candidate for the breast and ovarian cancer susceptibility gene BRCA1. Science 266:66–71.
5. Wooster R, Bignell G, Lancaster J, Swift S, Seal S, Mangion J, et al. (1995) Identification of the breast cancer susceptibility gene BRCA2. Nature 378:789–792.
6. Hoskins K, Weber BL (1995) Recent advances in breast cancer biology. Curr Opin Oncol 7:495–500.
7. Kinzler K, Vogelstein B (1997) Gatekeepers and caretakers. Nature 386:761–763.
8. Slamon D, Press M, Godolphin W, Ramos L, Haran P, Shek L, et al. (1989) Studies of the HER-2/neu oncogene in human breast cancer. Cancer Cells 7:371–378.
9. Anzick SL, Kononen J, Walker RL, Azorsa DO, Tanner MM, Guan X-Y, et al. (1997) AIB1, a steroid receptor coactivator amplified in breast and ovarian cancer. Science 277:965–968.
10. Reese DM, Slamon DJ (1997) HER-2/neu signal transduction in human breast and ovarian cancer. Stem Cells 15:1–8.
11. Hynes NE, Stern DF (1994) The biology of erbB-2/neu/HER-2 and its role in cancer. Biochim Biophys Acta 119:8:165–184.
12. Shih C, Padhy L, Murray M, Weinberg R (1981) Transforming genes of carcinomas and neuroblastomas introduced into mouse fibroblasts. Nature 260:261–264.
13. Bargmann C, Hung M, Weinberg R (1986) Multiple independent activations of neu oncogene by a point mutation altering the transmembrane domain of p185. Cell 45:649–657.
14. Slamon DJ, Clark GM, Wong SG, et al. (1987) Human breast cancer: correlation of relapse and survival with amplification of the HER-2/neu oncogene. Science 235:177–182.
15. Slamon DJ, Godolphin W, Jones LA, Holt J, Wong S, Keith D, et al. (1989) Studies of the HER-2/*neu* proto-oncogene in human breast and ovarian cancer. Science 244:707–712.
16. Pauletti G, Dandekar S, Smith K, Robbins P, Dawkins H, Papadimitriou J, et al. (1997) Chronology of HER-2/*neu* gene amplification in proliferative and malignant ductal lesions of the breast as determined by fluorescence *in situ* hybridization (FISH). Proc Am Assoc Cancer Res 38:414–415.
17. Liu E, Thor A, He M, Barcos M, Ljung B-M, Benz C (1992) The HER2 (c-erbB-2) oncogene is frequently amplified in *in situ* carcinomas of the breast. Oncogene 7:1027–1032.
18. Pauletti G, Godolphin W, Press MF, Slamon DJ (1996) Detection and quantitation of HER-2/*neu* gene amplification in human breast cancer archival material using fluorescence in situ hybridization. Oncogene 13:63–72.
19. Lonn U, Lonn S, Nylen U, Stenkvist B, Vennstrom B (1992) Detection and temporal appearance of multiple copies of c-erb-B2 genes in advanced mammary carcinoma using fine needle biopsies and the polymerase chain reaction. Breast Cancer Res Treat 23:191–200.
20. Iglehart JD, Kerns B-J, Huper G, Marks JR (1995) Maintenance of DNA content and erbB-2 alterations in intraductal and invasive phases of mammary cancer. Breast Cancer Res Treat 34:253–263.
21. Press MF, Bernstein L, Thomas PA, Meisner LF, Zhou J-Y, Ma Y, et al. (1997) HER-2/neu gene amplification characterized by fluorescence *in situ* hybridization: poor prognosis in node-negative breast carcinomas. J Clin Oncol 15:2894–2904.
22. Muss HB, Thor AD, Berry, D, Kute, T, Liu ET, Koerner F, et al. (1994) c-erbB2 expression and response to adjuvant therapy in women with node-positive early breast cancer. N Engl J Med 330:1260–1266.
23. Berns EMJJ, Foekens JA, van Staveren IL, van Putten WLJ, de Koning HYW, Portengen H, et al. (1995) Oncogene amplification and prognosis in breast cancer: relationship with systemic treatment. Gene 159:11–18.
24. Fehm T, Maimonis P, Weitz S, Teramoto Y, Katalinic A, Jager W (1997) Influence of circulating c-erbB-2 serum protein on response to adjuvant chemotherapy in node-positive breast cancer patients. Breast Cancer Res Treat 43:87–95.

25. Nicholson S, Wright C, Sainsbury J, Halcrow P, Kelly P, Angus B, Farndon J, Harris AL (1990) Epidermal growth factor receptor as a marker for poor prognosis in node-negative breast cancer patients: *neu* and tamoxifen failure. J Steroid Biochem 37:811–818.
26. Wright C, Nicholson S, Angus B, Sainsbury JR, Farndon J, Cairns J, et al. (1992) Relationship between c-erbB-2 protein product expression and response to endocrine therapy in advanced breast cancer. Br J Cancer 65:118–124.
27. Benz C, Scott G, Sarup J, Johnson R, Tripathy D, Coronado E, et al. (1993) Estrogen-dependent, tamoxifen-resistent tumorigenic growth of MCF-7 cells transfected with HER2/neu. Breast Cancer Res Treat 24:85–92.
28. Leitzel K, Teramoto Y, Konrad K, Chinchilli V, Volas G, Grossberg H, et al. (1995) Elevated serum c-erbB-2 antigen levels and decreased response to hormone therapy of breast cancer. J Clin Oncol 13:1129–1135.
29. Pietras RJ, Arboleda J, Reese DM, Wongvipat N, Pegram MD, Ramos L, et al. (1995) HER-2 tyrosine kinase pathway targets estrogen receptor and promotes hormone-independent growth in human breast cancer cells. Oncogene 10:2435–2446.
30. Pegram MD, Finn RS, Arzoo K, Beryt M, Pietras R, Slamon D (1997) The effect of HER-2/*neu* overexpression on chemotherapeutic drug sensitivity in human breast and ovarian cancer cells. Oncogene 15:537–547.
31. Borg A, Baldetorp B, Ferno M, et al. (1994) erb B2 amplification is associated with tamoxifen resistance in steroid-receptor positive breast cancer. Cancer Lett 81:137–144.
32. Pietras RJ, Fendly BM, Chazin VR, Pegram MD, Howell SB, Slamon DJ (1994) Antibody to HER-2/*neu* receptor blocks DNA repair after cisplatin in human breast and ovarian cancer cells. Oncogene 9:1829–1838.
33. Arteaga C, Winnier A, Poirier M, Lopez-Larraza D, Shawver L, Hurd S, et al. (1994) p185c-erbB-2 signaling enhances cisplatin-induced cytotoxicity in human breast carcinoma cells: association between an oncogenic receptor tyrosine kinase and drug-induced DNA repair. Cancer Res 54:3758–3765.
34. Pegram M, Lipton A, Pietras R, Hayes D, Weber B, Baselga B, et al. (1995) Phase II study of intravenous recombinant humanized anti-p185 HER-2 monoclonal antibody (rhuMAb HER-2) plus cisplatin in patients with HER-2/*neu* overexpressing metastatic breast cancer. Proc Am Soc Clin Oncol 14:106.
35. Carpenter, G, Wahl MI (1990) The epidermal growth factor family. Peptide Growth Factors Receptors 1:69–171.
36. Carraway KL III, Cantley LC (1994) A neu acquaintance for erbB3 and erbB4: a role for receptor heterodimerization in growth signaling. Cell 78:5–8.
37. Soltoff SP, Carraway KL III, Prigent SA, Gullick WG, Cantley LC (1994) erbB3 is involved in activation of phosphatidylinositol 3-kinase by epidermal growth factor. Mol Cell Biol 14:3550–3558.
38. Pawson T, Gish GD (1992) SH2 and SH3 domains: from structure to function. Cell 71:359–362.
39. Batzer A, Rotin D, Skolnik EY, Schlessinger JF (1994) Hierarchy of binding sites for Grb2 and Shc on the epidermal growth factor receptor. Mol Cell Biol 14:5192–5201.
40. Bollag G, McCormick G (1991) Regulators and effectors of ras proteins. Annu Rev Cell Biol 7:601–632.
41. Chardin P, Camonis JH, Gale NW, Van Aelst L, Schlessinger J, Wigler MH, et al. (1993) Human Sos1: a guanine nucleotide exchange factor for Ras that binds to GRB2. Science 260:1338–1346.
42. Earp HS, Dawson TL, Li X, Yu H (1995) Heterodimerization and functional interaction between EGF receptor family members: a new signaling paradigm with implications for breast cancer research. Breast Cancer Res Treat 35:115–132.
43. Klijn JGM, Berns PMJJ, Schmitz PIM, Foekens JA (1992) The clinical significance of epidermal growth factor receptor (EGF-R) in human breast cancer: a review on 5232 patients. Endocr Rev 13:3–17.
44. Normanno N, Ciardiello F, Brandt R, Salomon DS (1994) Epidermal growth factor-related peptides in the pathogenesis of human breast cancer. Breast Cancer Res Treat 29:11–27.
45. Sainsbury J, Farndon J, Needham G, Malcolm A, Harris A (1987) Epidermal growth factor receptor status as predictor of early recurrence of relapse and death from breast cancer. Lancet 1:1398–1402.
46. Klijn J, Berns P, Schmitz P, Foekens J (1993) Epidermal growth factor receptor (EGFR) in clinical breast cancer: update 1993. Endocr Rev Monogr 1:171–174.
47. Klijn J, Look M, Portengen H, Alexieva-Figusch J, van Putten W, Foekens J (1994) The prognostic value of epidermal growth factor receptor (EGFR) in primary breast cancer: results of a 10 year follow-up study. Breast Cancer Res Treat 29:73–83.

48. Nicholson R, McClelland R, Gee J, Manning D, Cannon P, Robertson J, et al. (1994) Epidermal growth factor receptor expression in breast cancer: association with response to endocrine therapy. Breast Cancer Res Treat 29:117–125.
49. Van Agthoven T, Portengen H, Foekens J, Dorssers L (1992) Ectopic expression of epidermal growth factor receptors induces hormone independence in ZR-75–1 human breast cancer cells. Cancer Res 52:5082–5088.
50. Long B, McKibben B, Lynch M, Van den Berg H (1992) Changes in epidermal growth factor receptor expression and response to ligand associated with acquired tamoxifen resistance or oestrogen independence in the ZR-75–1 human breast cancer cell line. Br J Cancer 65:865–869.
51. Dickstein BM, Wosikowski K, Bates S (1995) Increased resistance to cytotoxic agents in ZR75B human breast cancer cells transfected with epidermal growth factor receptor. Mol Cell Endocrinol 110:205–211.
52. Nass S, Dickson R (1997) Defining a role for c-myc in breast tumorigenesis. Breast Cancer Res Treat 44:1–22.
53. Dubik D, Dembinski T, Shiu R (1987) Stimulation of c-myc oncogene expression associated with estrogen-induced proliferation of human breast cancer cells. Cancer Res 47:6517–6521.
54. Davidson N, Prestigiacomo L, Hahm H (1993) Induction of jun gene family members by transforming growth factor a but not 17β-estradiol in human breast cancer cells. Cancer Res 53:291–297.
55. Leygue E, Gol-Winkler R, Gompel A, Louis-Sylvestre C, Soquet L, Staub S, et al. (1995) Estradiol stimulates c-myc proto-oncogene expression in normal human breast epithelial cells in culture. J Steroid Biochem Mol Biol 52:299–305.
56. Wenlu L, Park JW, Nuijens A, Sliwkowski MX, Gilbert A (1996) Heregulin is rapidly translocated to the nucleus and its transport is correlated with c-myc induction in breast cancer cells. Oncogene 10:2473–2477.
57. Dubik D, Shiu R (1992) Mechanism of estrogen activation of c-myc oncogene expression. Oncogene 7:1587–1594.
58. Shiu R, Watson P, Dubik D (1993) C-myc oncogene expression in estrogen-dependent and -independent breast cancer. Clin Chem 39:353–355.
59. Watson P, Pon R, Shiu R (1991) Inhibition of c-myc expression by phosphorothioate antisense oligonucleotide identifies a critical role for c-myc in the growth of human breast cancer. Cancer Res 51:3996–4000.
60. Fernandez-Pol J, Talkad V, Klos D,d Hamilton P (1987) Suppression of the EGF-dependent induction of c-myc proto-oncogene expression by transforming growth beta in human breast carcinoma cell line. Biochem Biophys Res Commun 144:1197–1205.
61. Spence M, Vestal R, Liu, J (1997) Oncostatin M-mediated transcriptional suppression of the c-myc gene in breast cancer cells. Cancer Res 57:2223–2228.
62. Valverius E, Ciardiello F, Heldin N, Blondel B, Merlino G, Smith G, et al. (1990) Stromal influences on transformation of human mammary epithelial cells overexpressing c-myc and SV40T. J Cell Physiol 145:207–216.
63. Schoenenberger C, Andres A, Groner B, van der Valk M, Lemeur M, Gerlinger P (1988) Targeted c-myc gene expression in mammary glands of trangenic mice induces mammary tumors with constitutive milk protein gene transcription. EMBO J 7:169–175.
64. Stewart T, Pattengale P, Leder P (1984) Spontaneous mammary adenocarcinomas in transgenic mice that carry and express MTV/myc fusion genes. Cell 38:627–637.
65. Leder A, Pattengale P, Kuo A, Stewart T, Leder P (1986) Consequences of widespread deregulation of the c-myc gene in trangenic mice: multiple neoplasms and normal development. Cell 45:485–495.
66. Amundadottir L, Johnson M, Merlino G, Smith G, Dickson R (1995) Synergistic interaction of transforming growth factor a and c-myc in mouse mammary and salivary gland tumorigensis. Cell Growth Differ 6:737–748.
67. Andres A, van der Valk M, Schonenberger C, Fluckiger F, LeMeur M, Gerlinger P, et al. (1988) Ha-ras and c-myc oncogene expression interferes with morphological and functional differentiation of mammary epithelial cells in single and double transgenic mice. Genes Dev 2:1486–1495.
68. Sinn E, Muller W, Pattengale P, Tepler I, Wallace R, Leder P (1987) Coexpression of MMTV/v-Ha-ras and MMTV/c-myc genes in transgenic mice: synergistic action of oncogenes in vivo. Cell 49:465–475.
69. Watson PH, Singh R, Hole A (1996) Influence of c-myc on the progression of human breast cancer. Curr Top Microbiol Immunol 213:267–283.
70. Kozbor D, Croce CM (1984) Amplification of the c-myc oncogene in one of five human breast carcinoma lines. Cancer Res 44:438–441.
71. Bonilla M, Ramirez M, Lopez-Cueto J, Gariglio P (1988) In vivo amplification and rearrangement of c-myc oncogene in human breast tumors. J Natl Cancer Inst 80:665–671.

72. Borg A, Baldetrop B, Ferno M, Olsson H, Sigurdsson H (1992) c-myc is an independent prognostic factor in postmenopausal breast cancer. Int J Cancer 51:687–691.
73. Bieche I, Champeme M, Lidereau R (1994) A tumor suppressor gene on chromosome 1p controls the amplification of myc family genes in breast cancer. Cancer Res 54:4274–4276.
74. Mizukami Y, Nonomura A, Takizawa T, Noguchi M, Michigishi T, Nakamura S, et al. (1995) N-myc protein expression in human breast carcinoma: prognostic implications. Anticancer Res 15:2899–2906.
75. Zhang F, Casey PJ (1996) Protein prenylation: molecular mechanisms and functional consequences. Annu Rev Biochem 65:241–69.
76. Tocque B, Delumeau I, Parker F, Maurier F, Multon M, Schweighoffer F (1997) Ras-GTPase activating protein (GAP): a putative effector for Ras. Cell Signal 9:153–158.
77. Clark G, Der C (1995) Aberrant function of the Ras signal transduction pathway in human breast cancer. Breast Cancer Res Treat 35:133–44.
78. Spandidos D (1987) Oncogene activation in malignant transfromation: a study of H-ras in human breast cancer. Anticancer Res 7:991–996.
79. Clair T, Miller W, Cho-Chung Y (1987) Prognostic significance of the expression of a ras protein with molecular weight of 21,000 in human breast cancer. Cancer Res 47:5290–5293.
80. Albini A, Graf J, Kitten G, Kleinman H, Martin G, Veillette A, et al. (1986) 17β-Estradiol regulates and v-Ha-ras transfection constitutively enhances MCF-7 breast cancer cell interactions with basement membrane. Proc Natl Acad Sci USA 83:8182–8186.
81. Basolo F, Elliott J, Tait L, Chen XQ, Maloney T, Russo I, et al. (1991) Transformation of human breast epithelial cells by c-Ha-ras oncogene. Mol Carcinog 4:25–35.
82. Conway K, Edmiston S, Fried DB, Hulka BS, Garrett PA, Liu ET (1995) Ha-ras rare alleles in breast cancer susceptibility. Breast Cancer Res Treat 35:97–104.
83. Migliaccio A, Di Domenico M, Castoria G, de Falco A, Bontempo P, Nola E, et al. (1996) Tyrosine kinase/p21ras/MAP-kinase pathway activation by estradiol-receptor complex in MCF-7 cells. EMBOJ 15:1292–300.
84. Archer S, Eliopoulos A, Spandidos D, Barnes D, Ellis I, Blamey R, Nicholson R, et al. (1995) Expression of ras p21, p53 and c-erbB-2 in advanced breast cancer and response to first line hormonal therapy. Oncogene 72:1259–1266.
85. Kohl N, Mosser S, deSolms S, Giuliani E, Ponpliano D, Graham S, et al. (1993) Selective inhibition of ras-dependent transformation by a farnesyltransferase inhibitor. Science 260:1934–1937.
86. Withers D, Harvey R, Faust J, Melnik O, Carey K, Meeker T (1991) Characterization of a candidate bcl-1 gene. Mol Cell Biol 11:4846–4853.
87. Rosenberg C, Kim H, Shows T, Kronenberg H, Arnold A (1991) Rearrangement and overexpression of D11S287E, a candidate oncogene on chromosome 11q13 in benign parathyroid tumors. Oncogene 6:449–453.
88. Schuuring E (1995) Involvement of the chromosome 11q13 region in human malignancy: cyclin D1 and EMS1 are two new candidate oncogenes—a review. Gene 159:83–96.
89. Sininski P, Liu-Donaher J, Parker SB, Li T, Fazeli A, Gardner H, Haslam SZ, et al. (1995) Cyclin D1 provides a link between development and oncogenesis in the retina and breast. Cell 82:621–630.
90. Wang T, Cardiff R, Zukerberg L, Lees E, Arnold A, Schmidt E (1994) Mammary hyperplasia and carcinoma in MMTV-cyclin D1 transgenic mice. Nature 369:669–671.
91. Lovec H, Grzeschiczek A, Kowalski M, Moroy T (1994) Cyclin D1/bcl-1 cooperates with myc genes in the generation of B-cell lymphoma in transgenic mice. EMBOJ 13:3487–3495.
92. Quelle D, Ashmun R, Shurtleff S, Kato J, Bar-Sagi D, Roussel M, et al. (1993) Overexpression of mouse D-type cyclins accelerates G1 phase in rodent fibroblasts. Genes Dev 7:1559–1571.
93. Dickson C, Fantl V, Gillett C, Brookes S, Bartek J, Smith R, et al. (1995) Amplification of chromosome band 11q13 and a role for cyclin D1 in human breast cancer. Cancer Lett 90:43–50.
94. van Diest P, Michalides R, Jannink I, van der Valk P, Peterse H, de Jong J, et al. (1997) Cyclin D1 expression in invasive breast cancer: correlations and prognostic value. Am J Pathol 150:705–711.
95. Michalides R, Hageman P, van Tinteren H, Houben L, Wientjens E, Klompmaker R, et al. (1996) A clinicopathological study on overexpression of cyclin D1 and of p53 in a series of 248 patients with operable breast cancer. Br J Cancer 73:728–734.
96. Courjal F, Louason G, Speiser P, Kataros D, Zeillinger R, Theillet C (1996) Cyclin gene amplification and overexpression in breast and ovarian cancers: evidence for the selection of cyclin D1 in breast and cyclin E in ovarian tumors. Int J Cancer 69:247–253.

97. Porter P, Malone K, Heagerty P, Alexander G, Gatti L, Firpo E, et al. (1997) Expression of cell-cycle regulators p27Kip1 and cyclin E, alone and in combination, correlate with survival in young breast cancer patients. Nature Med 3:222–225.
98. Nielsen N, Arnerlov C, Emdin S, Landberg G (1996) Cyclin E overexpression, a negative prognostic factor in breast cancer with strong correlation to oestrogen receptor status. Br J Cancer 74:874–880.
99. Rochefort H (1993) Response to PM Ravdin (Breast Cancer Res Treat 24:219–226, 1993), "Evaluation of cathepsin D as a prognostic factor in breast cancer." Breast Cancer Res Treat 26:107–111.
100. Himelstein B, Canete-Soler R, Bernhard E (1994) Metalloproteinases in tumor progression: the contribution of MMP-9. Invasion Metast 14:246–258.
101. Pietras RJ, Szego CM, Roberts JA, Seeler B (1981) Lysosomal cathepsin B-like activity: mobilization in prereplicative and neoplastic epithelial cells. J Histochem Cytochem 29:440–450.
102. Augereau P, Miralles F, Cavalles V (1994) Characterization of the proximal estrogen-responsive element of human cathepsin-D gene. Mol Endocrinol 8:693–703.
103. Rochefort H, Augereau P, Briozzo P (1988) Structure, function, regulation and clinical significance of 52k procathepsin D secreted by breast cancer cells. Biochimie 70:943–949.
104. Vignon F, Capony F, Chambon M (1986) Autocrine growth stimulation of the MCF-7 breast cancer cells by estrogen-regulated 52K protein. Endocrinology 118:1537–1545.
105. Pelizzola D, Gion M, Paradiso A, Dittadi R, Correale M, Mione R, et al. (1996) Cathepsin D versus other prognostic factors in breast cancer. Results and controversies of a multicenter study on 2575 cases. Int J Biol Markers 11:139–147.
106. Nadji M, Fresno M, Nassiri M, Gregory C, Herrero A, Morales A (1996) Cathepsin D in host stromal cells, but not in tumor cells, is associated with aggressive behavior in node-negative breast cancer. Hum Pathol 27:890–895.
107. Ravdin P, de Moor C, Hilsenbeck S, Samoszuk M, Vendely P, Clark G (1997) Lack of prognostic value of cathepsin D levels for predicting short term outcomes of breast cancer patients. Cancer Lett 116:177–183.
108. Gion M, Mione R, Dittadi R, Romanelli M, Pappagallo L, Capitanio G, et al. (1995) Relationship between cathepsin D and other pathological and biological parameters in 1762 patients with primary breast cancer. Eur J Cancer 31:A: 671–677.
109. Pietras R, Szego C (1990) Cathepsin D in breast cancer. N Engl J Med 322:1673–1674.
110. Thomas T, Thomas T (1993) Extradiol control of ornithine decarboxylase mRNA, enzyme activity, and polyamine levels in MCF-7 breast cancer cells: therapeutic implications. Breast Cancer Res Treat 29:189–210.
111. Pegg A, Secrist JA III, Madhubala R (1988) Properties of L1210 cells resistant to alpha-difluoromethylornithine. Cancer Res 48:2678–2682.
112. Martin R, Ilett K, Minchin R (1991) Cell cycle-dependent uptake of putrexcine and its importance in regulating cell cycle phase transition in culture adult mouse hepatocytes. Hepatology 14:1243–1250.
113. Manni A, Wechter R, Grove R, Wei L, Martel J, Demers L (1995) Polyamine profiles and growth properties of ornithine decarboxylase overexpressing MCF-7 breast cancer cells in culture. Breast Cancer Res Treat 34:45–53.
114. Huber M, Poulin R (1996) Post-translational cooperativity of ornithine decarboxylase induction by estrogens and peptide growth factors in human breast cancer cells. Mol Cell Endocrinol 117:211–218.
115. Manni A, Wright C (1984) Reversal of the antiproliferative effect of the antiestrogen tamoxifen by polyamines in breast cancer cells. Endocrinology 114:836–839.
116. Cohen F, Manni A, Glickman P, Bartholomew M, Demers L (1988) Involvement of the polyamine pathway in antiestrogen-induced growth inhibition of human breast cancer. Cancer Res 48:6819–6825.
117. Manni A, Wechter R, Wei L, Heitjan D, Demers L (1995) Phenotypic features of breast cancer cells overexpressing ornithine-decarboxylase. J Cell Physiol 163:129–136.
118. Persson L, Rosengren E (1988) Increased formation of N^1-acetylspermidine in human breast cancer. Cancer Lett 45:83–86.
119. Wagner AJ, Meyers C, Laimins LA, Hay N (1993) c-myc induces the expression and activity of ornithine decarboxylase. Cell Growth Differ 4:879–883.
120. Wrighton C, Busslinger M (1993) Direct transcriptional stimulation of the ornithine decarboxylase gene by fos in PC12 cells but not in fibroblasts. Mol Cell Biol 13:4657–4669.
121. Moshier J, Dosescu J, Skunca M, Luk G (1993) Transformation of NIH/3T3 cells by ornithine decarboxylase overexpression. Cancer Res 53:2618–2622.
122. Kingsnorth A, Wallace H, Bundred N, Dixon J (1984) Polyamines in breast cancer. Br J Surg 71:352–356.

123. Halmekyto M, Hyttinen J, Sinervirta R, Utrianen M, Myohanen S, Volpio H, et al. (1991) Transgenic mice aberantly expressing human ornithine decarboxylase gene. J Biol Chem 266:19746–19751.
124. Mesa-Tejada R, Keydar I, Ramanarayanan M, Ohno T, Fenoglio C, Spiegelman S (1978) Detection in human breast carcinomas of an antigen immunologically related to a group-specific antigen of mouse mammary tumor virus. Proc Natl Acad Sci USA 75:1529–1533.
125. Litvinov S, Golovkina T (1989) Expression of proteins immunologically related to murine mammary tumor virus (MMTV) core proteins in the cells of breast cancer continuous lines MCF-7, T47D, MDA-231 and cells from human mild. Acta Virol 33:137–142.
126. Day NK, Witkin SS, Sarkar NH, Kinne D, Jussawalla DJ, Levin A, et al. (1981) Antibodies reactive with murine mammary tumor virus in sera of patients with breast cancer: geographic and family studies. Proc Natl Acad Sci USA 78:2483–2487.
127. Callahan R, Drohan W, Tronick S, Schlom J (1982) Detection and cloning of human DNA sequences relaed to the mouse mammary tumor virus genome. Proc Natl Acad Sci USA 79:5503–5507.
128. Axel R, Schlom J, Spiegelman S (1972) Presence in human breast cancer of RNA homologous to mouse mammary tumor virus RNA. Nature 235:32–36.
129. de Ricqles D, Olomucki A, Gosselin F, Ridereau R (1993) Breast cancer and T-cell-mediated immunity to proteins of the mouse mammary tumour virus (MMTV). Eur Cytokine Netw 4:153–160.
130. Crepin M, Lidereau R, Chermann J, Pouillart P, Magdamenat H, Montagnier L (1984) Sequences related to mouse mammry tumor virus genome in tumor cells and lymphocytes from patients with breast cancer. Biochem Biophys Res Commun 118:324–331.
131. Al-Sumidaie AM, Hart CA, Leinster SJ, Green CD (1988) Particles with properties of retroviruses in monocytes from patients with breast cancer. Lancet 1:5–8.
132. Pogo BG-T, Holland JF (1997) Possibilities of a viral etiology for human breast cancer: a review. Biol Trace Element Res 56:131–142.
133. Rettig M, Ma H, Vescio R, Pold M, Schiller G, Belson D, et al. (1997) Kaposi's sarcoma-associated herpesvirus infection of bone marrow dendritic cells from multiple myeloma patients. Science 276:1851–1854.
134. Allred DC, Clark GM, Molina R, Tandon AK, Schnitt SJ, Gilchrist KW, et al. (1992) Overexpression of HER-2/*neu* and its relationship with other prognostic factors change during the progression of in situ to invasive breast cancer. Hum Pathol 23:974–979.
135. King M-C, Rowell S, Love SM (1993) Inherited breast and ovarian cancer. JAMA 269:1975–1980.
136. Bieche I, Lidereau R (1995) Genetic alterations in breast cancer. Genes Chromosom Cancer 14:227–251.
137. Ruppert JM, Wright M, Rosenfeld M, Grushcow J, Bilbao G, Curiel DT, et al. (1997) Gene therapy strategies for carcinoma of the breast. Breast Cancer Res Treat 44:93–114.
138. Collins K, Jacks T, Pavletich NK (1997) The cell cycle and cancer. Proc Natl Acad Sci USA 94:2776–2778.

11 Interactions Between Stroma and Epithelium in Breast Cancer

Implications for Tumor Genesis, Growth, and Progression

Kevin J. Cullen, MD, *Sahana S. Kaup, and Audrey A. Rasmussen*, MS

INTRODUCTION

Breast cancers are traditionally considered epithelial malignancies. In reality, breast cancers, like normal breast itself, are complex tissues with many interdependent components. Although it is the epithelial cell from ductal or lobular elements within the breast which undergoes malignant transformation, no breast cancer can grow beyond microscopic size and become clinically significant without a complex and dynamic interaction with the surrounding stroma. Stromal elements, consisting of matrix proteins, fibroblasts, vascular elements, and their myriad cellular products, are critical determinants of the growth and malignant behavior of a breast cancer. Ongoing growth and dissemination of a breast malignancy requires complex, but poorly understood, interactions between these elements.

Shortly after undergoing malignant transformation, a new tumor must acquire adequate blood supply to permit further growth. Future invasive or metastatic potential is determined by the ability of the tumor to degrade surrounding normal proteins including basement membrane and intercellular matrix permitting tumor cells access to lymphatic or vascular channels. The same cell-cell interactions are necessary for a metastatic focus to develop at a site distant from the primary tumor.

In the past, laboratory models of breast cancer have focused largely on analysis of the cellular and molecular biology of epithelial cells themselves. Increasingly, the interactions between tumor epithelium and stroma have been demonstrated to play an essential role in the progression of breast malignancies. This new insight has led to new avenues for therapeutic intervention and this disease as well as other malignancies.

STROMAL/EPITHELIAL INTERACTIONS IN NORMAL AND MALIGNANT BREAST

The growth and normal differentiation of breast epithelium is a dynamic process. Interacting signals from hormones, growth factors, and the epithelial microenvironment

From: *Contemporary Endocrinology: Endocrinology of Breast Cancer*
Edited by: A. Manni © Humana Press Inc., Totowa, NJ

regulate the profound changes in breast morphology and function throughout the stages of life. Structural and functional changes in the embryo, as well as the pubertal, lactating, premenopausal, and postmenopausal breast, also take place as a result of the influence of discrete autocrine, paracrine, and endocrine effects. The order and hierarchy of interactions between the complex mixture of cellular and extracellular components within the breast are incompletely understood, at best. Recent in vitro model systems have provided improved insight into these relationships.

An early demonstration of the importance of interactions between stroma and epithelium in the development of the breast was shown in rodent experiments, which demonstrated that for fetal mammary epithelium to develop normally into typical breast glands, interactions with a specific breast stromal matrix were required. Epithelial tissues from other sites did not undergo mammary differentiation when implanted in adult mammary fat pads *(1)*. However, converse experiments demonstrated that epithelium from other nonbreast sources including salivary gland would differentiate into mammary tissue when cultured in the presence of mesenchyme from mouse mammary fat pads. This mammary glandular differentiation was not observed when embryonic mesenchyme derived from embryonic lung pancreas or kidney was used *(2)*.

In vitro studies of breast epithelial differentiation have taken advantage of the expression of milk proteins such as β-casein by well-differentiated mammary epithelial cells. Complex in vitro three-dimensional model systems take advantage of this marker to evaluate specific stromal/epithelial interactions necessary to induce expression of this marker of terminal differentiation. Epithelial cells grown from pregnant rat mammary tissue produce β-casein when grown on Matrigel, an artificial basement membrane *(3)*. With this matrix, these cells form complex spherical structures resembling glands into which β-casein is secreted. Subsequent studies demonstrate that this differentiation is due to epithelial β_1-integrin subunit interactions with the extracellular matrix proteins *(4)*.

Whereas normal human breast epithelial cells in culture exhibit similar differentiation in response to culture on an artificial extracellular matrix construct (including production of β-casein, expression of basement membrane, and formation of glandular structures), malignant breast carcinoma cell lines do not show this response in vitro *(5)*. Neither immortal cell lines nor primary breast tumor cultures showed lumen formation, cellular polarity, or production of endogenous basement membrane when cultured on Matrigel. These experiments demonstrate that malignant breast epithelium has lost most of the differentiation responses to extracellular matrix components that characterize normal breast epithelium. Cancerous breast epithelium must therefore either have acquired an altered response to paracrine signals or developed its own autocrine modes of growth regulation.

Numerous studies indicate that soluble factors produced by stromal fibroblasts can exert distinct paracrine growth effects on normal and malignant breast epithelium. These effects appear to be specific to the site of origin of the stromal fibroblasts. Although some investigators have concluded that conditioned media from fibroblast derived from malignant lesions are mitogenic for malignant breast epithelial cells, and conditioned media from fibroblasts derived from benign breast tissues such as reduction mammoplasties are not *(6)*, other investigators have found that all fibroblasts exerted a mitogenic influence on human breast cancer epithelial cells when cultured in vitro *(7,8)*. The latter has been the experience in our laboratory as well.

Other lines of evidence strongly suggest that distinct populations of fibroblasts exist in normal as opposed to malignant breast. Several studies have shown that fibroblasts isolated from the stroma of malignant breast tissue exhibit migratory patterns in culture reminiscent of fetal fibroblasts. By contrast, fibroblasts from normal breast lack the ability to migrate into collagen gels when plated at confluent density *(9,10)*.

Furthermore, other studies suggest that skin fibroblasts from patients with breast cancer behave differently from skin fibroblasts in normals, suggesting an altered phenotype for fibroblasts outside the breast in cancer patients. Schor and others *(11–14)* have suggested that dermal fibroblasts from breast cancer patients have certain fetal phenotypic characteristics when compared with normal breast. These studies have largely evaluated patterns of cell proliferation in three-dimensional culture, but to date, no clear genotypic differences between skin fibroblasts in breast cancer patients and normals have been described.

STROMAL GENE PRODUCTS CRITICAL TO BREAST TUMOR GENESIS AND PROGRESSION

Matrix Proteins and Proteases

The extracellular matrix produced by breast stromal cells provides more than a simple passive scaffolding for epithelial cells. In addition to providing both boundaries and support for breast epithelial cells, these matrix proteins specifically influence the orientation and differentiation of normal breast epithelium. Again, coculture experiments demonstrate that mammary epithelial cells undergo significant morphologic and functional differentiation when grown in contact with the appropriate matrix *(15,16)*.

Although the stromal matrix exerts profound influences on tumor epithelium, in order for a tumor to grow and metastasize, tumor epithelium must be able to degrade and escape the extracellular matrix to gain access to lymphatic and vascular channels leading away from the primary tumor site. A large and expanding literature has emerged over the last decade describing the enzymes involved in degradation of matrix. Among these are the urokinase-type and tissue-type plasminogen activators, type IV collagenase, and others (for review, see ref. *17*). Not surprisingly, abundant recent studies have demonstrated that expression of these enzymes has critical prognostic importance in breast cancer as well as other malignancies *(18)*. In breast cancer, expression of these enzymes, including plasminogen activator, may be regulated by estrogen and presumably by other stromal interactions *(19–21)*. Whereas some components of the urokinase system are expressed in tumor epithelium, urokinase plasminogen activator is expressed by stromal myofibroblasts directly *(22)*.

In addition to widely studied collagenases and the plasminogen activator system, other stromal proteases may be important in the progression from in situ to invasive and metastatic breast cancer. Basset and coworkers *(23)* cloned a novel metalloproteinase based on subtractive hybridization comparing breast malignancy with fibroadenoma. Stromelysin-3 (ST-3) expression, although highly specific for tumors, is expressed not in tumor epithelium, but rather in surrounding stroma. Expression was specifically seen immediately surrounding malignant epithelial islands. No signal was detected in stroma surrounding in situ carcinomas. This line of evidence provides additional support for the hypothesis that the stroma surrounding malignant breast epithelium is phenotypically and functionally distinct from the stroma of normal breast. Interestingly, this protease is also expressed in fetal stromal tissues, where it may have an important role in the continuous process of gestational tissue remodeling *(23)*.

Peptide Growth Factors: IGF-II

A large body of research has developed in the last dozen years evaluating the expression and function of peptide growth factors in breast cancer. It has been apparent for some time that the stroma of normal and malignant breast is an active site of production of a number of these peptides, particularly the insulin-like growth factors, IGF-I and IGF-II.

Working in matched cultures of fibroblast derived from normal breast, breast tumor, and normal skin in patients undergoing surgery for breast cancer, we demonstrated that IGF expression differs significantly between normal and malignant breast stromal fibroblasts. Fibroblasts surrounding malignant breast epithelium preferentially expressed the potent mitogen IGF-II. By contrast, fibroblasts of normal breast predominantly express IGF-I. However, even though IGF-II expression was seen in malignant breast stroma but not normal stroma, no similar differences in expression of other peptide growth factors (transforming growth factor-α [TGF-α], fibroblast growth factors, and platelet-derived growth factors A and B) paralleled this change in gene expression *(24)*.

Since the differences in growth factor expression were seen in culture long after the stroma have been removed from the paracrine influences of surrounding malignant breast or normal breast epithelium, these changes in IGF expression appear to be the result of stable selection of stromal cells with an altered phenotype.

Subsequently, we demonstrated that stromal cells derived from normal breast, (IGF-II negative) showed marked induction of IGF-II expression when cultured in the presence of malignant breast epithelial cells (MCF-7). This response was seen only when stromal cells were plated at low density and permitted to proliferate through several cell divisions in the presence of malignant breast epithelium. When stromal cells were plated at high density and were largely contact inhibited, little induction of IGF-II expression was seen. These experiments were performed in a contact-independent coculture system in which fibroblasts and epithelial cells were separated by a porous membrane. This implies that soluble factors produced by breast epithelium were responsible for alteration in stromal phenotype *(25)*.

Coexpression of IGF-II and ST-3: Indicators of a Fetal Stromal Phenotype

Given the similarity in the pattern of expression reported for ST-3 and IGF-II, we asked whether these two genes were in fact coexpressed in the same cells. Analysis of stromal fibroblasts from normal breast confirmed that neither IGF-II or ST-3 was expressed, whereas fibroblasts derived from malignant breast tumors expressed both ST-3 and IGF-II. This provides further evidence of a tumor-specific stromal cell phenotype in breast cancer.

An understanding of the cellular origin of breast epithelium and stroma points out interesting relationships between expression of IGF-II and ST-3 in breast cancer and other malignancies. During fetal development, breast epithelium is derived from invagination of embryonic ectoderm, whereas stromal cells are derived from embryonic mesenchyme (mesoderm). In subsequent studies, we analyzed the expression of IGF-II and ST-3 and mesenchymal malignancies (sarcomas). In these tumors, we found a similar pattern of coexpression. Immunohistochemical analysis of IGF-II and ST-3 protein expression in sarcomas and breast tumors confirmed the mRNA data *(26,27)*.

ST-3 mRNA expression was also seen in most colon cancer cell lines, again matching reports of IGF-II gene expression. Since the two proteins are known to play an important role during fetal growth and development, their coexpression in fibroblasts from malignant tumors of ectodermal (breast cancer) and mesodermal (sarcoma) origin as well as in epithelial cells of endodermal origin (colon cancer) implies a more primitive cellular phenotype. The coordinated expression in a breast tumor of a growth factor and protease, which have important functions in regulating fetal growth and tissue remodeling, may be an important mechanism by which an adult malignancy can escape normal growth regulation.

ORIGINS OF STROMAL CELLS IN BREAST MALIGNANCIES

Although it appears clear that stromal fibroblasts within malignant breast tumors show specific, preferential expression of IGF-II (among other gene products), the origin of those stromal cells remains in question. Existing data may be interpreted as supporting a hypothesis in which IGF-II-expressing fibroblasts existed in the stroma before malignant transformation and that this IGF-II-expressing subpopulation, responding to paracrine signals from transformed breast epithelium, later migrated and became predominant in the cancer. In this model, IGF-II expression in the stroma could either predispose breast epithelium to become malignant or simply be the marker of another transforming event. By contrast, if all stromal fibroblasts in normal breast represent a precursor population capable of achieving one of several differentiated phenotypes in response to paracrine interactions, soluble factors from tumor epithelium could induce proximal stromal fibroblasts to upregulate IGF-II expression. As discussed above, our in vitro coculture model, which demonstrates a marked increase in IGF-II mRNA expression in fibroblast from normal breast cultured in the presence of MCF-7 cells, is most easily interpreted by the hypothesis that the upregulation of IGF-II message is the result of fibroblast selection by breast tumor epithelium rather than simply induction of IGF-II expression.

This selection of a subpopulation of stromal fibroblasts is distinct from the pattern of clonal epithelial cell expansion that has been demonstrated to occur in the progression from in situ to invasive cancer *(28)*. It appears likely that homogeneous populations of fibroblasts—each with distinctive phenotypes—can arise from an initially heterogeneous stromal cell population within the breast *(29)*. This hypothesis is supported by the observation that cultured fibroblast populations maintain their distinctive phenotypes, especially with regard to IGF or stromelysin expression long after they are removed from the influence of the tumor itself.

Coculture models utilizing collagen gels provide additional insight into these important stromal/epithelial interactions. Ronnov-Jensen and coworkers *(30)* have performed an extensive series of studies examining the origin of stromal myofibroblasts, which form a significant portion of the stromal reaction within breast tumors. These cells are characterized by the expression of smooth muscle-specific proteins including α-smooth muscle actin, smooth muscle myosin heavy chain, and calponin *(30)*. In contrast to myoepithelial cells, these myofibroblasts lack keratin expression. Coculture experiments in collagen gels by this group demonstrated that stromal fibroblasts grown in the presence of epithelial cells show significant upregulation of smooth muscle proteins, especially α-smooth muscle actin. The authors also demonstrated that vascular smooth muscle cells in proximity to malignant epithelium possess the ability to migrate toward tumor cells and alter their phenotype from vascular smooth muscle toward stromal myofibroblast *(30)*.

Staining of serial sections in our laboratory for IGF-II and α-smooth muscle actin demonstrate that these two proteins are coexpressed, implying that the IGF-II-expressing cells are derived from this myofibroblast population. Taken together, these studies suggest that paracrine soluble factors secreted by breast tumor epithelium induce selection of myofibroblasts, in part from vascular smooth muscle. They then populate the malignant breast stroma.

REGULATION OF STROMAL GENE EXPRESSION

Hormonal Regulation of Stromal Growth Factor Expression

Although estrogens are generally thought to act on breast tumor epithelium, estrogen may regulate expression of stromal proteins, including IGF-II, in very important ways. In human breast cancer, the best studied estrogen effects are mediated by estrogen receptor (ER) expressed in malignant tumor epithelium. Functional ER does not appear to be expressed in stromal tissues. Numerous studies have shown modulation of many IGF signaling components (ligands, receptors, and binding proteins) within epithelial cells as a result above estrogen stimulation, but the ability of these components to increase IGF-II in the stroma appears to be indirect, mediated by factors expressed by these ER-positive cells.

Evidence of estrogen regulation of fibroblast IGF-II expression in hormonally responsive mammary cancer stems from studies in rat NMU tumors. In this well-established tumor model system, Manni and coworkers *(31)* utilized mRNA in situ hybridization to identify the origin of IGF-related proteins in these tumors. They found that IGF-II expression was confined to the stroma and was under the positive regulation of estrogen. IGF-II levels decreased dramatically following ovariectomy (accompanied by tumor regression) and increased significantly with hormone replacement, resulting in the reactivation of tumor growth. Conversely, the levels of inhibitory binding protein IGFBP-6 dramatically increased with ovariectomy and fell with estrogen replacement, a change that could also increase estrogen-induced IGF-II effects *in vivo (31)*.

Genetic Regulation of Stromal Growth Factor Expression

A rapidly developing literature implicates imprinting as a critical regulatory mechanism for a number of growth-regulatory genes in breast cancer, including IGF-II. Genomic imprinting is defined as the epigenetic modification of a parental chromosome that regulates its expression *(32)*. In particular, DNA methylation of the promoter plays a role in imprinting, since it is specific to certain gene regions rich in cytosine and guanine residues known as CpG islands and is stably inherited for several generations *(33,34)*. These unique methylation patterns result in differential allelic expression of the parental chromosomes *(31–33)*. Expression of IGF-II (which maps to chromosome 11 [11p15.5]) in normal cells, is primarily from the unmethylated paternal allele; the methylated maternal allele remains "silent" *(31–35)*. IGF-II expression is driven by four successive promoters, P1–P4 *(36,37)*. The promoters P2, P3, and P4 are included in a CpG island and thus are regulated by methylation *(37)*. The P1 promoter is located 20 kb upstream of the CpG island and appears to be regulated independently *(36,37)*.

Methylation and Expression of IGF-II and H19 Genes

Regulation of IGF-II expression may not, however, be under the sole control of its cognate promoters. An adjacent locus on chromosome 11, H19, may contribute to the regulation of IGF-II expression in a tissue and developmentally specific fashion *(38,39)*. IGF-II loss of imprinting is associated with increased methylation of five *Hpa*II sites upstream of the H19 locus and a decrease in H19 expression *(40)*. The H19 promoter is normally hemimethylated; at the H19 promoter, the paternal allele is hypermethylated and the maternal allele is hemimethylated. Thus, the IGF-II and H19 loci are reciprocally imprinted *(41)*.

Loss of Imprinting of IGF-II in Fetal Development and Cancer

Although it appears that several combinations of IGF-II promoter activity are possible, ultimately the four promoter regions give rise to the same preprotein. In the liver, IGF-II expression is biallelic at P1 and monoallelic at P2–P4 *(37)*. However, promoter activity may differ in various tissues: P1 is expressed in most adult tissues, whereas P2–P4 are expressed in developing embryonic tissue *(42)*. Taking advantage of *Apa* I restriction fragment length polymorphism, Taniguchi et al. *(42)* demonstrated that the P1 promoter is expressed monoallelically in various tissues in early fetus. However, later in fetal development, imprinting of the P1 promoter is relaxed, or undergoes loss of imprinting (LOI), leading to biallelic expression of IGF-II from this promoter.

An example of this phenomenon occurs in fetal kidney; P1 promoter imprinting is relaxed, whereas the other three promoters maintain their imprinting throughout fetal development. In Wilms' tumor, a pediatric neoplasm of the kidney characterized by overexpression of IGF-II, there are three possible situations: imprinting may be relaxed at all four promoters (LOI); the promoters may undergo monoallelic expression; or, through loss of heterozygosity (LOH), IGF-II may be expressed from all four promoters on the remaining allele *(42)*. Loss of imprinting has been analyzed extensively in Wilms' tumor; out of 42 non-LOH Wilms' tumors screened for imprinting status, 77% of 16 informative tumors showed biallelic expression of IGF-II *(8)*. Other groups have shown similar LOI in this disease.

The involvement of H19 promoter methylation in IGF-II expression is demonstrated in an analysis of nine cases of Wilms' tumors exhibiting LOI of IGF-II *(40)*. These cases had reduced expression of H19 and increased expression of IGF-II from the maternal allele. In these tissues, the H19 promoter showed 90–100% methylation of the normally hemimethylated maternal allele, mimicking the paternal allele pattern *(40)*. This evidence is further supported by work done with DNA methyltransferase-deficient mice. In homozygous mutants, the paternal allele of the H19 gene was activated whereas the activated paternal allele of the IGF-II gene was repressed, demonstrating that methylation of the H19 promoter is required for IGF-II expression *(34)*. However, human choriocarcinoma cells and colon adenocarcinoma cells treated with a DNA methyltransferase inhibitor, 5-aza-2-deoxycytidine, undergo a reversal of LOI. The inhibitor switched both IGF-II and H19 from biallelic to monoallelic expression and activated H19 expression. The data also show that the effect of 5-aza-2-deoxycytidine was preferential to one allele *(43)*. Thus the cell context may determine the influence of methylation on IGF-II and H19 expression.

Loss of Imprinting of IGF-II in Breast Cancer

Recently, data have emerged suggesting that LOI may be important in determining IGF-II in breast cancer. A panel of tumor lines from various tissues including breast was examined to measure the level of methylation at the different IGF-II promoter regions:

there was increased methylation at promoters P2–P4 in the breast cell lines *(36)*. Recently it was demonstrated that out of 30 cases of sporadic breast carcinoma, 12 cases were heterozygous at an *Apa* I site of the IGF-II locus. Nine of these cases showed IGF-II expression from both alleles by cDNA polymerase chain reaction. Thus it was concluded that about 75% of informative cases studied exhibited loss of imprinting of IGF-II *(44)*. This data conflict with previous research that examined 18 fresh frozen breast tumors and normal adjacent tissue and 14 specimens of parrafin-embedded, formalin-fixed tissue. Imprinting of the IGF-II and H19 genes was maintained in practically all informative tissue, fresh frozen or fixed, leading to the authors' conclusion that LOI does not directly correlate with breast tumor progression *(45)*. This apparent controversy may be due to differing sensitivity of the assays used.

Work in our own laboratory suggests that LOI is present in IGF-II-expressing fibroblasts derived from breast cancers. However, significant further research will be required to define fully the role of imprinting in the regulation of IGF-II expression in breast cancer. However, since this mechanism may be amenable to pharmacologic manipulation (as discussed above, 5-azacytidine inhibits DNA methyltransferase, for example), this is an area with potential clinical impact.

PATHOPHYSIOLOGIC CONSEQUENCES OF STROMAL GROWTH FACTOR (IGF-II) EXPRESSION

Epithelial Cell Proliferation

Abundant evidence suggests that stromal growth factors, including IGF-II, can significantly enhance the growth of breast tumor epithelium and enhance its malignant behavior. The mitogenic effects of IGF-II are mediated by the IGF-I receptor, which is ubiquitously expressed in breast tumor epithelium. The IGF-I receptor serves as a critical cell cycle checkpoint. Activation of this receptor is critical for progression into S phase and can effectively inhibit apoptosis in many cell types. The mitogenic signaling cascades converge primarily on the activation of $p21^{ras}$ and its related network of mitogen-activated protein (MAP) kinases *(46)*, whereas the inhibition of apoptosis has recently been found to modulate key apoptotic proteins in human neural cell lines *(47)*. Although aberrant regulation of each of these processes might contribute to malignancy, IGF-IR-mediated transformation can also occur by independent signaling events. Studies in rodent fibroblast models have led to the conclusion that distinct regions of the IGF-IR control mitogenesis, transformation, and apoptosis *(48)*.

High levels of the IGF-IR are found on cultured breast epithelial cells, and paracrine and autocrine sources of IGF ligands are unusually high in breast tumors *(49–51)*. Also, elevated levels of IGF-IR and IGF-I binding sites have been reported in neoplastic breast epithelial cells, but not in benign epithelium or breast stroma *(52,53)*.

Numerous studies demonstrate that both IGF-I and IGF-II are mitogens for malignant breast epithelial cells. Furthermore, IGF-II overexpression in MCF-7 breast cancer cells produced clones with distinct alterations in morphology. These cells grew autonomously and adopted a more malignant phenotype, displaying a loss of contact inhibition and the ability to grow in soft agar and suspension cultures *(54)*. MCF-7 cells overexpressing IGF-II maintained their responsiveness to estrogen, but antibodies against the IGF-IR were unable to decrease this growth. These findings were confirmed in a similar study by Lee et al. *(55)* However, it is an oversimplification to imply that IGF-II is the predominant stromal mitogen in breast cancer. Media conditioned by breast tumor fibroblasts is strongly mitogenic for MCF-7 epithelial cells, but this stimulation is only partially blocked by saturating doses of IGFBP-1, an inhibitory binding protein that can completely abrogate the stimulatory effects of recombinant IGF-I or IGF-II in this model *(8)*.

In spite of its strong mitogenic effects, high levels of IGF-IR are generally correlated with a good prognosis. Retrospective studies positively correlate high IGF-I, IGF-II, and IGF-IR with longer disease-free periods and better overall survival, even in lymph node-positive patients *(56,57)*. Although this could reflect a beneficial effect of the IGFs, it may simply be that this better prognosis actually reflects an association between their expression and a cancer at an earlier stage of progression *(58)*. This notion is supported indirectly by the cellular localization of IGF-II-positive fibroblasts to areas adjacent to less invasive breast lesions and within highly desmoplastic stroma *(26)*. Additionally, the few malignant breast epithelial cell lines that express endogenous IGF-II were derived from well-differentiated, hormonally responsive tumors.

Invasive Potential

As discussed earlier, stromally expressed proteases serve to enhance the invasive and metastatic potential of a breast cancer. Directly and indirectly, IGF-II may enhance these effects. Among the IGF family members, the M6P/IGF-IIR is considered to have the greatest potential for influencing the degradation of the breast extracellular matrix. In this regard, the importance of the M6P/IGF-IIR in modulating the activity of IGF-II is superseded by its regulation of key M6P-bearing proteins. In many tissues, including the breast, trafficking of M6P-linked lysozomal enzymes and the activation of various M6P-bearing growth factors may increase the invasive potential of a tumor.

Analysis of breast tumor cytosols reveals a positive correlation between high levels of the M6P-tagged aspartyl protease, cathepsin D, and an increased risk of developing metastases *(59,60)*. However, there is no clear agreement in the the literature regarding the importance of cathepsin D as a prognostic indicator in breast cancer. High extracellular accumulations of cathepsin D could result from competition between IGF-II and M6P-bearing enzymes for binding to the M6P/IGF-IIR or from inactivating mutations to the M6P/IGF-IIR. There is evidence that both events occur in breast cancer. Overexpression of precursor IGF-II has been shown to alter the routing of cathepsin D from the lysozomal compartment to the extracellular space in a number of malignant cell types, including MCF-7 cells *(61,62)*. Furthermore, consistent with its role as a tumor suppressor gene, inactivating mutations in both alleles coding for the M6P/IGF-IIR have been identified in a significant percentage of primary breast tumors *(63)*.

The M6P/IGF-IIR also indirectly upregulates the activity of another protein important in extracellular matrix degradation, the urokinase-type plasminogen activator (uPA), by its involvement in the activation of the M6P-bearing TGF-β. This enzyme converts the zymogen plasminogen to plasmin, a serine protease with broad substrate specificity. Plasmin can cleave most extracellular matrix proteins, plus activate additional extracellular matrix degrading proteases and growth factors, including TGF-β itself *(64,65)*. In a potential positive feedback loop, TGF-β can also upregulate the levels of uPA mRNA and secretion by a number of separate mechanisms.

This may have significance in breast cancer progression. TGF-β is frequently secreted by cultured breast tumor epithelial cells *(66)*, and high levels of uPA have been shown to be significant in terms of the invasiveness of malignant breast epithelium. In breast cancer cell lines expressing different levels of uPA, there was a direct correlation to their ability to form plasmin and invade the artificial basement membrane Matrigel *(67)*. In the cell line that expressed the highest level of uPA, the hormone independent MDA-MB-231 cells, TGF-β was able to increase further the extent of uPA secretion *(68)*. Likewise, TGF-β has also been shown to increase the level of uPA expression in macrophages, a frequent stromal component of breast tumors *(69)*. Thus, the M6P/IGF-IIR is an essential component of the uPA activation pathway through its production of TGF-β.

Chemotaxis

Modified Boyden chamber and monolayer wounding assays have demonstrated chemotactic IGF effects in a number of normal and cancer cell lines *(70–73)*. Recently, this list has expanded to include cultured breast cancer cells *(74)*. Doerr and Jones *(74)* showed that MCF-7 breast cancer cells migrated specifically in response to 10 n*M* IGF-I, but only when plated on membranes coated with either vitronectin or type IV collagen. By contrast, the more aggressive MDA-MB-231 cells were less selective. They had the ability to traverse membranes coated with a wide variety of extracellular matrix components in response to several growth factors.

Some effort has focused on determining the receptors that mediate the IGF-I-induced motility response. Many studies have used αIR3 to demonstrate that IGF-IR signaling is a requirement for IGF chemotaxis *(75,76)*.

Angiogenesis

Angiogenesis is vital for the survival and propagation of a solid tumor. The increased network of blood vessels is used to deliver oxygen and nutrients to rapidly proliferating cells, remove metabolic waste, and provide a route for cancerous cells to propagate at distant metastatic sites. For the most part, high IGF expression does not directly correlate with an increase in metastatic growth, but the chemotactic effects of the IGFs on endothelial cells is a primary component of the literature that describes IGF effects on angiogenesis.

In vitro models have demonstrated that IGF-I can promote chemotaxis and induce tube formation of cultured vascular endothelial cells in a dose dependent manner *(77)*. Wound repair and corneal implant assays have also shown a modest in vivo angiogenic effect for IGF-I *(78,79)*. In these assays, the effects of this growth factor are frequently less pronounced than for highly angiogenic cytokines. In what may be a tissue-specific response, IGF-I neutralization in the ischemic central zone of injured mouse skeletal muscle paradoxically resulted in a notable increase in the number of capillaries *(80)*.

There is some suggestion that the M6P/IGF-IIR can mediate some IGF angiogenic effects through interactions with its IGF-II binding sites. Volpert et al. *(81)* extended their finding of M6P/IGF-IIR-induced endothelial cell migration to an angiogenic rat corneal implant model *(81)*. In this study, the implantation of pellets containing either IGF-I, IGF-II, or [Leu27]IGF-II generated a significant increase in neovascularization. The ability of M6P to inhibit the IGF-II and [Leu27]IGF-II effects reinforced the hypothesis that their effects were mediated by the M6P/IGF-IIR. By contrast, their conclusion that IGF-I acts through the M6P/IGF-IIR is unexpected since binding affinity data suggest that the biologic relevance of this interaction is negligible *(82)*. Furthermore, the finding that M6P was unable to compete away the IGF-I effects on angiogenesis, which were thought to be mediated by the M6P/IGF-IIR, was not addressed by the authors.

CONCLUSION

Stromal/epithelial interactions are critical at all stages of development and growth, in both the normal and malignant breast. Like the complex organ from which it arises, a breast cancer is a dynamic collection of varied cells and subcellular structures. Their interactions influence gene expression, cellular growth, morphology, and malignant potential. As the knowledge of the richness and complexity of these interactions increases, so too does the opportunity for targeted interventions, which may inhibit tumor growth in clinically useful ways.

REFERENCES

1. Sakakura T, Nishizuka Y, Dawe CJ (1979) Capacity of mammary fat pads of adult C3H/HeMs mice to interact morphogenetically with fetal mammary epithelium. J Natl Cancer Inst 63:733–736.
2. Sakakura T, Sakagami Y, Nishizuka Y (1979) Persistence of responsiveness to adult mammary gland to induction by embryonic mesenchyme. Dev Biol 72:201–210.
3. Streuli CH, Bailey N, Bissel MJ (1991) Control of mammary epithelial differentiation: basement membrane induces tissue-specific gene expression in the absence of cell-cell interaction and morphological polarity. J Cell Biol 115:1383–1391.
4. Streuli CH, Bissel MJ (1990) Expression of extracellular matrix components is regulated by substratum. J Cell Biol 110:1405–1415.
5. Petersen OW, Ronnov-Jessen L, Howlett AR, Bissell MJ (1992) Interaction with basement membrane serves to rapidly distinguish growth and differentiation pattern of normal and malignant human breast epithelial cells [published erratum appears in Proc Natl Acad Sci USA 1993; 90:2556]. Proc Natl Acad Sci USA 89:9064–9068.
6. Adams EF, Newton CJ, Braunsberg H, Shaikh N, Ghilchik M, James VHT (1988) Effects of human breast fibroblasts on growth and 17β-estradiol dehydrogenase activity of MCF-7 cells in culture. Breast Cancer Res Treat 11:165–172.
7. Ryan MC, Orr DJ, Horgan K (1993) Fibroblast stimulation of breast cancer cell growth in a serum-free system. Br J Cancer 67:1268–1273.
8. van Roozendaal KEP, Klijn JGM, van Ooijen B, Claassen C, Eggermont AMM, Henzen-Logmans SC, et al. (1996) Differential regulation of breast tumor cell proliferation by stromal fibroblasts of various breast sources. Int J Cancer 65:120–125.
9. Schor AM, Rushton G, Ferguson JE, Howell A, Redford J, Schor SL (1994) Phenotypic heterogeneity in breast fibroblasts: functional anomaly in fibroblasts from histologically normal tissue adjacent to carcinoma. Int J Cancer 59:25–32.
10. Brouty-Boye D, Mainguene C, Magnien V, Israel L, Beaupain R (1994) Fibroblast-mediated differentiation in human breast carcinoma cells (MCF-7) grown as nodules in vitro. Int J Cancer 56:731–735.
11. Azzarone B, Mareel M, Billard C, Scemama P, Chaponnier C, Maciera-Coelho A (1984) Abnormal properties of skin fibroblasts from patients with breast cancer. Int J Cancer 33:759–764.
12. Durning P, Schor SL, Sellwood RAS. (1984) Fibroblasts from patients with breast cancer show abnormal migratory behaviour *in vitro*. Lancet 2:890–892.
13. Schor SL, Haggie J, Durning P, Howell A, Sellwood RAS, Crowther D (1986) The occurrence of a foetal fibroblast phenotype in breast cancer. Int J Cancer 37:831–836.
14. Haggie J, Schor SL, Howell A, Birch JM, Sellwood RAS (1987) Fibroblasts from relatives of hereditary breast cancer display foetal-like behaviour *in vitro*. Lancet 1:1455–1457
15. Wicha MS, Lowrie G, Kohn E, Bagavandoss P, Mahn T (1982) Extracellular matrix promotes mammary epithelial growth and differentiation in vitro. Proc Natl Acad Sci USA 79:3213–3217.
16. Bissell MJ, Ram TJ (1989) Regulation of functional cytodifferentiation and histogenesis in mammary epithelial cells: role of the extracellular matrix. Environ Health Perspect 80:61–70.
17. Laiho M, Keski-Oja J (1989) Growth factors in the regulation of pericellular proteolysis: a review. Cancer Res 49:2533–2553.
18. Khokha R, Denhardt DT (1989) Matrix metalloproteinases and tissue inhibitor of metalloproteinases: a review of their role in tumorigenesis and tissue invasion. Invasion Metas 9:391–405.
19. Mira-y-Lopz R, Ossowski L (1987) Hormonal modulation of plasminogen activator: an approach to the prediction of human breast tumor responsiveness. Cancer Res 47:3558–3564.

20. Duffy MJ, O'Grady P, Simon J, Rose M, Lijnen HR (1986) Tissue-type plasminogen activator in breast cancer: relationship with estradiol and progesterone receptors. J Natl Cancer Inst 77:621–623.
21. Duffy MJ, Reilly D, O'Sullivan C, O'Higgans N, Fennelly JJ, Andreasen P (1990) Urokinase-plasminogen activator, a new and independent prognostic marker in breast cancer. Cancer Res 50:6827–6829.
22. Nielsen BS Sehested M, Timshel S, Pyke C, Dano K (1996) Messenger RNA for urokinase-plasminogen activator is expressed in myofibroblasts adjacent to cancer cells in human breast cancer. Lab Invest 74:168–177.
23. Basset P, Bellocq JP, Wolf C, Stoll I, Hutin P, Limacher JM, et al. (1990) A novel metalloproteinase gene specifically expressed in stromal cells of breast carcinomas. Nature 348:699–704.
24. Cullen KJ, Smith HS, Hill S, Rosen N, Lippman ME (1991) Growth factor messenger RNA expression by human breast fibroblasts from benign and malignant lesions. Cancer Res 51:4978–4985.
25. Singer C, Rasmussen A, Smith HS, Lippman ME, Lynch HT, Cullen KJ (1995) Malignant breast epithelium selects for insulin-like growth factor II expression in breast stroma: evidence for paracrine function. Cancer Res 55:2448–2454.
26. Giani C, Cullen KJ, Campani D, Rasmussen A (1996) IGF-II mRNA and protein are expressed in the stroma of invasive breast cancers: an in situ hybridization and immunohistochemistry study. Breast Cancer Res Treat 41:43–50.
27. Singer C, Rasmussen A, Lippman ME, Cullen KJ (1997) Coexpression of stromelysin-3 and insulin-like growth factor II in tumors of ectodermal, mesodermal, and endodermal origin: indicator of a fetal cell phenotype. J Clin Endocrinol Metab 82:1917–1922.
28. Zhuang Z, Merino MJ, Chuaqui R, Liotta LA, Emmert-Buck MR (1995) Identical allelic loss on chromosome 11q13 in microdissected in situ and invasive human breast cancer. Cancer Res 55:467–471.
29. Lazard D, Sastre X, Frid MG, Glukhova MA, Thiery JP, Koteliansky VE (1993) Expression of smooth muscle-specific proteins in myoepithelium and stromal myofibroblasts of normal and malignant human breast tissue. Proc Natl Acad Sci USA 90:999–1003
30. Ronnov-Jessen L, Petersen OW, Koteliansky VE, Bissell MJ (1995) The origin of the myofibroblasts in breast cancer. Recapitulation of tumor environment in culture unravels diversity and implicates converted fibroblasts and recruited smooth muscle cells. J Clin Invest 95:859–873.
31. Manni A, Badger B, Wei L, Zaenglein A, Grove R, Khin S, et al. (1994) Hormonal regulation of insulin-like growth factor II and insulin-like growth factor binding protein expression by breast cancer cells in vivo: evidence for stromal epithelial interactions. Cancer Res 54:2934–2942.
32. Lalande M (1997) Parental imprinting and human disease. Annu Rev Genet 30:173–195.
33. Razin A, Cedar H (1994) DNA methylation and genomic imprinting. Cell 77:473–476.
34. Li E, Beard C, Jaenisch R (1993) Role of DNA methylation in genomic imprinting. Nature 366:362–365.
35. Eden S, Cedar H (1995) Action at a distance. [News and Views]. Nature 375:16–17.
36. Issa JP, Vertino PM, Boehm CD, Newsham IF, Baylin SB (1996) Switch from monoallelic to biallelic human IGF-II promoter methylation during aging and carcinogenesis. Proc Natl Acad Sci USA 93:11757–11762.
37. Vu TH, Hoffman AR (1994) Promoter-specific imprinting of the human insulin-like growth factor-II gene. Nature 371:714–715.
38. Leighton PA, Ingram RS, Eggenschwiler, J, Efstratiadis A, Tilghman, SM (1995) Disruption of imprinting caused by deletion of the H19 gene region in mice. Nature 375: 34–39:1995.
39. Cui H, Hedborg F, Liangmei H, Nordenskjold A, Sandstedt B, Pfeifer-Ohlosson, S, et al. (1997) Inactivation of H19, an imprinted and putative tumor repressor gene, is a preneoplastic event during Wilms' tumorigenesis. Cancer Res 57:4469–4473.
40. Steenman MJC, Rainier S, Dobry CJ, Grundy P, Horon IL, Feinberg AP (1994) Loss of imprinting of IGF-II is linked to reduced expression and abnormal methylation of H19 in Wilms' yumour. Nature Genet 7:433–439.
41. Rainier S, Johnson LA, Dobry CJ, Ping AJ, Grundy PE, Feinberg AP (1993) Relaxation of imprinted genes in human cancer. Nature 362:747–749.
42. Taniguchi T, Schofield AE, Scarlett JL, Morison IM, Sullivan MJ, Reeve AE (1995) Altered specificity of IGF-II promoter imprinting during fetal development and onset of Wilms' Tumor. Oncogene 11:751–756.
43. Barletta JM, Rainier S, Feinberg AP (1997) Reversal of loss of imprinting in tumor cells by 5-aza-2ɜ-deoxycytidine. Cancer Res 57:48–50.
44. Wu HK, Squire JA, Catzavelos CG, Weksberg R (1997) Relaxation of imprinting of human insulin-like growth factor II gene, IGF-II, in sporadic breast carcinomas. Biochem Biophys Res Commun 235:123–129.
45. Yballe CM, Vu TH, Hoffman AR (1996) Imprinting and expression of insulin-like growth factor-II and H19 in normal breast tissue and breast tumor. J Clin Endocrinol Metab 81:1607–1612.

46. White MF, Kahn CR (1994) The insulin signaling system. J Biol Chem 269:1–4.
47. Singleton JR, Dixit VM, Feldman EL (1996) Type I insulin-like growth factor receptor activation regulates apoptotic proteins. J Biol Chem 271:31791–31794.
48. O'Connor R, Kauffmann-Zeh A, Liu Y, Lehar S, Evan GI, Baserga R, Blattler WA (1997) Identification of domains of the insulin-like growth factor I receptor that are required for protection from apoptosis. Mol Cell Biol 17:427–435.
49. Yee D, Cullen KJ, Paik S, Perdue JF, Hampton B, Schwartz A, et al. (1988) Insulin-like growth factor II mRNA expression in human breast cancer; insulin-like growth factor II mRNA expression in human breast cancer. Cancer Res 48:6691–6696.
50. Cullen KJ, Yee D, Sly WS, Perdue J, Hampton B, Lippman ME, et al. (1990) Insulin-like growth factor receptor expression and function in human breast cancer. Cancer Res 50:48–53.
51. Yee D, Brunner N, Rotwein P (1990) A novel insulin-like growth factor I messenger RNA is expressed in normal and tumor cells. Mol Endocrinol 4:1914–1920.
52. Pekonen F, Partanen S, Makinen T, Rutanen EM (1988) Receptors for epidermal growth factor and insulin-like growth factor I and their relation to steroid receptors in human breast cancer. Cancer Res 48:1343–1347.
53. Pollak MN, Huynh HT, Lefebvre SP (1992) Tamoxifen reduces serum insulin-like growth factor I (IGF-I). Breast Cancer Res Treat. 22:91–100.
54. Cullen KJ, Lippman ME, Chow D, Hill S, Rosen N, Zwiebel JA (1992) Insulin-like growth factor-II overexpression in MCF-7 cells induces phenotypic changes associated with malignant progression. Mol Endocrinol 6:91–100.
55. Lee AV, Darbre P, King RJ (1994) Processing of insulin-like growth factor-II (IGF-II) by human breast cancer cells. Mol Cell Endocrinol 99:211–220.
56. Toropainen E, Lipponen P, Syrjänen K (1995) Expression of insulin-like growth factor I (IGF-I) in female breast cancer as related to established prognostic factors and long-term prognosis. Eur J Cancer 31A:1443–1448:1995
57. Bonneterre J, Peyrat JP, Beuscart R, Demaille A (1990) Prognostic significance of insulin-like growth factor 1 receptors in human breast cancer. Cancer Res 50:6931–6935.
58. Toropainen EM, Lipponen PK, Syräjnen KJ (1995) Expression of insulin-like growth factor II in female breast cancer as related to established prognostic factors and long-term prognosis. Anticancer Res 15: 2669–2674.
59. Tandon AK, Clark GM, Chamness GC, Chirgwin JM, McGuire WL (1990) Cathepsin D and prognosis in breast cancer. N Engl J Med 322:297–302.
60. Spyratos F, Maudelonde T, Brouillet JP, Brunet M, Defrenne A, Andrieu C, et al. (1989) Cathepsin D: an independent prognostic factor for metastasis of breast cancer. Lancet 2:1115–1118.
61. Hoeflich A, Wolf E, Braulke T, Koepf G, Kessler U, Brem G, et al. (1995) Does the overexpression of pro-insulin-like growth factor-II in transfected human embryonic kidney fibroblasts increase the secretion of lysosomal enzymes? Eur J Biochem 232:172–178.
62. De Leon D, Terry C, Asmerom Y, Nissley P (1996) Insulin-like growth factor II modulates the routing of cathepsin D in MCF-7 breast cancer cells. Endocrinology 137:1851–1859.
63. Hankins GR, DeSouza A, Bently R, Patel M, Marks J, Iglehart J, et al. (1996) M6P/IGF2 receptor: a candidate breast tumor suppressor gene. Oncogene 12:2003–2009.
64. Mignatti P, Rifkin DB (1993) Biology and biochemistry of proteinases in tumor invasion. Physiol Rev 73:161–195.
65. Dennis PA, Rifkin DB (1991) Cellular activation of latent transforming growth factor β requires binding to the cation-independent mannose 6–phosphate/insulin-like growth factor II receptor. Proc Natl Acad Sci USA 88:580–584.
66. Dalal BI, Keown PA, Greenberg AH (1993) Immunocytochemical localization of secreted transforming growth factor-beta 1 to the advancing edges of primary tumors and to lymph node metastases of human mammary carcinoma. Am J Pathol 143:381–389.
67. Holst-Hansen C, Johannessen B, Høyer-Hansen G, Rømer J, Ellis V, Brünner N (1996) Urokinase-type plasminogen activation in three human breast cancer cell lines correlates with their in vitro invasiveness. Clin Exp Metast 14:297–307.
68. Arnoletti JP, Albo D, Granick MS, Solomaon MP, Castiglioni A, Rothman VL, et al. (1995) Thrombospondin and transforming growth factor-β 1 increase expression of urokinase-type plasminogen activator and plasminogen activator inhibitor-1 in human MDA-MB-231 breast cancer cells. Cancer 76:998–1005.

69. Falcone DJ, McCaffrey TA, Haimovitz-Friedman A, Garcia, M (1993) Transforming growth factor-1 stimulates macrophage urokinase expression and release of matrix-bound basic fibroblast growth factor. J Cell Physiol 155:595–605.
70. Minniti CP, Kohn EC, Grubb JH, Sly WS, Oh Y, Muller HL, et al. (1992) The insulin-like growth factor II (IGF-II)/mannose 6-phosphate receptor mediates IGF-II-induced motility in human rhabdomyosarcoma cells. J Biol Chem 267:9000–9004. .
71. Nakao-Hayashi J, Ito H, Kanayasu T, Morita I, Murota S (1992) Stimulatory effects of insulin and insulin-like growth factor I on migration and tube formation by vascular endothelial cells. Atherosclerosis 92:141- 149.
72. Klemke RL, Yebra M, Bayna EM, Cheresh DA (1994) Receptor tyrosine kinase signaling required for integrin alpha v beta 5–directed cell motility but not adhesion on vitronectin. J Cell Biol 127:859–866.
73. Jones JI, Prevette T, Gockerman A, Clemmons DR (1996) Ligand occupancy of the alpha-V-beta3 integrin is necessary for smooth muscle cells to migrate in response to insulin-like growth factor. Proc Natl Acad Sci USA 93:2482–2487.
74. Doerr ME, Jones JI (1996) The roles of integrins and extracellular matrix proteins in the insulin-like growth factor I-stimulated chemotaxis of human breast cancer cells. J Biol Chem 271:2443–2447.
75. Stracke ML, Engel JD, Wilson LW, Rechler MM, Liotta LA, Schiffmann E (1989) The type I insulin-like growth factor receptor is a motility receptor in human melanoma cells. J Biol Chem 264:21544–21549.
76. Grant MB, Guay C, Marsh R (1990) Insulin-like growth factor I stimulates proliferation, migration, and plasminogen activator release by human retinal pigment epithelial cells. Curr Eye Res 9:323–335.
77. Nakao-Hayashi J, Ito H, Kanayasu T, Morita I, Murota S (1992) Stimulatory effects of insulin and insulin-like growth factor I on migration and tube formation by vascular endothelial cells. Atherosclerosis 92:141–149.
78. Roesel JF, Nanney LB (1995) Assessment of differential cytokine effects on angiogenesis using an in vivo model of cutaneous wound repair. J Surg Res 58:449–459.
79. Grant MB, Mames RN, Fitzgerald C, Ellis EA, Aboufriekha M, Guy J (1993) Insulin-like growth factor I acts as an angiogenic agent in rabbit cornea and retina: comparative studies with basic fibroblast growth factor. Diabetologia 36:282–291.
80. Lefaucheur JP, Gjata B, Lafont H, Sebille A (1996) Angiogenic and inflammatory responses following skeletal muscle injury are altered by immune neutralization of endogenous basic fibroblast growth factor, insulin-like growth factor-1 and transforming growth factor-beta 1. J Neuroimmunol 70:37–44.
81 Volpert O, Jackson D, Bouck N, Linzer DI (1996) The insulin-like growth factor II/mannose 6-phosphate receptor is required for proliferin-induced angiogenesis. Endocrinology 137:3871–3876.
82 Jones JI, Clemmons DR (1995) Insulin-like growth factors and their binding proteins: biological actions. Endocr Rev 16:3–34.

12 Role of Angiogenesis in the Transition to Hormone Independence and Acquisition of the Metastatic Phenotype

Francis G. Kern, PHD

INTRODUCTION

Breast cancer becomes a life-threatening illness when the malignant tumor cells have acquired the capability of invading through the basement membrane and into the circulation, where they are then disseminated to distant sites in the body. Therefore it may seem intuitive that tumors that have acquired a capability of stimulating the growth of new blood vessels would possess a greater threat to the patient, and indeed a good amount of correlative clinical data now link tumors that have a higher number of microvessels with poor prognosis *(1–5)*. However, while neoangiogenesis is likely to be important in the dissemination of tumor cells, it is becoming more apparent that additional factors are required to allow proliferation of disseminated tumor cells at the distant sites.

When breast cancer presents as an invasive disease, it has been useful to use estrogen receptor (ER) content as a basis for choice of therapy. This relates to the fact that estrogen itself can stimulate the growth of breast cancer cells that contain ER through still unknown mechanism that involves binding of estrogen to nuclear ER and subsequent stimulation of its transcriptional activation functions. Consequently, a highly useful treatment for most patients with ER-positive tumors is hormonal therapy with antiestrogens, the most common being tamoxifen *(6–8)*. Although other ER-independent mechanisms may also contribute to the therapeutic effect of this agent *(9–11)*, it is commonly assumed that the benefit of this drug derives from its ability to bind to ER without stimulating the same type of transcriptional activity as an estrogen-bound receptor.

An invariable and unfortunate outcome of treatment of patients with tumors that initially respond to tamoxifen is the outgrowth of populations of cells that no longer respond to this treatment. In addition, some ER-positive tumors fail to show any initial response to this relatively benign form of treatment. What may not seem so intuitive is how expression of angiogenic growth factors might also be involved in either acquired or *de novo* antiestrogen resistance, yet recent studies with transfected breast cancer cell lines (discussed in greater detail below) raise this as a possibility. If this turns out to be

From: *Contemporary Endocrinology: Endocrinology of Breast Cancer*
Edited by: A. Manni © Humana Press Inc., Totowa, NJ

substantiated by clinical studies, then in the appropriate context, treatment with agents that inhibit angiogenesis may afford a means of restoring antiestrogen sensitivity to patients with acquired resistance or a means of conferring sensitivity to patients with *de novo* resistance.

CLINICAL DILEMMAS ASSOCIATED WITH TAMOXIFEN TREATMENT

A major dilemma for the clinician currently confronted with a patient with an ER-positive breast tumor is trying to make the best guess as to whether a patient will respond to this type of antiestrogen therapy in either an adjuvant or advanced breast cancer treatment setting. Since approximately 60% of patients with invasive ductal carcinoma present with ER-positive tumors, this particular question is relevant for a significant portion of women with breast cancer. It is also known that around 65–70% of patients with ER-positive tumors with advanced stage disease will show at least some response to tamoxifen *(12,13)*. Among those that eventually fail on this therapy, 50–70% of these patients still have tumors that contain ER when these sites are biopsied *(12–15)*. Therefore loss of ER is not the primary mechanism involved in the acquisition of antiestrogen resistance.

Two different types of second-line antihormonal therapies are currently in the final stages of clinical trials for use in patients who have failed on tamoxifen. One approach involves the use of inhibitors of the enzyme aromatase, which is involved in the biosynthesis of estradiol produced at extraovarian sites *(16–23)*. A second form of second-line therapy is the use of what have been called *pure antiestrogens (24)*. These are compounds that bind to the ER, result in no transcriptional activation, and may increase the degradation of the receptor *(25)*. They also do not possess any of the partial agonist properties of tamoxifen.

Various recent studies have shown that 20–40% of patients who have failed on tamoxifen therapy show some response to these second-line therapies and that an additional 30% show no immediate disease progression when switched to these forms of therapy *(19–23,26–28)*. Therefore these second-line approaches are likely to be of some value, but they also raise another dilemma for the oncologist. In addition to needing help from molecular oncologists and epidemiologists in determining who is most likely to respond initially to tamoxifen, the clinician will soon also need assistance in determining which patients who do not respond are likely to benefit from these alternative hormonal therapies.

MECHANISMS OF TAMOXIFEN RESISTANCE

A number of different mechanisms have been proposed for tamoxifen resistance. Based on what is known about some of these mechanisms, some educated guesses can be made as to whether the patient with a tamoxifen-resistant tumor that is due to one of these mechanisms is likely to respond to a second-line therapy. However, for many of these mechanisms for which a molecular basis for tamoxifen resistance has been demonstrated with cell lines or with in vitro assays, subsequent examination of patient samples has revealed that these types of alterations are unlikely to be responsible for most tamoxifen-resistant tumors. This includes point mutations in the hormone binding domain of the estrogen receptor, alterations in splicing of the ER mRNA that can result in constitutively active forms of the receptor, or metabolism of tamoxifen to metabolites with estrogenic activity *(8,29–35)*.

There is now recent evidence that the balance in the amounts of recently discovered steroid receptor coactivators and corepressors can influence whether tamoxifen will act as an antagonist or agonist of the estrogen receptor. At this point, work with in vitro systems suggests that the pure antiestrogens will still act as antagonists when tamoxifen is changed to an agonist as a result of alterations in the ratio of coactivators to corepressors *(36)*. Therefore other mechanisms are also probably responsible for those ER-positive tamoxifen-resistant breast tumors that fail to respond to second-line therapies.

Two potential mechanisms involve the downstream signaling events associated with activation of growth factor receptors. Work from a number of laboratories has demonstrated what has been termed cross talk between steroid receptors and either growth factor tyrosine kinase receptors or G-protein-coupled receptors *(37–44)*. In examples relevant to the question of tamoxifen resistance, phosphorylation of the estrogen receptor by MAP kinases, which are downstream effectors of a number of different signaling pathways including those mediated by growth factor receptors, or activation of G-protein-coupled receptors can result in tamoxifen acquiring agonistic properties *(37,38,43)*. However, the same studies show that the ER is not activated by these mechanisms when pure antiestrogens are present *(37–43)*.

Therefore at least one additional mechanism probably remains underlying the *de novo* or acquired tamoxifen resistance of ER-positive tumors that do not subsequently respond to a second-line treatment with the pure antiestrogens. Recent data suggest that one such mechanism may also involve growth factor signaling, which provides the breast tumor cell with an alternative pathway to the growth stimulation mediated by ER *(45)*. This would bypass the requirement for activation of the ER by an agonist for growth promotion to occur and would account for the failure of second-line antihormonal therapies.

ROLE OF GROWTH FACTORS IN THE ACQUISITION OF TAMOXIFEN RESISTANCE

It can now be seen that growth factor signaling can affect the resistance of a breast tumor cell to tamoxifen in a number of different ways, with two of these mechanisms potentially leading to tamoxifen acting as an agonist. In one scenario, growth factor signaling can affect the level of coactivators or corepressors. Although no experimental data currently exist indicating that this type of regulation is indeed occurring in breast cancer cells, the field is very new, the number of coactivators and corepressors being identified is continually expanding, and the experiments remain to be performed *(46)*. In a second scenario, growth factor signaling could result in activation of ER via phosphorylation, leading to increased agonistic activity for tamoxifen. In the third scenario, growth factor signaling could bypass the requirement for ER activation for growth. These three scenarios are not mutually exclusive, and all three mechanisms may be operating simultaneously within a cell to provide additive or perhaps synergistic growth-stimulatory effects. As such, these mechanisms may account for the clinical response observed in some patients when tamoxifen is withdrawn *(47,48)*. However the available evidence to date suggests that a better understanding is required of what particular growth factor signaling pathways can bypass the need for ER since these pathways may also be responsible for resistance to second-line therapies.

The initial indication of the potential importance growth factors might have in the process of the development of hormone independence came from work by Dickson and

Lippman *(49)*. These two investigators formulated the ideas that the genes for growth factors were part of the set of genes that were transcriptionally activated in ER-positive cells in response to estrogen treatment and that the subsequent growth stimulation of ER-positive breast cancer cell line xenografts in nude mice was the result of either the autocrine or paracrine effects of these factors *(49)*. This line of reasoning was supported by findings that continuous administration of epidermal growth factor (EGF) could facilitate the hormone-independent growth of an estrogen-dependent cell line as xenografts in ovariectomized athymic nude mice *(50)* and that transforming growth factor-α (TGF-α), another ligand for the EGF receptor, was induced by estrogen in the same cell line *(51–54)*.

Subsequently a number of laboratories have used a transfection approach to express constitutively growth factors or growth factor receptors whose overexpression was implicated by various clinical studies to be associated with estrogen-independent tumors or induced by estrogen in vitro *(39,55–66)*. Molecules such as protein kinase c (PKC)-α, ras^H, and raf-1, which are downstream effectors of many growth factor signaling pathways, have also been overexpressed in estrogen-dependent cell lines *(67–72)*. The transfected cell lines were then tested to determine whether the overexpression had any effect on the estrogen responsiveness or antiestrogen sensitivity in vitro or in vivo.

Many of these studies utilized the MCF-7 breast cancer cell line as a recipient since it is estrogen responsive in vitro and sensitive to treatment with antiestrogens *(73)*. In vivo, there is a strict estrogen dependence for tumor formation, and tumors will not develop in ovariectomized nude mice unless they are supplemented with estrogen *(74,75)*. Even though this cell line was derived from the pleural effusion of a patient with breast cancer *(76)*, the tumors that do develop with this cell line and most other breast cancer cell lines capable of in vivo growth are noninvasive and nonmetastatic *(69,77)*. This in vivo phenotype seen with MCF-7 cells is in line with the poor invasive ability seen in in vitro Matrigel basement membrane invasion assays *(78)*. Consequently, this cell also represents a useful model to determine the effects of overexpression on the metastatic and invasive phenotypes. To facilitate this process, we developed a clonal line of MCF-7 cells, designated as the ML-20 cell line, which stably expresses a transfected bacterial *lacZ* gene *(77,79)*. In many of our studies we have used this cell line as a recipient for retransfection since this allows a chromogenic substrate for β-galactosidase to be used to stain metastatic deposits of cells blue.

EFFECTS OF ANGIOGENIC GROWTH FACTOR OVEREXPRESSION ON THE METASTATIC PHENOTYPE

Varying degrees of increased estrogen-independent in vitro or in vivo growth can be conferred to ER-positive breast cancer cell lines by transfection with vectors for EGFR *(56,57,64)* HER-2/neu *(62,63)*, heregulin *(39,66)*, activated ras^H *(67–70)*, constitutively activated raf-1 *(71)*, PKC-α *(72)*, TGF-β *(61)*, insulin-like growth factor (IGF)-II *(59,60)*, fibroblast growth factor (FGF)-1 *(65)* and FGF-4 *(55)*. In those transfection studies in which estrogen-independent in vivo growth was a consequence of overexpression, it was only with the PKC-α and FGF-1 and FGF-4 transfectants that an increased metastatic phenotype was also consistently observed *(55,65,72)*. FGF-overexpressing cells acquire the ability to form tumors in ovariectomized athymic nude mice or beige mice without estrogen supplementation. They can also form tumors in either nude or beige mice treated with tamoxifen pellets. In either type of mice, and in either untreated or tamoxifen-treated mice, X-gal-stained cells can be readily detected in either the lungs or lymph nodes of tumor-bearing mice injected with FGF-1- or FGF-4 overexpressing cells *(45,65,77)*. By contrast, no cells are detected in lungs or lymph nodes of mice bearing control vector-transfected ML-20 cell tumors in estrogen-supplemented mice, even when these tumors are the same size as the tumors that form in mice injected with FGF-overexpressing cells *(65)*. However, if the same ML-20 cells are coinjected with FGF-4-overexpressing cells that do not themselves express β-galactosidase, X-gal-stained cells can be detected in the tumors of either untreated or tamoxifen-treated ovariectomized nude mice and in the lungs and lymph nodes of mice bearing tumors composed of the mixture *(55)*.

The underlying mechanism responsible for the increased metastatic phenotype associated with PKC-α overexpression remains to be elucidated. Both FGF-1 and FGF-4 are angiogenic growth factors and both can therefore stimulate the growth of new blood vessels in a tumor producing either factor *(80,81)*. Thus the mechanism likely to be responsible for the increased dissemination of tumor cells is likely to be related to the increased neoangiogenesis that is occurring in these tumors.

Although deposits of X-gal-stained cells can be seen in essentially 100% of the mice bearing tumors of either FGF-4- or FGF-1-overexpressing cells, we never observed the development of tumor nodules at either of these sites *(65,77)*. Since the disseminated tumor cells express the cDNAs for both hygromycin and G418, it is a relatively simple task to establish cell lines from the tumor cells present in the lungs or lymph nodes. These cells continue to express FGF and remain capable of forming tumors in either untreated or ovariectomized mice. However, these cells also do not appear to be able to develop into macrometastases. When inoculated via a tail vein route, these tumor cells disappear from the lungs with approximately the same kinetics as FGF-overexpressing cells that had not been established from lungs of tumor-bearing mice. With both cell types, X-gal-stained cells can no longer be detected by 96 h after injection *(82)*.

Long-lived angiogenic inhibitors produced by the primary tumor cells have been shown to be capable of inhibiting the development of macrometastases from cells that have been disseminated from the primary site. In these model systems, macrometastases are found when the primary tumor is resected *(83–86)*. However this was not the case when the primary tumors of FGF-1-overexpressing cells were resected. Tumors were allowed to develop for 3 weeks, at which point the tumors were of sufficient size that 100% of the animals sacrificed at this point had large numbers of disseminated cells present in both the lungs and lymph nodes. Tumors were resected from the remaining animals and after 3 weeks, this group of animals was sacrificed. Examination of the lungs and lymph nodes did not reveal any X-gal-stained cells in these organs *(82)*.

Taken together, these results indicate that the increased neoangiogenesis brought about by the production of an angiogenic growth factor facilitates the constant shedding of tumor cells into the circulation. However, the cells that accumulate within the lungs and lymph nodes of tumor-bearing mice do not possess any selective advantage at these distant sites compared with the cells remaining in the primary tumor. These cells are lacking in the ability to either attach, extravasate, or proliferate at these distant sites; as a consequence, they are cleared from these organs within a relatively short period. The mechanism of clearance remains to be elucidated but may involve an increased rate of apoptosis relative to tumor cells at the primary tumor site or attack by cells of the remaining immune system present in the athymic nude mice.

In addition to facilitating the spread of tumor cells, the production of an angiogenic growth factor would presumably confer some growth advantage over parental MCF-7 cells at these distant sites if the other missing components of the metastatic process were otherwise present. Consequently, the FGF-transfected cell lines are likely to be a useful model in determining the ability of the various proteases, attachment factors, apoptosis modulators, and other putative regulators of the metastatic process to facilitate the development of macrometastases in this system.

MECHANISMS MEDIATING ESTROGEN-INDEPENDENT GROWTH IN CELLS OVEREXPRESSING GROWTH FACTORS

A critical question is whether the estrogen-independent growth conferred by FGF overexpression is the result of a mechanism that activates ER or bypasses the need for an ER-regulated growth pathway. Heregulin overexpression can also confer on MCF-7 cells the ability to form tumors in ovariectomized nude mice *(39,66)*. Heregulin is a ligand for homodimers of erbB-3/HER-3 and erbB-4/HER-4 and heterodimers of erbB-2/HER-2/neu with either of these two transmembrane tyrosine kinase receptors *(87,88)*. Recent clinical evidence shows that patients with tumors overexpressing HER-2/neu respond poorly to tamoxifen therapy *(89)*, implying that activation of the erbB family of receptors is involved in resistance to this antiestrogen. In heregulin-overexpressing MCF-7 cells, the ER becomes tyrosine phosphorylated, and the numbers of ER are downregulated *(39,66)*. There is also evidence from transient expression assays with estrogen response element (ERE)-containing reporter constructs that the ER is constitutively activated in heregulin-overexpressing cells and that this effect can be reversed by treatment with the pure antiestrogen ICI 182,780 *(39)*. This raises the possibility that cells that have acquired resistance to tamoxifen through the activation of the erbB family of transmembrane tyrosine kinase receptors may be able to respond to this second-line antihormonal therapy.

By contrast, the evidence available to date suggests that signaling mediated by FGF receptors may instead confer on ER-positive breast cancer cells a mechanism that can bypass the need for ER activation. FGF-overexpressing cells have obtained the ability to form soft agar colonies with high efficiency in media depleted of estrogens. In media that contain estrogen, the effect of added 4-hydroxytamoxifen is diminished compared with control transfected cells. The same holds true in anchorage-dependent growth assays in which FGF-overexpressing cells have faster doubling times in estrogen-depleted media or in estrogen-containing media with added 4-hydroxytamoxifen *(65)*. The enhanced anchorage-dependent or anchorage-independent growth in estrogen-depleted media is not abrogated by treatment with the pure antiestrogen ICI 182,780, as might be expected if the effect were due to ligand-independent activation of ER mediated by FGF signaling pathways. Similarly, the FGF-transfected cells continue to show enhanced growth in either anchorage-dependent or anchorage-independent growth assays when ICI 182,780 is added to estrogen-containing media. There is no downregulation of ER in FGF-transfected cells, and there is no evidence from analysis of the basal levels of estrogen-induced genes or from transient assays with ERE-containing reporter constructs that FGF-overexpressing cells contain a constitutively activated ER. Furthermore, FGF-overexpressing cells continue to be able to form tumors in mice that have been treated with ICI 182,780 *(45)*.

ROLE OF PARACRINE AND AUTOCRINE EFFECTS OF FGF IN MEDIATING TAMOXIFEN RESISTANCE

Although FGF-4 is not expressed in human breast tumor tissues, there is considerable evidence that both FGF-1 and all four of the FGF transmembrane tyrosine kinase receptors are expressed in many breast tumor tissues *(65,90–100)*. The transfection studies discussed above certainly suggest a potential role for FGF expression in the acquisition of hormone independence or antiestrogen resistance in ER-positive breast tumors. Since FGF-1 can have both paracrine and autocrine or intracrine effects, it is important to dissect the relative contributions of these effects to the phenotypes observed in FGF-1-overexpressing cells. This process can be performed by retransfecting the FGF-1-overexpressing cells with a dominant-negative FGF receptor. Receptor dimerization is required for transmission of the signal resulting from FGF binding *(101,102)*. Therefore, a construct directing the expression of a transmembrane-anchored truncated FGF receptor lacking the cytoplasmic tyrosine kinase domain will effectively block the transmission of the growth signal through the formation of nonfunctional homo- and heterodimers. In such a pairing, the mutant lacking the tyrosine kinase domain will not be capable of phosphorylating the wild-type receptor on tyrosine residues in the cytoplasmic regulatory region of the receptor and thus will prevent the binding of downstream signaling molecules *(103–105)*.

FGF-1-overexpressing cells retransfected with the dominant negative FGF receptor no longer contained elevated levels of phosphorylated MAPKs in cell extracts, indicating that the dominant negative receptor was blocking FGF signaling. As expected, these cells were also no longer capable of forming soft agar colonies in either estrogen-depleted or antiestrogen-containing media, confirming that autocrine or intracrine effects of FGF were important in conferring this phenotype. In line with these in vitro results, when they are injected into ovariectomized nude mice, the retransfected cells are no longer capable of forming tumors without estrogen supplementation. However, the tumors that form in estrogen-supplemented animals are typically much larger than those formed by MCF-7 cells, suggesting that the paracrine effects of FGF-1 production can act in an additive or synergistic manner with the mitogenic effect of estrogen to stimulate tumor growth. An interesting finding from this study was the observation that in tamoxifen-treated animals, the FGF-overexpressing cell lines formed tumors at the same rate regardless of whether or not they were also expressing the dominant negative receptor. Thus the paracrine effects alone of FGF were capable of allowing antiestrogen-resistant in vivo tumor growth *(106)*. These results also indicate that tamoxifen resistance can be dissociated from estrogen independence.

It has been suggested that the partial agonistic properties of tamoxifen may be greater in the mouse than they are in the human *(107)*. When tamoxifen-treated mice are injected with MCF-7 cells that do not overexpress FGF, small tumors sometimes develop, but they usually remain static or regress *(75,108)*. Thus it is possible that the paracrine effects of FGF may cooperate with the weak mitogenic activity of tamoxifen to allow continued and progressive tumor development to occur. While this an intriguing possibility, it remains to be determined if these results seen in nude mice have any relevance to the tamoxifen resistance that occurs in human patients.

EFFECTS OF VEGF OVEREXPRESSION ON ANTIESTROGEN SENSITIVITY AND THE METASTATIC PHENOTYPE

As previously stated, FGF-1 is a strong angiogenic growth factor *(80)*. Therefore, one of the paracrine effects that is likely to be a strong contributor to the observed tumor growth of the dominant-negative receptor-transfected cell lines in tamoxifen-treated animals is the neoangiogenesis resulting from the continued production of this growth factor. To test the effect of neoangiogenesis directly, β-galactosidase-expressing MCF-7 cells were transfected with a vector directing the overexpression of the 165-amino acid form of vascular endothelial growth factor (VEGF). There is a considerable amount of evidence that expression of this particular isoform of this growth factor is an important determinant in the establishment of a neoangiogenic phenotype in many types of cancers. VEGF has been shown to be expressed in breast tumors *(93,109–113)*, and the extent of expression correlates with the number of microvessels present in the tumor *(109)*. This is a growth factor that is relatively specific for endothelial cells. There are two transmembrane tyrosine kinase receptors for VEGF. One is known as Flk1 in the mouse and as KDR in the human; the second is called Flt-1 *(114–117)*. Expression of both receptors is restricted to endothelial cells, hematopoietic stem cells, monocytes, megakaryocytes, and platelets *(116–120)*. mRNA for these receptors is strongly expressed in the endothelial cells of small vessels adjacent to infiltrating ductal carcinoma or metastatic ductal carcinoma cells as well as in the endothelial cells adjacent to comedo-type ductal carcinoma in situ. However, there is no evidence of expression of either receptor in endothelial cells in the normal areas of the breast *(113)*.

There are a few reports of ectopic expression of VEGF receptors in some types of tumor cells *(120–123)*, but an examination of the recipient ML-20 cell line using a sensitive reverse transcription polymerase chain reaction assay has failed to show any evidence of expression of either receptor in this MCF-7-derived breast cancer cell line. In line with this finding, cells overexpressing either the 121- or 165-amino acid forms of VEGF do not show any altered in vitro growth properties with regard to growth in either estrogen-depleted media or in antiestrogen-containing media *(124)*. Both types of VEGF transfectants are unable to form tumors in ovariectomized mice without estrogen supplementation. Overexpression of the 121-amino acid form of VEGF was reported to increase the in vivo growth rate in estrogen-supplemented animals *(125)*, but no statistical difference was observed between control transfectants and transfectants overexpressing the 165-amino acid form of VEGF in this treatment group *(124)*. This may relate to the fact that different sublines of MCF-7 cells have different in vivo growth rates in estrogen-supplemented mice and that the controls for the 121-amino acid transfection study grew poorly whereas the controls for the 165-amino acid study grew well in estrogen-supplemented mice, making any further stimulation due to VEGF overexpression difficult to observe.

No effect of overexpression of the 121-amino acid form of VEGF on either tamoxifen sensitivity or metastatic potential was seen in the one study. However, overexpression of the 165-amino acid form was found to increase the tumorigenicity of MCF-7 cells in tamoxifen-treated animals and to facilitate tumor cell dissemination. For the effect of tamoxifen to be observed, coinjection with Matrigel was required *(124)*. This is a mixture of basement membrane components that has been demonstrated to increase the tumorigenicity of a number of human cancer cell lines, including MCF-7 cells *(126,127)*. The 121-amino acid form of VEGF does not bind to heparin, whereas the 165-amino acid form is a heparin-binding growth factor *(128)*. It is difficult to compare studies with two different growth factor isoforms performed in two different laboratories. The difference in effects observed may simply relate to differences in expression levels. However, it is also possible that this difference in heparin binding capability may also explain the apparent difference between the 121- and 165-amino acid forms with regard to tamoxifen, since heparan-sulfate-containing proteoglycans present in the Matrigel mixture may protect the VEGF from inactivation due to binding to α2-macroglobulin *(129)*. Small amounts of other growth factors are present in the Matrigel mixture, and a cooperative effect of VEGF with these other factors cannot be excluded.

The apparent difference of the two forms in affect on metastatic potential may not necessarily be a contradictory result. The MCF-7 cells transfected with the 165-amino acid form of VEGF also expressed β-galactosidase, and therefore analysis of micrometastases could be readily performed. By contrast, the study examining the effect of the 121-amino acid form only looked for the presence of macrometastases *(125)*. In line with what was observed with MCF-7 cells overexpressing FGF-1, prior resection of the primary tumor also eliminated the ability to detect X-gal-stained VEGF-overexpressing cells as micrometastases in the lungs of mice that previously were bearing tumors *(124)*. Thus it appears that the both FGF-1 and VEGF can facilitate tumor cell dissemination, presumably by stimulating neoangiogenesis within the primary tumor, but both types of transfectants are still incapable of proliferating once disseminated to these distant sites.

In patients with breast cancer, the relationship between tamoxifen resistance or treatment failure with increased neoangiogenesis resulting from either FGF-1 expression, VEGF expression, or expression of any of a number of other angiogenic growth factors shown to be expressed in human breast tumors *(94)* remains to be critically evaluated. In one study a reduction in relapse-free survival was seen in patients with ER-positive patients receiving adjuvant tamoxifen therapy when they had high microvessel counts, but it has not yet been determined whether this phenotype is predictive for resistance to tamoxifen *(130)*.

POTENTIAL MECHANISMS FOR TAMOXIFEN RESISTANCE MEDIATED BY ANGIOGENIC GROWTH FACTORS

It also remains to be determined how neoangiogenesis can increase resistance to tamoxifen in these nude mouse models. It is possible that dividing endothelial cells may produce growth factors that can either directly stimulate the growth of estrogen-dependent breast tumor cells or increase the agonistic properties of tamoxifen as a downstream result of growth factor signaling. VEGF also increases the permeability of blood vessels. This increased permeability may be important in facilitating the development of a matrix capable of supporting a stromal network of fibroblasts, endothelial cells, and connective tissue *(131–133)*. Similarly, FGF-1 is a pleiotropic growth factor capable of stimulating fibroblasts as well as a number of other cell types *(134,135)*. It is possible that the increased stromal support that may result from expression of either growth factor may increase the mitogenic capability of tamoxifen. Others have observed an inverse relationship between the extent of apoptosis ongoing within a tumor and the degree of neovascularization measured by microvessel density *(86,136–138)*. It is therefore also possible that a reduced apoptotic index would have the net effect of allowing the weak mitogenic stimulus resulting from the agonistic properties of tamoxifen to result in observable tumor growth over time.

The ability of both the VEGF-overexpressing MCF-7 cells and the FGF-1-overexpressing cells retransfected with the dominant-negative FGFR to form tumors in tamoxifen-treated animals raises the possibility that treatment of patients with an angiogenesis inhibitor may be able to restore or convey some degree of tamoxifen sensitivity. Indeed, our own studies have shown that treatment of FGF-1-overexpressing cells with the angiogenesis inhibitor TNP-470, also known as AGM-1470, had the greatest antitumor effect in tamoxifen-treated animals. However, tumors still developed in this combined treatment group, and elimination of tumor-forming ability required treatment with an agent capable of inhibiting both the autocrine and paracrine effects of this growth factor *(139)*. Therefore, if the antiestrogen insensitivity is the combined effect of increased neoangiogenesis and an autocrine or intracrine growth signaling pathway that bypasses the need for ER, then a blockade of this pathway will also be required for restoration of antiestrogen sensitivity.

CONCLUDING REMARKS

The results with these models emphasize the importance of gaining a better understanding of the growth signaling pathways mediated by estrogen and growth factors such as FGF. It is becoming apparent that the growth signaling mechanisms in epithelial cells are likely to involve a network of branching and interacting pathways *(140,141)*. Signaling by fibroblast growth factors in breast epithelial cells is likely to be extremely complex. Ten different FGF family members and four FGF-related proteins have been identified thus far *(142–148)* as well as four different transmembrane tyrosine kinase receptors *(149,150)*. FGF signaling also appears to require the formation of a ternary complex of FGF, FGF receptor, and heparin *(151)*. Since members of the FGF family bind heparin with high affinity, the presence and spatial distribution of heparan sulfate proteoglycans on the cell surface and within basement membranes are also likely to influence the extent of FGF signaling that might occur within an individual tumor. Multiple receptors are likely to be expressed in individual cells with the resulting capability of heterodimer formation having still unknown effects with regard to receptor signaling and affinity for the various ligands. FGF-1, FGF-2, and FGF-7 are known to be expressed in breast tumor tissues, and each may have different signaling capabilities that may in part be modulated by the repertoire of receptors expressed on individual tumor cells *(152,153)*. There is also evidence that FGF receptors can be constitutively activated by mutations and that cell adhesion molecules and heparin can activate FGF receptors in a ligand-independent manner *(154–157)*.

Given this complexity, it may ultimately prove to be difficult to pinpoint one particular component of this system as a predictive indicator of a response to antiestrogen therapies. It therefore may be more useful to use pharmacologic and molecular approaches to dissect the downstream signaling events that occur in FGF-responsive breast cancer cells to assist in understanding how these pathways bypass the need for estrogen and where they also interact and converge. Although MAP kinases may be transiently activated in response to estrogen treatment of ER-positive breast cancer cells *(158,159)*, these cells remain capable of dividing in the presence of inhibitors of mevalonate synthesis such as lovastatin if estrogen is also supplied *(160,161)*. This suggests that pathways inhibited by this agent, which include those activated in response to growth factors, are not involved in growth signaling mediated by ER. However, both types of pathways are inhibited by microinjection with antibodies against cyclin D, suggesting that the two pathways converge at this point *(159)*.

While progress is being made in understanding how growth factor signaling pathways interact with those regulated by ER activation, it is obvious that our current state of knowledge is still in a rudimentary phase. Knowledge of the particular pathways activated by FGFRs is primarily limited to that gained from studies performed in rodent fibroblast or pheochromocytoma cell lines. It should be apparent that additional studies aimed at gaining a better understanding of these processes as they occur in normal and malignant breast epithelial cells are warranted.

ACKNOWLEDGMENTS

Some of the work described in this review was supported by NIH grants CA50376, CA09218, CA53185, and CA51008 and by the Susan G. Komen Foundation. I am indebted to my colleagues at the Lombardi Cancer Center at Georgetown University who collaborated on some of the studies mentioned in this review and for their helpful comments and discussions on the topics covered in this review, including Jamal Bullocks and Drs. Sandra McLeskey, Lurong Zhang, Anton Wellstein, Marc Lippman, Bob Dickson, and Dorraya El-Ashry. I would also like to thank Dr. El-Ashry for critically reading the manuscript.

REFERENCES

1. Weidner N, Semple JP, Welch WR, Folkman J (1991) Tumor angiogenesis and metastasis—correlation in invasive breast carcinoma. N Engl J Med 324:1–8.
2. Weidner N, Folkman J, Pozza F, Bevilacqua P, Allred EN, Moore DH, et al. (1992) Tumor angiogenesis: a new significant and independent prognostic indicator in early-stage breast carcinoma [see comments]. J Natl Cancer Inst 84:1875–1887.
3. Wellstein A (1994) Why monitor angiogenic factors in patients' urine. J Natl Cancer Inst 86:328–329.
4. Gasparini G, Harris AL (1995) Clinical importance of the determination of tumor angiogenesis in breast carcinoma: much more than a new prognostic tool. J Clin Oncol 13:765–782.
5. Fox SB, Leek RD, Weekes MP, Whitehouse RM, Gatter KC, Harris AL (1995) Quantitation and prognostic value of breast cancer angiogenesis: comparison of microvessel density, Chalkley count, and computer image analysis. J Pathol 177:275–283.
6. Furr BJ, Jordan VC (1984) The pharmacology and clinical uses of tamoxifen. Pharmacol Ther 25:127–205.
7. Jordan VC (1995) Third annual William L McGuire Memorial Lecture. Studies on the estrogen receptor in breast cancer—20 years as a target for the treatment and prevention of cancer. Breast Cancer Res Treat 36:267–285.
8. Wolf DM, Fuqua SA (1995) Mechanisms of action of antiestrogens. Cancer Treat Rev 21:247–271.
9. Gagliardi AR, Hennig B, Collins DC (1996) Antiestrogens inhibit endothelial cell growth stimulated by angiogenic growth factors. Anticancer Res 16:1101–1106.
10. McClay EF, Jones JA, Winski PJ, Albright KD, Christen RD, Howell SB (1996) Determinants of tamoxifen sensitivity control the nature of the synergistic interaction between tamoxifen and cisplatin. Cancer Res 56:3993–3997.
11. O'Brian CA, Liskamp RM, Solomon DH, Weinstein IB (1985) Inhibition of protein kinase C by tamoxifen. Cancer Res 45:2462–2465.
12. Johnston SR, Saccani-Jotti G, Smith IE, Salter J, Newby J, Coppen M, et al. (1995) Changes in estrogen receptor, progesterone receptor, and pS2 expression in tamoxifen-resistant human breast cancer. Cancer Res 55:3331–3338.
13. Johnston SR, Lu B, Dowsett M, Liang X, Kaufmann M, Scott GK, et al. (1997) Comparison of estrogen receptor DNA binding in untreated and acquired antiestrogen-resistant human breast tumors. Cancer Res 57:3723–3727.
14. Robertson JFR (1995) Oestrogen receptor—a stable phenotype in breast cancer. Br J Cancer in press.
15. Karnik PS, Kulkarni S, Liu XP, Budd GT, Bukowski RM (1994) Estrogen receptor mutations in tamoxifen-resistant breast cancer. Cancer Res 54:349–353.
16. Bajetta E, Zilembo N, Noberasco C (1995) Second-generation aromatase inhibitors. Tumori 81:77–80.
17. Mouridsen HT (1995) New endocrine agents in the treatment of breast cancer. Eur J Cancer 31A:826–827.
18. Plourde PV, Dyroff M, Dowsett M, Demers L, Yates R, Webster A (1995) Arimidex: a new oral, once-a-day aromatase inhibitor. J Steroid Biochem Mol Biol 53:175–179.

19. Bonnefoi HR, Smith IE, Dowsett M, Trunet PF, Houston SJ, da Luz RJ, et al. (1996) Therapeutic effects of the aromatase inhibitor fadrozole hydrochloride in advanced breast cancer. Br J Cancer 73:539–542.
20. Buzdar AU, Smith R, Vogel C, Bonomi P, Keller AM, Favis G, et al. (1996) Fadrozole HCl (CGS-16949A) versus megestrol acetate treatment of postmenopausal patients with metastatic breast carcinoma: results of two randomized double blind controlled multiinstitutional trials. Cancer 77:2503–2513.
21. Howell A, Downey S, Anderson E (1996) New endocrine therapies for breast cancer. Eur J Cancer 32A:576–588.
22. Miller WR (1996) Aromatase inhibitors—where are we now? [Editorial]. Br J Cancer 73:415–417.
23. Buzdar A, Jonat W, Howell A, Jones SE, Blomqvist C, Vogel CL, et al. (1996) Anastrozole, a potent and selective aromatase inhibitor, versus megestrol acetate in postmenopausal women with advanced breast cancer: results of overview analysis of two phase III trials. Arimidex Study Group. J Clin Oncol 14:2000–2011.
24. Wakeling AE, Dukes M, Bowler J (1991) A potent specific pure antiestrogen with clinical potential. Cancer Res 51:3867–3873.
25. Dauvois S, Danielian PS, White R, Parker MG (1992) Antiestrogen ICI 164,384 reduces cellular estrogen receptor content by increasing its turnover. Proc Natl Acad Sci USA 89:4037–4041.
26. Howell A, Robertson J (1995) Response to a specific antioestrogen (ICI 182780) in tamoxifen-resistant breast cancer. Lancet, 345:989–990.
27. Howell A, De Friend DJ, Robertson JF, Blamey RW, Anderson L, Anderson E, et al. (1996) Pharmacokinetics, pharmacological and anti-tumour effects of the specific anti-oestrogen ICI 182780 in women with advanced breast cancer. Br J Cancer 74:300–308.
28. Castiglione-Gertsch M (1996) New aromatase inhibitors: more selectivity, less toxicity, unfortunately, the same activity [Editorial; comment]. Eur J Cancer 32A:393–395.
29. Mahfoudi A, Roulet E, Dauvois S, Parker MG, Wahli W (1995) Specific mutations in the estrogen receptor change the properties of antiestrogens to full agonists. Proc Natl Acad Sci USA 92:4206–4210.
30. Roodi N, Bailey LR, Kao WY, Verrier CS, Yee CJ, Dupont WD, et al. (1995) Estrogen receptor gene analysis in estrogen receptor-positive and receptor-negative primary breast cancer. J Natl Cancer Inst 87:446–451.
31. Jiang SY, Langan-Fahey SM, Stella AL, McCague R, Jordan VC (1992) Point mutation of estrogen receptor (ER) in the ligand-binding domain changes the pharmacology of antiestrogens in ER-negative breast cancer cells stably expressing complementary DNAs for ER. Mol Endocrinol 6:2167–2174.
32. Catherino WH, Wolf DM, Jordan VC (1995) A naturally occurring estrogen receptor mutation results in increased estrogenicity of a tamoxifen analog. Mol Endocrinol 9:1053–1063.
33. Osborne CK, Coronado E, Allred DC, Wiebe V, DeGregorio M (1991) Acquired tamoxifen resistance: correlation with reduced breast tumor levels of tamoxifen and isomerizaion of trans-4-hydroxy-tamoxifen. J Natl Cancer Inst 83:1477–1482.
34. Tonetti DA, Jordan VC (1995) Possible mechanisms in the emergence of tamoxifen-resistant breast cancer. Anticancer Drugs 6:498–507.
35. Osborne CK, Fuqua SAW (1994) Mechanisms of tamoxifen resistance. Breast Cancer Res Treat 32:49–55.
36. Jackson TA, Richer JK, Bain DL, Takimoto GS, Tung L, Horwitz KB (1997) The partial agonist activity of antagonist-occupied steroid receptors is controlled by a novel hinge domain-binding coactivator L7/SPA and the corepressors N-CoR or SMRT. Mol Endocrinol 11:693–705.
37. Kato S, Endoh H, Masuhiro H, Kitamoto T, Uchiyama S, Sasaki H, et al. (1995) Activation of the estrogen receptor through phosphorylation by mitogen-activated protein kinase. Science 270:1491–1494.
38. Katzenellenbogen BS, Montano MM, Le Goff P, Schodin DJ, Kraus WL, Bhardwaj B, et al. (1995) Antiestrogens: mechanisms and actions in target cells. J Steroid Biochem Mol Biol 53:387–393.
39. Pietras RJ, Arboleda J, Reese DM, Wongvipat N, Pegram MD, Ramos L, et al. (1995) HER-2 tyrosine kinase pathway targets estrogen receptor and promotes hormone-independent growth in human breast cancer cells. Oncogene 10:2435–2446.
40. Ignar-Trowbridge DM, Teng CT, Ross KA, Parker MG, Korach KS, Mclachlan JA (1993) Peptide growth factors elicit estrogen receptor-dependent transcriptional activation of an estrogen-responsive element. Mol Endocrinol 7:992–998.
41. Ignar-Trowbridge DM, Pimentel M, Parker MG, Mclachlan JA, Korach KS (1996) Peptide growth factor cross-talk with the estrogen receptor requires the A/B domain and occurs independently of protein kinase C or estradiol. Endocrinology 137:1735–1744.

42. Bunone G, Briand P-A, Miksicek RJ, Picard D (1996) Activation of the unliganded estrogen receptor by EGF involves the MAP kinase pathway and direct phosphorylation. EMBO J 15:2174–2183.
43. Smith CL, Conneely OM, O'Malley BW (1993) Modulation of the ligand-independent activation of the human estrogen receptor by hormone and antihormone. Proc Natl Acad Sci USA 90:6120–6124.
44. El-Tanani MK, Green CD (1997) Two separate mechanisms for ligand-independent activation of the estrogen receptor. Mol Endocrinol 11:928–937.
45. McLeskey SW, Zhang L, El-Ashry D, Trock BJ, Lopez CA, Kharbanda S, et al. (1998) Tamoxifen-resistant FGF-transfected MCF-7 cells are cross-resistant *in vivo* to the antiestrogen, ICI 182,780 and two aromatase inhibitors. Clin Cancer Res 4:697–711.
46. Horwitz KB, Jackson TA, Bain DL, Richer JK, Takimoto GS, Tung L (1996) Nuclear receptor coactivators and corepressors. Mol Endocrinol 10:1167–1177.
47. Belani CP, Pearl P, Whitley NO, Aisner J (1989) Tamoxifen withdrawal response. Report of a case. Arch Intern Med 149:449–450.
48. Howell A, Dodwell DJ, Anderson H, Redford J (1992) Response after withdrawal of tamoxifen and progestogens in advanced breast cancer [see comments]. Ann Oncol 3:611–617.
49. Dickson R, Lippman ME (1987) Estrogenic regulation of growth and polypeptide growth factor secretion in human breast carcinoma. Endocr Rev 8:29–43.
50. Dickson RB, McManaway ME, Lippman ME (1986) Estrogen-induced factors of breast cancer cells partially replace estrogen to promote tumor growth. Science 232:1540–1543.
51. Dickson RB, Huff KK, Spencer EM, Lippman ME (1986) Induction of epidermal growth factor-related polypeptides by 17 beta-estradiol in MCF-7 human breast cancer cells. Endocrinology 118:138–142.
52. Bates SE, Valverius EM, Ennis BW, Bronzert DA, Sheridan JP, Stampfer MR, et al. (1990) Expression of the transforming growth factor-alpha/epidermal growth factor receptor pathway in normal human breast epithelial cells. Endocrinology 126:596–607.
53. Salomon DS, Kidwell WR, Kim N, Ciardiello F, Bates SE, Valverius E, et al. (1989) Modulation by estrogen and growth factors of transforming growth factor-alpha and epidermal growth factor receptor expression in normal and malignant human mammary epithelial cells. Recent Results Cancer Res 113:57–69.
54. Bates SE, Davidson NE, Valverius EM, Freter CE, Dickson RB, Tam JP, et al. (1988) Expression of transforming growth factor alpha and its messenger ribonucleic acid in human breast cancer: its regulation by estrogen and its possible functional significance. Mol Endocrinol 2:543–555.
55. McLeskey SW, Kurebayashi J, Honig SF, Zwiebel J, Lippman ME, Dickson RB, et al. (1993) Fibroblast growth factor 4 transfection of MCF-7 cells produces cell lines that are tumorigenic and metastatic in ovariectomized or tamoxifen-treated athymic nude mice. Cancer Res 53:2168–2177.
56. Valverius EM, Velu T, Shankar V, Ciardiello F, Kim N, Salomon D (1990) Over-expression of the epidermal growth factor in human breast cancer cells fails to induce an estrogen-independent phenotype. Int J Cancer 46:712–718.
57. van Agthoven T, van Agthoven TLA, Portengen H, Foekens JA, Dorssers, LCJ (1992) Ectopic expression of epidermal growth factor receptors induces hormone independence in ZR-75-1 human breast cancer cells. Cancer Res 52:5082–5088.
58. Clarke R, Brünner N, Katz D, Glanz P, Dickson RB, Lippman ME, et al. (1989) The effects of a constitutive expression of transforming growth factor-alpha on the growth of MCF-7 human breast cancer cells in vitro and in vivo. Mol Endocrinol 3:372–380.
59. Cullen KJ, Lippman ME, Chow D, Hill S, Rosen N, Zwiebel JA (1992) Insulin-like growth factor-II overexpression in MCF-7 cells induces phenotypic changes associated with malignant progression. Mol Endocrinol 6:91–100.
60. Daly RJ, Harris WH, Wang EY, Darbre PD (1991) Autocrine production of insulin-like growth factor II using and inducible expression system results in reduced estrogen sensitivity of MCF-7 human breast cancer cells. Cell Growth Differ 2:457–464.
61. Arteaga CL, Carty-Dugger T, Moses HL, Hurd SD, Pietenpol JA (1993) Transforming growth factor beta 1 can induce estrogen-independent tumorigenicity of human breast cancer cells in athymic mice. Cell Growth Differ 4:193–201.
62. Benz CC, Scott GK, Sarup JC, Johnson RM, Tripathy D, Coronado E, et al. (1993) Estrogen-dependent, tamoxifen-resistant tumorigenic growth of MCF-7 cells transfected with HER2/neu. Breast Cancer Res Treat 24:85–95.
63. Liu Y, El-Ashry D, Chen D, Ding IYF, Kern FG (1995) MCF-7 breast cancer cells overexpressing transfected c-erbB-2 have and in vitro growth advantage in estrogen-depleted conditions and reduced estrogen dependence and tamoxifen sensitivity in vivo. Breast Cancer Res Treat 34:97–117.

64. Miller DL, El-Ashry D, Cheville AL, Liu Y, McLeskey SW, Kern FG (1994) Emergence of MCF-7 cells overexpressing a transfected epidermal growth factor receptor (EGFR) under estrogen-depleted conditions: evidence for a role of EGFR in breast cancer growth and progression. Cell Growth Differ 5:1263–1274.
65. Zhang L, Kharbanda S, Chen D, Bullocks J, Miller DL, Ding IYF, et al. (1997) MCF-7 breast carcinoma cells overexpressing FGF-1 form vascularized, metastatic tumors in ovariectomized or tamoxifen-treated nude mice. Oncogene 15:2093–2108.
66. Tang CK, Perez C, Grunt T, Waibel C, Cho C, Lupu R (1996) Involvement of heregulin-beta2 in the acquisition of the hormone-independent phenotype of breast cancer cells. Cancer Res 56:3350–3358.
67. Kasid A, Lippman ME, Papageorge AG, Lowy DR, Gelmann EP (1985) Transfection of v-ras^{H} DNA into MCF-7 human breast cancer cells bypasses dependence on estrogen for tumorigenicity. Science 228:725–728.
68. Sommers CL, Papageorge A, Wilding G, Gelmann EP (1990) Growth properties and tumorigenesis of MCF-7 cells transfected with isogenic mutants of ras^{H}. Cancer Res 50:67–71.
69. Gelmann EP, Thompson EW, Sommers CL (1992) Invasive and maetastatic properties of MCF-7 cells and rasH-transfected MCF-7 cells. Int J Cancer 51:1–5.
70. Sukumar S, Carney WP, Barbacid M (1988) Independent molecular pathways in initiation and loss of hormone responsiveness of breast carcinomas. Science 240:524–526.
71. El-Ashry D, Miller DL, Kharbanda S, Lippman ME, Kern FG (1997) Constitutive Raf-1 kinase activity in breast cancer cells induces both estrogen-independent growth and apoptosis. Oncogene 15:423–435.
72. Ways DK, Kukoly CA, deVente J, Hooker JL, Bryant WO, Posekany KJ, et al. (1995) MCF-7 breast cancer cells transfected with protein kinase C-alpha exhibit altered expression of other protein kinase C isoforms and display a more aggressive neoplastic phenotype. J Clin Invest 95:1906–1915.
73. Levenson AS, Jordan VC (1997) MCF-7: the first hormone-responsive breast cancer cell line. Cancer Res 57:3071–3078.
74. Soule HD, McGrath CM (1980) Estrogen responsive proliferation of clonal human breast carcinoma cells in athymic mice. Cancer Lett 10:1140–1151.
75. Osborne CK, Hobbs K, Clark GM (1985) Effect of estrogens and antiestrogens on growth of human breast cancer cells in athymic nude mice. Cancer Res 45:584–590.
76. Engel LW, Young NA (1978) Human breast carcinoma cells in continuous culture: a review. Cancer Res 38:4327–4339.
77. Kurebayashi J, McLeskey SW, Johnson MD, Lippman ME, Dickson RB, Kern FG (1993) Quantitative demonstration of spontaneous metastasis by MCF-7 human breast cancer cells cotransfected with fibroblast growth factor 4 and lacZ. Cancer Res 53:2178–2187.
78. Sommers CL, Thompson EW, Torri JA, Kemler R, Gelmann EP, Byers SW (1991) Cell adhesion molecule uvomorulin expression in human breast cancer cell lines: relationship to morphology and invasive capacities. Cell Growth Differ 2:365–372.
79. McLeskey SW, Zhang L, Kharbanda S, Kurebayashi J, Lippman ME, Dickson RB, et al. (1996) Fibroblast growth factor overexpressing breast carcinoma cells as models of angiogenesis and metastasis. Breast Cancer Res Treat 39:103–117.
80. Thomas KA, Rios-Candelore M, Gimenez-Gallego G, DiSalvo S, Bennett C, Rodkey J, et al. (1985) Pure brain-derived acidic fibroblast growth factor is a potent angiogenic vascular endothelial cell mitogen with sequence homology to interleukin 1. Proc Natl Acad Sci USA 82:6409–6413.
81. Delli-Bovi P, Curatola AM, Newman KM, Sato Y, Moscatelli D, Hewick RM, et al. (1988) Processing, secretion, and biological properties of a novel growth factor of the fibroblast growth factor family with oncogenic potential. Mol Cell Biol 8:2933–2941.
82. Zhang L, Kharbanda S, Kern FG (1996) Characterization of the metastatic properties of FGF-1 transfected MCF-7 breast cancer cells. Proc Am Assoc Cancer Res 37:A418 abstract.
83. O'Reilly MS, Holmgren L, Shing Y, Chen C, Rosenthal RA, Moses M, et al. (1994) Angiostatin: a novel angiogenesis inhibitor that mediates the suppression of metastases by a Lewis lung carcinoma. Cell 79:315–328.
84. Chen C, Parangi S, Tolentino MJ, Folkman J (1995) A strategy to discover circulating angiogenesis inhibitors generated by human tumors. Cancer Res 55:4230–4233.
85. Folkman J (1995) Angiogenesis inhibitors generated by tumors. Mol Med 1:120–122.
86. O'Reilly MS, Boehm T, Shing Y, Fukai N, Vasios G, Lane WS, et al. (1997) Endostatin: an endogenous inhibitor of angiogenesis and tumor growth. Cell 88:277–285.
87. Karunagaran D, Tzahar E, Beerli RR, Chen X, Graus-Porta D, Ratzkin BJ, et al. (1996) ErbB-2 is a common auxiliary subunit of NDF and EGF receptors: implications for breast cancer. EMBO J 15:254–264.

88. Riese DJ, 2nd, van Raaij TM, Plowman GD, Andrews GC, Stern DF (1995) The cellular response to neuregulins is governed by complex interactions of the erbB receptor family [published erratum appears in Mol Cell Biol 1996;16:735]. Mol Cell Biol 15:5770–5776.
89. Carlomagno C, Perrone F, Gallo C, De Laurentiis M, Lauria R, Morabito A, et al. (1996) c-erb B2 overexpression decreases the benefit of adjuvant tamoxifen in early-stage breast cancer without axillary lymph node metastases. J Clin Oncol 14:2702–2708.
90. Smith J, Yelland A, Baillie R, Coombes RC (1994) Acidic and basic fibroblast growth factors in human breast tissue. Eur J Cancer 30A:496–503.
91. Anandappa SY, Winstanley JH, Leinster S, Green B, Rudland PS, Barraclough R (1994) Comparative expression of fibroblast growth factor mRNAs in benign and malignant breast disease. Br J Cancer 69:772–776.
92. Bansal GS, Yiangou C, Coope RC, Gomm JJ, Luqmani YA, Coombes RC, et al. (1995) Expression of fibroblast growth factor 1 is lower in breast cancer than in normal human breast. Br J Cancer 72:1420–1426.
93. Yoshiji H, Gomez DE, Shibuya M, Thorgeirsson UP (1996) Expression of vascular endothelial growth factor, its receptor, and other angiogenic factors in human breast cancer. Cancer Res 56:2013–2016.
94. Relf M, LeJeune S, Scott PA, Fox S, Smith K, Leek R, et al. (1997) Expression of the angiogenic factors vascular endothelial cell growth factor, acidic and basic fibroblast growth factor, tumor growth factor beta-1, platelet-derived endothelial cell growth factor, placenta growth factor, and pleiotrophin in human primary breast cancer and its relation to angiogenesis. Cancer Res 57:963–969.
95. Ding IY, McLeskey SW, Chang K, Fu YM, Acol JC, Shou MT, et al. (1992) Expression of fibroblast growth factors (FGFS) and receptors (FGFRS) in human breast carcinomas. Proc Am Assoc Cancer Res 33:A1610.
96. Coope RC, Browne PJ, Yiangou C, Bansal GS, Walters J, Groome N, et al. (1997) The location of acidic fibroblast growth factor in the breast is dependent on the activity of proteases present in breast cancer tissue. Br J Cancer 75:1621–1630.
97. Adnane J, Gaudray P, Dionne CA, Crumley G, Jaye M, Schlessinger J, et al. (1991) BEK and FLG, two receptors to members of the FGF family, are amplified in subsets of human breast cancers. Oncogene 6:659–663.
98. Theillet C, Adelaide J, Louason G, Bonnet-Dorion F, Jacquemier J, Adnane J, et al. (1993) FGFRI and PLAT genes and DNA amplification at 8p12 in breast and ovarian cancers. Genes Chromosom. Cancer 7:219–226.
99. Jacquemier J, Adelaide J, Parc P, Penault-Llorca F, Planche J, deLapeyriere O, et al. (1994) Expression of the FGFR1 gene in human breast-carcinoma cells. Int J Cancer 59:373–378.
100. Jaakkola S, Salmikangas P, Nylund S, Partanen J, Armstrong E, Pyrhonen S, et al. (1993) Amplification of fgfr4 gene in human breast and gynecological cancers. Int J Cancer 54:378–382.
101. Bellot F, Crumley G, Kaplow JM, Schlessinger J, Jaye M, Dionne CA (1991) Ligand-induced transphosphorylation between different FGF receptors. EMBO J 10:2849–2854.
102. Spivak-Kroizman T, Lemmon MA, Dikic I, Ladbury JE, Pinchasi D, Huang J, et al. (1994) Heparin-induced oligomerization of FGF molecules is responsible for FGF receptor dimerization, activation, and cell proliferation. Cell 79:1015–1024.
103. Ueno H, Gunn M, Dell K, Tseng A Jr, Williams L (1992) A truncated form of fibroblast growth factor receptor 1 inhibits signal transduction by multiple types of fibroblast growth factor receptor. J Biol Chem 267:1470–1476.
104. Amaya E, Musci TJ, Kirschner MW (1991) Expression of a dominant negative mutant of the FGF receptor disrupts mesoderm formation in *Xenopus* embryos. Cell 66:257–270.
105. Li Y, Basilico C, Mansukhani A (1994) Cell transformation by fibroblast growth factors can be suppressed by truncated fibroblast growth factor receptors. Mol Cell Biol 14:7660–7669.
106. Zhang L, Kharbanda S, Hanfelt J and Kern FG (1998) Both autocrine and paracrine effects of transfected acidic fibroblast growth factor are involved in the estrogen-independent and antiestrogen-resistant growth of MCF-7 breast cancer cells. Cancer Res, 58:352–361.
107. Jordan VC, Gottardis MM, Robinson SP, Friedl A (1989) Immune-deficient animals to study "hormone-dependent" breast and endometrial cancer. J Steroid Biochem 34:169–176.
108. Gottardis MM, Jordan VC (1988) Development of tamoxifen-stimulated growth of MCF-7 tumors in athymic mice after long-term antiestrogen administration. Cancer Res 48:5183–5187.
109. Toi M, Inada K, Suzuki H, Tominaga T (1995) Tumor angiogenesis in breast cancer: its importance as a prognostic indicator and the association with vascular endothelial growth factor expression. Breast Cancer Res Treat 36:193–204.

110. Anan K, Morisaki T, Katano M, Ikubo A, Kitsuki H, Uchiyama A, et al. (1996) Vascular endothelial growth factor and platelet-derived growth factor are potential angiogenic and metastatic factors in human breast cancer. Surgery 119:333–339.
111. Toi M, Kondo S, Suzuki H, Yamamoto Y, Inada K, Imazawa T, et al. (1996) Quantitative analysis of vascular endothelial growth factor in primary breast cancer. Cancer 77:1101–1106.
112. Toi M, Hoshina S, Takayanagi T, Tominaga T (1994) Association of vascular endothelial growth factor expression with tumor angiogenesis and with early relapse in primary breast cancer. Jpn J Cancer Res 85:1045–1049.
113. Brown LF, Berse B, Jackman RW, Tognazzi K, Guidi AJ, Dvorak HF, et al. (1995) Expression of vascular permeability factor (vascular endothelial growth factor) and its receptors in breast cancer. Hum Pathol 26:86–91.
114. de Vries C, Escobedo JA, Ueno H, Houck K, Ferrara N, Williams LT (1992) The fms-like tyrosine kinase, a receptor for vascular endothelial growth factor. Science 255:989–991.
115. Terman BI, Dougher-Vermazen M, Carrion ME, Dimitrov D, Armellino DC, Gospodarowicz D, et al. (1992) Identification of the KDR tyrosine kinase as a receptor for vascular endothelial cell growth factor. Biochem Biophys Res Commun 187:1579–1586.
116. Millauer B, Wizigmann-Voos S, Schmurch H, Martinez R, Miller NP, Risau W, et al. (1993) High affinity VEGF binding and developmental expression suggest Flk-1 as a major regulator of vasculogenesis and angiogenesis. Cell 72:835–846.
117. Quinn TP, Peters KG, de Vries C, Ferrara N, Williams LT (1993) Fetal liver kinase 1 is a receptor for vascular endothelial growth factor and is selectively expressed in vascular endothelium. Proc Natl Acad Sci USA 90:7533–7537.
118. Clauss M, Weich H, Breier G, Knies U, Rockl W, Waltenberger J, et al. (1996) The vascular endothelial growth factor receptor Flt-1 mediates biological activities. Implications for a functional role of placenta growth factor in monocyte activation and chemotaxis. J Biol Chem 271:17629–17634.
119. Barleon B, Sozzani S, Zhou D, Weich HA, Mantovani A, Marme D (1996) Migration of human monocytes in response to vascular endothelial growth factor (VEGF) is mediated via the VEGF receptor Flt-1. Blood 87:3336–3343.
120. Katoh O, Tauchi H, Kawaishi K, Kimura A, Satow Y (1995) Expression of the vascular endothelial growth factor (VEGF) receptor gene, KDR, in hematopoietic cells and inhibitory effect of VEGF on apoptotic cell death caused by ionizing radiation. Cancer Res 55:5687–5692.
121. Liu B, Earl HM, Baban D, Shoaibi M, Fabra A, Kerr DJ, et al. (1995) Melanoma cell lines express VEGF receptor KDR and respond to exogenously added VEGF. Biochem Biophys Res Commun 217:721–727.
122. Boocock CA, Charnock-Jones DS, Sharkey AM, McLaren J, Barker PJ, Wright KA, et al. (1995) Expression of vascular endothelial growth factor and its receptors Flt and KDR in ovarian carcinoma. J Natl Cancer Inst 87:506–516.
123. Charnock-Jones DS, Sharkey AM, Boocock CA, Ahmed A, Plevin R, Ferrara N, et al. (1994) Vascular endothelial growth factor receptor localization and activation in human trophoblast and choriocarcinoma cells. Biol Reprod 51:524–530.
124. Bullocks J, Zhang L, Ding IYF, McLeskey SW, Tobias CA, Miller DL, et al. (1997) Overexpression of vascular endothelial growth factor (VEGF) in MCF-7 breast carcinoma cells facilitates growth in tamoxifen-treated nude mice and tumor cell dissemination. Proc Am Assoc Cancer Res 38:A3521 abstract.
125. Zhang H, Craft P, Scott PAE, Ziche M, Weich HA, Harris AL, et al. (1995) Enhancement of tumor growth and vascular density by transfection of vascular endothelial cell growth factor into MCF-7 human breast carcinoma cells. J Natl Cancer Inst 87:213–219.
126. Noel A, De Pauw-Gillet M, Purnell G, Nusgens B, Lapiere C-M, Foidart J, -M. (1993) Enhancement of tumorigenicity of human breast adenocarcinoma cells in nude mice by Matrigel and fibroblasts. Br J Cancer 68:909–915.
127. Fridman R, Kibbey MC, Royce LS, Zain M, Sweeney TM, Jicha DL, et al. (1991) Enhanced tumor growth of both primary and estatblished human and murine tumor cells in athymic mice after coinjection with Matrigel. J Natl Cancer Inst 83:769–774.
128. Houck KA, Leung DW, Rowland AM, Winer J, Ferrara N (1992) Dual regulation of vascular endothelial growth factor bioavailability by genetic and proteolytic mechanisms. J Biol Chem 267:26031–26037.
129. Soker S, Svahn CM, Neufeld G (1993) Vascular endothelial growth factor is inactivated by binding to alpha 2–macroglobulin and the binding is inhibited by heparin. J Biol Chem 268:7685–7691.

130. Macaulay VM, Fox SB, Zhang H, Whitehouse RM, Leek RD, Gatter KC, et al. (1997) Breast cancer angiogenesis and tamoxifen resistance. Endocr Rel Cancer 2:97–103.
131. Senger DR, van de Water L, Brown LF, Nagy JA, Yeo K-T, Yeo T-K, Berse B, et al. (1993) Vascular permeability factor (VPF, VEGF) in tumor biology. Cancer Metastasis Rev 12:303–324.
132. Ferrara N (1995) The role of vascular endothelial growth factor in pathological angiogenesis. Breast Cancer Res Treat 36:127–137.
133. Klagsbrun M, D'Amore PA (1996) Vascular endothelial growth factor and its receptors. Cytokine Growth Factor Rev 7:259–270.
134. Gospodarowicz D, Ferrara N, Schweigerer L, Neufeld G (1987) Structural characterization and biological functions of fibroblast growth factor. Endocr Rev 8:95–114.
135. Burgess WH, Maciag T (1989) The heparin-binding (fibroblast) growth factor family of proteins. Annu Rev Biochem 58:575–606.
136. Holmgren L, O'Reilly MS, Folkman J (1995) Dormancy of micrometastases: balanced proliferation and apoptosis in the presence of angiogenesis suppression. Nature Med 1:149–153.
137. O'Reilly MS, Holmgren L, Chen C, Folkman J (1996) Angiostatin induces and sustains dormancy of human primary tumors in mice. Nature Med 2:689–692.
138. Lu C, Tanigawa N (1997) Spontaneous apoptosis is inversely related to intratumoral microvessel density in gastric carcinoma. Cancer Res 57:221–224.
139. McLeskey SW, Zhang L, Kharbanda S, Liu Y, Trock BJ, Gottardis MM, et al. (1996) Effects of AGM-1470 and pentosan polysulfate on tumorigenicity and metastasis of FGF-transfected MCF-7 cells. Br J Cancer 73:1053–1062.
140. Oldham SM, Clark GJ, Gangarosa LM, Coffey RJ Jr, Der CJ (1996) Activation of the Raf-1/MAP kinase cascade is not sufficient for Ras transformation of RIE-1 epithelial cells. Proc Natl Acad Sci USA 93:6924–6928.
141. Khosravi-Far R, Solski PA, Clark GJ, Kinch MS, Der CJ (1995) Activation of Rac1, RhoA, and Mitogen-Activated Protein Kinases is required for Ras transformation. Mol Cell Biol 15:6443–6453.
142. Miyamoto M, Naruo K, Seko C, Matsumoto S, Kondo T, Kurokawa T (1993) Molecular cloning of a novel cytokine cDNA encoding the ninth member of the fibroblast growth factor family, which has a unique secretion property. Mol Cell Biol 13:4251–4259.
143. Tanaka A, Miyamoto K, Minamino N, Takeda M, Sato B, Matsuo H, et al. (1992) Cloning and characterization of an androgen-induced growth factor essential for the androgen-dependent growth of mouse mammary carcinoma cells. Proc Natl Acad Sci USA 89:8928–8932.
144. Basilico C, Moscatelli D (1992) The FGF family of growth factors and oncogenes. Adv Cancer Res 59:115–165.
145. Yamasaki M, Miyake A, Tagashira S, Itoh N (1996) Strucure and expression of the rat mRNA encoding a novel member of the fibroblast growth factor family. J Biol Chem 271:15,918–15,921.
146. Beer HD, Florence C, Dammeier J, McGuire L, Werner S, Duan DR (1997) Mouse fibroblast growth factor 10: cDNA cloning, protein characterization, and regulation of mRNA expression. Oncogene 15:2211–2218.
147. Emoto H, Tagashira S, Mattei MG, Yamasaki M, Hashimoto G, Katsumata T, et al. (1997) Structure and expression of human fibroblast growth factor-10. J Biol Chem 272:23,191–23,194.
148. Smallwood PM, Munoz-Sanjuan I, Tong P, Macke JP, Hendry JH, Gilbert DJ, et al. (1996) Fibroblast growth factor (FGF) homologous factors: new members of the FGF family implicated in nervous system development. Proc Natl Acad Sci USA 93:9850–9857.
149. Givol D, Yayon A (1992) Complexity of FGF receptors: genetic basis for structural diversity and functional specificity. FASEB J 6:3362–3369.
150. Johnson DE, Williams LT (1993) Structural and functional diversity in the FGF receptor multigene family. Adv Cancer Res 60:1–41.
151. Kan M, Wang F, Xu J, Crabb JW, Hou J, McKeehan WL (1993) An essential heparin-binding domain in the fibroblast growth factor receptor kinase. Science 259:1918–1921.
152. Fenig E, Wieder R, Paglin S, Wang H, Resaud R, Haimovitz-Friedman A, et al. (1997) Basic fibroblast growth factor confers growth inhibition and mitogen-activated protein kinase activation in human breast cancer cells. Clin Cancer Res 3:135–142.
153. Wang H, Rubin M, Fenig E, DeBlasio A, Mendelsohn J, Yahalom J, et al. (1997) Basic fibroblast growth factor causes growth arrest in MCF-7 human breast cancer cells while inducing both mitogenic and inhibitory G_1 events. Cancer Res 57:1750–1757.

154. Green PJ, Walsh FS, Doherty P (1996) Promiscuity of fibroblast growth factor receptors. Bioessays 18:639–646.
155. Gao G, Goldfarb M (1995) Heparin can activate a receptor tyrosine kinase. EMBO J 14:2183–2190.
156. Webster MK, Donoghue DJ (1996) Constitutive activation of fibroblast growth factor receptor 3 by the transmembrane domain point mutation found in achondroplasia. EMBO J 15:520–527.
157. Neilson KM, Friesel RE (1995) Constitutive activation of fibroblast growth factor receptor-2 by a point mutation associated with Crouzon syndrome. J Biol Chem 270:26037–26040.
158. Migliaccio A, Di Domenico M, Castoria G, de Falco A, Bontempo P, Nola E, et al. (1996) Tyrosine kinase/p21Ras/MAP-kinase pathway activation by estradiol-receptor complex in MCF-7 cells. EMBO J 15:1292–1300.
159. Lukas J, Bartkova J, Bartek J (1996) Convergence of mitogenic signalling cascades from diverse classes of receptors at the cyclin D-cyclin-dependent kinase-pRB- controlled G1 checkpoint. Mol Cell Biol 16:6917–6925.
160. Addeo R, Altucci L, Battista T, Bonapace IM, Cancemi M, Cicatiello L, et al. (1996) Stimulation of human breast cancer MCF-7 cells with estrogen prevents cell cycle arrest by HMG-CoA reductase inhibitors. Biochem Biophys Res Commun 220:864–870.
161. Bonapace IM, Addeo R, Altucci L, Cicatiello L, Bifulco M, Laezza C, et al. (1996) 17 Beta-estradiol overcomes a G1 block induced by HMG-CoA reductase inhibitors and fosters cell cycle progression without inducing ERK-1 and -2 MAP kinases activation. Oncogene 12:753–763.

13 Role of the IGF System in Breast Cancer Proliferation and Progression

A. V. Lee, PHD *and D. Yee,* MD

INTRODUCTION

The insulin-like growth factor (IGF) family consists of two ligands (IGF-I and IGF-II), three receptors (IGFR1, IGFR2, and hybrid IGFR1/insulin receptor) and seven IGF binding proteins (IGFBP1–7). Similar to many other growth factor families such as epidermal growth factor (EGF) and platelet-derived growth factor (PDGF), the number and variety of effects that can be elicited by the IGF family are very diverse and continue to expand *(1)*. In particular, the ability of different ligands, receptors, and binding proteins to crossreact and the ensuing variety of biologic effects make assigning specific roles for each member difficult. This is especially true for the IGFBPs; several years of research have still failed to elucidate the true function of these proteins in IGF action *(2)*.

The IGFs, formerly known as somatomedins, were purified and sequenced in 1976 *(1)*; because of their close homology to proinsulin (approx 50%), they were termed insulin-like growth factors. Initial characterization concentrated on the production of IGF-I in the liver, as well as control of serum IGF-I levels by growth hormone (GH), which was thought to mediate bone elongation in an endocrine manner *(3)*. IGF-II, in contrast to IGF-I, is minimally GH responsive and is thought to be involved in fetal growth and development. Whereas early work concentrated on the endocrine function of IGFs, recent work has highlighted both autocrine and paracrine functions in growth, malignant transformation, and apoptosis *(4)*. These functions will be discussed throughout this review, mainly stemming from the pioneering gene knockout studies of Efstradiatis' group *(5,6)*.

IGF-I and IGF-II are single-chain polypeptides that interact with high-affinity receptors. IGFR1 is a classical tyrosine kinase receptor, normally found as a heterodimer consisting of two α- and β-subunits that span the plasma membrane *(7)*. The receptor can, however, also be found as a hybrid heterodimer with the structurally similar insulin receptor *(8–10)*. Unlike other classical tyrosine kinase receptors, such as EGF and PDGF receptors, IGFR1 activity is dependent on ligand binding; thus simple overexpression of IGFR1 does not result in ligand-dependent activation *(11)*. IGF-I and IGF-II have approximately equal affinity for IGFR1 in most systems, and IGFR1 is thought to transduce the effects of both ligands.

IGFR2, in contrast to IGFR1, has no tyrosine kinase activity, and its role in IGF signaling remains unclear at present. IGFR2 is a single-chain molecule *(12,13)* identical

From: *Contemporary Endocrinology: Endocrinology of Breast Cancer*
Edited by: A. Manni © Humana Press Inc., Totowa, NJ

to the mannose-6-phosphate (M-6-P) receptor, which is involved in sorting of M-6-P-bearing lysosomal enzymes in the Golgi apparatus and endoplasmic reticulum. At present there are conflicting data concerning a role for IGFR2 in IGF signaling. Nishimoto's group has shown IGF-II-mediated binding of a small molecular weight G-protein to the carboxy terminus of IGFR2 *(14)* and also defined mechanisms for inhibition of this binding *(15)*. However, the significance of this association and any possible downstream signaling events have yet to be elucidated. There are several anecdotal reports supporting a mitogenic role for IGFR2 in IGF-II-mediated proliferation, e.g., in cells that lack IGFR1 *(16,17)*. However, no studies have definitely proved a signaling mechanism, and detailed mutational analysis of IGFR2 has failed to find any signaling capability *(18)*. Of interest in breast cancer is the fact that IGFR2 can bind transforming growth factor-β (TGF-β) and procathepsin D *(17)*. The binding of this growth factor and protease is competed for by IGF-II, providing a complicated scenario of IGFR2 regulating a growth promoter (IGF-II), a growth inhibitor (TGF-β), and a protease (procathepsin D). The importance of all of these factors in breast cancer warrants further analysis of the role of this receptor in breast cancer growth. However, due to the failure to prove conclusively that IGFR2 has a signaling function, many have been led to hypothesize that it acts as an inactive "sink" by binding and inhibiting IGF-II-mediated action through the IGFR1. This hypothesis is substantiated by IGFR2 gene knockouts that had higher circulating IGF-II levels and were born larger than wild-type littermates *(5)*.

Whereas IGFR2 gene knockouts may have elucidated an important role for IGFR2 in controlling IGF-II action, the IGFR1 knockouts have been instrumental in defining a role for IGFR1 in growth, transformation, and apoptosis *(19)*. Mice lacking IGFR1 were born smaller than wild-type littermates and died soon after birth due to asphyxiation *(6)*. Necropsy revealed that the cause of death was lung hypoplasia, but also that almost every organ in the mouse suffered from a reduced number of cells. This places a role for IGFR1 in the growth of practically every cell in the developing embryo, confirming that IGFR1 is a critical regulator of the cell cycle. Of interest was the lack of developmental abnormalities, suggesting that IGFR1 is not an absolute requirement in this process. Fibroblasts obtained from IGFR1 null mice have been used to elucidate further the role of IGFR1 in the cell cycle. IGFR1-negative cells (R–) grow more slowly than wild-type controls in 10% serum and have an increase in each phase of the cell cycle *(20)*. Other growth factors fail to stimulate growth of R- cells *(21)*, and they are unable to be transformed by various oncogenes *(22,23)*. Substantiating the knockout studies, overexpression of IGFR1 in fibroblasts results in reduced growth factor requirements *(24)* with a decrease in susceptibility to apoptosis *(25)*. Mutational studies are defining the regions of the IGFR1 involved in physiologic events (growth, transformation, and apoptosis), thus defining the signal transduction pathways involved in these processes. For instance, transforming and mitogenic signals can clearly be dissected within the carboxy terminus of the receptor *(26)*.

The IGF blinding proteins (BPs) provide another level of control of IGF action, by binding the IGFs with higher affinity than IGFR proteins *(2)*. The IGFBPs are expressed in a complex tissue-specific pattern; this, and also the fact that a single IGFBP species is rarely expressed by itself, has hampered assignment of specific roles for IGFBPs. The IGFBPs seem to have four main functions: (1) to increase the half-life of bound IGFs by providing storage in the circulation and in the extracellular matrix; (2) to present IGFs to IGFRs and augment IGF action; (3) to sequester IGFs from IGFRs and inhibit IGF action; and (4) IGF-independent effects on other cellular processes, e.g., cell motility via the interaction of IGFBP-1 with the α5β1 integrin receptor *(27)*. The first role of IGFBPs, increasing IGF half-life, has been clearly shown for IGFBP-3, the binding protein species that binds the majority of IGF-I in human serum.

The role of IGFBPs in inhibiting and potentiating IGF action is less clear and depends on the biologic situation in which they are studied. For example, IGFBP-3 can be both stimulatory and inhibitory to IGF action when it is added exogenously to the same cell line, simply depending on whether it is added before or after IGF stimulation *(28)*. Transfection studies again showing an ability of IGFBP-3 either to augment growth or to inhibit growth confirm this confusing result *(29–31)*. An explanation for these conflicting data may arise from the studies of Oh et al., who have shown IGF and IGFR1-independent effects of IGFBP-3 on estrogen receptor (ER)-negative Hs578T breast cancer cells *(32)*, and the presence of a high-affinity binding protein for IGFBP-3 *(33)*. This is substantiated by inhibitory effects of IGFBP-3 in IGFR1 knockout cells that constitutively express IGFBP-3 *(34)*. We have shown that IGFBP-1 can inhibit IGF-mediated growth effects (discussed later in this chapter). However, phosphorylated IGFBP-1 binds IGF-I with high affinity and can block ligand/receptor interaction *(35)*, whereas unphosphorylated IGFBP-1 binds IGF-I with low affinity and has been shown to enhance IGF action *(36)*.

In summary, the IGF family acts in a complex manner to control cellular proliferation. Although IGF action is not an absolute requirement for embryonic development, it can clearly control the rate of proliferation within a number of organs. The autocrine, paracrine, endocrine, and possibly intracrine effects of the IGFs, and the strict control of IGF action, may provide us with a clue to importance of this growth factor family in both normal and neoplastic growth.

IGFS AND NORMAL BREAST DEVELOPMENT

Growth and development of normal mammary breast epithelium is controlled during puberty by a number of hormones. Thus rats that have been hypophysectomized and ovariectomized do not form mature mammary glands *(37)*. Studies delivering various hormone combinations back to these rats showed that in the absence of estrogen little or no mammary development occurred, while addition of GH and estrogen resulted in complete normal mammary development *(38)*. Further studies indicated that IGF-I could substitute for GH; thus IGF-I given systemically, or via implanted pellet in the mammary gland, induced mammary gland development in estrogen-treated hypophysectomized and ovariectomised rats *(39)*. IGF-I can not induce full mammary development on its own, suggesting a synergism between IGF and ER action.

The substantial body of evidence indicating that IGF-I is the mediator of local GH action, particularly on epipyseal plate growth *(40)*, has thus led to the hypothesis that IGF-I is responsible for GH-mediated normal mammary gland development. Studies have shown that IGF-I mRNA is present in the normal mammary epithelium *(41)* and that expression can be induced by GH *(42)*.

IGF-I may also be involved in lactational events within the normal breast. Thus two studies have shown that targeting of IGF-I overexpression to the lactating normal mammary epithelium, using the pregnancy-activated whey acidic protein promoter, resulted in ductal hypertrophy and an inhibition of postlactational mammary involution *(43,44)*. This may be a result of an inhibition of apoptosis within these cells. Thus the IGFs may be involved in the growth and development of normal mammary epithelium.

IGFS AND BREAST CANCER

IGF Ligands

IGF-I and -II are both potent mitogens for a number of breast cancer cell lines in vitro, with maximal proliferative effects at pico- to nanomolar concentrations *(45–48)*. Most breast cancer cells that respond to IGF-I are ER positive (e.g., MCF-7, ZR-75, or T47D), whereas ER-negative cells tend not to proliferate or have a minimal response to IGF stimulation (e.g., MDA-435, or MDA-231, MDA-468). Whether the ER is a requisite for IGF action or whether ER expression is simply representative of a cell with relatively intact growth signaling pathways (ER-positive breast tumors are more differentiated and less aggressive than ER-negative tumors) is not clear; however, the apparent synergism between the two signaling pathways (discussed later) may elucidate an important role for IGFs in breast cancer.

The initial measurement of IGF expression in breast cancer cells was technically hampered by the low levels of IGF expression and the interference of IGFBPs in radioimmunoassays *(49)*. Early reports of IGF-I-like immunoreactivity in MCF-7 conditioned media (CM) were probably owing to IGFBPs interfering with the assay; however, there are consistent reports of an IGF-like species being secreted by MCF-7 cells *(46,50,51)*. The inability to detect any IGF-I mRNA in any breast cancer cell line by a sensitive RNAse protection assay would seem, however, to confirm that breast cancer cells do not express IGF-I *(47)*.

IGF-II is expressed by a small number of breast cancer cell lines, but detection has again proved difficult *(47,52)*. We used a sensitive Western blotting technique to show IGF-II expression in CM, and the presence of IGF-II mRNA in the same cell lines expressing IGF-II peptide supports these data *(53)*. Thus we would expect that IGF-II could be an autocrine growth regulator in breast cancer, and this was confirmed by constitutive overexpression of IGF-II in MCF-7 cells, which led to autocrine proliferation that was inhibited by αIR3 *(54,55)*. Furthermore, in cells overexpressing IGF-II, we were able to use the Western blotting technique to show that large precursor forms of IGF-II are secreted, possibly as a result of saturation of the processing machinery *(53)*. In vivo studies with transgenic mice overexpressing IGF-II in the mammary gland have shown the development of breast cancer *(56)*, again confirming that IGF-II may be an important regulator of breast cell growth.

Breast cancer specimens have been examined for IGF expression by *in situ* hybridization. IGF-I is rarely expressed in breast epithelial tissue, but mainly in the stroma *(57,58)*, and IGF-II is expressed in breast stroma, but also in epithelial cells *(47,58)*. Recent immunohistochemistry (IHC) studies also support this observation *(59,60)*. Thus we expect that the IGFs may play a paracrine role in breast cancer proliferation. Supporting this hypothesis is the fact that IGF-II expression is increased in breast stroma associated with a malignancy, compared with benign and normal breast *(61)*. Additionally, in vitro studies have revealed that malignant breast epithelial cells can enhance expression of IGF-II from breast stroma *(62)*.

Although only a few studies have analyzed autocrine and paracrine IGF action within the breast, an increasing number of studies clearly show that serum IGF-I levels are increased in breast cancer patients, which could have an effect on endocrine and paracrine growth of breast tumors. Following the observation by Peyrat et al. *(63)* that breast cancer patients had higher serum IGF-I levels that age-matched controls, several reports indicated that either removal of the tumor or treatment with antiestrogens reduced serum IGF-I levels in patients (reviewed in ref. *64*). Although some groups have found no change in serum IGF-I levels *(65)*, and one report exists of an increase in serum IGF-I levels under tamoxifen treatment *(66)*, most data confirm the observation that antiestrogens lower circulating IGF-I levels. Interestingly, in some studies, the decrease in serum IGF-I levels is also associated with an increase in IGFBP-1 expression *(67,68)*. There are no data on the biologic significance of this result at present, but IGFBP-1 may increase the half-life of serum IGF-I, possibly negating the decrease in level, or IGFBP-1 may sequester IGF-I away from tumor cells to potentiate further the decrease in serum IGF-I levels.

While it is tempting to hypothesize that reduction of serum IGF-I levels may be in part responsible for the cytostatic/toxic effect of tamoxifen, presently no direct evidence shows that endocrine IGF regulates breast cancer cell growth. However, Pollack's group has studied potential mechanisms of how tamoxifen may decrease IGF-I levels and have found that tamoxifen can control GH secretion from the pituitary, thus controlling IGF-I production by the liver *(69,70)*. Additionally, IGF-I is an estrogen-responsive gene, and expression can be directly regulated by tamoxifen *(70)*. Further studies are needed to examine directly whether endocrine IGF-I can affect breast tumor growth and whether reduction of serum IGF-I may be a therapeutic target. Studies have been completed analyzing the effect of somatostatin analogs on lowering GH and IGF-I levels in breast cancer patients. A trial of lanreotide failed to lower GH levels in breast cancer patients *(71)*, whereas a trial of somatuline reduced IGF-I levels *(72)* but again had no effect on GH levels. The lack of clinical activity of these drugs justifies further evaluation of regimes aimed at lowering serum GH and IGF-I levels.

IGF Receptors

As mentioned previously, gene knockout studies have placed IGFR1 in a pivotal role in the growth and transformation of malignant cells *(19)*. It is not suprising, therefore, that all breast cancer cell lines express some level of IGFR1 mRNA and protein *(48)*. IGFR1 is thought to be the main mediator of both IGF-I and -II effects in breast cancer cells. However, overexpression of IGFR1 in MCF-7 cells does not result in dramatic phenotypic changes, with only slight changes in estrogen and IGF responsiveness *(73)*, as well as changes in E-cadherin association *(74)*.

Consistent with the expression of IGFR1 in all cell lines is the fact that most breast tumor specimens express IGFR1 mRNA *(48)*. IGFR1 is expressed at a higher level in breast tumor specimens compared with benign or normal tissue *(75)*, and protein analysis has indicated that a high number of breast tumors *(50–93%)* express IGFR1 *(75–77)*. Interestingly, higher IGFR1 levels are a favorable prognostic indicator (discussed later). Although IGFR1 levels are higher in breast cancer tissue compared with benign or normal breast tissue, IGFR1 gene copy number is rarely amplified. Berns et al. *(78)* found that only 19 (2%) of 975 breast tumors had gene amplification (between 3 and 56 copies).

Probably as a result of the lack of understanding of IGFR2 in breast cancer cells in culture, very few studies have examined IGFR2 expression in breast cancer. Even so, it has been shown that there is significant loss of heterozygosity (12/40 specimens) at the chromosomal locus of IGFR2 *(79)* and that this is associated with mutations in the other allele of IGFR2 (2/5 samples). Although it has yet to be shown whether these mutations disrupt IGFR2 function, e.g., IGF-II binding, it is tempting to hypothesize that loss of IGFR2 results in a release of previously bound IGF-II that can now act through the

IGFR1. Considering the potent mitogenic effect of IGFs in vitro, we would therefore expect this to result in enhanced tumor growth and a poor prognosis.

IGF Binding Proteins

Whereas the role of IGFBPs in IGF action is complex, they may actually be the controlling factor in IGF action *(2)*. Thus IGFBPs have the ability to augment, inhibit, or prolong IGF effects on a cell. Therefore, we and others have characterized IGFBP action and expression in breast cancer. Early studies of IGFBP expression in breast cancer cell lines, using a Western ligand blot assay with iodinated IGF-I, showed that all breast cancer cell lines secreted IGFBPs in CM and that IGFBP expression correlated with ER status *(80,81)*. Thus ER-positive cells expressed IGFBP-2, -4, and -5, and ER-negative cells expressed IGFBP-1 and 3. As with most generalizations, there are exceptions to this rule. The association of IGFBP expression with ER status is confirmed by the ability of estrogens and retinoids to modulate IGFBP expression *(35,82)*. Estrogen can induce IGFBP-2, -4, and -5 expression, whereas it inhibits IGFBP-3 expression. Interestingly, the increase in IGFBP-3 is associated with a decrease in proliferation, and studies have shown that IGFBP-3 can inhibit IGF-I- and estrogen-mediated growth when added exogenously to cells *(31)*, suggesting that IGFBP-3 may be one of the mediators of antiestrogen inhibition of growth. The same situation has recently been shown for IGFBP-5 *(83)*. Retinoic acid can also induce IGFBP-3 expression in MCF-7 cells, and this again results in a reduction in proliferation *(82)*

Analysis of IGFBP expression in primary breast cancer specimens substantiated the studies on cells in culture. Thus, all tumors expressed different patterns of IGFBP-2–6, and expression correlated with ER status *(84)*. IGFBP-3 was higher in ER-negative tumors, and IGFBP-4 and -5 were higher in ER-positive tumors. This was confirmed in other studies *(85)*. Clinical analysis of IGFBP expression revealed that IGFBP-4 expression was a favorable prognostic marker in a subset of small tumors *(86)* and that IGFBP-3 was associated with poor prognostic features *(87,88)*.

IGF Downstream Signaling Molecules

Recent studies have examined the role of IGFR1 downstream molecules in IGF action in breast cancer cells. Downregulation of IRS-1 expression in MCF-7 cells resulted in inhibition of serum-mediated growth but also cell death in serum-free media even when cells were stimulated with IGF-I *(89)*. Similar effects were seen in anchorage-independent growth. Reduction of another IGFR1 signaling molecule, SHC, also resulted in an inhibition of anchorage-dependent and -independent growth *(89)*. Substantiating these data is the observation that overexpression of IRS-1 in the same cells resulted in a decrease in estrogen responsiveness and an increase in autocrine-mediated growth *(90)*. The minimal effects of IGFR1 overexpression, seen in MCF-7 cells, but the dramatic effect of IRS-1 overexpression, may indicate that IRS-1 is the rate-limiting step in IGF action. For this reason we have analyzed IRS-1 expression in a series of primary human breast cancers *(88)*. IRS-1 was a poor prognostic indicator for a subset of breast cancer patients (discussed later).

ESTROGEN AND IGFS IN BREAST CANCER

It is well documented that estrogen is implicated in both the growth and progression of breast cancer, and this is substantiated by the expanding data confirming the successful

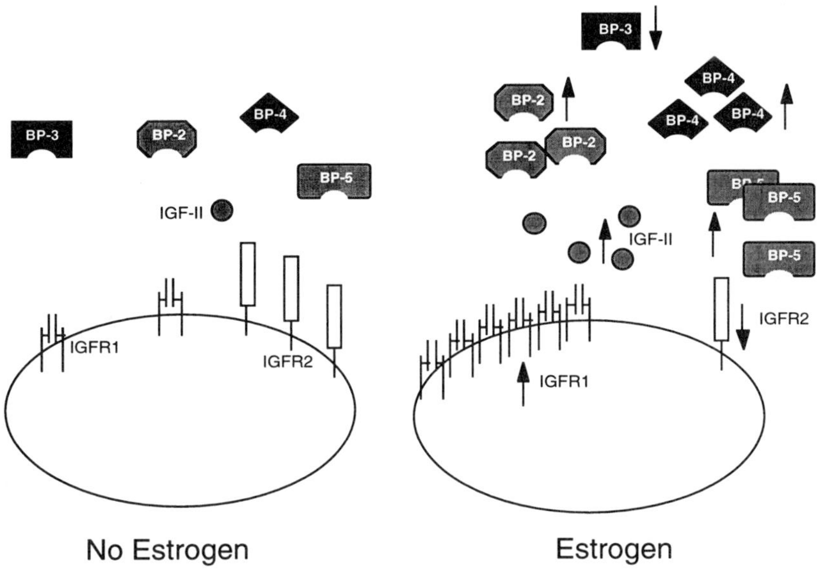

Fig. 1. Estrogen regulation of IGF family members in breast cancer. The figure is representative of data thus far concerning estrogen regulation of IGF system components in ER-positive breast cancer cells in vitro; however, a similar scenario is often seen in breast tumor specimens. In the presence of estrogen (right side) IGF-II, IGFR1, IGFBP-2, IGFBP-4, and IGFBP-5 expression are increased in breast cancer cells. By contrast, IGFR2 and IGFBP-3 expression are decreased. The result of estrogen treatment is an increase in IGF bioactivity within the cell.

use of tamoxifen, a nonsteroidal antiestrogen, in the treatment of the disease *(91)*. The discovery and cloning of the ER has increased the understanding of its mechanism of action, with recent discoveries of coactivators, corepressors, and interaction with the basal transcription machinery finally addressing the complex array of hormone effects within a cell and the body *(92)*. Despite this work, the mechanism of ER-mediated proliferation still remains unclear. The regulation of the IGF family by the ER (Fig. 1) and the regulation of ER action by the IGF family suggest that the IGFs may have a special role in this process *(93)*.

As mentioned previously, IGF-II is expressed by a number of breast cancer cell lines. IGF-II expression can be induced by estrogen in ER-positive cells, in xenograft MCF-7 tumors, and constitutive overexpression results in estrogen-independent autocrine growth. IGFR1 expression is increased by estrogen *(94)*, providing a scenario for IGF-mediated autocrine growth. Conversely, IGFR2 expression is decreased by estrogen *(95)*, and, as stated previously, this could result in release of previously bound IGF-II that can now act through IGFR1. Although it is tempting to hypothesize that IGF-II is the mediator of estrogen-regulated growth, the inability of blockade of IGFR1 by αIR3 to inhibit estrogen-mediated growth reduces the likelihood of this hypothesis *(96)*. However, antibody blockade experiments are complicated to perform and difficult to interpret, as IGF-II may be acting via other receptors. This is especially true considering the recent finding that IGF-II can cause proliferation in IGFR1 knockout cells through the insulin receptor *(97)* and through hybrid IGFR1/insulin receptors *(10)*. IGFBP expression is altered by estrogen; however, the role of IGFBPs in estrogen action remains unclear.

IGF-I and estrogen are both potent mitogens for most breast cancer cells and, when given together, cause additive growth *(48,94)*. Antiestrogens can specifically inhibit estrogen-mediated growth, but also significantly inhibit IGF-mediated proliferation *(98–101)*. Furthermore, inhibitors of IGF action not only inhibit IGF-I-mediated growth, but also significantly reduce estrogen-mediated growth *(31,101,102)*. The crossreactivity of these specific inhibitors again supports synergism between IGF and ER signaling pathways. There are several possible mechanisms for antiestrogen inhibition of IGF action. First, antiestrogens may inhibit IGF action by increasing expression of IGFBP-3 *(84,103)*, a binding protein with IGF-neutralization capabilities. Second, antiestrogens may affect phosphorylation of IGFR1 *(104)* or IRS-1 *(105)*, possibly by upregulation of protein tyrosine phosphatases *(106)*. Third, antiestrogens may downregulate expression of IGFR1 *(94)*, thus reducing the capacity of the cell to respond to IGF-I. Fourth, antiestrogens may inhibit ligand-independent activation of the ER by IGF-I *(101,107–109)*. Naturally, the mechanism is probably some combination of these scenarios.

In our studies inhibiting IGF-I action by ligand neutralization with IGFBP-1 (discussed in more detail later in the chapter), we have shown complete inhibition of IGF-mediated growth, but also a significant reduction of estrogen-mediated growth. This has also been shown for IGFBP-3 *(31)*. We hypothesize that some level of IGFR1 phosphorylation and IGF action is needed for maximal activation of the ER by estrogen. In transactivation studies, IGFBP-1 can inhibit ER-mediated transactivation not only by IGF-I, but also by estrogen, supporting our hypothesis. Furthermore, estrogen and IGF-I treatment resulted in enhanced ER-transactivational activity, suggesting that estrogen alone is insufficient to activate the ER fully. Thus there is considerable synergism between ER and IGF signaling pathways. Considering the importance of antiestrogens in breast cancer treatment, we believe that studies aimed at targeting IGFR1 in human breast cancer may provide a benefit to patients, possibly enhancing current antiestrogen therapies.

Of critical importance in the treatment of breast cancer patients is an understanding of resistance developed during antiestrogen treatment. While a greater understanding of ER action will eventually aid in this process, the effects of tamoxifen on IGF system components support a role for IGFs in this process. Thus IGF-II overexpression in MCF-7 cells results in tamoxifen-independent growth *(54,55)*. Furthermore, MCF-7 cells transfected with a mixed cDNA library and then selected for tamoxifen resistance were all found to overexpress IGF-II *(110)*. Tamoxifen resistance is also associated with increased IGFR1 levels in MCF-7 cells *(111)*, again providing an autocrine IGF-II/IGFR1 growth-regulatory drug-resistance scenario. Overexpression of IGFR1 results in a slight reduction in estrogen requirements *(73,74)*, and overexpression of IRS-1 results in autocrine-mediated growth with reduced estrogen requirements *(90)*. Finally, breast cancer cells showing varying phenotypic characteristics of estrogen independence and tamoxifen resistance show different patterns of IGFBP expression *(112)*.

In summary, there is a clear and convincing interrelationship between the IGFs and ER, shown both in in vitro and in vivo studies. On the one hand, IGF may enhance ER action by affecting ER function. However, it is also clear that estrogen enhances IGF function by altering expression of regulatory IGF system components (Fig. 1). The importance of the ER in breast cancer warrants further analysis of this synergism.

IGFS AS PROGNOSTIC MARKERS IN BREAST CANCER

Due to the importance of IGFs in breast cancer growth, and the role of IGFR1 in growth and transformation of malignant cells, many studies have been performed to analyze the

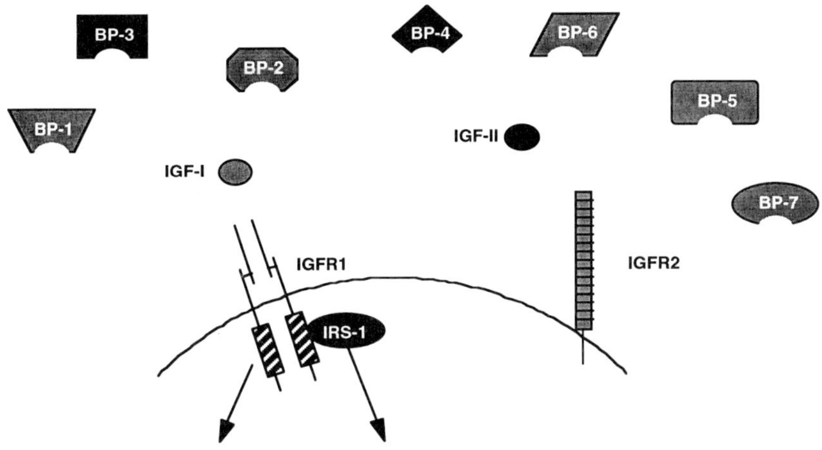

Fig. 2: The IGF system as a prognostic indicator in breast cancer. IGF system components that either are associated with poor prognostic markers or are themselves indicators of shorter disease-free survival are shown in black (BP-3, BP-4, IRS-1, and IGF-II). IGFR1 is a good prognostic marker (shaded). The other members of the IGF system have yet to be analyzed (shown in gray). Reprinted with permission from ref. *129*.

prognostic significance of IGF expression in breast cancer (Fig. 2). The IGF ligands have been measured by enzyme-linked immunosorbent assay (ELISA) assay on tumor cytosols *(113)*; IGF-II was found to be weakly associated with poor prognostic indicators (high p53, low ER, and low cathepsin D). Examination of IGF-II expression by IHC *(59)* also found expression to be weakly correlated with poor prognostic features (tumor grade, S-phase, and DNA ploidy). Even though circulating IGF-I levels are increased in breast cancer patients *(64)*, there is no correlation between serum IGF-I levels and several prognostic factors *(114)*, and IGF-I expression does not identify patients with better or worse short-term survival *(115)*.

Although most in vitro data suggest a role for IGFR1 in growth and transformation of cells, IGFR1 expression is associated with a better prognosis in both relapse-free survival and overall survival in breast cancer patients *(116,117)*. There are several possible reasons for this contradiction. It is known that IGFR1 is downregulated upon ligand binding and activation *(118)*, suggesting that the tumors that express low levels of IGFR1 and have a poor prognosis may have constitutively activated receptor. By contrast, the prognostic significance of IGFR1 may mirror that of the ER; thus, although the ER is a ligand-activated growth-promoting receptor in breast cancer cells in culture *(46)*, ER expression is a favorable prognostic indicator *(119)*, reflecting less aggressive well-differentiated tumors. As targeting of the ER is the most widely used chemostrategy in breast cancer at present *(91)*, it is possible that targeting IGFR1 may provide a similar benefit.

A recent study has shown that high levels of IGFR1 in breast cancer patients following lumpectomy and radiation therapy is associated with an increased risk of ipsilateral breast tumor recurrence *(120)*, and that this is strongly associated in those cases that relapsed before 4 years after treatment. Although no influence on overall survival was reported in these cases, high IGFR1 levels may identify a subset of radioresistant breast tumors, perhaps by protecting cells from apoptosis induced by ionizing radiation, thus warranting examination of anti-IGFR1 strategies in this subset of patients.

We have performed several studies examining the prognostic significance of IGFBP expression in primary breast cancer specimens. In summary, IGFBP-4 is an independent prognostic marker when patients were stratified by tumor size; patients with large tumors (>2 cm) and low IGFBP-4 expression had improved disease-free survival compared with patients with high IGFBP-4 expression and large tumors *(86)*. In a preliminary study we found that IGFBP-3 expression was associated with poor prognostic features *(87)*, and further analysis of a larger group of patients revealed again that IGFBP-3 was associated with poor prognostic features *(88)*, although IGFBP-3 levels were not an independent marker in multivariate analysis.

In an attempt to elucidate further the significance of IGF action in breast cancer, we performed the first study analyzing a major IGF downstream signaling molecule, IRS-I. Analysis of 200 breast tumor specimens indicated that IRS-I expression did not correlate with other prognostic factors *(88)*, but high expression predicted a shorter disease-free survival in patients with small tumors (<2 cm). In this group of patients, disease-free survival was similar to that in patients with large tumors (> 2cm); thus IRS-1 may identify patients with small tumors who will have an aggressive clinical course.

Compelling in vitro data concerning a role for IGFs in breast cancer cell proliferation has led to the analysis of IGF expression in breast cancer. Whereas some members of the IGF family actually do confer prognostic significance (Fig. 2), and thus presumably are affecting breast tumor progression, it is clear that measurement of a single member of the IGF family will not reveal the complicated interaction that occurs within the patient. It is therefore our goal to measure all the IGF family members in concert to provide a clearer picture of the role of IGF action in breast cancer and to elucidate possible new strategies for therapeutic intervention. It is this work that has led us and other to examine the possibility of targeting the IGFs in breast cancer; this will now be discussed.

INTERRUPTION OF IGF ACTION INHIBITS BREAST CANCER GROWTH

Due to the importance of IGFs, and in particular IGFR1, in breast cancer cell growth in vitro, we and others have attempted to block IGF signaling at the level of the ligand-receptor interaction. There are several mechanisms for achieving this: (1) blockade of IGFR1 binding, (2) neutralization of IGF ligand, and (3) inhibition of IGFR1 expression and signaling capability.

The earliest reports of inhibition of IGFR1 signaling came from antibody blocking experiments using a monoclonal antibody to the IGFR1 (αIR3). In vitro studies showed that incubation of αIR3 in CM of breast cancer cells inhibited IGF-I- and -II-mediated proliferation *(96)*. Arteaga et al. *(121)* then used the same antibody to inhibit MDA-MB-231 growth in vivo as a xenograft tumor. The same antibody can also affect an IGF-II autocrine growth loop in T61 xenograft tumors *(122)*, confirming the ability of the antibody to inhibit receptor function. However, since hybrid receptors or insulin receptor can also mediate IGF-stimulated growth, antibody blockade may not be sufficient to inhibit all the effects of IGFs.

We and others have exploited the fact that IGFBPs bind IGF ligand with higher affinity than IGFR1, to use IGFBPs as an IGF-neutralization strategy. Thus purified human IGFBP-1 can block IGF-I-mediated growth if added in twofold molar excess over IGF-I *(35)*. Similarly, the same effect can be seen with recombinant IGFBP-1; however, now an eightfold molar excess is needed for complete blockade *(102)*. Interestingly, IGFBP-1 also inhibited estrogen-mediated growth, substantiating the expanding data concerning synergism and crosstalk between IGF and ER signaling pathways (discussed in detail earlier in the chapter). Proof that IGFBP-1 specifically inhibited ligand-receptor interaction was shown by the ability of IGFBP-1 to reduce IGF-I-stimulated tyrosine phosphorylation of IGFR1. Transfection and overexpression of IGFBP-1 in MCF-7 cells achieved the same results *(123)*; we completely blocked IGF-I-mediated proliferation, and we could relieve this effect with an IGF analog that does not bind to IGFBPs (des 1-3 IGF-I). Similar in vitro studies have now been performed with IGFBP-3 *(70)*, again showing that IGF and estradiol effects can be blocked. Recently IGFBP-4 has been overexpressed in MCF-7 cells, and similar results seen, with inhibition of IGF responsiveness, but also inhibition of tumor growth *(124)*. Thus IGF neutralization is a feasible strategy for inhibition of IGF action in vitro. Although IGFBP-1 inhibited IGF, estrogen, and serum-mediated growth of MCF-7 cells in vitro, IGFBP-1 did not inhibit growth of MCF-7 cells in vivo. This may have been owing to the short-half life of IGFBP-1 when injected in the nude mouse ($t_{1/2}$ 2 h). Polyethylene glycol-conjugated IGFBP-1 (PegBP-1) had a longer half-life ($t_{1/2}$ 12 h) but lower tumor penetrance. However, PegBP-1 inhibited growth of MDA-231 flank xenograft tumors and MDA-435A ascites tumor formation *(125)*. We are now furthering these studies by examining the efficacy of smaller PegBP-1 conjugates.

One strategy for interruption of IGF action that has been used in a number of tumor model systems is direct targeting of IGFR1 expression *(126)*. Owing to the critical importance of IGFR1 in the growth and maintenance of malignant cells, inhibition of IGFR1 expression is not simple; however, results can be dramatic, as seen in glioblastoma cells treated with an antisense expression to IGFR1 *(127)*. These cells show little or no phenotype in vitro when they are treated with the oligonucleotides, but when injected in the rat they result in massive apotosis and complete tumor regression. Neuenschwander et al. *(128)* stably transfected MCF-7 cells with antisense to IGFR1 and saw a partial inhibition of receptor expression, correlated with a partial decrease in IGF-mediated growth. Unfortunately, constitutive expression of a vector that decreases IGFR1 may not be tolerated by cancer cells, and so complete inhibition of IGFR1 expression will be hard to establish.

CONCLUSIONS

Although many of the treatments of breast cancer are aimed at slowing the growth of the tumor, e.g., cytotoxic chemotherapy, many of these therapies are nonspecific and have severe unwanted side effects. In an attempt to determine the growth regulators of breast cancer, the IGF family has been shown to be an important mediator of breast cancer growth. Many studies have shown that the IGFs are potent mitogens for breast cancer cells and that interruption of IGF signaling can inhibit breast cancer growth in vitro and in vivo. Consistent with the proliferative effect of the IGFs in vitro, many of the IGF family members are indicators of the prognosis of breast cancer, with high expression of IGF family members generally being associated with poor prognostic indicators. The success of anti-IGF strategies in other cancers, and the importance of IGFs in breast cancer growth suggest that anti-IGF therapy may prove to be a beneficial treatment for breast cancer patients, particularly in conjunction with current antiestrogen therapies.

ACKNOWLEDGMENTS

The authors' work is supported by Public Health Service (PHS) grant P01CA30195 and PHS Cancer Center Support grant P30CA54174 from the National Cancer Institute, National Institutes of Health, Department of Health and Human Services.

REFERENCES

1. Schofield PN (1992) The Insulin-Like Growth Factors. Oxford University Press, Oxford.
2. Clemmons DR, Busby WH, Arai T, Nam TJ, Clark JB, Jones JI, et al. (1995) Role of insulin-like growth factor binding proteins in the control of IGF action. Prog Growth Factor Res 6:357–366.
3. Daughaday, W (1988) Insulin-like growth factors I and II. Peptide, messenger ribonucleic acid and gene structures, serum, and tissue concentrations. Endocr Rev 10:68–91.
4. Baserga, R (1995) The insulin-like growth factor I receptor: a key to tumor growth? Cancer Res 55:249–252.
5. Baker J, Liu J-P, Robertson EJ, Efstratiadis, A (1993) Role of insulin-like growth factors in embryonic and postnatal growth. Cell 75:73–82.
6. Liu J-P, Baker J, Perkins AS, Robertson, E, Efstratiadis, A (1993) Mice carrying null mutations of the genes encoding insulin-like growth factor I (igf-1) and type 1 IGF receptor (igf1r). Cell 75:59–72.
7. Ullrich A, Gray A, Tam A, Yang-Feng T, Tsubokawa M, Collins C, et al. (1986) Insulin-like growth factor I receptor primary structure: comparison with insulin receptor suggests structural determinants that define functional specificity. EMBO J 5:2503–2512.
8. Moxham CP, Duronio, V, Jacobs, S (1989) Insulin-like growth factor I receptor beta-subunit heterogeneity. Evidence for hybrid tetramers composed of insulin-like growth factor I and insulin receptor heterodimers. J Biol Chem 264:13238–13244.
9. Treadway JL, Fratalli AL, Pressin JE (1992) Intramolecular subunit interactions between insulin and insulin-like growth factor-1 αβH half-receptors induced by ligand and Mn/MgATP binding. Biochemistry 31:11801–11805.
10. Soos MA, Field CE, Siddle, K (1993) Purified hybrid insulin/insulin-like growth factor I receptors bind insulin-like growth factor-I, but not insulin, with high affinity. Biochem J 290:419–426.
11. Steele-Perkins G, Turner J, Edman J, Hari J, Pierce S, Stover C, et al. (1988) Expression and characterisation of a functional human insulin-like growth factor I receptor. J Biol Chem 23:11486–11492.
12. Morgan DO (1987) Insulin-like growth factor II receptor as a multi-functional binding protein. Nature 326:300–307.
13. MacDonald RG, Pfeffer S, Coussens L, Tepper M, Brocklebank C, Mole J, et al. (1988) A single receptor binds both insulin-like growth factor II and mannose-6-phosphate. Science 239:1134–1137.
14. Nishimoto, I (1993) The IGF-II receptor system—a G-protein-linked mechanism. Mol Reprod Dev 35:398–407.
15. Okamoto T, Katada T, Murayama Y, Ui M, Ogata, E, Nishimoto, I (1990) A simple structure encodes G protein-activating function of the IGF-II/mannose-6–phosphate receptor. Cell 62:709–717.
16. Blanchard M, Barenton B, Sullivan A, Foster B, Guyda, H, Posner, B (1988) Characterisation of the insulin-like growth factor (IGF) receptor in K562 erythroleukemia cells; evidence for a biological function for the type II IGF receptor. Mol Cell Endocrinol 56:235–244.
17. Mathieu M, Rochefort H, Barenton B, Prebois, C, Vignon, F (1990) Interactions of cathepsin-D and insulin-like growth factor-II (IGF-II) on the IGF-II/mannose-6-phosphate receptor in human breast cancer cells and possible consequences on mitogenic activity of IGF-II. Mol Endocrinol 4:1327–1335.
18. Korner C, Nurnberg B, Uhde, M, Braulke, T (1995) Mannose-6-phosphate/insulin-like growth factor II receptor fails to interact with G-proteins. J Biol Chem 270:287–295.
19. Rubin R, Baserga R (1995) Insulin-like growth factor-I receptor. Its role in cell proliferation, apoptosis and tumorigenicity. Lab Invest 73:311–331.
20. Sell C, Dumenil G, Deveaud C, Miura M, Coppola D, DeAngelis T, et al. (1994) Effect of a null mutation of the type 1 IGF receptor gene on growth and transformation of mouse embryo fibroblasts. Mol Cell Biol 14:3604–3612.
21. Coppola D, Ferber A, Miura M, Sell C, D'Ambrosio C, Rubin, R, et al. (1994) A functional insulin-like growth factor I receptor is required for the mitogenic and transforming activites of the epidermal growth factor receptor. Mol Cell Biol 14:4588–4595.

22. Sell C, Rubini M, Rubin R, Liu J-P, Efstratiadis, A (1993) Simian virus 40 large tumor antigen is unable to transform mouse embryonic fibroblasts lacking type-1 IGF receptor. Proc Natl Acad Sci USA 90:11217–112121.
23. Baserga R (1994) Oncogenes and the strategy of growth factors. Cell 79:927–930.
24. Pietrzkowski Z, Lammers R, Carpenter G, Soderquist AM, Limardo M, Philips PD, et al. (1992) Constitutive overexpression of insulin-like growth factor 1 and inslin-like growth facotr 1 receptor abrogates all requirements for exogenous growth factors. Cell Growth Differ 3:195–205.
25. Sell C, Baserga, R, Rubin, R (1995) Insulin-like growth factor I (IGF-I) and the IGF-I receptor prevent etoposide-induced apotosis. Cancer Res 55:303–306.
26. Miura M, Surmacz E, Burgaud J, Baserga, R (1995) Different effects on mitogenesis and transformation of a mutation at tyrosine 1251 of the insulin-like growth factor I receptor. J Biol Chem 270:22639–22644.
27. Jones JI, Gockerman A, Busby WH, Wright G, Clemmons DR (1993) Insulin-like growth factor binding protein 1 stimulates cell migration and binds to the $\alpha5\beta1$ integrins by means of its Arg-Gly-Asp sequence. Proc Natl Acad Sci USA 90:10553–10557.
28. De Mellow JS, Baxter RC (1988) Growth hormone-dependent insulin-like growth factor (IGF) binding protein both inhibits and potentiates IGF-stimulated DNA synthesis in human skin fibroblasts. Biochem Biophys Res Commun 156:199–204.
29. Cohen P, Lamson G, Okahima, T, Rosenfeld RG (1993) Transfection of the insulin-like growth factor binding protein-3 gene into Balb/C fibroblasts inhibits cellular growth. Mol Endocrinol 7:380–386.
30. Chen, J.-C., Shao Z-M, Sheikh, M (1994) Insulin-like growth factor binding protein enhancement of insulin-like growth factor-I (IGF-I) mediated DNA synthesis and IGF-I binding in a human breast carcinoma cell line. J Cell Physiol 158:69–78.
31. Pratt SE, Pollack MN (1994) Insulin-like growth factor binding protein 3 (IGFBP-3) inhibits estrogen-stimulated breast cancer cell proliferation. Biochem Biophys Res Commun 198:292–297.
32. Oh Y, Muller HL, Lee D, Fielder P, Rosenfeld RG (1993) Characterisation of the affinities of insulin-like growth factor (IGF)-binding proteins 1-4 for IGF-I, IGF-II, IGF-I/insulin hybrid, and IGF-I analogs. Endocrinology 132:1337–1344.
33. Oh Y, Muller HL, Pham H, Rosenfeld RG (1993) Demonstration of receptors for insulin-like growth factor binding protein-3 on HS578T human breast cancer cells. J Biol Chem 268:26045–26048.
34. Valentinis B, Bhala A, De Angelis T, Baserg, R, Cohen P (1995) The human insulin-like growth factor (IGF) binding protein-3 inhibits the growth of fibroblasts with a targeted disruption of the IGF-I receptor gene. Mol Endocrinol 9:361–367.
35. McGuire Jr, W, Jackson JG, Figueroa JA, Shimasaki SA, Powell DR, Yee D (1992) Regulation of insulin-like growth factor-binding protein (IGFBP) expression by breast cancer cells: use of IGFBP-1 as an inhibitor of insulin-like growth factor action. Natl Cancer Inst 84:1336–13411.
36. Jones JI, D'Ercole AJ, Camacho-Hubner C, Clemmons DR (1991) Phosphorylation of insulin-like growth factor binding protein 1 in cell culture and in vivo: effects on affinity for IGF-I. Proc Natl Acad Sci USA 88:7481–7485.
37. Lewis AA, Gomez ET, Turner CW (1942) Mammary gland development with mammogen I in the castrated and the hypophysectomized rat. Endocrinology 30:37–47.
38. Lyons WR (1993) Hormonal synergism in mammary growth. Proc R Soc 149:303–325.
39. Ruan W, Newman CB, Kleinberg DL (1992) Intact and aminoterminally shortened forms of insulin-like growth factor I induce mammary gland differentiation and development. Proc Natl Acad Sci USA 89:10872–10876.
40. Schlechter NL, Russell SM, Spencer EM, Nicoll CS (1986) Evidence suggesting that the direct growth-promoting effect of growth hormone on cartilage *in vivo* is mediated by local production of somatomedin. Proc Natl Acad Sci USA 83:7932–7934.
41. Murphy LJ, Bell GI, Friesen HG (1987) Tissue distribution of insulin-like growth factor I and II messenger ribonucleic acid in the adult rat. Endocrinology 120:1279–1282.
42. Ruan W, Catanese R, Wieczorek R, Feldman M, Kleinberg DL (1995) Estradiol enhances the stimulatory effect of insulin-like growth factor-I (IGF-I) on mammary development and growth-hormone-induced IGF-I messenger ribonucleic acid. Endocrinology 136:1296–1302.
43. Hadsell DL, Greenberg NM, Fligger JM, Baumrucker CR, Rosen JM (1996) Targetted expression of des (1–3) human insulin-like growth factor I (IGF-I) in transgenic mice influences mammary galnd development and IGF-binding protein expression. Endocrinology, in press.
44. Neuenschwander S, Schwartz A, Wood TL, Roberts CTJ (1996) Involution of the lactating mammary gland is inhibited by the IGF system in a transgenic mouse model. J Clin Invest 97:2225–2232.

45. Myal Y, Shiu RPC, Bhaumick B, M, B (1984) Receptor binding and growth-promoting activity of insulin-like growth factors in human breast cancer cells (T47D) in culture. Cancer Res 44:5486–5490.
46. Karey K, Sirbasku, D (1988) Differential responsiveness of human breast cancer cell lines to growth factors and 17β-estradiol. Cancer Res 48:4083–4092.
47. Yee D, Cullen K, Paik S, Perdue J, Hampton B, Schwartz A, et al. (1988) Insulin-like growth factor II mRNA expression in human breast cancer. Cancer Res 48:6691–6696.
48. Cullen K, Yee D, Sly W, Perdue J, Hampton B, Lippman M, et al. (1990) Insulin-like growth factor receptor expression and function in human breast cancer. Cancer Res 50:48–53.
49. Ahmed SR, Manni A, Gray G. Hammond JM (1990) Characterisation and hormonal regulation of radioimmunoassayable IGF-I (insulin-like growth factor I) like activity and IGF-binding proteins secreted by human breast cancer cells. AntiCancer Res 10:1217–1223.
50. Huff KK, Kaufman D, Gabbay KH, Spencer EM, Lippman ME, Dickson RB (1986) Secretion of an insulin-like growth factor-I-related protein by human breast cancer cells. Cancer Res 46:4613–4619.
51. Minuto F, Delmonte P, Barreca A, Nicolin A, Giordano G (1987) Partial characterisation of somatomedin C-like immunoreactivity secreted by breast cancer cells *in vitro*. Mol Cell Endocrinol 54:179–184.
52. Osborne CK, Coronado EB, Kitten LJ, Arteaga CR, Fuqua SAW, Ramasharma K, et al. (1989) Insulin-like growth factor-II (IGF-II): A potential autocrine/paracrine growth factor for human breast cancer acting via the IGF-I receptor. Mol Endocrinol 3:1701–1709.
53. Lee AV, Darbre P, King RJB (1994) Processing of insulin-like growth factor-II (IGF-II) by human breast cancer cells. Mol Cell Endocrinol 99:211–220.
54. Daly R, Harris W, Wang D, Darbre P (1991) Autocrine production of insulin like growth factor-II using an inducible expression system results in reduced estrogen sensitivity of MCF-7 human breast cancer cells. Cell Growth Differ 2:457–464.
55. Cullen K, Lippman M, Chow D, Hill S, Rosen N, Zwiebel, J (1992) Insulin-like growth factor-II over expression in MCF-7 cells induces phenotypic chances associated with malignant progression. Mol Endocrinol 6:91–100.
56. Bates P, Fisher R, Ward A, Richardson L, Hill DJ, Graham CF (1995) Mammary cancer in transgenic mice overexpressing insulin-like growth factor II (IGF-II). Br J Cancer 72:1189–1193.
57. Yee D, Paik S, Levovic GS, Marcus RR, Favoni RE, Cullen KJ, et al. (1989) Analysis of insulin-like growth factor I gene expression in malignancy: evidence for a paracrine role in human breast cancer. Mol Endocrinol 3:509–517.
58. Paik, S (1992) Expression of IGF-I and IGF-II mRNA in breast tissue. Breast Cancer Res Treat 22:31–38.
59. Toropainen EM, Lipponen PK, Syrjanen KJ (1995) Expression of insulin-like growth factor II in human breast cancer as related to established prognostic factors and long-term prognosis. AntiCancer Res 15:2669–2674.
60. Giani C, Cullen KJ, Campani D, Rasmussen A (1996) IGF-II mRNA and protein are expressed in the stroma of invasive breast cancers: an in situ hybridization and immunohistochemistry study. Breast Cancer Res Treat 41:43–50.
61. Singer C, Smith HS, Lippman ME, Cullen KJ (1992) IGF-I and IGF-II expression in fibroblasts derived from tumor, normal breast, and skin of breast cancer patients. Proc AACR 33, A1612.
62. Singer C, Rasmussen A, Smith HS, Lippman ME, Lynch T, Cullen KJ (1995) Malignant breast epithelium selects for insulin-like growth factor II expression in breast stroma: evidence for paracrine function. Cancer Res 55:2448–2454.
63. Peyrat JP, Bonneterre J, Hecquet B, Vennin P, Louchez MM, Fournier C, et al. (1993) Plasma insulin-like growth factor-1 (IGF-1) concentrations in human breast cancer. Eur J Cancer 29:492–497.
64. Pollack MN, Huynh HT, Lefebvre SP (1992) Tamoxifen reduces serum insulin-like growth factor I (IGF-I). Breast Cancer Res Treat 22:91–100.
65. Lahti EI, Knip M, Laatikainen TJ (1994) Plasma insulin-like growth factor I and its binding proteins 1 and 3 in postmenopausal patients with breast cancer receiving long-term tamoxifen. Cancer 74:618–624.
66. Lien EA, Johannessen DC, Aakvaag A, Lonning PE (1992) Influence of tamoxifen, aminoglutethimide and goserelin on human plasma IGF-I levels in breast cancer patients. J Steroid Biochem Mol Biol 41:541–543.
67. Lonning PE, Hall K, Aakvaag A, Lien EA (1992) Influence of tamoxifen on plasma levels of insulin-like growth factor I and insulin-like growth factor binding protein 1 in breast cancer patients. Cancer Res 52:4719–4723.
68. Reed MJ, Christodoulides A, Koistinen R, Seppala M, Teale JD, Ghilchik MW (1992) The effect of endocrine therapy with methoxyprogesterone acetate, 4-hydroxyandrostenedione or tamoxifen on

plasma concentrations of insulin-like growth factor (IGF)-I, IGF-II and IGFBP-1 in women with advanced breast cancer. Int J Cancer 52:208–212.
69. Malaab SA, Pollack MN, Goodyer CG (1992) Direct effects of tamoxifen on growth hormone secretion by pituitary cells in vitro. Eur J Cancer 28A, 788–793.
70. Huynh HT, Tetenes E, Wallace L, Pollack M (1993) *In vivo* inhibition of insulin-like growth factor I gene expression by tamoxifen. Cancer Res 53:1727–1730.
71. Di Leo A, Ferrari L, Bajetta E, Bartoli C, Vicario G, Moglia D, et al. (1995) Biological and clinical evaluation of lanreotide (BIM 23014), a somatostatin analogue, in the treatment of advanced breast cancer. A pilot study by the I.T.M.O. group. Italian Trials in Medical Oncology. Breast Cancer Res Treat 34:237–244.
72. Canobbio L, Cannata D, Miglietta L, Boccardo F (1995) Somatuline (BIM 23014) and tamoxifen treatment of postmenopausal breast cancer patients; clinical activity and effect on insulin-like growth factor-I (IGF-I) levels. AntiCancer Res 15:2687–2690.
73. Daws MR, Westley BR, May FE (1996) Paradoxical effects of overexpression of the type I insulin-like growth factor (IGF) receptor on the responsiveness of human breast cancer cells to IGFs and estradiol. Endocrinology 137:1177–1186.
74. Guvakova MA, Surmacz, E (1997) Overexpressed IGF-I receptors reduce estrogen growth requirements, enhance survival, and promote E-cadherin-mediated cell-cell adhesion in human breast cancer cells. Exp Cell Res 231:149–162.
75. Peyrat J-P, Bonneterre J, Beuscart J, Dijane J, Demaille A (1988) Insulin-like growth factor I receptors in human breast cancer and their relationship to estradiol and progesterone receptors. Cancer Res 48:6429–6433.
76. Pekonen F, Partanen S, Makinen T, Rutanen EM (1988) Receptors for epidermal growth factor and insulin-like growth factor I and their relation to steroid receptors in human breast cancer. Cancer Res 48:1343–1347.
77. Foekens JA, Portengen H, Jansen M, Klun G (1989) Insulin-like growth factor-I receptors and insulin-like growth factor-I-like activity in human primary breast cancer. Cancer (Phila) 63:2139–2147.
78. Berns EMJJ, Klijn JGM, van Staveren IL, Portegen, H, Foekens JA (1990) Sporadic amplification of the insulin-like growth factor 1 receptor gene in human breast tumors. Cancer Res 52:1036–1039.
79. Hankins GR, De Souza AT, Bentley RC, Patel MR, Marks JR, Iglehart JD, et al. (1996) M6P/IGF2 receptor: a candidate breast tumor supressor gene. Oncogene 12:2003–2009.
80. Clemmons DR, Camacho-Hubner C, Coronado E, Osborne CK (1990) Insulin-like growth factor binding protein secretion by breast cancer cell lines: correlation with estrogen receptor status. Endocrinology 127:2679–2686.
81. Yee D, Favoni R, Lippman M, Powell D (1991) Identification of insulin-like growth factor binding proteins in breast cancer cells. Breast Cancer Res Treat 18:3–10.
82. Fontana JA, Clemmons DR, LeRoith, D (1991) Retinoid modulation of insulin-like growth factor binding proteins and inhibition of breast carcinoma proliferation. Endocrinology 128:1115–1122.
83. Huynh H, Yang XF, Pollak, M (1996) A role for insulin-like growth factor binding protein 5 in the antiproliferative action of the antiestrogen ICI 182780. Cell Growth Differ 7:1501–1506.
84. Figueroa JA, Jackson JG, McGuire WL, Krywicki RF, Yee, D (1993) Expression of insulin-like growth factor binding proteins in human breast cancer correlates with estrogen receptor status. J Cell Biochem 52:196–205.
85. Shao, Z.-M., Sheikh MS, Ordonez JV, Feng P, Kute T, Chen J-C, et al. (1992) IGFBP-3 gene expression and estrogen receptor status in human breast carcinoma. Cancer Res 52:5100–5103.
86. Yee D, Sharma J, Hilsenbeck SG (1994) Prognostic significance of insulin-like growth factor-binding protein expression in axillary lymph node-negative breast cancer. Natl Cancer Inst 86:1785–1789.
87. Rocha R, Hilsenbeck SG, Jackson JG, Lee AV, Figueroa JA, Yee, D (1995) Insulin-like growth factor binding protein-3 (BP3) mRNA and protein expression are correlated in primary breast cancer tissue; higher levels are detected in tumors with poor prognostic features. Natl Cancer Inst 88:601–606.
88. Rocha RL, Hilsenbeck SG, Jackson JG, Van Den Berg CL, Weng C-N, Lee AV, et al. (1997) Insulin-like growth factor binding protein-3 and insulin receptor substrate-1 in breast cancer: correlation with clinical parameters and disease-free survival. Clin Cancer Res 3:103–109.
89. Nolan M, Jankowski L, Prisco M, Xu S, Guvakova M, Surmacz E (1997) Differential roles of IRS-1 and SHC signaling pathways in breast cancer cells. Int J Cancer, in press.
90. Surmacz, E, Burgard J-L (1995) Overexpression of IRS-1 in the human breast cancer cell line MCF-7 induces loss of estrogen requirements for growth and transformation. Clin Cancer Res 1:1429–1436.

91. Early Breast Cancer Trialists Collaborative Group. (1992) Systemic treatment of early breast cancer by hormonal, cytotoxic, or immune therapy: 133 randomized trials involving 31,000 recurrences and 24,000 deaths among 75,000 women. Lancet 339:1–15:71–85.
92. Horwitz KB, Jackson TA, Bain DL, Richer JK, Takimoto GS, Tung L (1996) Nuclear receptor coactivators and corepressors. Mol Endocrinol 10:1167–1177.
93. Westley BR, May FEB (1994) Role of insulin-like growth factors in steroid modulated proliferation. J Steroid Biochem Mol Biol 51:1–9.
94. Stewart A, Westley B, May F (1992) Modulation of the proliferative response of breast cancer cells to growth factors by oestrogen. Br J Cancer 66:640–648.
95. Mathieu M, Vignon F, Capony, F, Rochefort H (1991) Estradiol down regulates the mannose-6-phosphate/insulin-like growth factor-II receptor gene and induces cathepsin-D in breast cancer cells: a receptor saturation mechanism to increase the secretion of lysosomal proenzymes. Mol Cell Endocrinol 5:815–822.
96. Arteaga CL, Osborne CK (1989) Growth inhibition of human breast cancer cells *in vitro* with an antibody against the type I somatomedin receptor. Cancer Res 49:6237–6241.
97. Morrione A, Valentinis B, Xu SQ, Yumet G, Louvi A, Efstradiatis A, et al. (1997) Insulin-like growth factor II stimulates cell proliferation through the insulin receptor. Proc Natl Acad Sci USA 94:3777–3782.
98. Vignon F, Bouton M-M, Rochefort H (1988) Antiestrogens inhibit the mitogenic effect of growth factors on breast cancer cells in the total absence of estrogens. Biochem Biophys Res Commun 146:1502–1508.
99. Hasmann M, Rattel B, Loser R (1994) Preclinical data for droloxifene. Cancer Lett 84:101–116.
100. Newton CJ, Buric R, Trapp T, Brockmeier S, Pagotto U, Stalla G (1994) The unliganded estrogen receptor (ER) transduces growth factor signals. J Steroid Biochem Mol Biol 48:481–486.
101. Lee AV, Weng C-N, Jackson JG, Yee D (1997) Activation of estrogen receptor-mediated gene transcription by IGF-I in human breast cancer cells. J Endocrinol 152:39–47.
102. Figueroa JA, Sharma J, Jackson JG, McDermott MJ, Hilsenbeck SG, Yee D (1993) Recombinant insulin-like growth factor binding protein 1 inhibits IGF-I, serum and estrogen dependent growth of MCF-7 human breast cancer cells. J Cell Physiol 157:229–236.
103. Huynh H, Yang X, Pollak M (1996) Estradiol and antiestrogens regulate a growth inhibitory insulin-like growth factor binding protein 3 autocrine loop in human breast cancer cells. J Biol Chem 271:1016–1021.
104. Freiss G, Rochefort H, Vignon F (1990) Mechanisms of 4-hydroxytamoxifen anti-growth factor activity in breast cancer cells: alterations of growth factor receptor binding sites and tyrosine kinase activity. Biochem Biophys Res Commun 3:919–926.
105. Guvakova M, Surmacz E (1997) Tamoxifen interferes with the insulin-like growth factor I receptor (IGF-IR) signaling pathway in breast cancer cells. Cancer Res 57:2606–2610.
106. Freiss G, Vignon F (1994) Antiestrogens increase protein tyrosine phosphatase activity in human breast cancer cells. Mol Endocrinol 8:1389–1396.
107. Cho H, Aronica S, Katzenellenbogen BS (1994) Regulation of progesterone receptor gene expression in MCF-7 breast cancer cells: a comparison of the effects of cyclic adenosine 3'-5'-monophosphate, estradiol, insulin-like growth factor-I and serum factors. Endocrinology 134:658–664.
108. Ignar-Trowbridge DM, Pimentel M, Parker MG, McLachlan JA, Korach KS (1996) Peptide growth factors cross-talk with the estrogen receptor requires the A/B domain and occurs independently of protein kinase C or estradiol. Endocrinology 137:1735–1744.
109. Patrone C, Ma ZQ, Pollio G, Agrati P, Parker MG, Maggi A (1996) Cross-coupling between insulin and estrogen receptor in human neuroblastoma cells. Mol Endocrinol 10:499–507.
110. Lee AV, Toi M, Yee D (1994) Tamoxifen resistant MCF-7 cells exhibit increased expression of insulin-like growth factor-II. Breast Cancer Res Treat 32S, 57.
111. Wiseman LR, Johnson MD, Wakeling AE, Lykkesfeldt AE, May FE, Westley BR (1993) Type I IGF receptor and acquired tamoxifen resistance in oestrogen-responsive human breast cancer cells. Eur J Cancer 29A, 2256–2264.
112. McCotter D, van den Berg HW, Boylan M, McKibben B (1996) Changes in insulin-like growth factor-I receptor expression and binding protein secretion associated with tamoxifen resistance and estrogen independence in human breast cancer cells in vitro. Cancer Lett 99:239–245.
113. Yu H, Levesque MA, Khosravi MJ, Papanastasiou-Diamandi A, Clark GM, Diamandis EP (1996) Associations between insulin-like growth factors and their binding proteins and other prognostic indicators in human breast cancer. Br J Cancer 74:1242–1247.

114. Barni S, Lissoni P, Brivio F, Fumugalli, Merlini D, Cataldo M, Rovelli, F, et al. (1994) Serum levels of insulin-like growth factor-I in operable breast cancer in relation to the main prognostic variables and their perioperative changes in relation to those of prolactin. Tumori 80:212–215.
115. Bhatavedar JM, Patel DD, Karelia NH, Vora HH, Ghosh N, Shah NG, et al. (1994) Tumor markers in patients with advanced breast cancer as prognosticators: a preliminary study. Breast Cancer Res Treat 30:293–297.
116. Bonneterre J, Peyrat JP, Beuscart R, Demaille A (1990) Prognostic significance of insulin-like growth factor I receptors in human breast cancer. Cancer Res 50:6931–6935.
117. Papa V, Gliozzo B, Clark G, McGuire W, Moore D, Fujita-Yamaguchi Y, et al. (1993) Insulin-like growth factor-I receptors are overexpressed and predict a low risk in human breast cancer. Cancer Res 53:3736–3740.
118. Papa V, Hartmann KKP, Rosenthal SM, Maddux BA, Siiteri PK, Goldfine ID (1991) Progestins induce down-regulation of insulin-like growth factor-I (IGF-I) receptors in human breast cancer cells: potential autocrine role of IGF-II. Mol Endocrinol 5:709–717.
119. McGuire WL (1988) Estrogen receptor versus nuclear grade as prognostic factors in axillary node negative breast cancer. J Clin Oncol 6:1071–1072.
120. Turner BC, Haffty BG, Narayanan L, Yuan J, Havre PA, Gumbs AA, et al. (1997) Insulin-like growth factor-I receptor overexpression mediates cellular radioresistance and local breast cancer recurrence after lumpectomy and radiation. Cancer Res 57:3079–3083.
121. Arteaga CL, Kitten L, Coronado E, Jacobs S, Kull F, Allred DC, et al. (1989) Blockade of the type I somatomedin receptor inhibits growth of human breast cancer cells in athymic mice. J Clin. Invest 84:1418–1423.
122. Brünner N, Yee D, Kern FG, Spang-Thomsen M, Lippman ME, Cullen KJ (1993) Effect of endocrine therapy on growth of T61 human beast cancer xenografts is directly correlated to a specific down-regulaton of insulin-like growth factor II (IGF-II). Eur J Cancer 29A, 562–569.
123. Yee D, Jackson JG, Kozelsky TW, Figueroa JA (1994) Insulin-like growth factor binding protein 1 expression inhibits insulin-like growth factor I action in MCF-7 cells. Cell Growth Differ 5:73–77.
124. Huynh H, Beamer M, Pollack M (1997) Over-expression of insulin-like growth factor binding protein 4 in MCF-7 breast cancer cells is associated with reduced responsivity to insulin-like growth factors *in vitro* and reduced tumor growth *in vivo.* Proc Am Assoc Cancer Res 38, A3954.
125. Van Den Berg C, Cox GN, Stroh CA, Hilsenbeck SG, Weng C-N, McDermott MJ, et al. (1997) Polyethylene glycol conjugated insulin-like growth factor binding protein-1 (IGFBP-1) inhibits growth of breast cancer in athymic mice. Eur J Cancer 33:1108–1113.
126. Baserga, R (1996) Controlling IGF-receptor function: a possible strategy for tumor therapy. Trends Biotechnol 14:150–152.
127. Resnicoff M, Sell C, Rubini M, Coppola D, Ambrose D, Baserga R, et al. (1994) Rat glioblastoma cells expressing an antisense RNA to the insulin-like growth factor-1 (IGF-1) receptor are nontumorigenic and induce regression of wild-type tumors. Cancer Res 54:2218–2222.
128. Neuenschwander S, Roberts CT, Leroith D (1995) Growth inhibition of human breast cancer cells by stable expression of an insulin-like growth factor I receptor antisense ribonucleic acid. Endocrinology 136:4298–4303.
129. Lee AV, Yee D (1997) The IGF system as prognostic markers in breast cancer. Breast Cancer Res Treat 47:295–302.

14 Prognostic and Predictive Factors in Breast Cancer

Jan G. M. Klijn, MD, PHD,
Els M. J. J. Berns, PHD, *and John A. Foekens*, PHD

INTRODUCTION

The development of life-threatening cancers involves three important stages, which may or may not be temporally distinct (Fig. 1). First, normal cells have to undergo growth transformation, which is the result of a multistep process as a consequence of an accumulation of several genetic alterations. The multiple genetic alterations occur especially in two classes of cellular genes, the protooncogenes and the tumor suppressor genes, which are involved in the regulation of the cell cycle and the process of apoptosis. These genetic alterations can be inherited, but are mostly acquired. Once a carcinoma *in situ* has arisen, a second stage has enormous implications, i.e., the phase of invasion and metastasis. Also, tumor metastasis is a complex multistep process requiring the cooperation of molecules of different classes, functions, and types. Third, after having escaped the immune system, tumor cells must be or become resistant to therapeutic drugs before killing a patient. Therefore, in fact, many factors determine a patient's prognosis.

Over recent decades an increasing number of cell biological parameters, such as oncogenes/suppressor genes, hormone receptors, growth factors, and secretory proteins, appear to influence strongly the behavior of a tumor with respect to growth rate, apoptosis, extent of cellular differentiation, metastatic pattern, and development of resistance to therapy (Table 1). All these studies have provided a wealth of knowledge about the biology of breast cancer. In addition, most of these cell biological factors have been tested as prognostic parameters in patients with breast cancer, but less as a predictive factor for the type of response to therapy (Table 2). Thus far, only a few parameters have been investigated as targets for new treatment modalities, but this number is increasing. In this chapter we will review briefly the clinical significance of the most relevant classical and cell biological parameters, focusing on our own results.

From: *Contemporary Endocrinology: Endocrinology of Breast Cancer*
Edited by: A. Manni © Humana Press Inc., Totowa, NJ

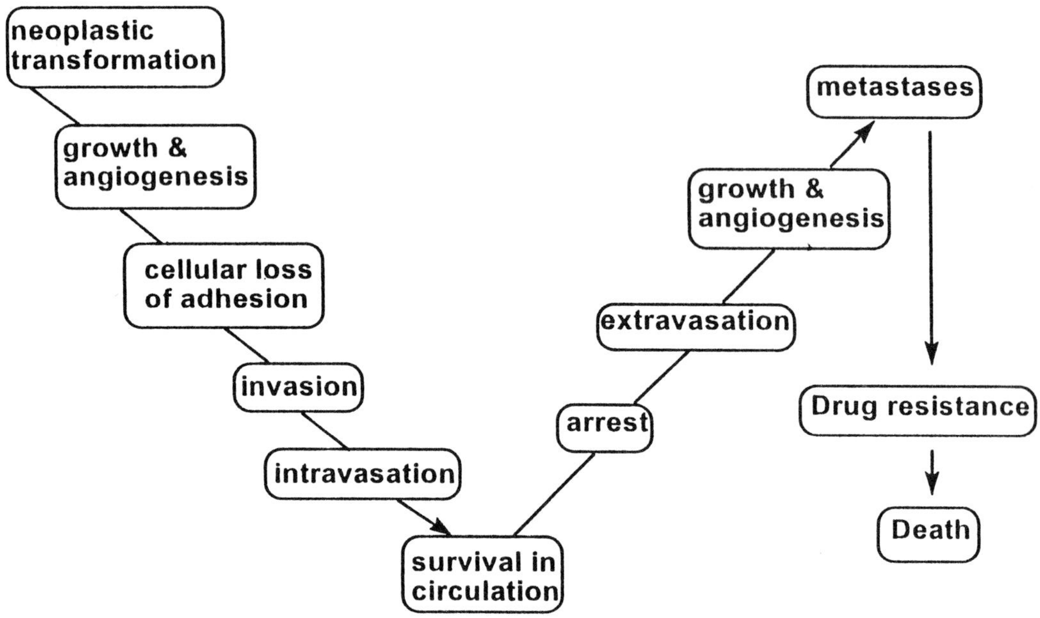

Fig. 1. Events in metastasis from neoplastic transformation to drug resistance and death.

RESULTS

Patient Characteristics

Race

In general black women have a worse prognosis than white women, even when corrected for type of surgery and stage of disease *(1–3)*. Confounding co-morbid conditions and socioeconomic factors also play a role.

Age and Menopausal Status

The possible prognostic influence of age at diagnosis of breast cancer has remained a matter of debate *(2,4–10)*. One of the reasons for this controversy could be that most studies did not take into account the menopausal status of the patient. In our own experience involving approximately 700 primary breast cancer patients, we showed that, when analyzing all patients, the combined age and premenopausal status was independently related with relapse-free and overall survival *(5,10)*. In addition, most studies have found a worse clinical outcome in younger patients, even after adjustment for other prognostic factors such as stage, grade, ER status, S-phase fraction, and p53 status. A matter of concern could be that some surgeons tend to treat larger tumors with breast-conserving therapy in younger women and take smaller lumps in order to ensure a better cosmetic result; however, this frequently results in cutting margins that are not free of tumor cells. In the younger age category the chance of a hereditary form of breast cancer also is greater, causing a higher risk of ipsilateral and contralateral secondary tumors *(11)*. Therefore, a more aggressive approach in the treatment of young breast cancer patients has to be considered.

Table 1
Classification of Prognostic Factors in Breast Cancer

A. Patient characteristics
   - Race
   - Age
   - Menopausal status
   - Performance status
   - Metabolic diseases

B. Variables determined in blood
   - Tumor marker levels (carcinoembryonic antigen, CA 15.3)
   - Hemoglobin, alkaline phosphatase, liver function tests
   - Fragment c receptor for Igτ (immunoglobulin τ) on mononuclear cells
   - Hormone levels
   - Growth factor levels

C. Tumor characteristics
   1. Histological features: type, grade, number of blood vessels, vascular invasion, necrosis
   2. Stage (tumor, node, metastasis), bone marrow micrometastases
   3. Cytoplasmic and nuclear steroid receptors: ER, PgR, AR, vitamin-D-receptor
   4. Membrane receptors for hormones and growth factors:
      - LHRHR
      - Prolactin receptor
      - IGF1R
      - EGFR
      - TGFBR
      - SSTR
      - VEGF
   5. Enzymes, proteins and other cytoplasmic factors:
      - Plasminogen activator expression
      - Plasminogen activator inhibitors (PAI1, PAI2) and receptor (uPAR)
      - Cathepsin B, D, and L
      - PS2 protein
      - Growth factor content (EGF, TGFA and B, IGF1)
      - Tyrosine kinase activities
      - Heat shock proteins
      - Aromatase activity
      - Haptoglobin-related protein (Hpr) epitope expression
      - Adhesion factors
      - Glutathione S transferase 3
      - Human milk fat globule antigens (HMFG-1)
      - Prostaglandin levels
   6. Chromosomal abnormalities:
      - Cytogenetic
      - Ploidy
      - Amplification, (over)expression of oncogenes (*c-myc*, *HER2/neu/c-erbB2*, *int2*, *ras*)
      - Deletion or mutation of suppressor genes (*TP53*, *RB*, *nm23*)
   7. Cell proliferation indices:
      - Labeling index
      - S-phase fraction
      - Ki-67 antigen
   8. Clonogenicity
   9. Immunological phenotypes

D. Response to treatment

[a]Modified from review of Klijn and Foekens 1990 *(2)*.

Table 2
Clinical Application of Modern Cell Biological Parameters in Patients with Breast Cancer

1.	For estimation of prognosis in patients with primary or metastatic breast cancer
2.	For selection of high- and low-risk patients with respect to treating or not treating
3.	For selection of type of therapy depending on tumour and patient characteristics
4.	As target for new treatment modalities

Performance Status and Metabolic Disease

A general phenomenon is that poor physical condition and metabolic or other diseases may also influence the prognosis of breast cancer patients *(2)*.

Variables Determined in Blood

A number of these variables (Table 1) such as tumor marker levels, growth factors, and receptors, as well as organ function tests, are associated with total tumor burden and stage. Therefore, a correlation of these factors with prognosis is not surprising. In addition, relatively high plasma levels of hormones and growth factors involved in the growth regulation of breast cancer, such as estrogens, growth hormone, prolactin, and IGF-1, have also been associated with poor prognosis *(2,12–15)*.

Tumor Characteristics

TNM Staging

Tumor stage is still the most powerful prognostic factor *(2,16)*. In all our studies on cell biological prognostic factors both nodal and tumor status repeatedly appear to be independent prognostic factors *(2,5,10,12–14)*. Patients with metastatic cancer, especially visceral disease, have the worse prognosis. The presence of micrometastasis determined by bone marrow biopsies at time of diagnosis of the primary tumor also indicates early relapse *(17)*.

Histological Features

Several histological features (Table 1) have prognostic significance *(2,10,18–20)*. Patients with tubular-, cribriform-, and mucinous-type breast carcinomas do better than patients with ductal carcinomas not otherwise specified (NOS). Poorly differentiated tumors are associated with early relapse. A concern with tumor-grading systems that has received considerable attention *(10)* has been the issue of subjective evaluation resulting in poor interobserver reproducibility. Some groups have used grade in combination with other prognostic factors as a prognostic index *(21)*. The number of blood vessels, i.e., microvessel density, reflecting neoangiogenesis, and vascular invasion also are important prognostic factors for poor prognosis *(22,23)*.

Steroid Hormone Receptors and Associated Factors

As demonstrated by many groups *(20,24–27)*, we found a clear prognostic value with respect to estrogen (ER) and progesterone receptor (PgR) levels as measured by dextran-coated charcoal (DCC) and enzyme immunoassays (EIA) *(5,10,28)*. However, in node-negative patients the differences regarding 5-yr relapse-free (RFS) and overall survival between the high- and low-risk groups are small, i.e., 8–10%. The prognostic value of ER and PgR even decreases with longer follow-up than 5 yr. With respect to site of relapse, patients with visceral disease have more frequently ER-negative tumors. Clark et al. *(26)* demonstrated that for each metastatic site, receptor-positive patients had longer survival than receptor-negative patients. With respect to adjuvant chemotherapy, Raemaekers et al. *(29)* found, in a CMF-treated group of patients, that PgR status was the most powerful predictor of recurrence, probably in relation to the castration effects of CMF. In general, steroid-receptor status is a good predictor for the efficacy of endocrine therapy in patients with primary and metastatic disease *(10,13,27,30)*. However, very high ER levels have been shown to be associated with a poorer prognosis *(31)*. Using immunohistochemical techniques a good correlation with the standard biochemical techniques was found (see reviews *10* and *27*). However, there are still some important technical issues involving the assessment of ER and PgR by immunohistochemical methods and the optimal cut-off values still remain to be determined *(10,27)*.

Receptors for androgens (AR) *(32,33)* and vitamin D *(34)* also have prognostic value. Patients with receptor-positive tumors had significantly longer disease-free survival than those with receptor-negative tumors. Patients with AR-positive tumors might benefit from treatment with (anti)androgens or high dose progestins, while in the future vitamin D analogs might be valuable in the treatment of patients with specific vitamin D receptor status.

Several estrogen-dependent factors have been investigated to assess their prognostic and predictive value. In our experience, the pS2 protein (with unknown function) is associated with good prognosis in case of high cytosolic tumor levels *(35,36)*. However, in immunohistochemical studies pS2 had no prognostic value *(13,14,27,36–38)*. With respect to prediction of response to endocrine therapy, pS2 might have some value in addition to ER and PgR *(37,38)*. The expression of tumor-associated 90K-antigen appeared to have no prognostic or predictive value *(39)*. On the other hand, we found recently that high tumor levels of the steroid receptor coactivator-1 (SRC-1) predict a favorable response to tamoxifen in patients with recurrent breast cancer *(40)*.

Proliferation Markers and DNA Content

The proliferative capacity of breast cancer is an important prognostic factor and can be determined by a variety of techniques, such as measuring of the mitotic index (MI), thymidine labeling index (TLI), thymidine kinase activity, bromodeoyuridine labeling, S-phase fraction (SPF), Ki67 antigen, MIB-1 antigen, PCNA nuclear protein, various cyclins, mitosin, and ki-S1, which recently has been shown to be identical to topoisomerase IIα *(2,10,21,27,41)*. In general, there is no consensus about the prognostic and predictive values of these parameters, and there are methodological differences among the various studies. For measuring of some of these parameters, extensive experience is warranted. Based on various reviews, it can be concluded that in most studies rapidly proliferating tumors are associated with a short relapse-free and overall survival. In three of four studies TLI was an independent prognostic factor *(27)*. Recently, a large study of 1800 node-negative breast cancer patients demonstrated an independent prognostic role for TLI *(42)*. Analysis of more than 127,000 breast cancer patients showed an increased incidence of higher SPF and aneuploidy in ER and PgR-negative tumors, larger tumors, node-positive tumors, and tumors from younger patients *(43)*. The difference in survival between patients with tumors having a high SPF as compared with those with a low SPF is, however, small. In a series of 9500 node-negative patients, and using different cut-off points for euploid and aneuploid tumors, the difference in 3-yr actuarial

RFS was only 6% in favor of those with a low proliferation index *(43)*. On the other hand, knowledge of the proliferation index of a tumor may be helpful in selecting patients for endocrine therapy (slowly proliferating tumors) or chemotherapy (rapidly proliferating tumors) *(41,44)*.

Peptide Hormones, Growth Factors, and Their Receptors

Many hormones, growth factors, and other agents are involved in the growth regulation of breast cancer *(12,45)*.

The epidermal growth factor receptor (EGFR), which belongs to the tyrosine kinase family of receptors, has been shown to be a marker of poor prognosis *(46)*. However there is no consensus about the relationship of EGFR with other prognostic factors and about the prognostic value as an independent factor determined by multivariate analysis *(10,12–14,47,48)*. We found only a tendency to a negative relationship between EGFR and RFS *(49,50)*. In our study on 214 patients with primary breast cancer (median follow-up 8.5 yr, maximum follow-up 15 yr), EGFR was negatively correlated to ER and PgR, whereas no association was found with age, lymph node status, and tumor size. Initially, after a follow-up of 5 yr, there was a tendency to a significant association between EGFR levels and tumor recurrence rate ($p = 0.08$). Patients with tumors containing intermediate levels of EGFR experienced a longer relapse-free survival than did patients with tumors possessing lower or higher levels of EGF-R. This effect was most pronounced in the subgroup of patients with positive axillary lymph nodes. However, after 10 yr follow-up, this association appears to be lost ($p = 0.28$). A similar phenomenon was observed for the ER. While at 5 yr follow-up ER status had significant prognostic value ($p = 0.01$), at 10 yr follow-up this significance also appears to be lost ($p = 0.40$). However, tumor size, lymph node status, grade, and PgR status maintained significant prognostic value by univariate analysis.

Based on 40 separate studies comprising 5232 patients *(47)*, the mean percentage of EGFR positivity reported in breast cancer is 45% (range 14–91%). Nine out of 15 different studies showed in some way a significant negative association between EGFR and RFS by univariate analysis *(48)*, and two others showed a tendency to such a relationship. Of seven studies applying multivariate analysis, two demonstrated an independent prognostic value of EGFR for RFS and two others demonstrated a tendency to a significant correlation, whereas three did not. It may be concluded that EGFR status has a more or less prognostic value in patients with primary breast cancer, but the prognostic power decreases with longer follow-up. Of great clinical significance is the association of EGFR with hormone resistance *(51)*. Therefore EGFR status can be used for selection of type of treatment. Finally, EGFR might be useful as a target for new treatment modalities.

The human homolog of the neu gene, called HER2 or C-erbB2, shares extensive homology with EGF-R (C-erbB1). HER2/neu or its protein p185$^{\text{C-erb-B-2}}$ is overexpressed in 10–35% of breast cancers. In a review of 11,408 cases (12) we calculated a mean HER2/neu positivity of 20% without finding any significant difference between the incidence of amplification (20.6%) and overexpression (19.2%). Many studies showed no or only minor prognostic value of HER2/neu in patients with primary breast cancer, especially in patients with uninvolved lymph nodes *(10,12–14,27,45,52)*. In our experience involving 1000 primary breast tumors, we observed a strong negative association between HER2/neu amplification and cytosolic levels of ER and PgR *(53)*. Patients with HER2/neu amplification showed a slightly poorer overall survival without a significant difference in RFS *(54)*. However, a recent prospective study indicated that HER2/neu amplification is an independent prognostic factor for risk of recurrence in node-negative patients *(55)*; there was some evidence that amplification was more important in patients who received chemotherapy compared with untreated patients. Indeed, HER2/neu might be of greater importance with respect to prediction of response to therapy and therapy resistance *(13,14,27,52)*. We *(56)* and others *(51)* found that patients with HER2/neu-positive tumors respond poorly to endocrine therapy for metastatic disease which is in agreement with the findings of Carlomagno et al. *(57)* indicating a lack of efficacy of adjuvant tamoxifen in early-stage breast cancer patients with overexpression of HER2/neu. Also, circulating levels of the extracellular domain of the HER2/neu protein appeared to predict a poor response to endocrine therapy *(58)*. However, a recent study found no association between HER2/neu and response to endocrine therapy in ER-positive patients *(59)*. With respect to chemotherapy, we reported previously that HER2/neu amplification was actually a predictor of good response to CMF chemotherapy in patients with metastatic disease *(13)*; these results were not in agreement with those of a study by Wright et al. *(60)* using mitoxanthrone. There is no agreement on the predictive value of HER2/neu with respect to the efficacy of adjuvant chemotherapy *(12–14,27,52)*. The apparent discrepancies between different trials can be explained by the use of different treatment regimens (dose and types of chemotherapy, but especially combination with endocrine therapy) and partially by the occurrence of chemocastration in the premenopausal patients group.

Within the context of a trial on triple endocrine therapy with tamoxifen, a somatostatin analog, and an antiprolactin, recently we reviewed *(15)* the role of growth hormone (GH), prolactin (PRL), and insulinlike growth factors (IGFs). Together with estradiol, insulinlike growth factors (IGF-1 and IGF-2) are the most potent mitogens for breast cancer cells *(45)*. The growth effects of both are mediated predominantly via IGF-1 receptors, which have been demonstrated in 67–93% of primary human breast cancers *(13,14,49,61)* at higher density than in normal or benign breast tissue *(62)*. In vivo, pituitary-derived GH regulates endocrinologically the secretion of IGF-1, and also possibly has a regulatory effect on local IGF-1 secretion within (tumor) tissues *(45)*. In addition, in breast cancer local production of GH with a potential paracrine function has been described. In vitro, physiological concentrations of the lactotrophic hormones GH and PRL can stimulate the growth of breast cancer cells *(63)*. In primary human breast cancers, receptors for these lactotrophic hormones have been demonstrated in 13–72% of series of tumors investigated, depending on the techniques used *(14)*. Furthermore, increased plasma levels of both GH and PRL as well as of IGF-1 have been found in patients with breast cancer. Therefore, suppression of GH, PRL, and IGF-1 secretion might be important in the treatment of breast cancer.

Suppression of GH and IGF-1 secretions can be induced by somatostatin and its analogs *(64,65)*. Interestingly, receptors for somatostatin (SSTR) have also been demonstrated in 36–67% of primary human breast cancers (14) and in even 75% by in vivo receptor scintigraphy, indicating that somatostatin analogs can directly affect tumor growth. Indeed, we and others have previously shown direct growth-inhibitory effects of somatostatin analogs on human breast cancer cell lines *(66)*. High expression of IGF-1-R has been reported to be associated with a poor prognosis, a favorable prognosis, and with a lack of a relationship with prognosis *(10)*. In the studies in which IGF-1-R was reported to be a favorable prognostic factor, only a very small subgroup consisting of 13% of the tumors was classified as positive. In our own experience, IGF-1-R could be a marker of poor prognosis in a very small subset of patients. This might be concluded from the analysis of IGF-1-R gene amplification, which sporadically was found in 2% of 975 tumors studied and appeared to be associated with poor survival *(67)*. In the studies reported so far, however, IGF-1-R was found not to be related with prognosis in node-negative breast cancer. In analogy with EGF-R, simultaneous measurement of IGF-1-R with its ligands *(61)* may prove to be more informative, in spite of the fact that IGF-1 on its own does not seem to be a valuable prognostic indicator in breast cancer. Combination treatment blocking estrogens, the GH/IGF-1 axis, and PRL might be worthwhile *(15)*.

The expression of a variety of other receptors and growth factors has also been studied in breast cancer biopsies. These, among others, involve TGF-B *(14,45,68,69)*, tumor necrosis factor-α *(70)*, basic fibroblast growth factor and its receptor *(14,45,71)* and luteinizing hormone-releasing hormone receptor (LHRH-R) *(14,72)*.

Because a number of growth factor receptors are tyrosine kinases *(45)*, a disturbance in the balance between tyrosine kinase and tyrosine phosphatase activities might be associated with tumor progression and/or prognosis. Studies have been undertaken to assess the prognostic value of total tyrosine kinase activity in breast cancer *(73)*, and to assess whether overexpression of an intracellular protein tyrosine phosphatase is associated with the overexpression of the $p185^{c\text{-}erbB\text{-}2}$ protein *(74)*. From a therapeutic point of view, the new class of tyrosine kinase inhibitors are of great interest. Of special interest could be the hepatocyte growth factor (HGF) *(45)*, also known as scatter factor; it is a fibroblast-derived growth factor, which affects epithelial cell proliferation, also from human breast, and has a major effect on cell motility (for review, see *75*). Recently, a high level of HGF in breast tumor extracts was found to be strongly related with a poor (relapse-free) survival, also in node-negative patients *(76)*. These observations still need confirmation, and future studies combining HGF with its receptor, the protein product of the c-met oncogene, may provide important information. Intriguingly, the c-met oncogene may also act as a metastasis suppressor gene since patients with LOH for the c-met locus on chromosome 7q13 experienced a poor prognosis *(77)*.

Oncogenes, Tumor Suppressor Genes and Apoptosis-Related Genes

The c-myc gene belongs to the myc family, which also includes N- and L-myc. This nuclear oncoprotein is important in cell growth and differentiation and essential for transition from $G_{0/1}$ to S-phase of the cell cycle; it is thought to be a transcription factor involved in DNA replication. High c-myc expression, when combined with a block in cell proliferation, induces apoptotic cell death. The c-myc gene has been found to be amplified in 1–56% of human primary breast tumors. In reviewing the literature *(14,78)*, we calculated the incidence of c-myc amplification to be approximately 20% (in 2493 breast cancers), including our series in which we found a frequency of amplification of 17.1% in 1000 tumors analyzed *(53)*. Regarding the prognostic significance of c-myc amplification in node-negative breast cancer, only very few studies are currently available *(10)*.

The amplicon FGF3/int-2;FGF4/hst-2;bcl-1;PRAD1;cyclinD;EMS-1;GST-pi has been found to be amplified in 9–23% of human breast tumors (for a review, see *79*). In our series involving 1000 breast tumor biopsies, we found an incidence of amplification of 14.1% *(53)*. Several studies have shown that amplification of the amplicon at 11q13 is associated with a poor prognosis in breast cancer, also in node-negative disease *(79)*.

Regarding its prognostic value in node-negative breast cancer, however, controversy exists. We recently reported that about half of the breast tumors that showed an amplification of the amplicon at 11q13 also showed an amplification of either the c-myc or the HER-2/neu gene *(56)*. Because c-myc amplification has been shown to be strongly related with a poor prognosis, studies relating the amplicon at 11q13 with poor prognosis should be interpreted with caution and the observed relation may have been caused by the existence of frequent coamplification with the c-myc gene. Preliminary data suggest that another amplicon, involving 20q13, may also be of prognostic importance in node-negative breast cancer as suggested by Tanner et al. *(80)*.

The human tumor suppressor gene p53 is located on chromosome 17p13.1. In about half of all cancers, alterations in p53 or its pathway are observed *(81)*. Genetic alterations of p53 are mostly acquired during life, but in a small minority of cancers the p53 gene defects are hereditary, resulting in the Li–Fraumeni syndrome. The gene appeared to be involved in cell cycle control, DNA repair, apoptosis, cellular differentiation, senescence, and angiogenesis. The main function of normal p53 is to preserve genome integrity, and the gene has therefore been designated "guardian of the genome" by Lane et al. in 1992. About 30% of breast cancers show p53 mutations *(10,14,27,52,81)*. Once mutated, most of the p53 proteins have a prolonged half-life resulting in a nuclear accumulation of nonfunctional p53 that can be detected by immunohistochemistry. More than 40 studies of p53 as a prognostic indicator for breast cancer have been reported *(52,81)*. Although there are discrepancies in results, in general p53 mutations or overexpression are associated with a poor outcome, also in node-negative disease. Also in our experience, using different methods, p53 alterations are an indication for poor prognosis *(82–87)*. Especially mutations in residues of p53 that directly contact DNA predict poor outcome *(85)* independent of myc gene alterations *(86)*. Recently we showed that the presence of a p53 protein alteration predicts poor response to tamoxifen therapy of patients with recurrent breast cancer *(84,87)*. Mutations of p53 might also predict clinical resistance to chemotherapy *(88,89)*. The application of taxanes hopefully may overcome this therapeutic problem *(89)*. In breast cancer, an inverse relation between the expression of bcl-2 and p53 has been found. High levels of bcl-2 correlated with favorable prognosis and may be associated with type of response to systemic therapy *(10,27)*. Regarding other tumor suppressor genes, we found no significant role with respect to prognosis for both the retinoblastoma gene *(13,90)* and MTS-I gene, encoding an inhibitor of cyclin-dependent kinase 4 *(91)*. Recently we found that patients with BRCA1-associated breast cancers had a similar prognosis as patients with sporadic breast cancers *(11)*. On the other hand, there are several reports showing that reduced nm23 expression is associated with aggressive tumor behavior *(10,13,92)*.

The Metastatic and Proteolytic Cascade

The metastatic cascade (Fig. 1) involves many important processes, induced by mutations of genes controlling metastasis. Growth-transformed cells must subsequently be able to detach from themselves and extracellular substratum within the primary tumor (for instance, by loss expression of cadherins and integrins), to degrade the extracellular matrix and membranes by proteolysis, to move away with help of scatter or autocrine motility factors, to invade lymph or blood vessels, to survive our immune clearance (it is estimated that <0.1% of circulating tumor cells will form productive metastasis), to adhere to the endothelium, to extravasate from the lumen of the vessels into the surrounding tissue, to proliferative in the new organ environment, and to induce new stroma and angiogenesis as soon as a tumor deposit of about 1 mm^3 has been reached. From this tumor deposit the metastatic cascade can restart. Many molecular events, adhesion factors, growth factors, motility factors, proteases, and inhibitors are involved in this metastatic process. However, at present it is unclear how many genetic "hits" must occur to convert a nonmetastatic tumor cell into its malignant offspring.

Invasion is an active process which involves reciprocal communication between tumor cells and the target organ tissue. This process is the balance of the expression of invasion promotor and suppressor genes particularly affecting the microecosystem in which the cancer cells are located. Malignant cells have a great heterogeneity of effector systems upon which they can call to achieve their ultimate goal of dissemination and colonization of distant metastases. One of these effector systems is the proteolytic cascade. A large number of publications showed a significant relationship between metastasis-related factors and final clinical outcome (such as disease-free, post-relapse and overall survival) and prediction of response to several types of systemic therapy.

The components of the urokinase plasminogen activator system are especially important with respect to clinical outcome *(10,13,14)*. In a pilot study involving 52 patients with primary breast cancer, Duffy et al. *(93)* have shown that an increased enzymatic activity of uPA in the primary breast tumor was associated with a shorter relapse-free survival. Owing to the complexity of the urokinase system of plasminogen activation, it was hypothesized that this important finding could be substantiated by measurement of the uPA antigen level. Indeed, in a first prospective study on uPA antigen by Jänicke et al. *(94)*, it was shown that uPA was an independent prognostic factor for relapse for the whole group of patients consisting of 50 node-negative and 54 node-positive breast cancer patients. This finding of a relationship between a high level of uPA antigen and a poor relapse-free, metastasis-free, and/or overall survival in primary breast cancer, also for node-negative patients, has since been confirmed in their later reports and by several independent groups of investigators *(10,27,95–100)* including ours *(13,14,101–104)*. Moreover, we recently established that a high level of uPA in the primary breast tumors is independently associated with a poor response to tamoxifen therapy in patients with recurrent breast cancer, i.e., the first study connecting the urokinase system of plasminogen activation with clinical endocrine resistance *(13,14,104)*. As may have been expected, in a collaborative study involving 505 patients we recently observed that a high level of uPAR is related with a poor prognosis in primary breast cancer *(98)*. Duggan et al. *(97)* also reported that a high level of uPAR in breast cancer cytosols was associated with a poor prognosis. Also, as may have been expected, a high level of the inhibitor PAI-2 in the primary breast tumor was related with a more favorable prognosis *(96,103)*, particularly in patients with high tumor levels of uPA *(103)*. However, it was an unexpected finding of Jänicke et al. *(99)* that a high level of the inhibitor PAI-1 in tumor extracts was associated with a poor prognosis in breast cancer. These initial observations were recently confirmed by us *(102)* and others *(96,98)*. It has been speculated that PAI-1 may be involved in the protection of the tumor tissue against uPA-directed degradation. A high PAI-1 level could also be a biochemical measure of the degree of neovascularization, or could be important for the reimplantation of circulating tumor cells at the metastatic site. In our recent analysis, including more patients and refined subgroup analysis, it appeared that one or more of the factors can be strong prognostic factors in specific subgroups, while they are of no or limited prognostic value in other patients *(10,98)*. These results show the need for performing studies on larger numbers of patients to enable powerful statistical analyses in clinically important subgroups of patients and to establish the risk for individual patients. In this respect, our most recent data on the prognostic value of uPA and PAI-1 in 940 node-negative primary breast cancer patients, using their previously established cut-off points *(101,102)*, confirm their significance as markers to identify node-negative patients at high risk for relapse *(10)*. Concerning the presence of a relationship between components of the urokinase system and response to tamoxifen therapy in recurrent breast cancer, similar to what we observed for uPA, high levels of uPAR and PAI-1 were found to be related with a poor response and a short duration of response, while a high level of PAI-2 was related with a more favorable response *(104)*. These data were confirmed recently in a larger series of more than 500 hormono-naive patients who received tamoxifen as first-line therapy for recurrent disease *(10)*. Interestingly, in patients who progressed on hormonal therapy and subsequently were treated with chemotherapy, no relationship of uPA or PAI-1 with response to chemotherapy was observed.

In summary, there is accumulating evidence that the components of the urokinase system of plasminogen activation are related with prognosis in primary—also node-negative—breast cancer, and with the efficacy of response to tamoxifen therapy in recurrent disease, without being related with the efficacy of response to chemotherapy. Within the proteolytic cascade, cathepsin D *(13,14,27,36)*, and cathepsin B and L *(105)* also play an important role and have prognostic value.

CONCLUSIONS

Many classical and modern cell biological factors are currently available to estimate the prognosis of patients with primary and metastatic breast cancer. In addition, some of these factors are useful to predict response especially to endocrine therapy, but fewer of them to chemotherapy *(106–108)*. More important, in the near future an increasing number of these factors will be used as targets for new treatment modalities, such as protease inhibitors, monoclonal antibodies, specific tyrosine kinase inhibitors, and statins of angiogenesis.

REFERENCES

1. Bain RP, Greenberg RS, Whitaker JP. Racial differences in survival of women with breast cancer. J Chron Dis 1986;39:631–642.
2. Klijn JGM, Foekens JA. Prognostic factors in breast cancer. In: Goldhirsch A, ed. Endocrine Treatment of Breast Cancer IV. Monograph Series of the European School of Oncology, 1990, pp. 17–25.
3. Moormeier J. Breast cancer in black women. Ann Intern Med 1996;124:897–905.
4. Langlands O, Kerr GR. Prognosis in breast cancer, the effect of age and menstrual status. Clin Oncol 1979;5:123–133.
5. Alexieva-Figusch J, van Putten WLJ, Blankenstein MA, Blonk-van der Wijst J. Klijn JGM. The prognostic value and relationships of patient characteristics, progestin receptor, estrogen receptor, and site of relapse in primary and metastatic human breast cancer. Cancer 1988;61:758-768.
6. De la Rochefordiere A, Assalain B, Campana F, et al. Age as a prognostic factor in premenopausal breast carcinoma. Lancet 1993;341:1039–1043.
7. Nixon AJ, Neuberg D, Hayes DF, et al. Relationship of patient age to pathologic features of the tumor and prognosis for patients with stage I or II breast cancer. J Clin Oncol 1994;12:888–894.
8. Albain KS, Allred DC, Clark GM. Breast cancer outcome and predictors of outcome: are there age differentials? Monogr Natl Cancer Inst 1994;16:35–42.
9. Chung M, Chang HR, Bland KI, Wanebo HJ. Younger women with breast carcinoma have a poorer prognosis than older women. Cancer 1996;77:97–103.

10. Foekens JA, Berns PMJJ, Look MP, Klijn JGM. Prognostic factors in node-negative breast cancer. In: Pasqualini JR, Katzenellenbogen BS, eds. Molecular and Clinical Endocrinology. Hormone Dependent Cancer, vol. 1, Marcel Dekker Inc, New York, 1996, pp. 217–253.
11. Verhoog LC, Brekelmans CTM, Seynaeve C, van den Bosch LMC, Dahmen G, van Geel AN, Tilanus-Linthorst MMA, Bartels CCM, Wagner A, van den Ouweland A, Devilee P, Meijers-Heijboer EJ, Klijn JGM. Survival and tumour characteristics of breast-cancer patients with germline mutations of BRCA1. Lancet 1998;351:316–321.
12. Klijn JGM, Berns PMJJ, Bontenbal M, Alexieva-Figusch J, Foekens JA. Clinical breast cancer, new developments in selection and endocrine treatment of patients. J Steroid Biochem Molec Biol 1992;43:211–221.
13. Klijn JGM, Berns PMJJ, Bontenbal M, Foekens JA Cell biological factors associated with the response of breast cancer to systemic treatment. Cancer Treatm Rev 1993;19(suppl. B):45–63.
14. Klijn JGM, Berns PMJJ, Foekens JA. Prognostic factors and response to therapy in breast cancer. Cancer Surveys 1993;18:165–198.
15. Bontenbal M, Foekens JA, Lamberts SWJ, de Jong FH, van Putten WLJ, Braun HG, Burghouts JThM, van der Linden GHM, Klijn JGM. Feasibility, endocrine and anti-tumour effects of a triple endocrine therapy with tamoxifen, a somatostatin analogue and an antiprolactin in post-menopausal metastatic breast cancer: a randomized study with long-term follow-up. Br J Cancer 1998;77:115–122.
16. Carter CL, Allan C, Henson DE. Relation of tumor size, lymph node status, and survival in 24,740 breast cancer cases. Cancer 1989;63:181–187.
17. Coombes RC, Berger U, Mansi J, Redding H, Powles TJ, Neville AM, McKinna A, Nash AG, Gazet J-C, Ford HT, Ormerod M, McDonnel T. Prognostic significance of micrometastases in bone marrow in patients with primary breast cancer. NCI Monogr 1986;1:51–53.
18. Simpson FJ, Page DL. Prognostic value of histopathology in the breast. Semin Oncol 1992;19:254–262.
19. Elston CW, Ellis IO. Pathologic prognostic factors in breast cancer: experience from a large study with long-term follow-up. Histopathology 1991;19:403–410.
20. Fisher B, Redmond C, Fisher ER, Caplan R. Relative worth of estrogen or progesterone receptor and pathologic characteristics of differentiation as indicators of prognosis in node negative breast cancer patients: findings from National Surgical Adjuvant Breast Cancer and Bowel Project Protocol B-06. J Clin Oncol 1988;6:1076–1087.
21. van der Linden JC, Lindeman J, Baak JPA, et al. The multivariate prognostic index and nuclear DNA content are independent prognostic factors in primary breast cancer patients. Cytometry 1989;10:56–62.
22. Folkman J. Tumorangiogenesis: In Mendelsohn J, Howly PM, Israel MA, Liotta LA, eds. The Molecular Basis of Cancer. W.B. Saunders Company, Philadelphia, 1995, pp. 206–232.
23. Harris AL. Antiangiogenesis for cancer therapy. Lancet 1997;349:13–15.
24. Jensen EV. Hormone dependency of breast cancer. Cancer 1981;47:2319–2326.
25. Horwitz KB, Wei LL, Sedlacek SM, d'Arville CN. Progestin action and progesterone receptor structure in human breast cancer: a review. Recent Prog Horm Res 1985;41:249–316.
26. Clark GM, Sledge GW, Osborne CK, McGuire WL. Survival from first recurrence: relative importance of prognostic factors in 1,015 breast cancer patients. J Clin Oncol 1987;5:55–61.
27. Ravdin PM. Prognostic factors in breast cancer: In Bonadonna G, Hortobagyi GN, Gianni AM, eds. Textbook of Breast Cancer, A Clinical Guide to Therapy. Martin Dunitz Ltd, London, 1997, pp. 35–64.
28. Foekens JA, Portengen H, van Putten WLJ, Peters HA, Krijnen HLJM, Alexieva-Figusch J, Klijn JGM. Prognostic value of estrogen and progesterone receptors measured by enzyme immunoassays in human breast tumor cytosols. Cancer Res 1989;49:5823–5828.
29. Raemaekers JMM, Beex LVAM, Pieters GFFM, Smals AGH, Benraad ThJ, Kloppenborg PWC, the Breast Study Group. Progesterone receptor activity and relapse-free survival in patients with primary breast cancer: the role of adjuvant chemotherapy. Breast Cancer Res Treatm 1987;9:191–199.
30. Santen RJ, Manni A, Harvey H, Redmond C. Endocrine therapy of breast cancer in women. Endocr Rev 1990;11:221–265.
31. Thorpe SM, Christensen IJ, Rasmussen BB, Rose C. Short recurrence-free survival assocatiated with high oestrogen receptor levels in the natural history of postmenopausal, primary breast cancer. Eur J Cancer 1993;29A:971–977.
32. Teulings FAG, Van Gilse HA, Henkelman MS, Portengen H, Alexieva-Figusch J. Estrogen, androgen, glucocorticoid and progesterone receptors in progestin-induced regression of human breast cancer. Cancer Res 1980;40:2557–2561.

33. Kuenen-Bouwmeester V, van der Kwast ThJ, Claassen CC, Look MP, Liem GS, Klijn JGM, Henzen-Logmans SC. The clinical significance of androgen receptors in breast cancer and their relation to histological and cell biologial parameters. Eur J Cancer 1996;32:1560–1565.
34. Colston KW, Berger U, Coombes RC. Possible role for vitamin D in controlling breast cancer cell proliferation. Lancet 1989;i:188–191.
35. Foekens JA, Rio M-C, Sequin P, van Putten WLJ, Fauque J, Nap M, Klijn JGM, Chambon P. Prediction of relapse and survival in breast cancer patients by pS2 protein status. Cancer Res 1990;50:3832–3837.
36. Foekens JA, van Putten WLJ, Portengen H, de Koning HYWCM, Thirion B, Alexieva-Figusch J, Klijn JGM. Prognostic value of pS2 and cathepsin D in 710 human primary breast tumors: multivariate analysis. J Clin Oncol 1993;11:899–908.
37. Foekens JA, Portengen H, Look MP, Van Putten WLJ, Thirion B, Bontenbal M, Klijn JGM. Relationship of pS_2 with response to tamoxifen therapy in patients with recurrent breast cancer. Br J Cancer 1994;70:1217–1223.
38. Jansen RLH, Hupperets PSGJ, Arends JW, et al. PS2 is an independent prognostic factor for post-relapse survival in primary breast cancer. Anticancer Res 1998;18:577–582.
39. Foekens JA, Klijn JGM, Natoli C, van Putten WLJ, Di Stefano P, Look MP, Portengen H, Iacobelli S. Expression of tumor-associated 90K-antigen in human breast cancer: no correlation with prognosis and response to first-line therapy with tamoxifen. Int J Cancer 1995;64:130–134.
40. Berns EMJJ, van Staveren IL, Klijn JGM, Foekens JA. Predictive value of SRC-1 for tamoxifen response of recurrent breast cancer. Breast Cancer Res Treatm 1998;48:87–92.
41. Silvestrini R, Daidone MG. Review of proliferative variables and their predictive value: In Senn HJ, Gelber RD, Goldhirsch A, Thürlimann B, eds. Adjuvant Therapy of Breast Cancer IV; Recent Results in Cancer Research 127. Springer-Verlag, Heidelberg, 1993, pp. 71–77.
42. Silvestrini R, Daidone MG, Luise A, et al. Biological and clinicopathologic factors as indicators of specific relapse types in node-negative breast cancer. J Clin Oncol 1995;13:697–704.
43. Wenger CR, Beardslee S, Owens MA, et al. DNA ploidy, S-phase, and steroid receptors in more than 127,000 breast cancer patients. Breast Cancer Res Treatm 1993;28:9–20.
44. Muss HB. Endocrine therapy for advanced breast cancer: a review. Breast Cancer Res Treatm 1992;21:15–26.
45. Dickson RB, Lippman ME. Growth factors in breast cancer. Endocrine Rev 1995;16:559–590.
46. Sainsbury JRC, Needham GK, Farndon JR, Malcolm AJ, Harris AL. Epidermal-growth-factor receptor status as predictor of early recurrence and of death from breast cancer. Lancet 1987;I:1398–1402.
47. Klijn JGM, Berns PMJJ, Schmitz PIM, Foekens JA. The clinical significance of epidermal growth factor receptor (EGF-R) in human breast cancer: a review on 5232 patients. Endocrine Rev 1992;13:3–18.
48. Klijn JGM, Berns PMJJ, Schmitz PIM, Foekens JA. Epidermal growth factor receptor (EGF-R) in clinical breast cancer: update 1993. Endocrine Rev Monogr 1993;1:171–174.
49. Foekens JA, Portengen H, van Putten WLJ, Trapman AMAC, Reubi J-C, Alexieva-Figusch J, Klijn JGM. Prognostic value of receptors for insulin-like growth factor 1, somatostatin, and epidermal growth factor in human breast cancer. Cancer Res 1989;49:7002–7009.
50. Klijn JGM, Look MP, Portengen H, Alexieva-Figusch J, van Putten WLJ, Foekens JA. The prognostic value of epidermal growth factor receptor (EGF-R) in primary breast cancer: results of a 10 year follow-up study. Breast Cancer Res Treat 1994;29:73–83.
51. Nicholson S, Wright C, Sainsbury JRC, et al. Epidermal growth factor receptor (EGFr) as a marker for poor prognosis in node-negative breast cancer patients: neu and tamoxifen failure. J Steroid Biochem Molec Biol 1990;37:811–814.
52. The American Society of Clinical Oncology Clinical practice guidelines for the use of tumor markers in breast and colorectal cancer. J Clin Oncol 1996;14:2843–2877.
53. Berns PMJJ, Klijn JGM, van Staveren IL, Portengen H, Noordegraaf E, Foekens JA. Prevalence of amplification of the oncogenes c-myc, HER2/neu and int-2 in one thousand human breast tumours: correlation with steroid receptors. Eur J Cancer 1992;28:697–700.
54. Berns PMJJ, Klijn JGM, van Putten WLJ, van Staveren IL, Portengen H, Foekens JA. C-myc amplification is a better prognostic factor than HER2/neu amplification in primary breast cancer. Cancer Res 1992;52:1107–1113.
55. Andrulis IL, Bull SB, Blackstein ME, et al. Neu/erbB-2 amplification identifies a poor-prognosis group of women with node-negative breast cancer. J Clin Oncol 1998;16:1340–1349.

56. Berns EMJJ, Foekens JA, Van Staveren IL, Van Putten WLJ, De Koning HYWCM, Portengen H, Klijn JGM. Oncogene amplification and prognosis in breast cancer: relationship with systemic treatment. Gene 1995;159:11–18.
57. Carlomagno C, Perrone F, Gallo C, et al. C-erbB2 overexpression decreases the benefit of adjuvant tamoxifen in early-stage breast cancer without axillary lymph node metastases. J Clin Oncol 1996;14:2702–2708.
58. Yamauchi H, O'Neill A, Gelman R, et al. Prediction of response to antiestrogen therapy in advanced breast cancer patients by pretreatment circulating levels of extracellular domain of the HER-2/c-neu protein. J Clin Oncol 1997;15:2518–2525.
59. Elledge RM, Green S, Ciocca D, Pugh R, Allred DC, Clark GM, Hill J, Ravdin P, O'Sullivan J, Martino S, Osborne CK. HER-2 expression and response to tamoxifen in estrogen receptor-positive breast cancer: a Southwest Oncology Group Study. Clin Cancer Res 1998;4:7–12.
60. Wright C, Cairns J, Cantwell BJ, Cattan AR, Hall AG, Harris AL, Horne CHW. Response to mitoxantrone in advanced breast cancer: correlation with expression of c-erbB-2 protein and glutathione S-transferases. Br J Cancer 1992;65:271–274.
61. Foekens JA, Portengen H, Janssen M, Klijn JGM. Insulin-like growth factor-1 receptors and insulin-like growth factor-1-like activity in human primary breast cancer. Cancer 1989;63:2139–2147.
62. Peyrat JP, Bonneterre J, Laurent JC, Louchez MM, Amrani S, Leroy-Martin B, Vilain MO, Delobelle A, Demaille A. Presence and characterization of insulin-like growth factor-I receptors in benign breast diseases. Eur J Cancer Clin Oncol 1988;24:1425–1431.
63. Manni A, Wright C, Davis G, Glenn J, Joehl R, Feil P. Promotion by prolactin of the growth of human breast neoplasms cultured in vitro in the soft agar clonogenic assay. Cancer Res 1986;46:1668–1672.
64. Manni A, Boucher AE, Demers LM, Harvey HA, Lipton A, Simmonds MA, Bartholomew M. Endocrine effects of combined somtatostatin analog and bromocriptine therapy in women wtih advanced breast cancer. Breast Cancer Res Treat 1989;14:289–298.
65. Lamberts SWJ, van der Lely AJ, de Herder WW, Hofland LJ. Octreotide. N Engl J Med 1996;334:246–254.
66. Setyono-Han B, Henkelman MS, Foekens JA, Klijn JGM. Direct inhibitory effects of somatostatin (analogues) on the growth of human breast cancer cells. Cancer Res 1987;47:1566–1570.
67. Berns PMJJ, Klijn JGM, van Staveren IL, Portengen H, Foekens JA. Sporadic amplification of the insulin-like growth factor 1 receptor gene in human breast tumors. Cancer Res 1992;52:1036–1039.
68. Murray PA, Barrett-Lee P, Travers M, Luqmani Y, Powles T, Coombes RC. The prognostic significance of transforming growth factors in human breast cancer. Br J Cancer 1993;67:1408–1412.
69. Thompson AM, Kerr DJ, Steel CM. Transforming growth factor β1 is implicated in the failure of tamoxifen therapy in human breast cancer. Br J Cancer 1991;63:609–614.
70. Bebök Z, Márkus B, Németh P. Prognostic relevance of transforming growth factor alpha (TGF-α) and tumor necrosis factor alpha (TNF-α) detected in breast cancer tissues by immunohistochemistry. Breast Cancer Res Treatm 1994;29:229–235.
71. McLeskey SW, Zhang L, El-Ashrey D, et al. Tamoxifen-resistant fibroblast growth factor-transfected MCF-7 cells are cross-resistant in vivo to the antiestrogen ICI 182, 780 and two aromatase inhibitors. Clin Cancer Res 1998;4:697–711.
72. Baumann GH, Kiesel L, Kaufmann M, Bastert G, Runnebaum B. Characterization of binding sites for a GnRH-agonist (buserelin) in human breast cancer biopsies and their distribution in relation to tumor parameters. Breast Cancer Res Treatm 1993;25:37–46.
73. Romain S, Chinot O, Klijn JGM, Van Putten WLJ, Guirou O, Look M, Martin PM, Foekens JA. Prognostic value of cytosolic tyrosine kinase activity in 249 node-positive breast cancer patients. Br J Cancer 1994;70:304–308.
74. Wiener JR, Kerns BLM, Harvey EL, et al. Overexpression of the protein tyrosine phosphatase PTB1B in human breast cancer: association with $p185^{c\text{-}erbB\text{-}2}$ protein expression. J Natl Cancer Inst 1994;86:372–378.
75. Jiang WG, Hallett MB, Puntis MCA. Hepatocyte growth factor/scatter factor, liver regeneration and cancer metastasis. Br J Surg 1993;80:1368–1373.
76. Yamashita JI, Ogawa M, Yamashita SI, et al. Immunoreactive hepatocyte growth factor is a strong and independent predictor of recurrence and survival in human breast cancer. Cancer Res 1994;54:1630–1633.
77. Bieche, I, Champème, M.H, Matifas, F, Hacène, K, Callahan, R, Lidereau, R. Loss of heterozygosity on chromosome 7q and aggressive primary breast cancer. Lancet 1992;339:139–143.

78. Berns PMJJ, Foekens JA, van Putten WLJ, van Staveren IL, Portengen H, de Koning WCH, Klijn JGM. Prognostic factors in human primary breast cancer: comparison of c-myc and HER2/neu amplification. J Steroid Biochem Molec Biol 1992;43:13–19.
79. Borg A. Gene alterations in human breast cancer. In: Spandidos DA, ed. Current Perspectives on Molecular Oncology, Vol 1 (part B): Cancer Genes and Their Clinical Implications. JAI Press LTD, London, 1992, pp. 21–79.
80. Tanner MM, Tirkkonen M, Kallioniemi A, et al. Increased copy number at 20q13 in breast cancer: defining the critical region and exclusion of candidate genes. Cancer Res 1994;54:4257–4260.
81. Klijn JGM, ed. Prognostic and Predictive Value of p53. In: ESO Scientific Updates. Elsevier Science, Amsterdam, vol. 1, 1997, pp. 1–163.
82. de Witte HH, Foekens JA, Lennerstrand J, Smid M, Look MP, Klijn JGM, Benraad ThJ, Berns EMJJ. Prognostic significance of TP53 accumulation in human primary breast cancer: comparison between a rapid quantitative immunoassay and SSCP analysis. Int J Cancer 1996;69:125–130.
83. Berns EMJJ, de Witte HH, Klijn JGM, Willman K, Look MP, Meijer-van Gelder ME, Benraad ThJ, Foekens JA. Prognostic value of TP53 protein accumulation in human primary breast cancer: an analysis by luminometric immunoassay on 1491 tumor cytosols. Anticancer Res 1997;17:3003–3006.
84. Berns PMJJ, Klijn JGM, Foekens JA. Prognostic and predictive significance of p53 protein accumulation in human primary breast cancer analysed with a luminometric immunoassay (LIA) on tumour cytosols. In: Klijn JGM, ed. Prognostic and Predictive Value of p53. ESO Scientific Updates, Elsevier Science B.V, Amsterdam, 1997, Vol. 1, pp. 51–63.
85. Berns EMJJ, van Staveren IL, Look MP, Smid M, Klijn JGM, Foekens JA. Mutations in residues of TP53 that directly contact DNA predict poor outcome in human primary breast cancer. Br J Cancer 1998;77:1130–1136.
86. Berns EMJJ, Klijn JGM, Smid M, van Staveren IL, Look MP, van Putten WLJ, Foekens JA. TP53 and myc gene alterations independently predict poor prognosis in breast cancer patients. Gene Chromosom Cancer 1996;16:170–179.
87. Berns EMJJ, Klijn JGM, van Putten WLJ, de Witte HH, Look MP, Meijer-van Gelder ME, Willman K, Portengen H, Benraad ThJ, Foekens JA. p53 Protein accumulation predicts poor response to tamoxifen therapy of patients with recurrent breast cancer. J Clin Oncol 1998;16:121–127.
88. Elledge RM, Allred DC. p53 status: impact on breast tumour biology and response to therapy. In: Klijn JGM, ed. Prognostic and Predictive Value of p53 ESO Scientific Updates, Elsevier Science, Amsterdam, 1997, Vol. 1, pp. 63–76.
89. Börresen-Dale AL. Subgroups of p53 mutations may predict the clinical behaviour of cancers in the breast and colon and contribute to therapy response. In: Klijn JGM, ed. Prognostic and Predictive Value of p53. ESO Scientific Updates, Elsevier Science, Amsterdam, 1997, Vol. 1, pp. 23–33.
90. Berns EMJJ, de Klein A, van Putten WLJ, van Staveren IL, Bootsma A, Klijn JGM, Foekens JA. Association between the RB-1 gene alterations and factors of favourable prognosis in human primary breast cancer without effect on survival. Int J Cancer 1995;64:140–145.
91. Berns EMJJ, Klijn JGM, Smid M, van Staveren IL, Gruis NA, Foekens JA. Infrequent CDKN2 (MTS-1/p16) gene alterations in human primary breast cancer. Br J Cancer 1995;72:964–967.
92. Steeg PS, De La Rosa A, Flatow U, MacDonald NJ, Benedict M, Leone A. Nm23 and breast cancer metastasis. Breast Cancer Res Treatm 1993;25:175–187.
93. Duffy MJ, O'Grady P, Devaney D, O'Siorain L, Fennelly JJ, Lijnen HJ. Urokinase plasminogen activator, a marker for aggressive breast carcinomas: preliminary report. Cancer 1988;62:531–533.
94. Jänicke F, Schmitt M, Hafter R, Hollreider A, Babic R, Ulm K, Gössner W, Graeff H. Urokinase-type plasminogen activator (u-PA) antigen is a predictor of early relapse in breast cancer. Fibrinolysis 1990;4:69–78.
95. Spyratos F, Martin PM, Hacène K, Romain S, Andrieu C, Ferrero-Poüs C, Detieux S, Le Doussal V, Tubiana-Hulin M, Brunet M. Multiparametric prognostic evaluation of biological factors in primary breast cancer. J Natl Cancer Inst 1992;84:1266–1272.
96. Bouchet C, Spyratos F, Martin PM, Hacène K, Gentile A, Oglobine J. Prognostic value of urokinase-type plasminogen activator (uPA) and plasminogen activator inhibitors PAI-1 and PAI-2 in breast carcinomas. Br J Cancer 1994;69:398–405.
97. Duggan C, Maguire T, McDermott E, O'Higgins N, Fennelly JJ, Duffy MJ. Urokinase plasminogen activator and urokinase plasminogen activator receptor in breast cancer. Int J Cancer 1995;61:597–600.

98. Grφndahl-Hansen J, Peters HA, van Putten WLJ, Look MP, Pappot H, Rφnne E, Danφ K, Klijn JGM, Brünner N, Foekens JA. Prognostic significance of the urokinase type plasminogen activator receptor in breast cancer. Clin Cancer Res 1995;1:1079–1087.
99. Jänicke F, Pache L, Schmitt M, Ulm K, Thomssen C, Prechtl A, Graeff H. Both the cytosols and detergent extracts of breast cancer tissues are suited to evaluate the prognostic impact of the urokinase-type plasminogen activator and its inhibitor, plasminogen activator inhibitor type 1. Cancer Res 1994;54:1–4.
100. Fernö M, Bendahl P-O, Borg A, Brundell J, Hirschberg L, Olsson H, Killander D. Urokinase plasminogen activator, a strong independent prognostic factor in breast cancer, analysed in steroid receptor cytosols with a luminometric immunoassay. Eur J Cancer 1996;32A:793–801.
101. Foekens JA, Schmitt M, van Putten WLJ, Peters HA, Bontenbal M, Jänicke F, Klijn JGM. Prognostic value of urokinase-type plasminogen activator in 671 primary breast cancer patients. Cancer Res 1992;52:6101–6105.
102. Foekens JA, Schmitt M, van Putten WLJ, Peters HA, Kramer MD, Jänicke F, Klijn JGM. Plasminogen activator inhibitor-1 and prognosis in primary breast cancer. J Clin Oncol 1994;12:1648–1658.
103. Foekens JA, Buessecker F, Peters HA, Krainick U, van Putten WLJ, Look MP, Klijn JGM, Kramer MP. Plasminogen activator inhibitor-2: prognostic relevance in 1012 patients with primary breast cancer. Cancer Res 1995;55:1423–1427.
104. Foekens JA, Look MP, Peters HA, van Putten WLJ, Portengen H, Klijn JGM. Urokinase-type plasminogen activator (uPA) and its inhibitor PAI-1 predict poor response to tamoxifen therapy in recurrent breast cancer. J Natl Cancer Inst 1995;87:751–756.
105. Foekens JA, Kos J, Peters HA, Krašovec M, Look MP, Cimerman N, Meijer-van Gelder ME, Henzen-Logmans SC, van Putten WLJ, Klijn JGM. Prognostic significance of cathepsins B and L in primary human breast cancer. J Clin Oncol 1998;16:1013–1021.
106. Nooter K, Brutel de la Rivière G, Klijn JGM, Stoter G, Foekens JA. Multidrug resistance protein in recurrent breast cancer. Lancet 1997;349:1885–1886.
107. Nooter K, Brutel de la Riviere G, Look MP, van Wingerden KE, Henzen-Logmans SC, Scheper RJ, Flens MJ, Klijn JGM, Stoter G, Foekens JA. The prognostic significance of expression of the multidrug resistance-associated protein (MRP) in primary breast cancer. Br J Cancer 1997;76:486–493.
108. Romain S, Martin PM, Klijn JGM, van Putten WLJ, Look MP, Guirou O, Foekens JA. DNA synthesis enzyme acitivity: a biological tool useful for predicting anti-metabolic drug sensitivity in breast cancer. Int J Cancer 1997;74:156–161.

15 Role of the Polyamine Pathway in the Natural History of Breast Cancer

Andrea Manni, MD

INTRODUCTION

The diamine putrescine and the polyamines spermidine and spermine are small, aliphatic amines that play a major role in multiple cellular functions affecting proliferation and differentiation *(1–3)*. The biosynthesis and metabolism of these compounds are quite complex and highly regulated. A simplified scheme of the polyamine metabolic pathway is illustrated in Fig. 1. Three enzymes are of critical importance in the regulation of cellular polyamine pools because of their short half-life and rapid inducibility upon exposure of a target cell to an appropriate stimulus *(2,3)*. Ornithine decarboxylase (ODC) catalyzes the formation of putrescine from ornithine, the first and rate-limiting step in polyamine biosynthesis. Inhibition of this enzyme, particularly with the irreversible inhibitor α-difluoromethylornithine (DFMO), has been extensively used to probe basic biochemical and biological issues of polyamine physiology. S-adenosylmethionine decarboxylase (SAMDC) promotes the formation of the more distal polyamines, spermidine and spermine. Since spermidine may be the most critical polyamine controlling cell proliferation *(4)*, regulation of the activity of this enzyme is likely to have major biological importance. Spermidine/spermine N^1acetyl transferase (SSAT) is involved in the back conversion pathway and is the rate-limiting enzyme in polyamine catabolism. Induction of this enzyme by polyamine analogs has recently been shown to correlate with the antitumor activity of these compounds *(5)*. The intracellular polyamine milieu of normal tissues is tightly regulated by the modulation of these critical enzymes involved in polyamine synthesis and catabolism. Derangements in the polyamine metabolic pathway are likely to play a major role in cancer since the cellular levels of polyamines and their metabolic enzymes are higher in tumors than in surrounding normal tissue *(6,7)*. These observations point to polyamines as potential targets for anticancer therapy and chemoprevention. In this chapter, we will summarize up-to-date information on polyamine involvement in breast cancer biology with particular emphasis on their role in cell proliferation, tumor progression, and mammary carcinogenesis.

From: *Contemporary Endocrinology: Endocrinology of Breast Cancer*
Edited by: A. Manni © Humana Press Inc., Totowa, NJ

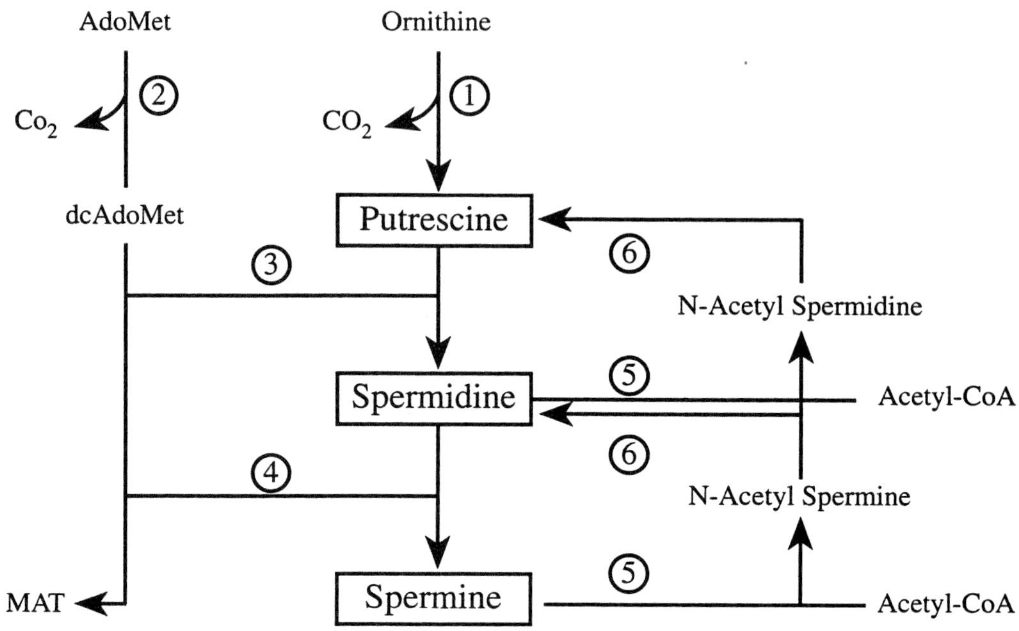

Fig. 1. Polyamine metabolic pathway. The three critical enzymes include ornithine decarboxylase (1), S-adenosylmethionine decarboxylase (2), and spermine/spermidine *N1*-acetyltransferase (5). Additional enzymes involved in the pathway are spermidine synthase (3), spermine synthase (4), and polyamine oxidase AdoMet, adenosylmethionine; dcAdoMet, decarboxylated adenosylmethionine; MAT, 5'-methylthioadenosine (6). (From ref. *57*, with permission.)

POLYAMINE INVOLVEMENT IN BREAST CANCER CELL PROLIFERATION

Considerable evidence provided by our *(8–10)* and other laboratories *(11,12)* has demonstrated that polyamines play a critical role in breast cancer cell proliferation. Using a variety of in vitro and in vivo experimental breast cancer systems, we and others have shown that administration of the ODC inhibitor DFMO exerts a potent antitumor action, which can be reversed by exogenous polyamine administration *(8,9,13,14)*. Recently, we have also shown that effective suppression of SAMDC with a newly developed inhibitor of this enzyme had a marked antiproliferative effect in several human breast cancer cell lines in culture *(15)*. A potential major advantage of SAMDC inhibitors over DFMO is represented by their ability to suppress profoundly the cellular levels of spermine, which is usually not affected in a major way by DFMO administration. Initial preliminary data indicated that at least some hormone-independent breast cancer cell lines may be less responsive than the hormone-dependent ones to DFMO administration *(14,16)*. Subsequent data, however, have failed to substantiate the differential sensitivity of breast cancer cells to antipolyamine therapy based upon their hormonal responsiveness *(13,17)*.

In hormone-responsive breast cancer cells, polyamine biosynthesis is under estrogen control since estradiol has been found to stimulate ODC and to increase cellular polyamine content *(18)*. Conversely, administration of the antiestrogen tamoxifen has been shown to induce moderate suppression of cellular polyamine pools *(19)*. The relevance, however, of this effect to the antiproliferative action of tamoxifen remains uncertain since attempts to reverse antiestrogen-induced growth inhibition with exogenous polyamine administration have met with variable success *(11,12,20,21)*. In any event, administration of DFMO consistently inhibits estradiol-stimulated ODC activity as well as estrogen-stimulated tumor growth in a variety of experimental systems *(8,18,22)*. Interestingly, other estrogen-regulated events (assessed concomitantly with tumor growth) such as induction of progesterone receptor synthesis in mammary tumors and stimulation of uterine growth in tumor-bearing rats have not been found to be affected by DFMO administration *(23,12)*. These observations highlight the selectivity of polyamine involvement in hormone action and point to a critical role of these compounds as distal effectors of estradiol-stimulated breast cancer cell proliferation.

The importance of the interaction between estrogen and polyamines in supporting tumor growth is reinforced by our observation that manipulation of the polyamine pathway significantly enhances hormonally induced synchronization of experimental breast cancer growth in vivo *(24)*. The practical implication of these findings is that combined hormone/polyamine manipulation may improve the implementation of kinetically designed chemotherapy.

Data from our own and other laboratories suggest that polyamines may influence hormone action in breast cancer cells at multiple steps. These include the association kinetics of the estrogen receptor with specific DNA sequences *(25)*, the synthesis of estradiol-regulated cell cycle-specific genes *(26)*, and the synthesis and/or action of hormonally regulated growth factors *(22,27,28)*. These findings led us to hypothesize that constitutive activation of the polyamine pathway may provide breast cancer cells with a growth advantage no longer requiring the presence of estrogens and may thus be at least one factor involved in the transition of hormone-dependent breast cancer to a hormone-independent and more aggressive phenotype.

POLYAMINE INVOLVEMENT IN TUMOR PROGRESSION

To test directly the influence of activation of the polyamine pathway on tumor progression to hormone independence, we employed a transfection approach to induce overexpression of ODC in the hormone-responsive MCF-7 breast cancer cell line. We were, indeed, able to induce marked ODC overexpression in transiently *(29)* as well as stably transfected cells *(30)*; it was associated with a selective increase in cellular putrescine content, whereas spermidine and spermine levels were not altered. In the aggregate, our results were consistent with the notion that ODC overexpression confers a modest (although statistically significant) growth advantage to breast cancer cells in liquid culture. By contrast, and surprisingly, anchorage-independent growth in soft agar was significantly reduced in ODC overexpressing MCF-7 breast cancer cells compared with controls *(30)*. The reason for this finding is unknown but may be related to cellular toxicity resulting from excessive accumulation of putrescine *(31)*. Interestingly, we observed that ODC-transfected MCF-7 clones manifested a reduction (mean 33%, range 13–68%, $p<0.0001$) in the proliferative response to increasing concentrations of estradiol *(30)*, thus suggesting that activation of polyamine biosynthesis may contribute in part to the acquisition of estrogen independence by breast cancer cells. This contention is further supported by recent data reported by us using an in vivo model of mammary tumor progression *(32)*. In this system, we observed that tumor progression to hormone independence as well as a less differentiated and more metastatic phenotype was associated with increased cellular expression of ODC activity.

Since induction of ODC overexpression by transfection selectively increased cellular putrescine content without altering spermidine and spermine levels, we next transfected MCF-7 cells with SAMDC, the rate-limiting enzyme in the formation of these two distal polyamines *(33)*. This was, indeed, the first successful attempt to generate SAMDC overexpressing cells using a transfection approach in any experimental system. Biochemical analysis of these cells revealed an approx fivefold increase in SAMDC activity. ODC activity was markedly suppressed (to approx 20% of the level detected in control cells), whereas SSAT levels were increased, although to a variable extent. Analysis of cellular polyamine pools revealed a selective accumulation of spermine (approx 80% increase over control); both putrescine and spermidine contents were decreased (approx 15% and approx 48% of control, respectively). Evaluation of the biologic properties of these cells revealed that, in contrast to ODC overexpressing MCF-7 cells (see above), SAMDC-overproducing breast cancer cells exhibited a significant growth advantage in soft agar *(33)*. This difference probably reflects the different polyamine profiles induced by ODC versus SAMDC overexpression. While ODC-overexpressing clones were characterized by selective accumulation of putrescine, SAMDC-overproducing breast cancer cells manifested a selective increase in spermine. Since clonogenicity in soft agar correlates with tumor aggressiveness, these data suggest that spermine may be selectively involved in conferring a more invasive phenotype to breast cancer cells.

Limited information is currently available on the importance of polyamine in the progression of clinical breast cancer. Glickman et al. *(34)* observed that high ODC activity was associated with high cellularity, low histologic differentiation, and high nuclear aplasia, thus suggesting that increased polyamine biosynthetic activity may lead to a more aggressive breast cancer phenotype. Kingsnorth et al. *(35)* observed that increased intracellular polyamine levels were positively correlated with factors known to have an adverse effect on survival, such as high histologic grade and estrogen receptor negative status. Furthermore, these authors reported that tumors recurring within 2 years of mastectomy had significantly higher levels of spermidine and spermine than those that did not. However, a formal survival analysis that takes into account the contribution of other prognostic variables was not performed. In a recently published pilot study involving a cohort of 50 primary human breast cancers *(36)*, we have correlated cellular levels of ODC, SAMDC, and SSAT activities to disease-free survival and overall survival. The major finding of our study was that ODC activity was a strong negative independent prognostic factor for both end points. With regard to overall survival, the adverse influence of ODC expression was superior even to that provided by the number of positive nodes (Table 1). Figure 2 depicts the effect of a 10-fold difference in ODC activity on overall survival after adjustment for other prognostic factors. In the aggregate, these findings provide strong support for the notion that activation of the polyamine metabolic pathway adversely impacts on breast cancer behavior, leading to a more aggressive phenotype.

POLYAMINE INVOLVEMENT IN MAMMARY CARCINOGENESIS

Considerable evidence points to a major role for ODC and polyamines in carcinogenesis. ODC activity, which is transiently increased on growth factor exposure, becomes constitutively activated during cell transformation by chemical carcinogens *(37)*, viruses *(38)*, and oncogenes *(39)*. Elevated levels of ODC are frequently detected in transformed

Table 1
Evaluation of Prognostic Factors According to Multivariate Analysis

	Overall survival (39 patients, 31 deaths)		
Variable	*Risk ratio*	*95% CI*	p *value*
Age	1.03	0.99–1.06	0.12
ER	1.26	0.58–2.74	0.56
Number of positive nodes	1.08	1.01–1.16	0.03
Tumor size (cm)	1.02	0.85–1.23	0.82
Log (ODC)	3.11	1.60–6.04	0.0008
Log (SSAT)	3.11	0.81–11.9	0.10
Log (SAMDC)	0.32	0.06–1.63	0.17

Abbreviations: ER, estrogen receptor; ODC, ornithine decarboxylase; SSAT, spermidine/spermine N^1 acetyl transferase; SAMDC, *S*-adenosylmethionine decarboxylase.
(Adapted from ref. *36*, with permission.)

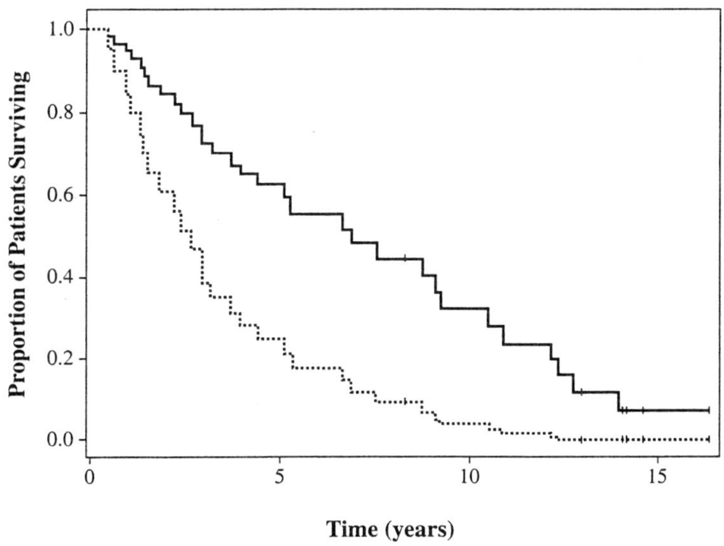

Fig. 2. Influence of a 10–fold difference in ODC activity (solid line, ODC 10 pmol/mg; dashed line, ODC 100 pmol/mg) on survival after adjustments were introduced for estrogen receptor and lymph node status. (From ref. *36*, with permission.)

cell lines *(40)*, animal tumors *(41)*, and some preneoplastic lesions *(42)*. In addition, induction of ODC activity and polyamine biosynthesis is critical in several experimental animal models of carcinogenesis *(43,44)*. A direct role of polyamines in mammary carcinogenesis has not yet been shown. However, the observation that breast cancer specimens have higher levels of polyamines and their metabolic enzymes than the surrounding normal breast tissue *(45)* suggests the possible involvement of these compounds in mammary tumor development. In addition, DFMO administration exerts a protective effect in the promotion stage of chemically induced rat mammary tumors *(46,47)*. This protection is associated with suppressed ODC activity and polyamine levels and is blocked by addition of putrescine to the diet in conjunction with DFMO treatment *(46)*. Collectively, these results suggest that polyamines may play an important role in mammary tumorigenesis.

To test this hypothesis directly, we induced ODC overexpression in the spontaneously immortalized MCF-10A human mammary epithelial cell line *(48)*. The potential clinical relevance of this experimental system is highlighted by the resemblance of its progressive stages of transformation (following oncogenic activation) to those of the human disease, i.e., hyperplasia without and with atypia, carcinoma *in situ*, and invasive cancer *(49)*. We observed that induction of ODC overexpression in MCF-10A cells conferred anchorage-independent growth, whereas growth in liquid culture was either unaffected or actually decreased *(48)*. This finding indicates that the increased clonogenicity in soft agar is not a nonspecific consequence of a growth advantage provided by ODC overexpression, but reflects the specific involvement of polyamines in transformation.

It was apparent, however, that the degree of clonogenicity conferred to MCF-10A cells by ODC overexpression alone was quite modest *(48)*. Furthermore, ODC overexpressing MCF-10A cells were unable to form tumors in nude mice (unpublished observations). These findings are not surprising, since acquisition of the fully transformed phenotype by normal breast epithelial cells is known to require multiple genetic aberrations. In recent experiments conducted in MCF-10A cells *(50)*, we have, indeed, observed that ODC overexpression, while having a modest effect on its own, markedly potentiated the colony-stimulating effect induced by activation of HER2-neu, a reasonably well-established oncogene involved in human mammary carcinogenesis. These findings are in line with similar observations made in different experimental systems. For instance, induction of ODC overexpression alone, while able to transform NIH-3T3 cells *(51)*, cannot by itself transform normal diploid keratinocytes or fibroblasts *(52)*, rather, those studies indicate that ODC primarily cooperates with other oncogenic pathways such as ras signaling to induce transformation.

The mechanisms by which ODC overexpression leads to malignant transformation remain largely unknown. Control of protein phosphorylation has been suggested as a potential critical event *(53)*. We have shown that induction of ODC overexpression in MCF-10A cells leads to activation of ERK *(48,50)*, a critical kinase in the mitogen-activated protein kinase (MAPK) signalling cascade, a final common pathway activated by various growth factors (including HER-2neu), tumor promoters, and differentiating agents (Fig. 3). Our recent preliminary results also point to an important role of the MAPK cascade as a mediator of the above-mentioned cooperativity between polyamines and HER2-neu in inducing transformation of MCF-10A cells *(50)* (Fig. 3). The significance of this finding has recently been strengthened by the report of Sivaraman et al. *(54)*, who demonstrated 5–10-fold increases in MAPK activity and expression in human breast cancer specimens over benign conditions. These data strongly implicate this family of enzymes in breast cancer development in women. Our results also emphasize the specificity of the influence of ODC overexpression on activation of the MAPK cascade since the activities of the stress-activated protein kinases, p38 and SEK, were not modified *(50)*. In the aggregate, our results suggest that increased polyamine biosynthetic activity critically interacts with HER2-neu in promoting human mammary cell transformation in culture and that the MAPK cascade is an important mediator of this interaction. It will be important to determine whether the cooperativity between ODC and HER2-neu extends beyond conditions of growth in soft agar to in vivo tumorigenicity in nude mice.

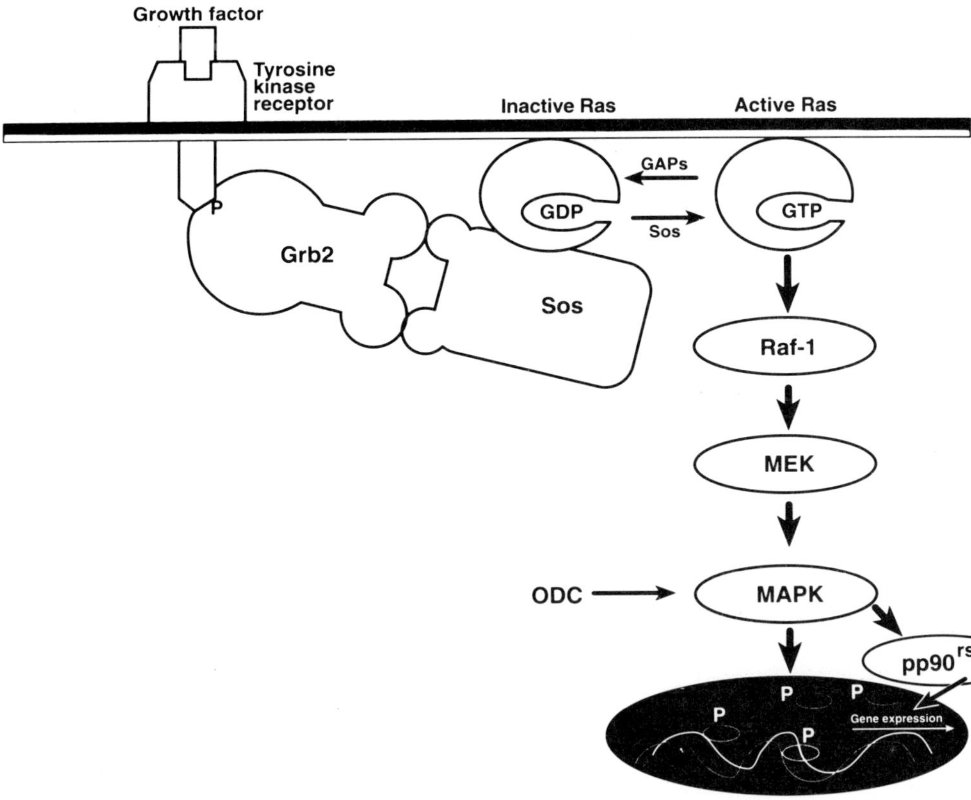

Fig. 3. A simplified scheme of the MAPK signaling cascade. Ras proteins (by direct interaction with Raf-1) are critical intermediates between receptor tyrosine kinases (such as HER-2neu) and downstream serine/threonine kinases (Raf-1, MEK, MAPK). Our data indicate that ODC overexpression feeds into this signaling cascade by increasing MAPK activity.

CLINICAL PERSPECTIVES

On the basis of the data reviewed above, there is sufficient rationale to test antipolyamine therapy in the treatment of human breast cancer. Carefully performed phase I studies have shown that it is safe to administer DFMO to humans with modest and transient toxicity *(55)*. We are currently in the process of initiating a phase II clinical trial of DFMO in women with metastatic breast cancer progressing after an initial endocrine therapy. There is concern that the usefulness of DFMO as an effective antitumor agent in vivo may be limited by the lack of major suppression of the distal polyamines, spermine and spermidine. This is due to the well-known occurrence of multiple compensatory events aimed at preserving cellular polyamine pools *(3)*, including transport of exogenous polyamines from host tissues into the tumor cells *(56)*. This problem may be circumvented by the recent development of polyamine analogs *(57)* and the new inhibitors of SAMDC *(15)*. Both classes of compounds have been shown to be effective in suppressing cellular spermidine and spermine levels. It is the author's opinion that antipolyamine therapy in breast cancer is most likely to be effective in patients with a low tumor burden. If the role of ODC in mammary carcinogenesis is confirmed in future studies, polyamine biosynthesis inhibitors could play a significant role as chemopreventive agents. A small pilot study supported by the National Cancer Institute is actually under way testing the feasibility of DFMO administration in breast cancer prevention in women.

Finally, it is possible that antipolyamine therapy could be found to be most useful in the treatment of breast cancer when used in combination with hormonal therapy and/or chemotherapy. Definition of the molecular mechanisms subserving polyamine action in breast cancer will obviously be critical for the rational design of combination treatments. For instance, inhibitors of HER2-neu *(58)* and MEK (the upstream kinase responsible for activation of MAPK) *(59)* are currently available, and some of them are being tested as antitumor agents in clinical trials. If confirmed by additional studies, our data discussed above would provide a strong rationale for combining these compounds with polyamine biosynthesis inhibitors in the treatment and chemoprevention of human breast cancer.

REFERENCES

1. Tabor CW, Tabor H (1984) Polyamines. Annu Rev Biochem 53:749–790.
2. Pegg AE (1986) Recent advances in the biochemistry of polyamines in eukaryotes. Biochem J 234:249–262.
3. Pegg AE (1988) Polyamine metabolism and its importance in neoplastic growth and as a target for chemotherapy. Cancer Res 48:759–774.
4. Shantz LM, Holm I, Janne OA, Pegg AE (1992) Regulation of S-adenosylmethionine decarboxylase activity by alterations in the intracellular polyamine content. Biochem J 288:511–518.
5. Casero RA, Mank AR, Xiao L, Smith J, Bergeron RJ, Celano P (1992) Steady-state messenger RNA and activity correlates with sensitivity to N^1, N^{12}-bis(ethyl)spermine in human cell lines representing the major forms of lung cancer. Cancer Res 52:5359–5363.
6. Janne J, Poso H, Raina A (1978) Polyamines in rapid growth and cancer. Biochemi Biophysi Acta 473:242–293.
7. Takami H, Romsdahl MM, Nishioka K (1979) Polyamines in blood cells as a cancer marker. Lancet 2:912–914.
8. Manni A, Wright C (1984) Polyamines as mediators of estrogen action on the growth of experimental breast cancer in rats. J Natl Cancer Inst 73:511–514.
9. Manni A, Wright C (1985) Polyamines as mediators of the effect of prolactin and growth hormone on the growth of N-nitroso-N-methylurea-induced rat mammary tumor cultured *in vivo* in soft agar. J Natl Cancer Inst 74:941- 944.
10. Manni A, Badger B, Luk G, Wright C, Caplan R, Rockette H, et al. (1988) Role of polyamines in the growth of hormone-responsive experimental breast cancer in vivo. Breast Cancer Res and Treat 11:231- 240.
11. Hoggard N, Green CD (1986) Polyamines and growth regulation of cultured human breast cancer cells by 17β-estradiol. Mol Cell Endocrinol 46:71–78.
12. Kendra KL, Katzenellenbogen BS (1987) An evaluation of the involvement of polyamines in modulating MCF-7 human breast cancer cell proliferation and progesterone receptor levels by estrogen and antiestrogen. J Steroid Biochem 28:123–128.
13. Glikman P, Manni A, Demers L, Bartholomew M (1989) Polyamine involvement in the growth of hormone-responsive and -resistant human breast cancer cells in culture. Cancer Res 49:1371–1376.
14. Lima G, Shiu RPC (1985) Role of polyamines in estradiol-induced growth of human breast cancer cells. Cancer Res 45:2466–2470.
15. Manni A, Badger B, Wechter R, Kunselman S, Rossini A, Demers L (1995) Biochemical and growth-modulatory effects of the new S-adenosylmethionine decarboxylase inhibitor CGP 48664 in malignant and immortalized normal human breast epithelial cells in culture. Int. J Cancer 62:485–491.
16. Thomas T, Kiang DT, Janne OA, Thomas TJ (1991) Variations in amplification and expression of the ornithine decarboxylase gene in human breast cancer cells. Breast Cancer Res and Treat 19:257–267.
17. Manni A, Badger B, Martel J, Demers L (1992) Role of polyamines in the growth of hormone-responsive and -resistant human breast cancer cells in nude mice. Cancer Lett 66:1–9.
18. Thomas T, Thomas TJ (1993) Estradiol control of ornithine decarboxylase mRNA, enzyme activity, and polyamine levels in MCF-7 breast cancer cells: therapeutic implications. Breast Cancer Res and Treat 29:189–201.

19. Cohen FJ, Manni A, Glikman P, Bartholomew M, Demers L (1990) Interactions between growth factor secretion and polyamines in MCF-7 breast cancer cells. Eur J Cancer 5:603–608.
20. Thomas T, Kiang DT (1987) Additive growth-inhibitory effects of DL-α-difluoromethylornithine and antiestrogens on MCF-7 breast cancer cell line. Biochem Biophys Res Commun 148:1338–1345.
21. Cohen FJ, Manni A, Glikman P, Bartholomew M, Demers L (1988) Involvement of the polyamine pathway in antiestrogen-induced growth inhibition of human breast cancer. Cancer Res 48:6818–6825.
22. Glikman PI, Manni A, Bartholomew M, Demers L (1990) Polyamine involvement in basal and estradiol stimulated insulin-like growth factor I secretion and action in breast cancer cells in culture. J Steroid Biochem Mol Biol 37:1–10.
23. Manni A, Badger B, Lynch J, Demers L (1990) Selectivity of polyamine involvement in hormone action on normal and neoplastic target tissues of the rat. Breast Cancer Res and Treat 17:187–196.
24. Manni A, Khin S, Biser N, English H, Badger B, Martel J, et al. (1992) Synchronization of breast cancer cell proliferation *in vivo* by combined hormonal and polyamine manipulation. Cancer Res 52:5720–5724.
25. Thomas T (1989) Structural specificity of polyamines in facilitating the high affinity binding of estrogen receptor to specific DNA sequences. FASEB J 3:A1192.
26. Thomas T, Thomas TJ (1994) Regulation of cyclic B_1 by estradiol and polyamines in MCF-7 breast cancer cells. Cancer Res 54:1077–1084.
27. Manni A, Wright C, Feil P, Baranao L, Demers L, Garcia M, et al. (1986) Autocrine stimulation by estradiol-regulated growth factors of rat hormone-responsive mammary cancer: interaction with the polyamine pathway. Cancer Res 46:1594–1598.
28. Manni A, Wright C, Luk GD, Davis G, Demers L (1987) Role of polyamines in the synthesis of estradiol-regulated growth factors in rat mammary cancer in culture. Breast Cancer Res and Treat 9:45–51.
29. Manni A, Wechter R, Grove R, Wei L, Martel J, Demers L (1995) Polyamine profiles and growth properties of ornithine decarboxylase overexpressing MCF-7 breast cancer cells in culture. Breast Cancer Res and Treat 34:45–53.
30. Manni A, Wechter R, Wei L, Heitjan D, Demers L (1995) Phenotypic features of breast cancer cells overexpressing ornithine-decarboxylase. J Cell Physiol 163:129–136.
31. Tome ME, Fiser SM, Gerner EW (1994) Consequences of aberrant ornithine decarboxylase regulation in rat hepatoma cells. J Cell Physiol 158:237–244.
32. Manni A, Grove R, Kunselman S, Aldaz M (1995) Involvement of the polyamine pathway in breast cancer progression. Cancer Lett 92:49–57.
33. Manni A, Badger B, Grove R, Kunselman S, Demers L (1995) Isolation and characterization of human breast cancer cells overexpressing S-adenosylmethionine decarboxylase. Cancer Lett 95:23–28.
34. Glikman P, Vegh I, Pollina MA, Mosto AH, Levy CM (1987) Ornithine decarboxylase activity, prolactin blood levels, and estradiol and progesterone receptors in human breast cancer. Cancer (Phila.) 60:2237–2243.
35. Kingsnorth AN, Wallace HM, Bundred NJ, Dixon JMJ (1984) Polyamines in breast cancer. Br J Surg 71:352–356.
36. Manni A, Mauger D, Gimotty P, Badger B (1996) Prognostic influence on survival or increased ornithine decarboxylase activity in human breast cancer. Clin Cancer Res 2:1901–1906.
37. Gilmour SK, Verma AK, Madara T, O'Brien TG (1987) Regulation of ornithine-decarboxylase gene expression in mouse epidermis and epidermal tumors during two-stage tumorigenesis. Cancer Res 47:1221–1225.
38. Haddox MK, Magun BE, Russell DH (1980) Ornithine decarboxylase induction during GI progression of normal and Rous-sarcoma-virus-transformed cells. Cancer Res 40:604–608.
39. Sistonen L, Hölttä E, Lehvaslaiho H, Lethola L, Alitalo KJ (1989) Activation of a chimeric EGF-R/neu tyrosine kinase induces the FOS/JUN transcription factor complex, glucose transporter and ornithine decarboxylase. J Cell Biol 109:1911–1919.
40. Scalabrino G, Ferioli ME (1982) Polyamines in mammalian tumors: part II. Adv Cancer Res 36:1–102.
41. Scalabrino G, Ferioli ME (1981) Polyamines in mammalian tumors: part I Adv Cancer Res 35:151–268.
42. Luk GD, Baylin SB (1984) Ornithine decarboxylase as a biological marker in familial colonic polyposis. N Engl J Med 311:80–83.
43. O'Brien TG (1976) The induction of ornithine decarboxylase as an early, possibly obligatory, event in mouse skin carcinogenesis. Cancer Res 36:2644–2653.
44. Kingsnorth AN, King WWK, Diekema KA, McCann PP, Ross JS, Malt RA (1983) Inhibition of ornithine decarboxylase with 2-difluoromethylornithine: reduced incidence of dimethylhydrazine-induced colon tumors in mice. Cancer Res 43:2545–2549.

45. Persson L, Rosengren E (1989) Increased formation of N^1-acetylspermidine in human breast cancer. Cancer Lett 45:83–86.
46. Thompson HJ, Meeker LD, Herbst EJ, Ronan AM, Minocha R (1985) Effect of concentration of D,1-2-difluoromethylornithine on murine mammary carcinogenesis. Cancer Res 45:1170–1173.
47. Thompson HJ, Ronan AM, Ritacco KA, Meeker LD (1986) Effect of tamoxifen and D,1-2-difluoromethylornithine on the growth, ornithine decarboxylase activity and polyamine content of mammary carcinomas incuded by 1-methyl-1-nitrosurea. Carcinogenesis 7:837–840.
48. Manni A, Wechter R, Gilmour S, Verderame MF, Mauger D, Demers LM (1997) Ornithine decarboxylase over-expression stimulates mitogen-activated protein kinase and anchorage-independent growth of human breast epithelial cells. Int J Cancer 70:175–182.
49. Miller FR, Soule HD, Tait L, Pauley RJ, Wolman SR, Dawson PI, et al. (1993) Xenograft model of progressive human proliferative breast disease. J Natl Cancer Inst 85:1725–1731.
50. Manni A, Wechter R, Verderame M (1997) Cooperativity between ornithine decarboxylase (ODC) and HER-2neu in transformation of human mammary epithelial cells. Program of the American Association of Cancer Res Annual Meeting, April 12–16, 1997, San Diego CA, p. 146, abstract #2493.
51. Moshier JA, Dosescu J, Skunca M, Luk GD (1993) Transformation of NIH/3T3 cells by ornithine decarboxylase overexpression. Cancer Res 53:2618–2622.
52. Clifford A, Morgan D, Yuspa SH, Soler AP, Gilmour S (1995) Role of ornithine decarboxylase in epidermal tumorigenesis. Cancer Res 55:1680–1686.
53. Hölttä E, Auvinen M, Paasinen A, Kangas A, Andersson LC (1994) Ornithine-decarboxylase-induced cellular transformation: the involvement of protein tyrosine kinase(s) and pp130. Biochem Soc Trans 22:853–859.
54. Sivaraman VS, Wang H-Y, Nuovo GJ, Malbon CC (1997) Hyperexpression of mitogen-activated protein kinase in human breast cancer. J Clin Invest 99:1478–1483.
55. Love RR, Carbone PP, Verma AK, Gilmore D, Carey P, Tutsch KD, et al. (1993) Randomized phase I chemoprevention dose-seeking study of α-difluoromethylornithine. J Natl Cancer Inst 85:732.
56. Hessels J, Kingma AW, Ferwerda H, van den Berg GA, Keig J, Muskiet FAJ (1989) Microbial flora in the gastrointestinal tract abolishes cytostatic effects of α-difluoromethylornithine in vivo. Int J Cancer 43:1155–1164.
57. Porter CW, Sufrin JR (1986) Interference with polyamine biosynthesis and/or function by analogs of polyamines or methionine as a potential anticancer chemotherapeutic strategy. AntiCancer Res 6:525–542.
58. Bacus SS, Kiguchi K, Chin D, King R, Huberman E (1990) Differentiation of cultured human breast cancer cells (AU-565 and MCF-7) associated with loss of cell surface HER-2/neu antigen. Mol Carcinog 3:350–362.
59. Simon C, Juarez J, Nicolson GL, Boyd D (1996) Effect of PD 098059, a specific inhibitor of mitogen-activated protein kinase kinase, on urokinase expression and *in vitro* invasion. Cancer Res 56:5369–5374.

IV

Estrogen, Progestins, and Prolactin in Breast Cancer Biology: *Targets for Treatment*

16 Aromatase Inhibitors in Breast Carcinoma

Harold A. Harvey, MD

INTRODUCTION

At different times during a woman's life such as puberty, menstruation, pregnancy, and menopause, the breast epithelium undergoes dramatic changes. These changes in epithelial cell function, growth, and differentiation are orchestrated by the interaction of different peptide hormones such as insulin, IgF-1, prolactin, growth hormone and steroid hormones including estrogens and progestins. However, in the case of breast malignancy, estrogens appear to be the major hormones that initiate malignant transformation of the duct epithelial cells and regulate their further growth. The pioneering work of George Beatson eventually established the concept of estrogen dependency of some human breast cancers *(1)*. Hormone-dependent breast cancers are characterized by the presence of an intact and functional estrogen receptor. Hormonal manipulations employed in the treatment of breast cancer are intended to either block the estrogen receptor or else reduce the synthesis of estrogens. Antiestrogens, such as tamoxifen or toremifene, are the mainstay of palliative endocrine therapy in women with metastatic hormone-dependent breast cancer. Patients who respond but later progress on this form of therapy will frequently respond to second-line endocrine treatment. It is therefore important to develop effective second-line therapies that interfere with hormonal action through mechanisms other than blockade of the estrogen receptor. The aromatase inhibitors are a newer class of compounds, which provide just such an approach to the endocrine treatment of breast cancer. Increasing use of these agents has essentially eliminated the need for major endocrine ablative procedures such as adrenalectomy or hypophysectomy as palliative therapy for metastatic breast cancer.

SIGNIFICANCE OF AROMATASE

A major mechanism of estrogen biosynthesis depends on the function of the aromatase enzyme system. This enzyme catalyzes tine conversion of androgens into estrogens. The major substrates for this enzymatic conversion are androstenedione and testosterone both

From: *Contemporary Endocrinology: Endocrinology of Breast Cancer*
Edited by: A. Manni © Humana Press Inc., Totowa, NJ

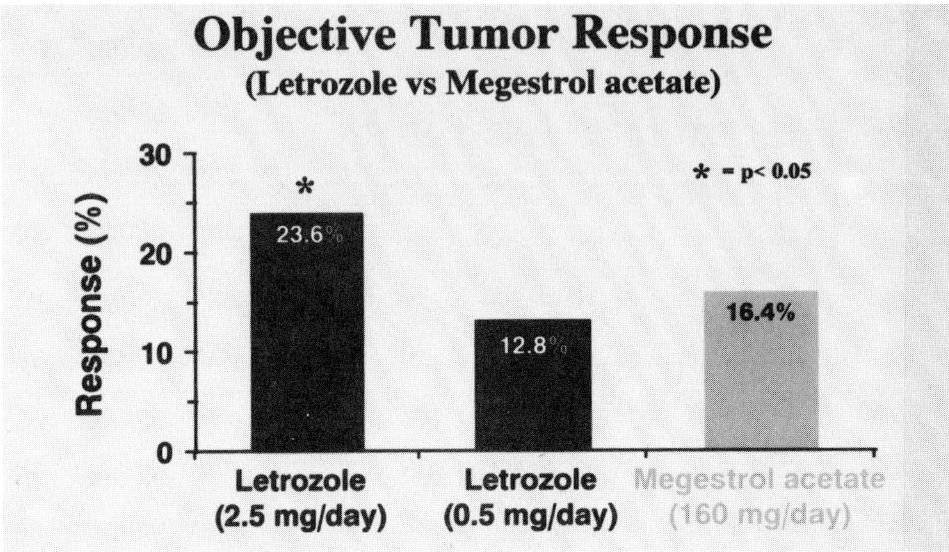

Fig. 1. Objective tumor response (Letrozole vs Megestrol acetate). Reprinted from ref. *25*.

of which are produced in the adrenal glands, and to a lesser extent, in the ovaries *(2,3)*. In the postmenopausal state, the ovarian contribution is negligible and the adrenal gland is the major source of androgens. The aromatase enzyme acts to convert androstenedione to estrone at peripheral sites such as fat, liver and muscle (Fig. 1). In addition, some breast carcinomas contain high levels of aromatase activity and appear to be capable of synthesizing *in situ* estrogen sufficient to sustain their own growth *(4)*.

Aromatase consists of a complex containing a cytochrome P-450nm protein as well as the flavoprotein nicotinamide adenine dinucleotide phosphate (NADPH) cytochrome P-450nm reductase *(5)*. The gene coding for the cytochrome P-450nm protein (P-450nm AROM) exceeds 70 kilobases and is the largest of the cytochrome P-450nm family *(6)*. The cDNA of the aromatase gene contains 3.4 Kb and encodes a polypeptide of 503 amino acids with a molecular weight of 55. Approximately 30% homology exists with other cytochrome P-450nm proteins. Because its overall homology to other members of the P-450nm super family is low, aromatase belongs to a separate genc-family designated CYP19. Aromatase expression occurs in many organs, including ovary, placenta, hypothalamus, liver, muscle, adipose/issue, and breast cancer tissue itself.

Aromatase catalyzes three separate steroid hydroxylations involved in the conversion of androstenedione to estrone. The first two give rise to 19-hydroxy and 19-aldehyde structures and the third, although still controversial, probably also involves the C-19 methyl group with the release of formic acid *(7)*. This enzyme action results in the saturation of the A-ring of the steroid molecule to produce an aromatic structure, hence the term aromatization.

A preponderance of evidence now suggests that some breast cancers have the capacity to synthesize intratumoral estrogen via aromatase activity *(8)*. The expression of aromatase is highest in the stromal compartment of these tumors *(9)*. In the breast itself, it is the peritumoral adipose tissue that contains the highest amount of aromatase activity that can be detected by biochemical assay or immunohistochemical staining *(10)*. In any event, the clinical significance of these observations is that some breast cancer tissues contain biologically relevant amounts of aromatase activity and thus may be an important target for action by aromatase inhibitors used to treat the disease. Newly available potent aromatase inhibitors are capable of further decreasing the already low levels of circulating estrogens in postmenopausal women with hormone-dependent breast cancer. Some of these agents may, as well, reduce levels of intratumoral aromatase activity. Thus, they provide a clinically important alternative therapeutic option after failure of antiestrogens.

CLINICAL EVOLUTION OF AROMATASE INHIBITORS

A convenient classification divides inhibitors into the mechanism based or "suicide inhibitors" (Type 1) and the competitive inhibitors (Type 11). Suicide inhibitors initially compete with the natural substrate (i.e., androstenedione and testosterone) for binding to the active site of the enzyme. The enzyme, then, specifically acts upon the inhibitor to yield reactive alkylating species which form covalent bonds at or near the active site of the enzyme. Through this mechanism, the enzyme is irreversibly inactivated. Competitive inhibitors, on the other hand, bind reversibly to the active site of the enzyme and prevent product formation only as long as the inhibitor occupies the catalytic site. Whereas mechanism-based inhibitors are exclusively steroidal in type, competitive inhibitors consist both of steroidal and nonsteroidal compounds *(11)*.

The first aromatase inhibitor to be widely used in the treatment of metastatic breast cancer in postmenopausal women was the drug aminoglutethimide. When combined with a corticosteroid such as hydrocortisone, the regimen produced durable clinical responses in 30–50% of patients *(l2)*. This approach, however, had several important drawbacks. First, aminoglutethimide was associated with a number of troublesome side effects including drowsiness, skin rash, and ataxia. Second, it soon became apparent that in the standard doses of 1000 mg daily, aminoglutethimide could also inhibit other cytochrome-P-450 mediated steroid hydroxylations, particularly those involving the cholesterol side-chain cleavage enzymes *(13)*. This nonselectivity for aromatase could lead to some inhibition of the biosynthesis of other steroid hormones such as cortisol, aldosterone and also thyroid hormone. Third, it was possible to develop newer drugs which were 10- to 1000-fold more potent inhibitors of aromatase in vitro than was aminoglutethimide.

Nevertheless, the successful clinical use of aminoglutethimide provided an impetus to investigate further the concept of inhibiting estrogen biosynthesis as a means of treating breast cancer. The problem of the multiple actions of aminoglutethimide, its associated side effects, and the need for exogenous glucocorticoid spurred interest in the development of second- and third-generation aromatase inhibitors *(14–18)*.

Thus, the clinical evolution of therapeutically useful aromatase inhibitors has been characterized by progressive improvements in their toxicity profile, specificity, and potency when compared to aminoglutethimide. Several new agents in this class are now clinically available. Most are orally administered nonsteroidal competitive (Type II) inhibitors of aromatase and include the agents anastrazole and letrozole (Table 1).

Clinical efficacy of these new compounds has now been demonstrated in large, randomized prospective trials, the more important of which are discussed below.

CLINICAL TRIALS

Anastrozole

Anastrozole (Arimidex®) (ICI-D 1033; 2, 2'-[5-(1 H- 1 ,2,4-triazol- 1-ylmethyl)1,3-phenylene]bis(2-methyl-propiononitrile) is a potent and selective benzyltriazole deriva-

Table 1
Currently Available Aromatase Inhibitors

Drug/Type	*Potency*	*Selectivity*	*Toxicity*	*Dose*	*Approval Status*
Nonsteroidal					
Aminogiutethimide	–+	+	+++	250 po bid	Non-USA
Fadrozole	+++	++	+	2 mg po bid	Japan
Letrozole	++++	+++	+	2.5 mg po qd	USA
Anastrozole	+++	+++	+	1 mg po qd	USA
Steroidal					
Formestane (4-OHA)	+	+++	++	500 mg im q2w	Europe
Exemestane	++	++	++	Investigational	

tive. At a concentration of 15 nmoL/L, this compound will inhibit aromatase enzyme activity by 50%. Maximal hormonal suppression was achieved with an oral dose of 0.1 mg/kg. In rats, this activity was assayed as inhibition of ovulation and androstenedione-induced uterine hypertrophy, and in monkeys, as suppression of plasma estradiol. The estimated elimination half-life is 32.2 h.

Anastrozole was the first aromatase inhibitor to be approved in the United States for the management of advanced breast carcinoma in postmenopausal women. This approval was based on results of two pivotal trials that, together, accrued a total of 764 patients randomized to receive either anastrozole 1 mg po qd or anastrozole 10 mg qd or megestrol acetate 40 mg qid. These patients had metastatic disease that was progressing following therapy with tamoxifen given either in the adjuvant setting or as first-line endocrine therapy for metastatic disease. Patients in the three arms of the trial had similar prognostic characteristics such as age, estrogen receptor status, disease-free interval, and sites of metastases. Results from this important trial showed similar overall response rates of about 25% (objective response rate 12.5%). However, anastrozole was better tolerated and it was associated with less undesirable weight gain, dyspnea, and fewer thromboembolic events when compared to megestrol acetate *(19)*. As there was no differences between the two doses of anastrozole, the drug was approved at a dose of 1 mg daily. Further analysis of this trial revealed that anastrozole 1 mg conferred a survival advantage compared to the progestin (median of 26.7 vs 22.5 mo). The 2-yr survival was 56.1% for the group of patients receiving anastrozole 1 mg compared to 46.3% for patient treated with megestrol acetate *(20)*.

LETROZOLE

The second aromatase inhibitor to gain approval in the United States with the indication for management of postmenopausal women with metastatic breast cancer was letrozole (Femara®). Letrozole ([4,4'-(lH-1,2,4-tiiazol-1-yl-methylene) -bis-benzonitrile]) is also a potent nonsteroidal competitive aromatase inhibitor. This agent possesses considerable selectivity for aromatase. In preclinical studies, for example, letrozole caused inhibition of aldosterone production in vitro only at concentrations 10,000 times higher than those required for inhibition of estrogen production. Letrozole is a remarkably potent and selective aromatase inhibitor. When administered orally to adult female rats at a dose of 1 mg/kg/day for 14 days, letrozole decreases uterine weight to that observed after a surgical ovariectomy. At doses greater than 1000 times higher than the concentration required to cause a 50% inhibition of the aromatase enzyme, letrozole does not significantly suppress either aldosterone or corticosterone in rats. Letrozole also causes significant regression of dimethylbenzanthracene (DMBA)-induced rat mammary tumors *(21)*.

Clinical studies in normal healthy volunteers as well as dose-seeking Phase I trials in postmenopausal women with advanced breast cancer showed that letrozole in a dose as little as 0.25 mg po daily caused maximal suppression of plasma and urinary estrogens. These studies also established the fact that letrozole in women was quite selective for the inhibition of aromatase because, over a wide dose range, there were no significant changes in the levels of gonadotropins, adenocorticotropic hormone (ACTH), cortisol, aldosterone, or thyroid-stimulating hormone (TSH) *(22,23)*. Phase 11 trials of letrozole in heavily pretreated postmenopausal women with metastatic breast cancer demonstrated both clinical efficacy and lack of significant toxicity *(24)*.

Approval of this agent was based on the results of two large, multicenter, randomized trials similar in design to the studies involving anastrozole. In a pivotal trial, 555 postmenopausal women with metastatic breast carcinoma progressing after treatment with tamoxifen were randomized to receive either letrozole 0.5 mg daily, letrozole 2.5 mg daily, or standard doses of megestrol acetate. The women in the three treatment groups were comparable in all respects. The two doses of letrozoole caused similar prompt and profound suppression of plasma and urinary estrogens. This suppression of estrogens was significantly greater than was seen with megestrol acetate. Letrozole 2.5 mg yielded an overall response rate of 33% compared to 25% for letrozole 0.5 mg and 32% for megestrol acetate. However, the median duration of response for letrozole 2.5 mg was 33 months compared to 18 months for both megestrol acetate and the lower dose of letrozole. Similarly, there is a trend in time to tumor progression and survival that favors the letrozole 2.5-mg dose. As with anastrozole, this trial also demonstrated that the aromatase inhibitor was better tolerated. Side effects reported on letrozole were low grade and infrequent and included mild headache, nausea, diarrhea, and hot flashes. Significantly, letrozole was associated with less weight gain, dyspnea, thromboembolic events, and vaginal bleeding when compared to megestrol acetate *(25)*. Letrozole is prescribed at a dose of 2.5 mg daily. It is somewhat unclear as to why the higher dose is the more effective dose clinically, despite similar degrees in estrogen suppression. A possible explanation for this apparent dose response is that letrozole 2.5 mg may inhibit intratumoral aromatase as well as being a potent inhibitor of peripheral enzyme action (Figs. 1 and 2).

In a second study involving 555 postmenopausal patients with advanced breast cancer progressing after tamoxifen therapy, letrozole was compared to aminoglutethimide 250 mg bid and cortisone. Letrozole 2.5 mg daily produced an objective response rate of 18% vs 12% for aminoglutethimide. The median response duration was 23 months for letrozole compared to 15 mo for aminoglutethimide and there was a statistically significant improvement in survival for the patients receiving letrozole. Moreover, letrozole produced less somnolence and skin rash *(26)*. The results of these large, well-conducted, randomized trials suggest that the side-effect profile and the dosing schedules of both anastrozole and letrozole are superior to megestrol acetate and aminoglutethimide. Both of these aromatase inhibitors are highly specific and potent. It is probable that in clinical practice, either of these agents will now replace megestrol acetate or other progestins as second-line therapy in postmenopausal women with metastatic breast carcinoma who are no longer responding to treatment with antiestrogens but yet remain candidates for further hormonal therapy.

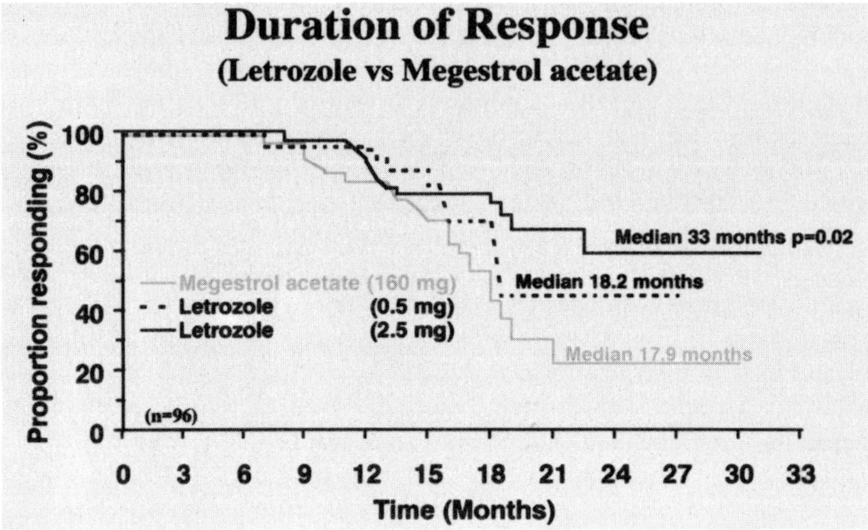

Fig. 2. Duration of response (Letrozole vs Megestrol acetate). Reprinted from ref. *25.*

Fadrozole

Fadrozole (CGS 16949A; 4-(5,6,7,8-tetrahydroimidazol[1,Sa]-pyridin-Syl) benzonitrile monohydrochloride) is a fairly potent inhibitor of aromatase with a K_i of 0.19 n*M* (vs 600 n*M* for aminoglutethimide) *(27,28)*. Cholesterol side-chain cleavage activity is minimal, but C-11 hydroxylase inhibitory effects are observed in vitro at high drug concentrations.

Initial dose-seeking studies conducted in patients demonstrated effective aromatase inhibition at doses of 1.8–4.0 mg daily *(27)*. A Phase II study then compared doses of 0.6 mg three times daily, 1 mg twice daily, and 2 mg twice daily. Maximal suppression of plasma and urinary estrogens occurred at a dose of 1.0 mg twice daily and minimal effects on cortisol secretion were observed. Basal cortisol and ACTH levels were unaffected and cortisol levels increased appropriately after exogenous synthetic ACTH (Cortrosyn) administration in all patients. Basal levels of aldosterone also remained stable following administration of all three drug doses. There were no changes in urinary or plasma sodium or potassium nor in standing blood pressure to suggest a clinical state of aldosterone deficiency. However, Cortrosyn-stimulated aldosterone levels were significantly blunted at all three doses *(29)*. Based on several Phase 11 trials, toxicity attributed to this agent was mild and consists mainly of nausea, anorexia, fatigue, and hot flashes. The potency of the compound, its relatively specific effects on aromatase, and its lack of toxicity suggested that it might provide a major improvement over aminoglutethimide for treatment of patients with breast cancer.

Two large multicenter Phase III trials in the United States comparing fadrozole hydrochloride to megesterol acetate in patients who had received only tarnoxifen as prior hormonal therapy have now been completed. These two studies accrued a total of 682 patients. Final clinical results show that there were no significant differences between the two treatment arms of the trials with respect to time to progression, objective response rates (12–14%), response duration or survival. Fadrozole was generally well tolerated in a dose of 2 mg. po bid *(30)*. Fadrozole has been approved for the treatment of advanced breast cancer in postmenopausal women in Japan. This agent is not likely to be further developed in the United States, as both anstrozole and letrozole appear to be more potent and selective aromatase inhibitors.

4-OH Androstenedione

Formestane (Lentaron®, 4-OHA; 4-hydroxyandrost-4-ene-3,1 7-dione) is a structural analog of androstenedione and is thus a highly specific aromatase inhibitor. It was the first steroidal suicide-type (Type 1) aromatase inhibitor to enter clinical trials and is now commercially available in Europe.

Using the in vitro placental aromatase assay system, 4-OHA was shown to be 60-fold more potent than aminoglutethimide ($K_i = 4.1 \times 10^{-3}$). Extensive studies revealed no estrogenic, antiestrogenic, or antiandrogenic properties *(31)*. However, transformation to 4-hydroxytestosterone occurs and androgenic effects can be demonstrated under certain circumstances *(32)*.

4-Hydroxyandrostenedione (Lentaron) has been studied extensively in Europe in postmenopausal women with breast cancer. Data from four Phase II clinical trials of 4-OHA demonstrated a 33% objective regression rate of breast cancer in postmenopausal patients previously treated with multiple endocrine therapies. Toxicity included six patients with sterile abscesses due to intramuscular injections, two of sufficient severity to warrant discontinuation of therapy. No androgenic effects were observed *(33)*.

Hoffken and colleagues conducted a large trial of 4-OHA in postmenopausal women *(34)*. Patients initially received 500 mg intramuscularly every 2 weeks for 6 weeks and then 250 mg every 2 weeks thereafter. Plasma estradiol levels fell from baseline values of 10–11 pa/mL to levels of approximately 4 pa/mL for up to 7 months of therapy. The drug appeared specific, as no reduction of cortisol or symptoms of cortisol deficiency were observed. Of 86 evaluable patients, there were 2 complete and 19 partial remissions (24%) and 26 with disease stabilization (30%). Side effects included minor systemic symptoms in 11% (hot flashes, constipation, alopecia, and pruritus) and local symptoms in 8% (pruritus, local pain, and erythema). These side effects resulted in discontinuation of therapy in only 2% of patients. Phase III trials are now ongoing to compare this inhibitor with standard endocrine therapies. In general, 4-OHA is better tolerated than aminoglutethimide. This agent is not available in the United States.

EXEMESTANE

Another aromatase under active investigation is exemestane. Exemestane (6-methyleneandrosta-1,4-diene-3, 1 7-dione) is an irreversible (Type I or mechanism based) aromatase inhibitor. Single-dose administration reveals a major reduction of plasma estrogens with this compound *(35)*. Phase III trials are underway but results have not yet been reported.

SELECTION OF PATIENTS FOR AROMATASE INHIBITION THERAPY

Endocrine therapy is usually offered to patients with metastatic disease who have receptor positive (ER+ or PR+) or receptor-unknown disease. In addition to the level of receptors, clinical features that might suggest a favorable response include a long disease-free interval after initial surgery or the presence of nodal, soft tissue, bone, pleural or nodular lung metastases. Patients with central nervous system (CNS) involvement, extensive liver disease, Iymphangitic spread of tumor in the lungs or rapidly progressing and life threatening disease are not ordinarily considered candidates for hormonal

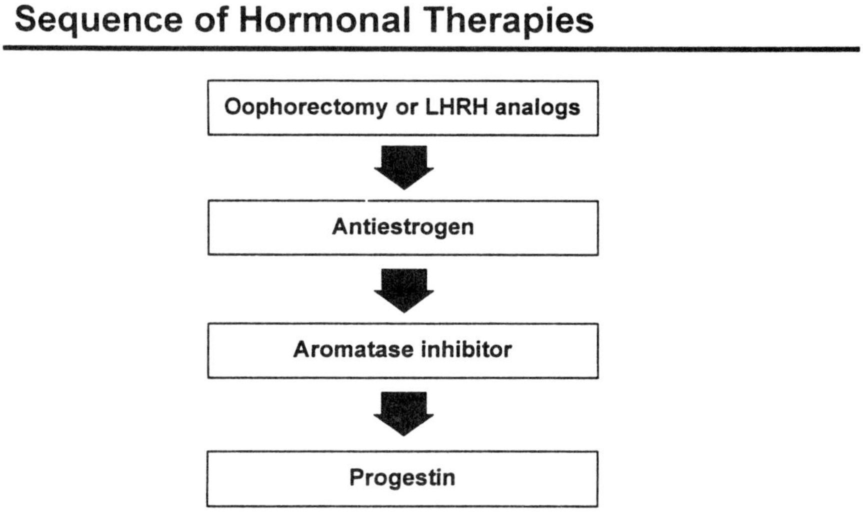

Fig. 3. Sequence of hormonal therapies.

therapy. Considerable clinical experience and data from the literature suggest that most endocrine therapies with the possible exceptions of androgens and glucocorticoids, are equally effective. The decision to choose one endocrine therapy over another depends on the menopausal status of the patient, considerations of efficacy, ease of administration, cost, and side effects. Historically, of all the endocrine therapies, tamoxifen was associated with the fewest side effects. This aspect still favors tarnoxifen as the endocrine therapy of first choice. Aromatase inhibitors are then considered either as second- or third-line endocrine approaches. More recently, however, the widespread use of tamoxifen as adjuvant therapy, frequently administered for long periods of time, presents the clinician with a new therapeutic dilemma. A practical approach is to rely on tamoxifen as first-line therapy for patients with metastatic disease who have not received this agent in the adjuvant setting or have discontinued tarnoxifen for a period of greater than 1 year. For other patients who are still candidates for hormone therapy, the major choices at present are between progestins such as megestrol acetate or medroxyprogesterone acetate and aromatase inhibitors. Given their equal or greater efficacy and better tolerability, aromatase inhibitors should now replace progestins as second-line hormonal therapy for metastatic breast cancer (Fig. 3).

It has been speculated that the determination of aromatase content of a particular tumor by either biochemical measurement or immunohistochemistry might aid in selecting patients who are likely to respond to therapy with aromatse inhibitors *(36,37)*. Preliminary evidence also suggests that breast cancers that overexpress the Her-2/neu protein may be relatively resistant to hormonal therapies including tamoxifen and aromatase inhibitors *(38,39)*. If confirmed, this information together with other considerations might well assist the clinician in selecting patients better for these forms of therapy.

PREMENOPAUSAL PATIENTS

Considerations of efficacy, cost, toxicity and ease of administration also dictate the choice of endocrine therapy in premenopausal patients. Based on these considerations, first-line therapy would include either tamoxifen or oophorectomy. Effective castration can be accomplished either by surgery, pelvic irradiation, or the use of LH–RH analogs. In humans, the premenopausal ovary has generally been considered to be resistant to the blockade of estrogen production by aromatase inhibitors because any lowering of plasma estrogens would lead to reflex increases in both follicle-stimulating hormone (FSH) and LH. These increased gonadotropin levels would then respectively induce increased ovarian production of estradiol and of androstenedione, the major substrate for aromatase action. On the other hand, the activity of the very potent third-generation inhibitors makes it possible that these compounds might also inhibit ovarian steroidogenesis and therefore may be of value in the treatment of breast cancer in premenopausal women. However, there are no supporting clinical studies and the use of aromatase inhibitors should be restricted to the treatment of breast cancer in postmenopausal patients.

FUTURE PERSPECTIVES

As discussed earlier, several new potent and highly specific aromatase inhibitors are now available for the treatment of breast cancer. They offer several distinct advantages over some older forms of endocrine therapy, including a well-understood mechanism of action, good toxicity profile, convenient dosing schedules, and the absence of estrogen effects on the endometrium. On the other hand, their long-term effects on bone mineral density and serum lipids are unknown *(18)*.

New clinical trials with these promising agents are either underway or are planned in order to address several questions, including their role in the treatment of premenopausal women as discussed above. Although presently approved only as second-line therapies after tamoxifen failure, aromatase inhibitors are now being tested as first-line endocrine treatment for metasatic breast cancer in direct comparison to antiestrogens. Moreover, nonsteroidal aromatase inhibitors would not be expected to induce endometrial carcinoma in women and so could be investigated both as adjuvant hormonal therapy as well as in the chemoprevention of human breast cancer. If either anastrozole or letrozole agents should prove to be effective as first-line endocrine therapy, then it would, indeed, be prudent to examine their role in the adjuvant setting, especially in older patients with breast cancer. Recent reports suggest that antiestrogens (tamoxifen, raloxifene) might be effective chemoprevention of breast cancer in healthy women considered to be at an increased risk for developing this disease. A possible role for aromatase inhibitors in the chemoprevention of breast cancer has also been proposed considering the potential for aromatase to mediate strogen production in the breast *(40)*. Coombes et al. have reported that 4-OHA prevents NMU-induced rat mammary carcinoma *(41)*. Similar observations with other aromatase inhibitors and animal models, suggest that inhibitors of estrogen biosynthesis can prevent breast cancer.

A few clinical studies have attempted to combine different classes of endocrine agents but there are few clinical data to support this approach as being superior to using these agents in sequence to treat metastatic breast cancer (e.g., tamoxifen followed by an aromatase inhibitor, followed by a progestin). In clinical practice, the sequential use of hormonal agents can produce long-term palliation of hormone-dependent breast cancer. Eventually, however, the problem of hormone resistance is encountered The mechanism by which tumors become resistant to hormones in general are only partially understood. Refractoriness to therapy with aromatase inhibitors is related not to the failure of these agents to suppress estradiol levels as might be seen if there were upregulation of aromatase, but rather is likely due to some other mechanism of hormone resistance.

The paracrine production of aromatase, specific growth factors, and cytokines within the microenvironment of a breast tumor require further study. A greater understanding of the biologic interaction of these factors could lead, for example, to the development of new therapeutic strategies. In summary, recently reported clinical studies of highly potent aromatase inhibitors have shown that it is possible to develop specific, nontoxic compounds which reduce serum estradiol concentrations to undetectable levels in postmenopausal patients with advanced breast cancer. Some of these compounds may also in fact, effectively target intratumoral synthesis of estrogen by aromatase. These compounds are emerging as a valuable approach to the treatment of hormone-dependent breast cancer.

REFERENCES

1. Beatson GT. On the treatment of inoperable cases of carcinoma of the mamma. Suggestions for a new method of treatment, with illustrative cases. Lancet 1896;Il:104–107.
2. Grodin JM, Sitteri PK, MacDonald PC. Sources of estrogen production in postmenopausal women. J Clin Endocrinol Metab 1973;36:207–214.
3. Hemsell Dl, Grodin G, Breuner PF et al. Plasma precursors of estrogen II. Correlation of the extent of conversion of plasma androstenedione to estrone with age. J Clin Endocrinol Metab 1974;38:476–479.
4. Reed MH. The role of aromatase in breast tumors. Breast Cancer Res Treat 1994;30:7–17.
5. Simpson ER, Merrill JC. Hollub AJ et al. Regulation of estrogen biosynthesis by human adipose cells. Endocr Rev 1989;10:136–148.
6. Simpson ER, Mahendroo MS, Means GD et al. Tissue specific promoters regulate aromatase cytochrome P450 expression. Clin Chem 1993;39:317–324.
7. Fishman J, Hahn EF. The nature of the final oxidative step in the aromatization sequence. Steroids 1987;50:339–345.
8. Abul-Hajj, Iverson R, Kiang DT. Aromatization of androgens by human breast cancer. Steroids 1979;33:205–222.
9. Santen RJ, MartelJ, Hoagland M et al. Stromal spindle cells contain aromatase in human breast tumors. J Clin Endocrinol Metab 1994;79:627–632.
10. Miller WR, O'Neil JS. The importance of local synthesis of estrogen within the breast. Steroids 1998;50:537–548.
11. Brodie AM. Aromatase, its inhibitors and their use in breast cancer treatment. Pharmacol Ther 1993;60:501–515.
12. Santen RJ, Worgul TJ, Lipton A, Harvey HA et al. Aminoglutethimide as treatment of postmenopausal women with advanced breast carcinoma: Correlation of clinical and hormonal responses. Ann Intern Med 1982;96:94–101.
13. Cocconi G. First generation aromatase inhibitors-aminoglutethimide and testolatone Breast Cancer Res Treat.1994;30:57–80.
14. Harvey HA. Emerging role of aromatase inhibitors in the treatment of breast cancer. Oncology 998:12(3 suppl 5):32–35
15. Miller WR. Aromatase inhibitors and breast cancer. Cancer Treat Rev 1997:23(3):171–187.
16. Blamey RW. The role of selective non-steroidal aromatase inhibitors in future treatment strategies. Oncol 1997:54(Suppl 2):27–31.
17. Roseman BJ, Buzdar AU, Singletary SE. Use of aromatase inhibitors in postmenopausal women with advanced breast cancer. J Surg Oncol 1997;66(3):215–220.
18. Harvey HA. Aromatase inhibitors in clinical practice: current status and a look to the future. Semin Oncol 1996;23:33–38.
19. Buzdar AU, Jonat W, Howell A et al. Anastrozole, a potent and selective aromatase inhibitor, versus megestrol acetate in postmenopausal women with advanced breast cancer: Results of overview analysis of two phase III trials. J Clin Oncol 1996;19:2000–2011.
20. Buzdar AU. Anastrozole: a new addition to the armamentarium against advanced breast cancer. Am J Clin Oncol 1998 21(2):161–166.

21. Schiweck K, Bhatnagar AS, Batzl CH, Lang M. Anti-tumor and endocrine effects of non-steroidal aromatase inhibitors on estrogendependent rat mammary tumors. J Steroid Biochem Moi Biol 1993;44:633–636.
22. Demurs LM, Lipton A, Harvey HA et al. The efficacy of CGS 20267 in suppressing estrogen biosynthesis in patients with advanced stage breast cancer. J Steroid Biochem Molec Biol 1993;44:687–691.
23. Iveson TJ, Smith IE, Ahern J et al. Phase I study of the oral nonsteroidal aromatase inhibitor CGS 20267 in postmenopausal patients with advanced breast cancer. Cancer Res 1993;53:266–270.
24. Lipton A, Demers LM, Harvey HA et al. Letrozole (CGS 20267): Phase I study of a new potent oral aromatase inhibitor in breast cancer. Cancer 1995; 75:2132–2138.
25. Dombernowsky P, Smith I, Falkson G et al. Letrozole, a new oral aromatase inhibitor for advanced breast cancer: double blind randomized trial showing a dose effect and improved efficacy and tolerability compared with megestrol acetate. J Clin Oncol 998;16(2):453–461.
26. Marty M, Gershanovich M et al. Letrozole, a new potent, selective aromatase inhibitor superior to aminoglutethimide in postmenopausal women with advanced breast cancer previously treated with antiestrogrns. Proc Am Soc Clin Oncol 1997;16:544.
27. Santen RJ, Demers LM, Lynch J, Harvey HA et al. Specificity of low dose fadrozole hydrochloride (CGS 16949A) as an aromatase inhibitor. J Clin Endocrinol Metab 1991;73:99–106.
28. Steele RE, Mellor LB, Sawyer WK et al. In vitro and in vivo studies demonstrating potent and selective estrogen inhibition with the nonsteroidal aromatase inhibitor CGS 16949A. Steroids 1987;50:147–161.
29. Harvey HA, Lipton A, Santen RJ et al. Phase I and phase II clinical trials of fadrozole hydrochloride in postmenopausal women with metastatic breast cancer. Adv Clin Oncol 1994;2:155–158.
30. Buzdar AU, Smith R, Vogel C et al. Fadrozole HCL (CGS-16949A) versus megestrol acetate treatment of postmenopausal patients with metastatic breast carcinoma: results of two randomized double blind controlled multi-institutional trials. Cancer 1996;77(12):2503–2513.
31. Brodie AMH, Longcope C: Inhibition of peripheral aromatization by aromatase inhibitors 4-hydroxy and 4-acetoxy-androstene-3,17-dione.
32. Brodie AMH, Romanoff ID, Williams KIH: Metabolism of the aromatase inhibitor 4-hydroxy-4-androstenedione,3,17-dione by male rhesus monkeys. J Steroid Biochem 1981;14:693–696.
33. Goss PE, Powles TJ, Dowsett M et al. Treatment of advanced postmenopausal breast cancer with an aromatase inhibitor, 4-hydroxyandrostenedione: Phase II report. Cancer Res 1986;46:4823–4826.
34. Hoffken K, Jonat W, Possinger K et al. Aromatase inhibition with 4-hydroxyandrostenedione in the treatment of postmenopausal patients with advanced breast cancer. A phase 11 study. J Clin Oncol 1990;8:875–880.
35. Evans TRJ, diSalle E, Ornati G et al. Phase I and endocrine study of exemestane (FCE 24304), a new aromatase inhibitor, in postmenopausal women. Cancer Res 1992;52:5933–5939.
36. Bezwoda WR, Mansoor N, Dansey R. Correlation of breast tumor aromatase activity and response to aromatase inhibition with aminoglutethimide. Oncology 1987;44:345–349.
37. Miller WR, Hawkins RA, Miller P et al. Aromatase inhibition: determinants of response and resistance. Endocr Related Cancer 1995;2:73–85.
38. Yamauchi H, O'Neill A, Gelman R et al. Prediction of response to antiestrogen therapy in advanced breast cancer patients by pretreatment circulating levels of extracellular domain of the HER-2/c-neu protein. J Clin Oncol 1997;15(7):2518–2525
39. Leitzel K, Teramoto Y, Konrad K et al. Elevated serum c-erbB-2 antigen levels and decreased response to hormone therapy of breast cancer. J Clin Oncol 1995;13:1129–1135.
40. Kelloff GJ, Lubet RA, Lieberman R et al. Aromatase inhibitors as potential cancer chmemopreventives. Cancer Epidemiol Biomarkers Prevent 1998;7(1):65–78.
41. Coombes RC, Wilkinson JR, Bliss JM et al. 4-hydroxyandrostenedione in the prophylaxis of N-methyl-N-nitrosourea induced mammary tumourigenesis. Br J Cancer 1991;64:247–250.

17 Role of Progestins and Progesterone Receptors in Breast Cancer Biology

Anne Guiochon-Mantel, MD, PhD
and Edwin Milgrom, MD, PhD

INTRODUCTION

Progesterone is a major component in the regulation of normal female reproductive function. Its main physiologic role in the mammary gland is the lobular-alveolar development in preparation for milk secretion and suppression of milk protein synthesis prior to parturition *(1)*. Its role in the proliferation of the normal mammary gland and in the initiation of breast cancer is the subject of controversy (for review, see ref. *2*).

The mechanism of progesterone action in target tissues is complex, and a distinction has to be made between the direct targets of progesterone action and indirect consequences of progesterone regulation. For instance, as the effects of progesterone are mediated by its receptor and this receptor is induced by estradiol in most target tissues, the delineation of specific progesterone effects is not clear. The recent development of a mouse model carrying a null mutation of the progesterone receptor (PR) gene *(3,4)* has been used to answer many of the complex questions of progesterone action in vivo, particularly its action in mammary gland development. Moreover, it has confirmed the importance and diversity of roles of progesterone in normal female development and reproduction.

PROGESTINS AND MAMMARY CELL PROLIFERATION

The hormonal control of mammary gland development and function has been the subject of extensive investigations over several decades (for review, see refs. *2*, *5*, and *6*). Although mammary epithelial development involves complex interactions between a number of different hormones, the principal role of progesterone appears to be in promoting lobular-alveolar development in the adult gland *(1,3,4)*. The mechanism through which progesterone exerts its action in the normal breast is difficult to study because of the paucicity of models. Most of the data are derived from studies on breast cancer cells in culture. The validity of extending this information to the normal breast has yet to be fully tested. For instance, the effects of progesterone on the prolactin receptor are opposite in breast cancer cells and in normal mammary gland; in breast cancer cells, like T47D, progestins increase prolactin receptor levels *(7)*, whereas in the normal mammary gland progestins antagonize prolactin induction of prolactin receptors *(8)*. Moreover, a

From: *Contemporary Endocrinology: Endocrinology of Breast Cancer*
Edited by: A. Manni © Humana Press Inc., Totowa, NJ

decrease in PR levels is associated with exposure to progestins *(9,10)* in breast cancer cell lines, whereas in the normal breast during the luteal phase, there is a persistence of the PR level *(11,12)*.

Progesterone and Cell Proliferation in Normal Breast

Mammary glands in PR null mice develop ductal structures that are relatively similar to those described in wild-type mice. However, there is a failure to form interductal lobular-alveolar structures upon exposure to estradiol and progesterone *(3,4,13)*. The influence of progesterone is likely to be proliferative in this process, mediated by progesterone regulation of genes expressed during cell cycle progression *(14)*, growth factors *(14,15)*, and growth factor receptors *(16)*. Progesterone also exerts a differentiating effect on the breast through its role in preparing for lactation *(17)*. The role of progesterone in differentiation at other times has not been extensively explored.

The human breast is known to respond to the fluctuations in serum hormone levels during the menstrual cycle with cyclical changes in breast volume and cellular morphology. An increase in DNA synthesis in normal breast epithelium has been consistently observed during the late luteal phase *(18)*. The increase in DNA synthesis correlates with an increase in the number of epithelial mitoses and is followed by an increase in apoptotic activity *(19)*. These results support a role for progesterone in the induction of a cyclical proliferation of normal breast epithelium. They are in contradiction to pharmacologic studies of the proliferation of breast epithelium in patients who had received estradiol and progesterone prior to surgery. In this situation, epithelial mitoses and expression of proliferative cell nuclear antigen were lowest in progesterone-treated patients *(20)*. In vitro data obtained with cultures of normal breast epithelial cells have produced inconsistent results *(2)*.

Progesterone and Human Mammary Carcinoma Proliferation

Synthetic progestins are effective agents in the treatment of metastatic breast cancer. Despite the widespread clinical use of progestins, and in contrast to their well-defined antiproliferative effects on normal and neoplastic endometrium, relatively little is known concerning the molecular mechanisms of action of progestins as antitumor agents in breast cancer. This is because only a few studies have addressed the effects of progestins on cell proliferation in human breast tumors *(21,22)*. Most of the data has been obtained from studies with human mammary carcinoma cell lines. In these cells, the growth-inhibitory effect of progestins was observed only when growth was stimulated by estradiol *(23)*. The question of whether or not progestins can only inhibit estradiol-induced cell proliferation remains controversial. However, several lines of evidence show that as long as PR is present, progestins inhibit cell proliferation, even in the absence of estradiol *(24,25)*. Conversely, there are several reports showing a proliferative effect of progestins on breast carcinoma cell lines. However, this proliferative effect of progestin is always markedly less than the proliferative effect of estradiol *(26)* and may be explained by a biphasic effect of progestins on the progression of the cell cycle in T47D cells. There is an initial stimulatory effect with a transient shortening of the G_1 phase, and a later inhibitory effect resulting from a delayed progression through the G_1 phase *(14,27)*.

Markers of Progestins Action in Breast

Genes independently regulated by progestins in the mammary gland have been sought for their potential therapeutic or prognostic value in breast cancer. A non-tissue-specific alkaline phosphatase activity is induced by progestins in T47D cells *(28)*. This induction correlates with the acquisition of a differentiated secretory phenotype in T47D *(29)*. However, the induction of this activity by progestins has not been characterized in vivo. Its clinical significance in breast cancer remains to be determined.

Progestins rapidly induce fatty acid synthase transcriptionally and posttranscriptionally *(30)*. This enzyme is postulated to be a marker of differentiation and progestin responsiveness in breast cancer *(31)*. However, its level in breast cancer tissues is not correlated with estradiol receptor (ER) or PR level *(31)*.

Progestin Therapy and Breast Cancer Risk

The use of exogenous hormone clearly has an impact on the risk of certain cancers, and in some cases hormonal "chemoprevention" is already occurring as a result of such use. We will discuss the impact on cancer incidence of the two forms of exogenous hormones widely used today: oral contraceptives and hormone replacement therapy of menopause (for review, see ref. *32*).

Oral Contraceptives

The use of combination oral contraceptives during the past 30 years has led to a dramatic decline in the incidence of cancer of the ovary and of the endometrium *(33,34)*. Conversely, the incidence of breast cancer has not been substantially affected. Epidemiologic studies of combination oral contraceptive and breast cancer have produced mixed results. There is evidence of a modest increase in breast cancer risk in women diagnosed under age 45. The few studies in women diagnosed over age 45 find no change in risk with the previous use of oral contraceptives *(35)*. The basis of this discrepancy by age of diagnosis is not understood. Oral contraceptives inhibit gonadotropin secretion and thus reduce ovarian steroidogenesis to low levels. This ovarian steroid loss is compensated for by the synthetic estrogen and progestin. As a result, the simultaneous presence of estrogen and progestins in oral contraceptives does not appear to modify the relative risk of breast cancer significantly.

Hormone Replacement Therapy of Menopause

There is a strong correlation between estradiol replacement therapy and endometrial cancer risk. The benefit of adding a progestin to estradiol replacement therapy in reducing endometrial mitotic activity has been clearly established *(36,37)*. However, there is an ongoing controversy about the effect of progestin on breast cancer risk *(38–40)*. It has now been established by several meta-analyses that the addition of progestin does not modify the risk of breast cancer induced by the estrogen replacement therapy *(41–44)*. Moreover, this risk is not changed in the case of existence of familial antecedents of breast cancer. Hormonal replacement therapy of menopause can be prescribed for at least 10 years, without significantly increasing the risk of breast cancer *(42)*.

MOLECULAR MECHANISMS OF PROGESTERONE ACTION

Progesterone effects are mediated by its nuclear receptor. In the absence of ligand, the receptor is "inactive" and complexed to a series of proteins of the heat-shock and immunophilin families *(43)*. The interaction with the ligand elicits a series of events: the dissociation from the heat-shock proteins, the "activation" of the receptor, and its high-affinity binding to specific DNA elements (hormone responsive elements [HRE]) located in the regulatory region of genes (for review, see ref. *46*). This specific interaction of "activated" receptor with the DNA allows its interaction with the transcription machinery complex, inducing the modulation of transcription of the gene located in the region and thus the modulation of the synthesis of the corresponding protein. The progress in the knowledge of transcriptional control in animal cells during the last 5 years has established a solid foundation for the reformulation of the mechanisms of transcriptional control by steroid hormone receptors (for review, see refs. *47* and *48*). Transcription requires two classes of transcription factors. One class comprises general factors (TFIIA, -B, -D, -E, -F and -H) and is responsible for basal promoter activity. The other class comprises modulators that either activate (coactivators, for instance SRC-1) or repress (corepressors, for instance SMRT, N-CoR) transcription. Cointegrators, like CBP/p300, have also recently been identified *(49)*. They coordinate the transcriptional effects of simultaneous signals emanating from cell surface receptors and from nuclear receptors. Thus they act as cointegrators of multiple competing, and perhaps conflicting, signals that can impact one promoter. The basal level of transcription of most genes appears to be maintained by histone deacetylation. Acetylation of chromatin in vivo is coupled to transcription, and specific histone acetyltransferases target histones bound to DNA and overcome the inhibitory effect of chromatin on gene expression. There is an equilibrium between histone acetylation and histone deacetylation toward the progressive accumulation of nucleosomes containing acetylated histones. The cointegrator CBP/p300 and the coactivator SRC-1 possess intrinsic histone transferase activity *(50,51)*. Furthermore, CBP/p300 recruits to promoters histone acetylases, for instance P/CAF *(52)*. N-CoR and SMRT recruit histone deacetylases *(53)*. Besides these transcription factors, proteins modifying the structural organization of the chromatin (for instance, proteins of the SWI/SNF family) have been shown to regulate transcription.

Steroid hormone receptors act at all these levels. A direct interaction has been demonstrated in vitro between steroid hormone receptors and general transcription factors like TFIIB or TFIID *(47)*. Steroid hormone receptors recruit some coactivators in the presence of ligand *(54–57)*. Moreover a cooperation between certain steroid hormone receptors and proteins of the SWI/SNF family has been identified *(58)*.

Structure of the Progesterone Receptor

PR is a member of a superfamily of transcription factors including receptors for steroid hormones, thyroid hormones, retinoic acid, products of the intermediary metabolism as well as other known transcription factors, and proteins of unknown function (orphan receptors). These proteins are characterized by an organization into specific functional domains that are conserved between species and family members (for review, see refs. *59* and *60*). The most highly conserved region is in the center of the protein and corresponds to a two zinc fingers DNA binding motif. The carboxy-terminal domain is less conserved and is the ligand binding domain. This domain behaves like a molecular switch *(61)*. It contains the activation function 2 (AF-2). In the absence of ligand, it binds the 90-kDa heat-shock protein. After binding the ligand, it mediates the dimerization and the interaction with coactivators, allowing the modulation of transcription.

The amino-terminal domain of PR contains a ligand-independent activation function (AF-1). Both AF-1 and AF-2 activate transcription in a different promoter- and cell-specific fashion *(62)*. They work in a synergistic manner and are required for full receptor activity in most cellular contexts.

PR has been cloned in different species, including human, rabbit, and chick *(63–65)*. The chromosomal gene structure has been elucidated in the human and is a single copy of more than 90 kbp composed of 8 exons *(66)*. It has been mapped to chromosome 11q22-23 *(67)*. In the human, two PR proteins, PR-A (85 kDa) and PR-B (115 kDa), have been described *(68,69)*. PR-B differs from PR-A only in that it contains an additional amino-terminal fragment of 164 amino acids *(70)*. Recently, a third activation domain (AF-3), which appears to function only in a restricted cell and promoter context, has been found *(71)*. It is located within this PR-B-specific amino-terminal domain. PR-A and PR-B are encoded by a single gene, under the control of distinct promoters, each of which gives rise to a distinct subgroup of PR mRNA *(70)*. An equimolar expression of PR-A and PR-B is observed in human breast cancer cells in culture *(69)*. In human breast tumors the ratio of expression of PR-A and PR-B proteins differs markedly between patients *(72)*. The biologic importance of these different ratios of PR expression has not been extensively explored, and little is known of their relative modulation in vivo.

Regulation of Progesterone Receptor Expression

PR is under the dual control of estradiol and progesterone, which act sequentially to regulate the cellular concentration of PR and therefore the likely cellular responsiveness to progestins. Estradiol increases PR transcriptionally in most target tissues. Conversely, progesterone downregulates PR transcriptionally and posttranscriptionally. This downregulation of PR by progesterone is not observed in all cell types. In the uterus, it is observed only in epithelial cells and not in stromal and myometrial cells. Moreover, PR levels do not decrease in the normal breast between the follicular and luteal phases.

The main regulatory site in the rabbit PR gene is an intragenic estradiol-responsive element (ERE) overlapping the initiation of translation *(73)*. The same ERE confers progesterone downregulation. PR does not interact directly with this ERE, but through an interaction with ER *(73)*. In the case of the rat PR, four imperfect ERE have been identified by in vitro techniques *(74)*. One of these ERE appears to be biologically active *(75)*. In the case of human PR, the two PR isoforms are under the control of different promoters, both of which are estrogen inducible. No classical ERE was detected in the corresponding sequence *(70)*.

In addition to sex steroids, other regulators of PR gene expression have been described. Retinoic acid has been shown to decrease the transcription of the PR gene. Growth factors and phorbol esters have been reported to decrease or increase PR mRNA concentration in a cell-specific manner. In the rabbit PR, repression by retinoic acid and AP1 is mediated by the same ERE as repression by progesterone. It is achieved by protein-protein interaction and not by a direct contact with the ERE *(76)*. In the rat PR, induction by thyroid hormones is mediated by the same ERE as estradiol induction *(75)*.

Progestin regulation of PR level is likely to vary among cell types, between species, and more importantly in different physiologic situations in order to regulate cellular sensitivity to progestins.

Intracellular Traffic of Progesterone Receptor

Immunohistochemical Localization of Progesterone Receptor

Steroid hormone receptors are intracellular proteins that may be found in both the cytosolic and nuclear fractions of a tissue homogenate. Until 1984–1986, the classical model of action of steroid hormones proposed that a cytoplasmic receptor protein undergoes nuclear translocation after interaction with its ligand *(77,78)*. In 1984–1986, the development of monoclonal antibodies against steroid receptors *(79,80)* allowed immunocytochemical studies to be undertaken. This technology avoids the problem of the receptor redistribution during cell homogenization. Immunocytochemistry showed exclusive nuclear localization of the ER *(81)*, and of the PR *(82)*, even in the absence of endogenous hormone. The nuclear localization of PR and ER have been demonstrated in a wide number of target tissues and in different species.

Nuclear Localization Mechanism

The nuclear localization of large proteins like steroid hormone receptors is an active process: it is temperature dependent, requires adenosine triphosphate, and displays saturation kinetics. Active transport into the nucleus requires that proteins contain suitable nuclear localization signals (NLS) (for review, see ref. *83*). They are mostly short basic sequence motifs, rich in arginines and lysines. Active nuclear import of proteins takes place in at least two steps. The first step is the interaction between the protein and the nuclear pore complex through the NLS. The second step is the translocation to the nucleus. Only this second step is an active process. The development of in vitro transport assays has recently allowed characterization of the proteins involved in these different steps and the proposal of a model (for review, see ref. *84*). An NLS-containing protein binds in the cytosol to the NLS receptor with the aid of a 97-kDa protein. This NLS protein-NLS receptor-p97 complex next binds to the nuclear pore via nucleoporins. A complex composed of the small guanosine triphosphatase Ran/TC4 and of a B2-p10 dimer acts at a subsequent step to allow translocation through the pore. Cloning of the receptors and in vitro mutagenesis studies led to the description of karyophilic signals for steroid hormone receptors *(85–88)*.

The NLS of PR is a complex signal. It is formed of two subsignals, constitutive and hormone dependent. It encompasses the hinge region between the DNA and the ligand binding domains (containing the constitutive signal) and the second zinc finger of the DNA binding region (containing the hormone-dependent signal). It bears several stretches of basic amino acids. It is worth mentioning that all steroid hormone receptor NLSs are complex signals. If these receptors are aligned through their DNA binding regions, sequences homologous to the PR constitutive NLS are found. These sequences are always implicated in the nuclear localization of these receptors.

Nucleocytoplasmic Shuttling

There is indirect evidence that the nuclear localization of PR was the result of an equilibrium between the nucleus and the cytoplasm. The first indication was the observation of an in vivo interaction between receptor monomers during nuclear transport *(86)*. This hormone-induced oligomerization between a cytoplasmic and a nuclear monomer, in the absence of protein synthesis, implies that both monomers are not rigidly confined to their respective compartments, rather, a dynamic situation must exist in which they may contact each other. Further evidence is the result of energy depletion experiments. In these conditions, an efflux of the receptor from the nucleus was observed *(89)*. These experiments suggested that steroid hormone receptors, despite their size, exit continuously from the nucleus to the cytoplasm and are constantly and actively transported back into the nucleus.

The existence of a nucleocytoplasmic shuttling of the receptor was confirmed directly by the study of the migration of PR between nuclei in interspecies heterokaryons. A mouse L cell line permanently expressing PR was fused with human 293 cells devoid of receptor, in the presence of protein synthesis inhibitors. The presence of the receptor in human nuclei was observed 12 h after the fusion; the receptor had migrated from one nucleus to the other, indicating a shuttle through the cytoplasm *(89)*.

Thus the residency of the PR in the nucleus is a dynamic phenomenon resulting from the continuous active transport into the nucleus conterbalanced by diffusion into the cytoplasm. Similar experiments have been performed on ligand-bound-glucocorticoid receptors (GR) *(90)* and on ER *(91)*, showing the same results.

This mechanism of nuclear localization of the receptor explains some previous observations: ligand-free PR or ER, which reside in the nucleus, are found in the cytosol after homogenization even when nuclear structures have been preserved. In these conditions, active transport is blocked by dilution and low temperature. Under these conditions, the exit of receptors from the nucleus to the cytoplasm is not counterbalanced by active entry into the nucleus. Incidentally, association of receptors with nuclei after homogenization of cells at 25°C has been described *(92)*. Moreover, localization of ligand-free GR in cytoplasm or both cytoplasm and nuclei has been considered as completely different from that of ER or PR, which are located in the nucleus. However, if the receptor continually shuttles between nucleus and cytoplasm, the case of the GR may be only quantitatively and not qualitatively different from that of sex steroid receptors. A less effective or masked constitutive karyophilic signal would lead to an increased time of residency of the receptor in the cytoplasm and to an apparent distribution between cytoplasmic and nuclear compartments.

The understanding of receptor function may also be modified by the fact that receptors shuttle between the nucleus and cytoplasm. Receptors could thus interact with cytoplasmic components. Moreover, this mechanism is compatible with receptors exerting biologic activities in the cytoplasm.

The mechanism by which proteins enter the nucleus is well understood (see above), but the outward movement of nuclear proteins involved in the shuttling process is not. Using the same type of energy depletion and heterokaryons experiments, it has been shown that NLSs are also implicated in the outward movement of PR through the nuclear envelope *(93)*.

BREAST CANCER AND PROGESTERONE RECEPTOR

Determination of PR and ER in breast cancer have two interests: for prognosis and for the estimation of the effectiveness of hormonal therapy. ER is an indicator of the degree of tumoral differentiation. PR is an indicator of the functionality of ER, as its synthesis is induced by estradiol.

Receptor Determination: Biochemical and Immunohistochemical Methods

Steroid receptors are very sensitive to the action of endogenous proteases. Samples have thus to be quickly put in liquid nitrogen and transported to the laboratory. The standard assay is performed on the supernatant of the homogenate after ultracentrifigation (cytosol). In the case of premenopausal patient or the use of exogenous steroid, a whole cellular extract may be necessary to have access to the totality of the receptor sites. It is thus critical to know the hormonal status of the patient to interpret the result. Indeed, in the case of physiologic or pharmacologic levels of hormones, steroid receptors are strongly bound to the nucleus and their concentration in the cytosolic fraction does not reflect their total concentration in the cell. Initially, isotopic methods were used. The binding of a radioactive steroid with a high affinity for the receptor was studied. These techniques measure only functional receptors. The availability of monoclonal antibodies allowed the development of enzyme-linked immunosorbent assays *(94)*. These methods allow the detection of mutant receptors that do no longer bind the ligand. Moreover, they are not disturbed by the presence of endogenous ligand. They can also be used on a very small amount of tissue.

These antibodies can also detect the receptors on paraffin-embedded breast tumors or on fine-needle aspirates. Immunohistochemical techniques have several advantages, compared with biochemical detection: they are more rapid and need less equipment, they allow the detection of receptors in a very small amount of tissue, they can be used to evaluate tumoral heterogeneity, and other histologic parameters can be tested on the same section. However, they give mainly a qualitative result. Much effort has been expended during the past few years to produce quantitative results. The different steps have been standardized: fixation, antigen retrieval, antibody controls, analysis and interpretation of immunostaining, and report and quality assurance parameters. Based on correlations with biochemical studies, a threshold of 10% positive cells, whatever the intensity of the labeling, has been proposed for receptor positivity *(95,96)*. Immunohistochemical determinations now tend to replace biochemical techniques, but the problem of whether the biopsy is representative of the entire tumor remains.

Prognostic Value of Progesterone and Estradiol Receptors

Receptor determination in tumors has been performed for more than 15 years. Several prospective studies have been performed to evaluate the pronostic value of receptor measurement. Approximately 60–80% of the tumors contain ER. However, only 40–50% of the tumors contain PR. In the case of invasive adenocarcinomas, there is a strong correlation between the presence of steroid receptors and the degree of differentiation. Tumors containing ER have a better prognosis *(97)*. The presence of ER and PR improves this prognosis. The presence of PR in the tumor is an element of good prognosis, notably in the absence of node invasion *(98)*.

Hormone Dependence of Breast Cancer: Therapeutic Use of Steroid Receptor Assays

Essential consequences of the presence of ER in the tumor resides in the possibility of hormonal withdrawal therapy. Diminution of cellular proliferation by blocking hormonal action is the basis of hormone therapy of hormone-dependent cancers. Antiestrogen therapy by tamoxifen has demonstrated its efficiency in the treatment of ER-positive tumors *(99)*. Moreover, it presents a cytotoxic effect, responsible for a certain action in ER-negative women. In addition, there is an associated 40% decrease in controlateral breast cancer during adjuvant tamoxifen therapy. Tamoxifen maintains bone density and reduces fatal myocardial infarction *(99)*, reflecting the fact that this product also has an estrogen agonistic activity. It induces the synthesis of PR and it doubles the normal risk of developing endometrial cancer *(99)*. A new strategy is being developed to exploit the target site-specific action of antiestrogens. The use of raloxifene, an antiestrogen with high affinity for ER but only weak estrogenicity for the uterus, is being evaluated. The effect of aromatase inhibitors is also under study. These molecules act by inhibiting the production of estradiol.

Hormonal Phase and Breast Cancer Surgery

The influence of the timing of surgery in relation to the menstrual cycle on the survival of breast cancer patients has been both advocated and disputed. Eight years ago, it was suggested that the timing of surgery (during the follicular or corpus luteum phase of the menstrual cycle) could substantially influence the survival time in premenopausal breast cancer patients *(100)*. However, since then, several researchers have analyzed their data, and in general they could not confirm this observation *(101)*. Thus consensus on the menstrual phase related to the expected best prognostis is still required *(102)*.

PROGESTINS AND ANTIPROGESTIN THERAPY OF BREAST CANCER

Mechanisms of Antiprogestin Action

There is a great interest in the study of antiprogestins for two main reasons. First, they have been shown to have a great therapeutic potential such as interruption of early pregnancy, postcoital contraception, triggering of labor, and treatment of hormone-dependent tumors. Second, antiprogestins have also been used as potent tools to investigate the molecular mechanisms of action of the hormone.

After binding to the receptor, antihormones can act at all the steps of hormone action including "activation," dimerization, or binding of the dimers to hormone-responsive elements (HREs). In the case of antiestrogens, two types of antihormones have been described *(103,104)*: type I, which allows binding of the "activated" receptor to the HRE, and type II (or pure antiestrogens), which prevents this binding. In the case of antiprogestins, this type of classification has also been proposed. RU 486 (mifepristone) is the only antiprogestin used therapeutically. Its molecular mechanism of action on the PR has been largely studied by in vitro and in vivo experiments and is the object of a quasi-consensus, i.e., it "activates" PR, it induces its in vivo oligomerization *(86,105)* and RU 486-wild-type PR complexes bind in vivo to HREs *(106,107)*. Thus RU 486 acts at a distal step of hormone action (failure of transactivation by RU 486-receptor complexes bound to HREs). Moreover, an agonistic effect of RU 486 has been described in certain cell and promoter configurations *(107)*. This attests to the capacity of binding to HREs of RU486-PR complexes. By performing limited protease digestion of in vitro synthetised PR in the absence or presence of ligands, it was demonstrated that progesterone and RU 486 induce distinct conformational changes within the receptor protein. With the use of specific monoclonal antibodies, these conformational changes were shown to occur at the extreme carboxy terminus of the receptor *(108)*. The 42 amino acids located in the carboxy-terminal region of PR are required for the receptor to bind progesterone *(109)*. However, a mutant PR with these 42 amino acids deleted still binds RU486 and fully activates transcription in the presence of RU486 *(109)*. Thus, the conformation of the receptor bound to the HRE is influenced by the nature of the ligand.

Recently, a different antiprogestin molecule, ZK 98299 (onapristone), has been characterized. Studies of ZK 98299-PR complexes failed to detect in vitro binding to HRE *(110)*. This has led to the suggestion that ZK 98299 may be an example of a second class of antiprogestins that act by preventing the formation of DNA-PR complexes. In vivo experiments have shown that it "activates" PR and that it induces its oligomerization *(105,111)*. The results of in vivo competition with a constitutive PR for the binding to a progesterone responsive element (PRE) have shown that ZK 98299-PR complexes do bind the PRE. In these experiments ZK 98299 differs only quantitatively and not qualitatively from RU 486, the latter being 10-fold more potent than ZK 98299. This is correlated with their difference in affinity for the receptor, measured in vivo *(111)*. However, the results of in vivo genomic footprinting experiments are completely the opposite in that neither ZK 98299-PR complexes nor RU 486-PR complexes bind PRE *(112)*. Proteolytic fragment analysis studies show that ZK 98299 induces a fragment pattern intermediate between that induced by R5020 and by RU486 *(113)*. Thus it seems that, contrary to antiestrogens, it is difficult to identify two clear types of antiprogestins.

Progestins and Antiprogestin Therapy of Breast Cancer

The synthetic progestins, megestrol acetate and medroxyprogestrone acetate, are effective agents in the treatment of metastatic breast cancer. Response rates similar to those observed with the antiestrogen tamoxifen and similarly predicted by the presence of ER and PR have been observed *(114,115)*. Clinical data relating objective response after progestin treatment to steroid hormone receptor status reveal that, in both ER-positive and ER-negative tumors, the additional presence of PR ensures a significantly greater response to therapy *(115)*. This effect seems to be caused both by a direct effect on tumor cells (see above) and by indirect effects on the hypothalamo-pituitary-adrenal axis. Indeed, a potential mechanism for progestins to modulate the effect of estrogens on cellular proliferation is by regulating the concentration of the active estrogen, 17β-estradiol. Inhibition of estradiol synthesis is thought to be a major effect of treatment of postmenopausal breast cancer patients with medroxyprogesterone acetate. Evidence that high-dose medroxyprogesterone acetate suppresses the hypothalamo-pituitary-adrenal axis, and in turn the synthesis of adrenal androgens, supports this conclusion *(116)*.

Based on pharmacologic results, antiprogesterone therapy of PR-positive tumors has also been proposed. Indeed, these agents possess a potent antitumor activity in hormone-dependent experimental breast cancer models *(117,118)*. Although the underlying mechanism is not clear, induction of functional differentiation seems to be a major event *(119)*. This treatment is currently under investigation. Preliminary studies have shown good tolerance for antiprogesterone, and partial and transient remissions have been reported *(120,121)*. One problem that must be considered when using these agents is the antiglucocorticoid effect when they are used at high concentration for a long period.

REFERENCES

1. Topper YJ, Freeman CS (1980) Multiple hormone interactions in the developmental biology of the mammary gland. Physiol Rev 60:1049–1106.
2. Clarke CL, Sutherland RL (1990) Progestin regulation of cellular proliferation. Endocr Rev 11:266–301.
3. Lydon JP, DeMayo FJ, Funk CR, Mani SK, Hughes AR, Montgomery CA, et al. (1995) Mice lacking progesterone receptor exhibit pleiotropic reproductive abnormalities. Genes Dev 9:2266–2278.
4. Lydon JP, DeMayo FJ, Conneely OM, O'Malley BW (1996) Reproductive phenotypes of the progesterone receptor null mutant mouse. J Steroid Biochem Mol Biol 56:67–77.
5. Bossler R (1970) The morphology of hormonal induced structural changes in the female breast. Curr Top Pathol 53:1–89.
6. Banerjee MR (1976) Responses of mammary cells to hormones. Int Rev Cytol 47:1–97.

7. Murphy LJ, Murphy LC, Stead B, Sutherland RL, Lazarus L (1986) Modulation of lactogenic receptors by progestins in cultured human breast cancer cells. J Clin Endocrinol Metab 62:280–287.
8. Djiane J, Durand P (1977) Prolactin-progesterone antagonism in self-regulation of prolactin receptors in the mammary gland. Nature 266:641–643.
9. Read LD, Snider CE, Miller JS, Greene GL, Katzenellenbogen BS (1988) Ligand-modulated regulation of progesterone receptor messenger ribonucleic acid and protein in human breast cancer cell lines. Mol Endocrinol 2:263–271.
10. Alexander IE, Clarke CL, Shine J, Sutherland RL (1989) Progestin inhibition of progesterone receptor gene expression in human breast cancer cells. Mol Endocrinol 3:1377–1386.
11. Battersby S, Robertson BJ, Anderson TJ, King RJB, McPherson K (1992) Influence of menstrual cycle, parity and oral contraceptive use on steroid hormone receptors in normal breast. Br J Cancer 65:601–607.
12. Söderqvist G, Von Schoultz B, Tani E, Skoog L (1993) Estrogen and progesterone content in breast epithelial cells from heathly women during the menstrual cycle. Am J Obstet Gynecol 168:874–879.
13. Shyamala G (1997) Roles of estrogen and progesterone in normal mammary gland development. Insights from progesterone receptor null mutant mice and in situ localization of receptor. Trends Endocrinol Metab 8:34–39.
14. Musgrove EA, Hamilton JA, Lee CS, Sweeney KJ, Watts CK, Sutherland RL (1993) Growth factor, steroid, and steroid antagonist regulation of cyclin gene expression associated with changes in T-47D human breast cancer cell cycle progression. Mol Cell Biol 13:3577–3587.
15. Murphy LC, Murphy LJ, Dubik D, Bell GI, Shiu RPC (1988) Epidermal growth factor gene expression in human breast cancer cells: regulation of expression by progestins. Cancer Res 48:4555–4560.
16. Murphy LJ, Sutherland RL, Stead B, Murphy LC, Lazarus L (1986) Progestin regulation of epidermal growth factor receptor in human mammary carcinoma cells. Cancer Res 46:728–734.
17. Houdebine LM, Teyssot B, Devinoy E, Ollivier-Bousquet M, Djiane J, Kelly PA, et al. (1983) Role of progesterone in the development and the activity of the mammary gland, In: *Progesterone and Progestins* (Bardin CW, Milgrom E, Mauvais-Jarvis P, eds.), Raven Press, New York, pp. 297–319.
18. Masters JRW, Drife JO, Scarsbrick JJ (1977) Cyclic variation of DNA synthesis in human breast epithelium. J Natl Cancer Inst 58:1263–1265.
19. Anderson TJ, Ferguson DJP, Raab GM (1982) Cell turnover in the "resting" human breast: influence of parity, contraceptive pill, age and laterality. Br J Cancer 46:376–382.
20. Chang KJ, Lee, TTY, Linares-Cruz G, Fournier S, de Lignières B (1995) Influences of percutaneous administration of estradiol and progesterone on human breast epithelial cell cycle *in vivo*. Fertil Steril 63:785–791.
21. Dao TL, Sinha DK, Nemoto T, Patel J (1982) Effect of estrogen and progesterone on cellular replication of human breast tumors. Cancer Res 42:359–362.
22. Jones B, Russo J (1987) Influence of steroid hormones on the growth fraction of human breast carcinomas. Am J Clin Pathol 88:132–138.
23. Vignon F, Bardon S, Chalbos D, Rochefort H (1983) Antiestrogenic effect of R5020, a synthetic progestin in human breast cancer cells in culture. J Clin Endocrinol Metab 56:1124–1130.
24. Sutherland RL, Hall RE (1988) Effect of medroxyprogesterone acetate on proliferation and cell cycle kinetics of human mammary carcinoma cells. Cancer Res 48:5084–5091.
25. Horwitz KB, Freidenberg GR (1985) Growth inhibition and increase of insulin receptors in antiestrogen-resistant $T47D_{co}$ human breast cancer cells by progestins: implications for endocrine therapies. Cancer Res 45:167–173.
26. Hissom JR, Bowden RT, Moore MR (1989) Effects of progestins, estrogens and anti-hormones on growth and lactate dehydrogenase in the human breast cancer cell line T47D. Endocrinology 125:418–423.
27. Musgrove EA, Lee CS, Sutherland RL (1991) Progestins both stimulate and inhibit breast cancer cell cycle progression while increasing expression of transforming growth factor α, epidermal growth factor receptor, c-*fos*, and c-*myc* genes. Mol Cell Biol 11:5032–5043.
28. Di Lorenzo D, Albertini A, Zava D (1991) Progestin regulation of alkaline phosphatase in the human breast cancer cell line T47D. Cancer Res 51:4470–4475.
29. Di Lorenzo D, Gianni M, Savoldi GF, Ferrari F, Albertini A, Garattini E (1993) Progesterone induced expression of alkaline phosphatase is associated with a secretory phenotype in T47D breast cancer cells. Biochem Biophys Res Commun 192:1066–1072.
30. Joyeux C, Rochefort H, Chalbos D (1989) Progestin increases gene transcription and messenger ribonucleic acid stability of fatty acid synthetase in breast cancer cells. Mol Endocrinol 4:681–686.

31. Chalbos D, Joyeux C, Galtier F, Rochefort H (1992) Progestin-induced fatty acid synthetase in human mammary tumours from molecular to clinical studies. J Steroid Biochem Mol Biol 43:223–228.
32. Henderson BE, Ross RK, Pike MC (1993) Hormonal chemoprevention of cancer in women. Science 259:633–638.
33. Henderson BE, Casagrande JT, Pike MC, Mack T, Rosario I, Duke A (1983) The epidemiology of endometrial cancer in young women. Br J Cancer 47:749–756.
34. Weiss NS, Sayvetz TA (1980) Incidence of endometrial cancer in relation to the use of oral contraceptives. N Engl J Med 302:551–554.
35. Spicer DV, Pike MC, Pike A, Rude R, Shoupe D, Richardson J (1993) Pilot trial of a gonadotropin hormone agonist with replacement hormones as a prototype contraceptive to prevent breast cancer. Contraception 47:427–444.
36. Gal D, Edman CD, Vellios F, Forney JP (1983) Long-term effect of megestrol acetate in the treatment of endometrial hyperplasia. Am J Obstet Gynecol 146:316–322.
37. Gambrell RD (1982) Clinical use of progestins in the menopausal patient: dosage and duration. J Reprod Med 27:531–538.
38. Sherman BM, Korenman SG (1974) Inadequate corpus luteal function: a patho-physiological interpretation of human breast cancer epidemiology. Cancer 33:1306–1312.
39. Henderson BE, Ross KK, Judd HJ, Krailo M, Pike MC (1985) Do regular onvulatory cycles increase breast cancer risk. Cancer 56:1206–1214.
40. Potten CS, Watson RJ, William GT, Tickle S, Roberts SA, Harris M, et al. (1988) The effect of age and menstrual cycle upon proliferative activity of the normal human breast. Br J Cancer 58:163–170.
41. Armstrong BK (1988) Oestrogenotherapy after the menopause—boon or bane? Med J Aust 148:213–214.
42. Dupont WD, Page DL (1991) Menopausal estrogen replacement therapy and breast cancer. Arch Intern Med 151:67–72.
43. Steinberg KK, Thacker SB, Smith SJ, Stroup DF, Zack MM, Flanders WD, et al. (1991) A meta-analysis of the effect of estrogen replacement therapy on the risk of breast cancer. JAMA 265:1985–1990.
44. Colditz GA, Egan KM, Stampfer MJ (1993) Hormone replacement therapy and risk of breast cancer: results from epidemiologic studies. Am J Obstet Gynecol 168:1473–1480.
45. Smith D, Toft D (1993) Steroid receptors and their associated proteins. Mol Endocrinol 7:4–11.
46. Truss M, Beato M (1993) Steroid hormone receptors: interaction with deoxyribonucleic acid and transcription factors. Endocr Rev 14:459–479.
47. Beato M, Sanchez-Pacheco A (1996) Interaction of steroid hormone receptors with the transcription initiation complex. Endocr Rev 17:587–609.
48. Horwitz KB, Jackson TA, Bain DL, Richer JK, Takimoto GS, Tung L (1996) Nuclear receptor coactivators and corepressors. Mol Endocrinol 10:1167–1177.
49. Kamei Y, Xu L, Heinzel T, Torchia J, Kurokawa R, Gloss B, et al. (1996) A CBP integrator complex mediates transcriptional activation and AP-1 inhibition by nuclear receptors. Cell 85:403–414.
50. Bannister AJ, Kouzarides T (1996) The CBP co-activators is a histone acetyltransferase. Nature 384:641–643.
51. Spencer TE, Jenster G, Burcin MM, Allis CD, Zhou J, Mizzen CA, et al. (1997) Steroid receptor coactivator-1 is a histone acetyltransferase. Nature 389:194–198.
52. Yang XY, Ogrysko VV, Nishikawa J, Howard BH, Nakatani YA (1996) A p300/CBP-associated factor that competes with the adenoviral oncoprotein E1A. Nature, 382:319–324.
53. Pazin MJ, Kadonaga JT (1997) What's up and down with histone deacylation and transcription? Cell 89:325–328.
54. Cavaillès V, Dauvois S, Danielian PS, Parker MG (1994) Interaction of proteins with transcriptionally active estrogen receptors. Proc Natl Acad Sci USA 91:10009–10013.
55. Le Douarin B, Zechel C, Garnier JM, Lutz Y Tora L, Pierrat B, et al. (1995) The N-terminal part of TIF1, a putative mediator of the ligand-dependent activation function (AF-2) of nuclear receptors, is fused to B-raf in the oncogenic protein T18. EMBO J 14:2020–2033.
56. Halachmi S, Marden E, Martin G, MacKay H, Abbondanza C, Brown M (1994) Estrogen receptor-associated proteins: possible mediators of hormone-induced transcription. Science 264:1455–1458.
57. Onate SA, Tsai SY, Tsai MJ, O'Malley BW (1995) Sequence and characterization of a coactivator for the steroid hormone receptor superfamily. Science 270:1354–1357.
58. Muchardt C, Yaniv M (1993) A human homologue of *Saccharomyces cerevisiae SNF2/SWI2* and *Drosophila brm* genes potentiates transcriptional activation by the glucocorticoid receptor. EMBO J 12:4279–4290.

59. Gronemeyer H, Laudet V (1995) Transcription factors. 3. Nuclear receptors. *Rev Protein Profile* 2:1173–1308.
60. Carson-Jurica MA, Schrader WT, O'Malley BW (1990) Steroid receptor family: structure and functions. Endocr Rev 11:201–220
61. Bourguet W, Ruff M, Chambon P, Gronemeyer H, Moras D (1995) Crystal structure of the ligand-binding domain of the human nuclear receptor RXR-alpha. Nature 375:377–382.
62. Bocquel MT, Kumar V, Stricker C, Chambon P, Gronemeyer H (1989) The contribution of the N-and C-terminal regions of steroid receptors to activation of transcription is both receptor and cell-specific. Nucleic Acids Res 17:2581–2595.
63. Loosfelt H, Atger M, Misrahi M, Guiochon-Mantel A, Meriel C, Logeat F, et al. (1986) Cloning and sequence analysis of rabbit progesterone-receptor complementary DNA. Proc Natl Acad Sci USA 83:9045–9049.
64. Misrahi M, Atger M, d'Auriol L, Loosfelt H, Meriel C, Fridlansky F, et al. (1987) Complete amino acid sequence of the human progesterone receptor deduced from cloned cDNA. Biochem Biophys Res Commun 143:740–748.
65. Gronemeyer H, Turcotte B, Quirin-Stricker C, Bocquel MT, Meyer ME, Krozowski Z, et al. (1987) The chicken progesterone receptor: sequence, expression and functional analysis. EMBO J 6:3985–3994.
66. Misrahi M, Venencie PY, Saugier-Veber P, Sar S, Dessen P, Milgrom E (1993) Structure of the human progesterone receptor gene. Biochem Biophys Acta 1216:289–292.
67. Rousseau-Merck MF, Misrahi M, Loosfelt H, Milgrom E, Berger R (1987) Localization of the human progesterone receptor gene to chromosome 11q22–11q23. Hum Genet 77:280–282.
68. Lessey BA, Alexander PS, Horwitz KB (1983) The subunit structure of human breast cancer progesterone receptors: characterization by chromatography and photoaffinity labeling. Endocrinology 112:1267–1274.
69. Horwitz KB, Alexander PS (1983) In situ photolinked nuclear progesterone receptors of human breast cancer cells: subunit molecular weights after transformation and translocation. Endocrinology 113:2195–2201.
70. Kastner P, Krust A, Turcotte B, Stropp U, Tora L, Gronemeyer H, et al. (1990) Two distinct estrogen-regulated promoters generate transcripts encoding the two functionally different human progesterone receptor forms A and B. EMBO J 9:1603–1614.
71. Sartorius CA, Melville MY, Hovland AR, Tung L, Takimoto GS, Horwitz KB (1994) A third transactivation function (AF3) of human progesterone receptors located in the unique N-terminal segment of the B-isoform. Mol Endocrinol 8:1347–1360.
72. Graham JD, Yeates C, Balleine RL, Harvey SS, Milliken JS, Bilous AM, et al. (1996) Progesterone receptor A and B protein expression in human breast cancer. J Steroid Biochem Mol Biol 56:93–98.
73. Savouret JF, Bailly A, Misrahi M, Rauch C, Redeuilh G, Chauchereau A, et al. (1991) Characterization of the hormone responsive element involved in the regulation of the progesterone receptor gene. EMBO J 10:1875–1883.
74. Kraus WL, Montano MM, Katzenellenbogen S (1994) Identification of multiple, widely spaced estrogen-responsive regions in the rat progesterone receptor gene. Mol Endocrinol 8:952–969.
75. Scott R.E.M., Wu-Peng XS, Yen PM, Chin WW, Pfaff DW (1997) Interactions of estrogen-and thyroid hormone receptors on a progesterone receptor estrogen response element (ERE) sequence: a comparison with the vitellogenin A2 consensus ERE. Mol Endocrinol 11:1581–1592.
76. Savouret JF, Rauch M, Redeuilh G, Sar S, Chauchereau A, Woodruff K, et al. (1994) Interplay between estrogens, progestins, retinoic acid and AP-1 on a single regulatory site in the progesterone receptor gene. J Biol Chem 269:28955–28962.
77. Jensen T, Suzuki T, Kawashima T, Stumpf WE, Jungblut PW, DeSombre ER (1968) A two-step mechanism for the interaction of oestradiol with the rat uterus. Proc Natl Acad Sci USA 59:632–638.
78. Gorski J, Toft D, Shyamala G, Smith D, Notides A (1968) Hormone receptors: studies on the interaction of estrogen with the uterus. Recent Prog Horm Res 24:45–81.
79. Greene GL, Fitch FW, Jensen EV (1980) Monoclonal antibodies to estrophilin: probes for the study of estrogen receptors. Proc Natl Acad Sci USA 77:157–161.
80. Logeat F, Vu Hai MT, Fournier A, Legrain P, Buttin G, Milgrom E (1983) Monoclonal antibodies to rabbit progesterone receptor: crossreaction with other mammalian progesterone receptors. Proc Natl Acad Sci USA 80:6456–6459.
81. King WJ, Greene GL (1984) Monoclonal antibodies localize oestrogen receptor in the nuclei of target cells. Nature 30:7745–7747.

82. Perrot-Applanat M, Logeat F, Groyer-Picard MT, Milgrom E (1985) Immunocytochemical study of mammalian progesterone receptor using monoclonal antibodies. Endocrinology 116:1473–1484.
83. Dingwall C, Laskey RA (1991) Nuclear targeting sequences—a consensus? Trends Biochem Sci 16:478–481
84. Gorlich D, Mattaj IW (1996) Nucleocytoplasmic transport. Science 271:1513–1518.
85. Picard D, Yamamoto KR (1987) Two signals mediate hormone-dependent nuclear localization of the glucocorticoid receptor. EMBO J 6:3333–3340.
86. Guiochon-Mantel A, Loosfelt H, Lescop P, Sar S, Atger M, Perrot-Applanat M, et al. (1989) Mechanisms of nuclear localization of the progesterone receptor: evidence for interaction between monomers. Cell 57:1147–1154.
87. Ylikomi T, Bocquel MT, Berry M, Gronemeyer H, Chambon P (1992) Cooperation of proto-signals for nuclear accumulation of estrogen and progesterone receptors. EMBO J 11:3681–3694.
88. Picard D, Kumar V, Chambon P, Yamamoto KR (1990) Signal transduction by steroid hormones: nuclear localization is differentially regulated in estrogen and glucocorticoid receptors. Cell Regul 1:291–299.
89. Guiochon-Mantel A, Lescop P, Christin-Maitre S, Loosfelt H, Perrot-Applanat M, Milgrom E (1991) Nucleocytoplasmic shuttling of the progesterone receptor. EMBO J 10:3851–3859.
90. Madan AP, De Franco DB (1993) Bidirectional transport of glucocorticoid receptors across the nuclear envelope. Proc Natl Acad Sci USA 90:3588–3592.
91. Dauvois S, White R, Parker MG (1993) The antiestrogen ICI182780 disrupts estrogen receptor nucleocytoplasmic shuttling. J Cell Sci 106:1377–1388.
92. Molinari AM, Medici N, Armetta I, Nigro V, Montcharmont B, Puca GA (1985) Particulate nature of the unoccupied uterine estrogen receptor. Biochem Biophys Res Commun 128:634–642.
93. Guiochon-Mantel A, Delabre K, Lescop P, Milgrom E (1994) Nuclear localization signals also mediate the outward movement of proteins from the nucleus. Proc Natl Acad Sci USA 91:7179–7183.
94. Leclercq G, Bojar H, Goussard J, Nicholson RI, Pichon MF, Piffanelli A, et al. (1986) Abbott monoclonal enzyme immunoassay measurement of estrogen receptors in human breast cancer: a European multicenter study. Cancer Res 46:4233S-4236S.
95. Esteban JM, Ahn C, Battifora H, Felder B (1994) Quantitative immunohistochemical assay for hormonal receptors: technical aspects and biological significance. J Cell Biochem suppl 19:138–145.
96. Gray DJ, Pace GE, Deegs CS (1994) Immunohistochemical detection of steroid receptors in paraffin-embedded tissues comparison with biochemical method and rationale for a changeover in a community hospital. Am J Clin Pathol 102:257–262.
97. Knight WA, Livingston RB, Gregory EJ, Mc Guire NL (1977) Estrogen receptor as an independant pronostic factor for early reccurence in breast cancer. Cancer Res 37:4669–4671.
98. Pichon MF, Pallud C, Hacene F, Milgrom E (1992) Pronostic value of progesterone receptor after long-term follow-up in primary breast cancer. Eur J Cancer 28A, 1676–1680.
99. Jordan VC (1995) Third annual William L McGuire memorial lecture. Studies on the estrogen in breastcancer—20 years as a target for the treatment and prevention of cancer. Breast Cancer Res Treat 36:267–285.
100. Hrushesky WJ, Bluming AZ, Gruber SA, Sothern RB (1989) Menstrual influence on surgical cure of breast cancer. Lancet 2:949–952.
101. Jager W, Sauerbrei W (1995) Effect of timing of surgery during the menstrual cycle of premenopausal breast cancer patients. Breast Cancer Res Treat 34:279–287.
102. Mondini G, Decian F, Sorice G, Friedman D, Spirito C, Costantini M, et al. (1997) Timing of surgery related to menstrual cycle and prognosis of premenopausal women with breast cancer. Anticancer Res 17:787–790.
103. Reese JC, Katzenellenbogen BS (1991) Differential DNA binding abilities of estrogen receptor occupied with two classes of antiestrogens: studies using human estrogen receptor overexpressed in mammalian cells. Nucleic Acids Res 19:6595–6602.
104. Gronemeyer H, Benhamou B, Berry M, Bocquel MT, Gofflo D, Garcia T, et al. (1992) Mechanisms of antihormone action. J Steroid Biochem Mol Biol 41:217–221.
105. Bocquel MT, Ji J, Ylikomi T, Benhamou B, Vergezac A , Chambon P, et al. (1993) Type II antagonists impair the DNA binding of steroid hormone receptors. J Steroid Biochem Mol Biol 45:205–215.
106. Guiochon-Mantel A, Loosfelt H, Ragot T, Bailly A, Atger M, Misrahi M, et al. (1988) Receptors bound to antiprogestin form abortive complexes with hormone responsive elements. Nature 336:695–698.

107. Meyer ME, Pornon A, Jingwei J, Bocquel MT, Chambon P, Gronemeyer H (1990) Agonistic and antagonist activities of RU486 on the functions of the human progesterone receptor. EMBO J 12:3923–3932.
108. Allan GF, Tsai SY, Tsai MJ, O'Malley BW (1992) Ligand-dependent conformational changes in the progesterone receptor are necessary for events that follow DNA binding. Proc Natl Acad Sci USA 89:11750–11754.
109. Vegeto E, Allan GF, Schrader WT, Tsai MJ, McDonnell DP, O'Malley BW (1992) The mechanism of RU486 antagonism is dependent on the conformation of the carboxy-terminal tail of the human progesterone receptor. Cell 69:703–713.
110. Klein-Hitpass L, Cato ACB, Henderson D, Ryffel GU (1991) Two types of antiprogestins identified by their differential action in transcriptionally active extracts from T47D cells. Nucleic Acids Res 19:1227–1234.
111. Delabre K, Guiochon-Mantel A, Milgrom E (1993) In vivo evidence against the existence of antiprogestins disrupting receptor binding to DNA. Proc Natl Acad Sci USA 90:4421–4425.
112. Truss M, Bartsch J, Beato M (1994) Antiprogestins prevent progesterone receptor binding to hormone responsive elements *in vivo*. Proc Natl Acad Sci USA 91:11333–11337.
113. Allan GF, Lombardi E, Haynes-Johnson D, Palmer S, Kiddoe M, Kraft P, et al. (1996) Induction of a novel conformation in the progesterone receptor by ZK299 involves a defined region of the carboxyl-terminal tail. Mol Endocrinol 10:1206–1213.
114. McGuire WL, Cavalli F, Bonomi P (1985) Progestin therapy for breast cancer: a panel discussion. Breast Cancer Res Treat 6:213–220.
115. Sedlacek SM, Horwitz KB (1984) The role of progestins and progesterone receptors in the treatment of breast cancer. Steroids 44:467–483.
116. Dogliotti L, Mussa A, Di Carlo F (1983) Medroxyprogesterone acetate high dose and bromocriptine: results of a 4 year study in stage IV breast cancer, In: *Role of Medroxyprogesterone in Endocrine Related Tumors*, vol. 2 (Campo L, Robustelli Della Cuna G, Taylor RW, eds.), Raven Press, New York, pp. 115–129.
117. Bakker GH, Setyono-Han B, de Jong FH, Klijn JGM (1987) Mifepristone in treatment of experimental breast cancer in rats, In: *Hormonal Regulation of Cancer: Peptides, Growth Factors and New (Anti) Steroidal Agents* (Klijn JGM, Paridiens R, Foekens JA, eds.), Raven Press, New York, pp. 39–48.
118. Schneider MR, Michna H, Nishino Y, El Etr MF (1989) Antitumor activity of the progesterone antagonists ZK98299 and RU486 in the hormone dependent MXT mammary tumor model of the mouse and the DMBA- and MNU-induced mammary tumor model of the rat. Eur J Cancer Clin Oncol 25:691–701.
119. Klijn JG, de Jong FH, Bakker GH, Lamberts SW, Rodenburg CJ, Alexieva-Figush J (1989) Antiprogestins, a new form of endocrine therapy for human breast cancer. Cancer Res 49:2851–2856.
120. Romieu G, Maudelonde T, Ulmann A, Pujol H, Grenier J, Cavalie G, et al. (1987) The antiprogestin RU 486 in advanced breast cancer: preliminary clinical trial. Bull Cancer 74:455–461.
121. Li M, Spitzer E, Zschiesche W, Binas B, Parczyk K, Grosse R (1995) Antiprogestins inhibit growth and stimulate differentiation in the normal mammary gland. J Cell Physiol 164:1–8.

18 Prolactin and Its Receptors in Human Breast Cancer

Barbara K. Vonderhaar, PHD

PROLACTIN AS A MITOGEN IN BREAST CANCER

The peptide hormone prolactin (PRL) plays a key role in normal growth, development, and differentiation of the mammary gland. Induction of milk protein synthesis both in vivo and in vitro is dependent on PRL *(1)*. Less well recognized is the mitogenic action of PRL. Although the ovarian steroids, estrogen and progesterone, are involved in mammary ductal growth and branching, strong evidence suggests that lobuloalveolar development and extensive growth of the alveolar cells require PRL *(1,2)*. Progesterone acts synergistically with PRL to induce mitogenesis during mammary gland development, possibly by increasing the PRL receptor levels in these glands *(3)*.

Prolactin in Rodent Mammary Cancer

The same hormones that are important for normal growth are also involved to varying degrees in the development of breast cancer. PRL's role in breast cancer is well established in rodent model systems. In mice, multiple pituitary isografts, which secrete large amounts of PRL, significantly increased the incidence of spontaneous mammary tumors *(4)*. Boot et al. *(5)* obtained more tumors in animals given daily injections of PRL, suggesting a key role in mammary tumor development. Similarly, a body of evidence in rats suggests a key role of PRL in induction of mammary tumors *(6,7)*. There is a direct correlation between serum PRL levels and susceptibility of various rat strains to induction of tumors by chemical carcinogens *(8)*. Both nitrosomethylurea- and 7,12-dimethylbenz[a]anthracene-induced tumors in rats are dependent on PRL for sustained growth *(9)*. There is a direct correlation between drug-induced hyperprolactinemia and increased tumor growth as well as between hypoprolactinemia and retarded tumor growth in rodents *(6,10)*.

Prolactin in Human Breast Cancer

In contrast to the rodent model system, the function of PRL in the etiology and progression of human breast cancer is not clear. Holtkamp et al. *(11)* reported that hyperprolactinemia occurred in 44% of patients with metastatic breast disease during the course of the disease. Studies of human breast biopsies showed more than 70% to be positive for PRL receptors, whereas approximately 80% of breast cancer cells in

From: *Contemporary Endocrinology: Endocrinology of Breast Cancer*
Edited by: A. Manni © Humana Press Inc., Totowa, NJ

culture respond to PRL's mitogenic signal *(12)*. Several studies have shown that basal serum PRL levels are significantly elevated in a subset of women at risk for familial breast cancer *(13,14)* and that the circadian rhythm of PRL secretion from the pituitary differs between groups at high vs low risk of breast cancer *(15)* with no seasonal variations *(16)*. In one study *(17)*, hyperprolactinemia and/or *p53* were associated with aggressiveness of the tumor, early disease relapse or metastases, and poor overall survival in patients with node-negative breast cancer. By contrast, Lissoni et al. *(18)* reported that a surgery-induced rise in PRL, despite its potential stimulation of cancer cell growth, was paradoxically associated with a longer disease-free survival in operable breast carcinoma in patients both with and without axillary node involvement. Surgery-induced hyperprolactinemia was associated with a significant decline in the serum level of IGF-I *(19)*.

Effects of Prolactin In Vivo

Immunologically detectable PRL appears in 60–85% of human breast cancer biopsies *(20,21)*, and specific PRL receptors have been demonstrated in more than 70% of biopsy samples *(22–25)*. However, there is no clear correlation between circulating PRL levels and the etiology or prognosis of breast cancer *(14,26,27)*. When patients were treated with PRL-inhibiting ergot drugs that significantly diminish circulating pituitary PRL, no change in disease state was observed *(28,29)*. Operating on the assumption that the lack of effect may have been due to the presence of human growth hormone (hGH), which is also a lactogen, Manni et al. *(30)* administered a combination therapy of bromocriptine and a somatostatin analog to a group of women with advanced breast cancer. Circulating levels of PRL, detected by a single assay, were abolished nearly completely in eight of nine patients, whereas hGH levels were suppressed in seven of nine patients during treatment. Although overall antitumor effects could not be assessed reliably because the patients entering the study had been pretreated heavily with chemotherapeutic agents, only one patient experienced disease stabilization. In a similar study, Anderson et al. *(31)* treated patients long term with bromocriptine and the long-acting, superpotent somatostatin analog octretide; they found that there was no evidence of disease progression for periods of up to 6 months in four of six patients with advanced breast cancer who had failed first- and second-line endocrine therapies. Whereas immunoreactive PRL, GH, and insulin-like growth factor-I (IGF-I) in 24-h profiles of serum were greatly reduced by these treatments, diurnal peaks of bioreactive lactogenic hormone as well as GH levels were still apparent although much reduced.

Effects of Prolactin In Vitro

In contrast to the lack of convincing data in vivo, investigations in vitro using human breast tumor tissue and cells show clear responses to PRL. These responses include increased DNA *(32–35)*, protein *(36)*, and α-lactalbumin *(37)* synthesis; colony formation *(38,39)*; and changes in shape, adhesion, lipid accumulation *(40)*, and estrogen receptor (ER) content *(41)*. Primary breast biopsy samples grown in nude mice respond to lactogenic hormones with increased growth *(42)*. Malarkey et al. *(38)* found that physiologic levels of human PRL (hPRL) and hGH increased the population doubling of primary breast tumor cultures. We have shown that most human breast cancer cell lines, both ER positive and ER negative, express PRL receptors, and more than 80% of human breast cancer cell lines tested respond to PRL's mitogenic signal *(12,43)*. Both T47D and MCF-7 human breast cancer cells respond to lactogenic stimulation when grown as solid tumors in nude mice *(7)*. Direct effects of PRL on growth of the ER-positive cell lines MCF-7, T47D, and ZR75.1 can be demonstrated only under proper growth conditions in the presence of charcoal-stripped serum (CSS). PRL-stimulated growth of MCF-7 cells was greater in the presence of 1% CSS compared with 10% *(43)*. The maximal effect was observed at 100–250 ng/mL hPRL. Growth was also stimulated by hGH, human placental lactogen, and ovine PRL but required higher concentrations to achieve the same effect. Thus MCF-7 cells were more sensitive to the mitogenic effect of hPRL than to other lactogens. Bovine PRL had no effect on the growth of these human breast cancer cells. The ER-negative cell line T47Dco also responds to PRL as a mitogen in the presence of CSS *(44)* or in serum-free conditions *(45)*. Lemus-Wilson et al. *(46)* also showed that PRL acts as a mitogen in MCF-7 and ZR75.1 when grown in serum-free media.

Effects of PRL on the growth of breast cancer cells are modulated by the presence of other growth factors and hormones. Melatonin, the primary hormone from the pineal gland, completely blocks hPRL-induced growth of MCF-7 and ZR75.1 *(46)*. Bovine PRL, when added simultaneously with hPRL, blocked the effect of hPRL on the growth of MCF-7 cells *(12,43)*. As little as 50–100 ng/mL of bovine PRL was able to block the hPRL-induced growth of these cells. By contrast, bovine PRL is an effective mitogen in normal mouse mammary cell lines. The ability of bovine PRL to act as an antagonist of hPRL may be unique to the mitogenic action of PRL in human breast cancer cells.

PROLACTIN SYNTHESIS AND SECRETION BY BREAST CANCER CELLS

In breast cancer, the lack of correlation between clinical data and in vitro responses may be explained, in part, by our recent observation that breast cancer cells themselves synthesize and secrete PRL. Extrapituitary production of PRL by breast tumors has long been suspected. Following surgical removal of the pituitary in humans the circulating levels of all pituitary hormones become undetectable except for PRL. Circulating levels of PRL remained at 30–80% of the presurgical levels for as long as 10 months in breast cancer patients who received a total hypophysectomy *(47)*. Patients given bromocriptine plus a somatostatin analog persistently maintained low levels of circulating bioactive PRL *(31)*. Although these data could result from other PRL-like molecules circulating in the blood, it was also possible that PRL itself was produced by peripheral tissues. Both normal tissue and tumors appear to generate this hormone. The placenta is the richest extrapituitary source *(48)*. The high concentrations of PRL in human amniotic fluid result from the decidua. PRL is also produced by the brain, uterus, dermal fibroblasts, and immune system *(48–51)*. Recently our laboratory and several others have provided evidence that PRL is produced by both normal and malignant mammary epithelial cells and thus may be an autocrine factor in this tissue *(52)*. Steinmetz et al. *(53)* showed by *in situ* hybridization that PRL gene transcripts are present in secretory mammary epithelial cells in pregnant rats. PRL mRNA has also been demonstrated by both Northern analysis and PCR in mammary glands from lactating rats *(54)*, goats, and sheep *(55)*, suggesting local synthesis of PRL by this gland. More recently, the presence of PRL was demonstrated by polymerase chain reaction (PCR) in some primary human breast carcinomas *(56)* and in human breast cancer cells in culture in our laboratory *(52)*.

We determined that PRL is synthesized by human breast cancer cells and acts in an autocrine manner to stimulate cell proliferation with a panel of anti-PRL monoclonal

Table 1
Synthesis of PRL as a function of ER and PRL Receptor Status

Cell line	*ER status*	*PRL R status*	*PRL mRNA*
ZR 75-1	+	+	+
T47D	+	+	+
MCF-7	+	+	+
T47Dco	–	+	+
MCF 10a	–	+	+
BT20	–	+	–
MDA MD-231	–	–	–
MDA MB-468	–	+	+
MDA MB-453	–	+	+
Hs578t	–	+	+
SK-BR-3	–	not done	+
A1N4	–	+	+

Abbreviations: PRL, prolactin; ER, estrogen receptor; R, receptor.

antibodies and by use of the antisense technique. Using a panel of monoclonal antibodies against human PRL, proliferation of both T47Dco and MCF-7 human breast cancer cell lines was inhibited by 20–90% *(52)*. In addition, when T47Dco cells were treated with antisense RNA directed against the gene encoding for pituitary PRL, significant growth inhibition (>50%) was obtained *(57)*. Reverse transcription (RT)-PCR, followed by Southern analysis using hPRL cDNA as the probe, confirmed the presence of the message in T47Dco and MCF-7 cells *(52)*. In addition, 82% of all breast cancer cell lines tested contained mRNA for PRL *(58)*.

That the protein is actually synthesized and secreted by the cells in culture was confirmed by metabolically labeling T47Dco cells with ^{35}[S]cysteine. Conditioned media and cell extracts both contain a 22-kDa protein precipitated by anti-hPRL monoclonal antibody. Conditioned media prepared from T47Dco cells stimulated the PRL-responsive Nb2 rat lymphoma cells to grow in a concentration-dependent manner. These cells respond to picogram quantities of lactogens. The level of biologic activity in the conditioned media is equivalent to 0.7 μg/mL (14.5 pg PRL/cell) of pituitary PRL as measured by the Nb2 assay and is approximately 30% of the amount normally produced by the rat pituitary cell line, GH3 *(59,60)*. By using a specific radioimmunoassay RIA for human pituitary PRL, 0.35 μg/mL of PRL protein was detected. The activity in the conditioned media, like that of the human pituitary PRL, was abolished when the media were pretreated with anti-PRL antibody *(52)*.

More than 80% of all breast cancer cell lines contain mRNA for PRL (Table 1). There is no correlation of ER status with PRL receptors or with the ability to synthesize PRL. When human breast cancer cells were grown as solid tumors in nude mice, the resulting tumors contained PRL gene transcripts *(57)*. Immunologically detectable PRL was present in 60–85% of human breast cancer biopsies *(20,21)*. In addition, we found that 73% of primary breast cancer surgical samples also contained mRNA for PRL. In most cases, the amount of mRNA for PRL and its receptors is significantly elevated in cancerous vs the adjacent, noninvolved tissue from the same patient. There was no correlation between the presence of PRL mRNA and ER status *(58)*.

Posttranslational Modifications of PRL

PRL achieves its many diverse activities through different posttranslational modifications. Glycosylation and phosphorylation alter immunoreactivity and biologic activity of PRL *(61,62)*. Phosphorylated forms of PRL have been demonstrated in murine, bovine, and avian species *(63)*. Wicks and Brooks *(64)* have shown that phosphorylated PRL has less activity compared with the nonphosphorylated form. The phosphorylated form of PRL is unable to bind to the receptor owing to conformational change in the hormone. Dephosphorylation of PRL restored its biologic activity. The biologic activity of glycosylated PRL in the Nb2 mitogenesis assay and in mammary casein synthesis is similar to or lower than that of the nonglycosylated PRL *(65,66)*. However, receptor binding activity and immunologic crossreactivity are greatly reduced as a result of glycosylation. Hoffman et al. *(67)* suggested that glycosylation may selectively downregulate PRL action in target tissues. Recombinant human PRL, in both glycosylated and nonglycosylated forms, was purified from the murine C127 cell expression system. The 23-kDa nonglycosylated form of the PRL was three to four times more active in the Nb2 mitogenesis bioassay compared with the 25-kDa glycosylated form *(68)*. The physiologically diverse effects of PRL on target tissues is suggested to be due to changes in the ratio of glycosylated and nonglycosylated forms of PRL *(69)*.

The nature of the posttranslational alteration of PRL synthesized by the mammary gland and breast cancer cells is unknown. Our observations that a panel of monoclonal antibodies directed against pituitary PRL vary in their ability to recognize the PRL produced by breast cancer cells *(52)* suggests that there are marked differences in posttranslational modifications between the pituitary and the mammary gland.

Regulation of Expression of Prolactin

The hormones and growth factors that regulate expression of PRL by human breast cancer cells in vivo and in vitro are currently unknown. Recent studies *(70)* have shown that PRL synthesis is regulated in T47D cells by the distal promoter used by decidua and lymphocytes rather than the proximal promoter used by the pituitary.

PROLACTIN RECEPTORS

The presence of specific receptors for PRL has been demonstrated in both normal and malignant mammary glands. PRL receptors belong to the cytokine hematopoietic family of receptors *(71)*. The members of this superfamily are single membrane-spanning receptors organized into three domains, comprising an extracellular ligand binding domain, a hydrophobic transmembrane domain and an intracellular domain containing a proline-rich motif. The three different forms of the PRL receptor differ in their cytoplasmic domain. The long (90-kDa) and short (40-kDa) forms of the receptor are generated by differential splicing of a single gene and differ only in the length of the cytoplasmic domain *(72)*. The intermediate form of the receptor is a deletion mutant of the long form, lacking 198 amino acids in its cytoplasmic region. This form of the receptor is more sensitive to PRL compared with the other forms, is the predominant form in Nb2 rat lymphoma cells *(73)*, and may be present in some human breast cancers *(56)*. Both the long and the intermediate forms of the PRL receptor are able to induce differentiation as measured by induction of milk protein gene expression *(74)*. Both forms have also been shown to induce mitosis *(75)*. We have shown that the short form of the mouse PRL receptor is also able to induce mitosis but not differentiation *(76)*.

Mammary cells, both normal and malignant, contain both long and short forms of the receptor. Interaction of PRL with its receptor induces dimerization of the membrane-associated receptor *(77)*. Because the receptors exist in multiple charged forms (Ziska and Vonderhaar, unpublished data) as well as different sizes, a variety of dimeric combinations are possible. The physiologic significance of homo- vs heterodimerization is an open question.

In human breast cancer, the correlation of disease parameters with ER and PR is quite clear. However, it is less clear for the PRL receptor because of its multiple size and charged forms. Specific PRL receptors have been demonstrated in >70% of the biopsy samples by specific binding assays *(22–25)*. In our study *(58)*, >90% of breast cancer surgical samples were positive for PRL receptor mRNA, but the amount varied considerably. The ratio of long and short forms is unknown. No message for the intermediate form of the receptor has been detected in our samples, in contrast to the report by Clevenger et al. *(56)*. No correlation has been found between the presence of PRL receptors and ER status. The majority of cancerous tissue contained significantly more mRNA for the PRL receptor than did adjacent, noninvolved tissue from the same patient *(58)*.

PROLACTIN MITOGENIC SIGNALING PATHWAYS

Kinases Associated with the PRL Receptor

PRL receptors do not have intrinsic kinase activity. They recruit several different kinases that could transduce its mitogenic signal. JAK2, a member of the Janus family of kinases, is associated with the PRL receptor constitutively. It is phosphorylated upon PRL binding in rat lymphoma *(78, 79)*, mouse mammary explants *(80)*, and murine lymphoid BAF-3 cells *(81)*. JAK1 also is associated with the PRL receptor and is phosphorylated upon ligand binding in murine lymphoid BAF-3 cells transfected with the long form of the PRL receptor *(81)* The PRL receptor is also phosphorylated in response to PRL within 1 min of the hormone treatment both in vivo in rabbit mammary gland and in vitro in CHO cells transfected with the long form of PRL receptor cDNA *(82)*. Receptor dimerization is hypothesized to result in JAK transphosphorylation, thereby activating its intrinsic protein tyrosine kinase activity. Phosphorylation of the JAK proteins may be one of the earliest cellular events in response to the hormone, which ultimately triggers a chain of events in the PRL signaling pathway (Fig. 1). PRL receptors induce phosphorylation of cytoplasmic transcription factors, the STAT proteins, mainly STAT1, STAT3, and STAT5 *(83)*. STAT5 is activated for PRL's differentiation signal *(84)*. Recently two different STAT5 proteins have been isolated from mouse mammary tissue (STAT5a and STAT5b). Both of the transcription factors recognize GAS sequences. Their expression is concurrent during mammary gland development, increasing from the virgin state, reaching a maximum at day 16 of pregnancy, and declining during lactation *(85)*. STAT5a is essential for full lobuloalveolar development and lactation, as demonstrated by use of knockout mice *(86)*; STAT5b knockout mice lactate normally. The phosphorylation of STAT proteins has also been reported in Nb2 cells *(79)* and in normal mammary epithelial cells (HC11) *(84)*. We have reported activation of STAT5 upon PRL treatment in T47D breast cancer cells *(87)*. DaSilva et al. *(83)* also reported the phosphorylation of STAT1, STAT3, and STAT5 in T47D cells upon 15 min of PRL treatment. Activation of STAT

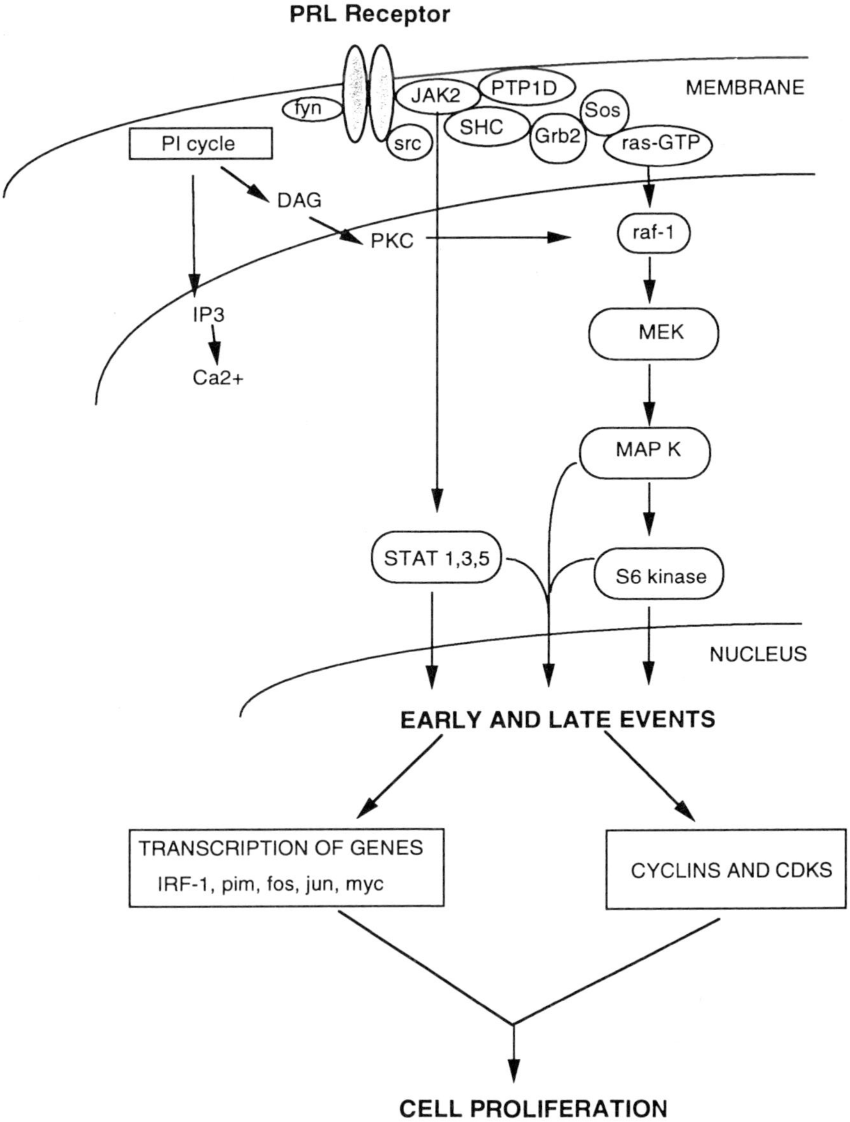

Fig. 1. Signaling pathways for PRL-induced cell proliferation.

proteins results in translocation of the transcription factors to the nucleus and activation of gene transcription *(88)*.

PRL induces the association of PRL receptors with pp60 c-src and activation of its tyrosine kinase activity in hepatocytes of lactating rats *(89)* in which the short form of the receptor is predominant. PRL stimulation in rat lymphoma Nb2 cells induces the association and activation of src family protein tyrosine kinase p59 fyn *(90)* and also guanine nucleotide releasing factor-vav *(91)*. Recently a protein tyrosine phosphatase PTP1D was reported to be associated with the PRL receptor-JAK2 complex in Nb2 cells, which was essential for PRL signal transduction for induction of β-casein *(92)*. In CHO cells transfected with the rabbit PRL receptor, herbimysin A and tyrphostin, two tyrosine kinase inhibitors, were able to decrease the expression of a β-lactoglobin promoter/CAT construct by over 50%. Orthovanadate, an inhibitor of tyrosine phosphatase, was able to substitute for PRL in inducing CAT responses in these cells *(93)*. This suggests an intricate role of both kinases and phosphatases for PRL signal transduction.

The ras-MAPK Pathway

A variety of growth factors and cytokines mediate proliferation by activating the ras-MAP kinase pathway of signal transduction. Activation of ras p21 protein by PRL has been reported in a variety of cell systems by measuring the guanine nucleotides bound to the protein *(94,95)*. Raf-1, MEK, and MAP kinase are downstream kinases in the ras-MAPK pathway that are activated for mitosis induced by PRL (Fig. 1). In Nb2 cells, PRL rapidly phosphorylates c-raf-1 *(96)*. Raf-1 is closely associated with the PRL receptor in these cells. We have reported the activation of these enzymes in mammary cells in response to 5 min of PRL treatment *(87)*. PRL activates these enzymes in a rapid and transient manner in both normal and breast cancer cells as they respond to the hormone as a mitogen. Tyrosine kinase inhibitors have been able to block MAP kinase activity and PRL-induced growth in these mammary cells *(87)*. Cells transfected with the long or the short form of the PRL receptor cDNA were also able to activate MAP kinase. There was a rapid activation of MAP kinase reaching a peak within 5 min of PRL treatment in both of the transfectants *(76)*, suggesting that both the long form and the short form of the PRL receptor are able to induce mitosis through a common signaling pathway. PRL also activates MAP kinase in rat liver, in vivo, and in Nb2 cells *(97,98)*. Activation and nuclear translocation of PKC and MAP kinase have been reported during PRL-induced proliferation of Nb2 cells *(98,99)*. A preliminary report in Nb2 cells has shown PRL activation of 40S ribosomal protein S6 kinase *(100)*, an enzyme downstream from MAP kinase in this signal cascade. The activation of S6 kinase reached its peak at 1.5–2 h after PRL treatment. Rapamycin, a specific inhibitor of S6 kinase, inhibited PRL-induced mitogenesis *(100)*.

The PKC Pathway

The PKC pathway of signal transduction is important for PRL-induced cell proliferation *(101)*. The phosphoinositide cycle plays a role in signal transduction for PRL, which then activates PKC. Endogenously added phospholipase C, an enzyme that hydrolyzes L-α-phosphoinositol 4,5-diphosphate (PIP2) to D-myo-inositol trisphosphate and diaclglycerol, elicited PRL-like effects on ornithine decarboxylase activity and RNA synthesis in pregnant mouse mammary gland explants in culture *(102)*. We have reported in NOG-8 mammary cells that PRL activates and translocates PKC to the membranes within 5–10 min *(103)*. In addition, activation of PKC by PRL occurs in splenocytes, liver, hypothalamus, and Nb2 cells *(104,105)*. Waters and Rillema *(106)*, using explants from mouse mammary glands, showed translocation of PKC upon PRL treatment. In addition, activation of nuclear PKC by PRL has been reported in Nb2 cells *(99,104,107)*. The phosphorylation and activation of PI3-kinase for signal transduction of PRL in Nb2 cells have been reported *(108)*.

The SHC-Grb Pathway

Growth hormone receptor, which is a member of the same receptor family as the PRL receptor, activates the JAK-SHC pathway in 3T3-F442A cells *(109)*. The association of JAK2 with SHC occurs in a rapid and transient manner. JAK2 is associated with SHC proteins in Nb2 cells upon 15 min of PRL treatment *(94)*. In breast cells, both normal and malignant, we have shown that PRL can phosphorylate SHC proteins within 1 min of hormone treatment followed by association with the Grb2-Sos complex in these cells. Also JAK2 is phosphorylated and associated with SHC protein upon PRL activation in these mammary epithelial cells *(110)*. Thus, for PRL signal transduction, both the JAK-STAT and the SHC-ras-MAP kinase pathways (Fig. 1) are operative for induction of the mitogenic response in human breast cancer cells. Possible crosstalk between the MAP kinase pathway and the JAK-STAT pathway has been suggested *(111)*.

Early Response Genes

Modulation of early response genes and late response genes in the signaling pathways of a mitogen results in an increase in cell growth. PRL has been shown to induce transcription of early genes in a number of systems. Ovine PRL, which is known to be involved in proliferation of cells, stimulates expression of c-*myc (112)*. Recently Berlanga et al. *(89)* showed that in hepatocytes, after 30 min of PRL treatment, there is a rapid induction of the expression of the proto-oncogenes c-*fos*, c-*jun*, and c-*src* even in the presence of cyclohexamide. This suggests that PRL stimulates the expression of genes with AP-1 or SRE sequences in their promoter regions. *Pim-1*, an early response gene, is stimulated by PRL during mitogenesis of Nb2 cells *(113)*. Peak expression occurs at 2–4 h of PRL treatment and is not affected by cyclohexamide. *Pim-1*, a proto-oncogene that encodes a conserved cytosolic serine/threonine protein kinase, is rapidly induced in hematopoietic cells upon mitogen stimulation. Another early activation gene induced over 20-fold in Nb2 cells by PRL is interferon regulatory factor-1 (IRF-1). This gene is induced twice by PRL in a single cell cycle, first during G1 at 30–60 min and again during early S phase at 10–12 h of hormone treatment *(114)*. The second peak of IRF-1 mRNA expression in early S phase is dependent on the continuous presence of PRL throughout G_1 and is correlated tightly with DNA synthesis and subsequent cell proliferation. The GAS site in the IRF-1 promoter is thought to act as a PRL-responsive element that responds to the mitogenic signal of PRL in T-cells. Its activation in breast cells has not been established.

Late Response Genes

Cyclins play an important role in the progression of the cell cycle *(115)*. Several cyclins are amplified in malignant cells compared with their normal counterparts. *Cyclin D1* is among the most commonly overexpressed oncogenes in breast cancer. *Cyclin D1* knockout mice have abnormal mammary gland development; they are devoid of PRL-dependent lobuloalveolar structures in the mature gland *(116)*. In addition, following PRL stimulation of quiescent Nb2 cells, *cyclin D2* mRNA level increases in mid-G_1 phase and decreases sharply before S phase. Cyclin D3 level increases in late G_1/early S phase and gradually decreases during S phase *(117)*. Hosokawa et al. *(117)* cloned both *cyclin D2* and *D3* genes but were unable to identify *cyclin D1* in these rat lymphoma cells. Further elucidation of the activation of specific late response genes should help to clarify the distinguishing events in PRL-induced mitogenesis vs differentiation.

THE ANTILACTOGEN BINDING SITE (ALBS)

That the mammary gland can make its own PRL and that the majority of human breast tumors contain PRL receptors suggest that antagonists of PRL, acting directly at the

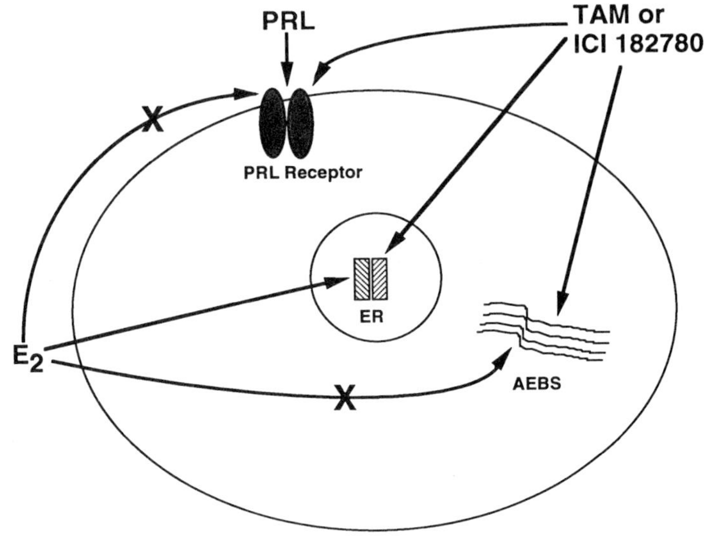

Fig. 2. Interactions at the antilactogen binding site (ALBS) on the PRL receptor.

receptor level, might present an alternate clinical approach to controlling this disease in PRL-responsive tumors. Included among these are mutants of hGH and hPRL, some of which have been shown to have antilactogenic activity in vitro under defined growth conditions *(107,118–122)*. In addition, tamoxifen (TAM), the first line of therapy in pre- and postmenopausal ER-positive breast cancer patients, is also an antilactogen *(123)*. TAM therapy has been shown to be effective in 14–30% of ER-negative breast cancer patients *(124–126)*. Frequently, inhibition of cell proliferation in vitro with lower concentrations of TAM can be reversed by estrogens. However, the growth rates cannot be restored by estradiol in the presence of higher concentrations of the antiestrogen *(127)*. Micromolar concentrations of TAM inhibit the growth of several ER-negative human breast cancer cell lines *(45,128,129)*. Besides the ER, there are several other cellular proteins that may be directly affected by TAM *(123)*. Pollak et al. *(130)* have suggested that during TAM therapy, there is a decrease in circulating IGF-I, which could account for the estrogen-independent response in some patients. Others have suggested that direct interaction of TAM with PKC may be responsible *(131)*. We have shown that the antilactogenic activity of TAM results from interaction with the antilactogen binding site (ALBS) *(132)*, which is located on the PRL receptor.

The ALBS is a member of the family of high-affinity membrane-associated binding sites called antiestrogen binding sites (AEBS) *(133,134)*, which have been identified in a variety of tissues *(135,136)*. Faye et al. *(137)* isolated a clone of MCF-7 cells, RTx6, that was TAM resistant. This resistant clone differed from the parent MCF-7 cells in having no AEBS but was identical to the parent cells with respect to the ER content and affinity. These cells could not be inhibited by TAM, whereas MCF-7 cells were. Antiestrogens, acting through the ALBS, inhibit the growth of PRL-responsive cells, even in the absence of ER *(45,138)*. We showed that the ALBS, located on cellular membranes, binds TAM and related non-steroidal antiestrogens with high affinity but does not bind estrogens (Fig. 2) *(123,139)*. It is through the ALBS that TAM inhibits PRL-induced growth of ER negative Nb2 rat lymphoma cells *(140)*; the effects are not reversed by estradiol. The order of affinities of the various antiestrogens (TAM, 4-OH-TAM, nafoxidine, -2-(4-tert-butyl-phenoxy)ethyl-diethylamine hydrochloride, LY156758, and LY117018) for the ALBS parallels the order of their potencies as growth and lactogen binding inhibitors. We have also shown that binding of lactogenic hormones to particulate and solubilized microsomal membranes isolated from normal mammary glands of lactating mice was inhibited by direct addition of 10^{-10} *M* or greater concentrations of TAM to the binding assays *(139)*. Estradiol and other antiestrogens such as BPEA, LY117018, and LY156758 did not have this effect. Maximal inhibition of PRL binding by TAM was observed in the light microsomes that contain the plasma membranes.

In studies to characterize the relationship of the ALBS to the PRL receptor *(132)*, we found that TAM acts by inhibiting the binding of PRL to its receptor rather than promoting dissociation of the hormone-receptor complex. TAM decreases the number of binding sites without changing the receptor's affinity for PRL. The ALBS and PRL receptor copurify on either PRL-Sepharose or TAM-Sepharose affinity columns; both are recognized by the anti-PRL receptor monoclonal antibody B6.2 *(132)*. Both the ER-positive T47D and the ER-negative T47Dco cell lines bind lactogenic hormones specifically, and this binding was inhibited by 30–50% when 10^{-11} *M* TAM was added directly to the T47D live cell binding reaction *(45)*. At 10^{-9} *M*, TAM inhibited binding by 70–90% with complete inhibition at 10^{-7} *M* TAM. TAM at 10^{-7} *M* completely inhibited PRL-induced growth for both cell lines. Thus, we concluded that the ALBS is on the PRL receptor, and TAM and other related, nonsteroidal, triphenylethylene antiestrogens can inhibit growth of ER-negative human breast cancer cells through this mechanism.

Unfortunately, TAM retains estrogen agonist activity through the ER in some tissues, and some human breast cancers develop resistance to TAM over time. Therefore, another class of novel steroidal antiestrogens with no intrinsic agonist activity was developed *(141,142)*. Members of this class of "pure" antiestrogens, such as ICI 182780, a 7α-alkylsulfinyl analog of estradiol, are up to two orders of magnitude more potent than the triphenylethylene compounds in terms of inhibition of ER-positive human breast cancer cell growth in culture. In addition, treating nude mice with ICI 182780 inhibited the growth of ER-positive MCF-7 human breast tumor implants that had acquired TAM resistance *(143)*. These data suggest an additive effect of the steroidal and nonsteroidal antiestrogens in ER-positive breast cancer. Phase I clinical trials with the "pure" antiestrogen have given promising results. Patients who had received adjuvant TAM and subsequently recurred, or who had relapsed following an initial favorable response to the antiestrogenic drug, gained further benefit from ICI 182780 treatment *(144)*. Thus these "pure" antiestrogens appear to have a role as a second-line therapy in ER-positive patients who fail primary TAM treatment.

In our studies *(45)*, ICI 182780 was able to block PRL binding in both ER-positive and ER-negative cells at much lower concentrations when compared with TAM; 10^{-11} *M* ICI 182780 inhibited PRL binding by more than 85%, and at 10^{-9} *M* there was 100% inhibition of PRL binding. ICI 182780 was also able to inhibit PRL-induced growth in the ER-negative cells, but at a much lower concentration (10^{-11} *M*) than TAM. The effect of ICI 182780 was specific for the PRL-induced growth. Growth of the cells resumed after removing TAM or ICI 182780 from the media at 3 d of culture, indicating that they are cytostatic agents. Their effects were neither additive nor synergistic, suggesting a similar mode of action. When specific TAM binding was performed in the presence of the anti-PRL receptor MAb B6.2, binding was inhibited in a concentration-dependent manner.

This suggests a direct interaction of TAM with the PRL receptor in these cells and supports the idea that both TAM and, by inference, ICI 182780 act through the ALBS on ER-negative breast cancer cells.

Work from several laboratories *(145,146)* supports the involvement of transforming growth factor-β (TGF-β) in TAM-mediated inhibition of ER-positive cancer cells. Several human breast cancer cell lines secrete active TGF-β into the medium. The expression of mRNA for TGF-β1, -β2, or -β3 varied with the different cell lines studied *(147)*. Knabbe et al. *(145)* reported that treatment of the ER-positive breast cancer cell line MCF-7 with growth-inhibitory concentrations of TAM induced an 8–27-fold increase in secreted TGF-β. The secreted TGF-β was in the active form and inhibited the growth of an ER-negative breast cancer cell line, MDA-MB 231. In addition, Warri et al. *(148)* reported elevated TGF-β1 gene expression in association with the appearance of apoptosis in ER-positive breast cancer cells treated with the antiestrogen toremifene. Chen et al. *(149)* showed upregulation of TGF-β production and secretion in conjunction with apoptosis in MCF-7 breast cancer cells treated with TAM. Perry et al. *(150)* reported that TAM induced morphological and biochemical changes typical of apoptosis in ER-positive and ER-negative breast cancer cells. By contrast, Arrick et al. *(147)* reported no effect of either estrogen or TAM on expression of mRNA for any members of the TGF-β family in ER-negative MDA-MB-231 cells.

Since we demonstrated that 10^{-9} *M* TAM inhibited PRL-induced proliferation of ER-negative T47Dco cells by 87% under serum-free conditions *(45)*, we considered the possibility that this effect may be due to autocrine TGF-β. We demonstrated that these cells contain the 70-kDa type II TGF-β receptor, which is crucial for transmembrane signaling *(151,152)* and that exogenously added TGF-β1 is capable of significantly reducing their proliferation even in the presence of PRL. Our results *(153)* also showed that TAM, in the absence of PRL, induced TGF-β1 but not TGF-β2 or TGF-β3 synthesis and secretion by these cells. However, the mitogen PRL inhibited TAM's induction of TGF-β1 even while TAM was inhibiting PRL-induced proliferation. No protein was secreted in the presence of PRL ± TAM. In contrast to ER-positive cells, the ER-negative cells secrete TGF-β1 in a biologically inactive form. Therefore, it appears that inhibition of PRL-induced growth of this ER-negative human breast cancer cell line by TAM is not mediated by members of the TGF-β family in vitro. The data do not rule out the possibility that, in vivo, an activated TGF-β may be involved in TAM-induced growth inhibition of ER-negative breast cancer. It is possible that a paracrine TGF-β results from cells associated with the breast epithelial cells. Several laboratories reported that stromal fibroblasts secrete negative growth modulators, including TGF-β, which act upon neighboring cancer cells, irrespective of ER status *(154,155)*.

Using the ER-negative, mouse mammary epithelial cell line NOG-8, we showed that TAM inhibited PRL binding *(138)*. Subsequently, TAM at concentrations as low as 10^{-9} *M*, rapidly inhibited PRL signal transduction through raf-1, MEK, and MAP kinase. This, in turn, led to inhibition of PRL-induced growth of these PRL-responsive mammary cells. Thus it appears that TAM acts primarily by inhibiting PRL's binding to its receptor and subsequently blocking the hormone's signal transduction pathways.

CONCLUSIONS

The role of PRL in human breast cancer is still largely undefined. The ability of this hormone to stimulate growth of human breast cancer cells in culture coupled with the presence of active receptors for PRL on the majority of breast carcinomas suggests that this peptide hormone is an active player in this disease. Understanding its role is complicated by the fact that human breast cancer cells synthesize and secrete significant amounts of biologically active PRL. These data suggest that clinically useful reagents should be sought that act at the level of the target tissue. The drug tamoxifen, in addition to its action as an antiestrogen, is also an antilactogen and hence may have clinical usefulness in patients whose tumors are PRL receptor positive even if they are ER negative.

REFERENCES

1. Vonderhaar BK (1987) Prolactin: transport, function, and receptors in mammary gland development and differentiation, In: *The Mammary Gland* (Neville MC, Daniel CW, eds.), Plenum, New York, pp. 383–438.
2. Vonderhaar BK (1984) Hormones and growth factors in mammary gland development, In: *Control of Cell Growth and Proliferation* (Veneziale CM, ed.), Van Nostrand, Reinhold, New York, pp. 11–33.
3. Nagasawa H, Miur K, Niki K, Namiki H (1985) Interrelationship between prolactin and progesterone in normal mammary gland growth in SHN virgin mice. Exp Clin Endocrinol 86:357–360.
4. Muhlbock O, Boot LM (1959) Induction of mammary cancer in mice without the mammary tumor agent by isografts of hypophyses. Cancer Res 19:402–412.
5. Boot LM, Muhlbock O, Ropcke G (1962) Prolactin and the induction of mammary tumors in mice. Gen Comp Endocrinol 2:601–602.
6. Welsch C, Nagasawa H (1977) Prolactin and murine mammary tumorigenesis: a review. Cancer Res 37:951–963.
7. Vonderhaar BK, Biswas R (1987) Prolactin effects and regulation of its receptors in human mammary tumor cells, In: *Cellular and Molecular Biology of Mammary Cancer* (Medina D, Kidwell W, Hepner G, Anderson E, eds.), Plenum, New York, pp. 205–219.
8. Boyns AR, Buchan R, Cole EN, Forrest APM, Griffiths K (1973) Basal prolactin blood levels in three strains of rat with differing incidence of 7, 12-dimethylbenzanthracene-induced mammary tumors in rats. Eur J Cancer 9:169–171.
9. Mershon J, Sall W, Mitchner N, Ben-Jonathan N (1995) Prolactin is a local growth factor in rat mammary tumors. Endocrinology 136:3619–3623.
10. Welsch CW, Gribler C (1973) Prophylaxis of spontaneously developing mammary carcinoma in C3H/HeJ female mice by suppression of prolactin. Cancer Res 33:2939–2946.
11. Holtkamp W, Nagel GA, Wander HE, Rauschecker HF, VonHeyden D (1984) Hyperprolactenemia is an indicator of progressive disease and poor prognosis in advanced breast cancer. Int J Cancer 34:323–328.
12. Das R, Vonderhaar BK (1997) Prolactin as a mitogen in mammary cells. J Mammary Gland Biol Neoplasia 2:29–39.
13. Love RR, Rose DP (1985) Elevated bioactive prolactin in women at risk for familial breast cancer. Eur J Cancer Clin Oncol 21:1553–1554.
14. Love RR, Rose DR, Surawicz TS, Newcomb PA (1991) Prolactin and growth hormone levels in premenopausal women with breast cancer and healthy women with a strong family history of breast cancer. Cancer 68:1401–1405.
15. Haus E, Lakatua DJ, Halberg F, Halberg E, Cornelissen G, Sackett LL, et al. (1980) Chronobiological studies of plasma prolactin in women in Kyushu, Japan and Minnesota, USA. J Clin Endocrinol Metab 51:632–640.
16. Holdaway IM, Mason BH, Gibbs EE, Rajasoorya C, Lethaby A, Hopkins KD, et al. (1997) Seasonal variation in the secretion of mammotrophic hormones in normal women and women with previous breast cancer. Breast Cancer Res Treat 42:15–22.
17. Patel DD, Bhatavdekar JM, Chikhlikar PR, Ghosh N, Suthar TP, Shah NG, et al. (1996) Node negative breast carcinoma: hyperprolactinemia and/or overexpression of p53 as an independent predictor of poor prognosis compared to newer and established prognosticators. J Surg Oncol 62:86–92.
18. Lissoni P, Barni S, Cazzaniga M, Ardizzoia A, Rovelli F, Tancici G, et al. (1995) Prediction of recurrence inoperable breast cancer by postoperative changes in prolactin secretion. Oncology 52:439–442.
19. Barni S, Lissoni P, Brivio F, Fumagalli L, Merlini D, Cataldo M, et al. (1994) Serum levels of insulin-like growth factor-I in operable breast cancer in relation to the main prognostic variables and their perioperative changes in relation to those of prolactin. Tumori 80:212–215.

20. Purnell DM, Hillman EA, Heatfield BM, Trump BF (1982) Immunoreactive prolactin in epithelial cells of normal and cancerous human breast and prostate detected by the unlabeled antibody peroxidase-antiperoxidase method. Cancer Res 42:2317–2324.
21. Agarwal PK, Tandon S, Agarwal AK, Kumar S (1989) Highly specific sites of prolactin binding in benign and malignant breast disease. Indian J Exp Biol 27:1035–1038.
22. Codegone ML, DiCarlo R, Muccioli G, Bussolati G (1981) Histology and cytometrics in human breast cancers assayed for the presence of prolactin receptors. Tumori 67:549–552.
23. Peyrat JP, DeWailly D, Djiane J, Kelly PA, Vandewalle B, Bonneterre J, et al. (1981) Total prolactin binding sites in human breast cancer biopsies. Breast Cancer Res Treat 1:369–373.
24. Bonneterre J, Peyrat JP, Vandewalle B, Beuscart R, Vie MC, Cappelaere P (1982) Prolactin receptors in human breast cancer. Eur J Cancer Clin Oncol 18:1157–1162.
25. L'Hermite-Baleriaux M, Casteels S, Vokaer A, Loriaus C, Noel G, L'Hermite M (1984) Prolactin and prolactin receptors in human breast disease. Prog Cancer Res Ther 31:325–334.
26. Wang DY, Hampson S, Kwa HG, Moore JW, Bulbrook RD, Fentiman IS, et al. (1986) Serum prolactin levels in women with breast cancer and their relationship to survival. Eur J Cancer Clin Oncol 22:487–492.
27. Ingram DM, Nottage EM, Roberts AN (1990) Prolactin and breast cancer risk. Med J Austr 153:469–473.
28. Henson JC, Coune A, Staquet M (1972) Clinical trial of 2-Br-a-ergocryptine (CB154) in advanced breast cancer. Eur J Cancer 8:155–156.
29. Pearson OH, Manni A (1978) Hormonal control of breast cancer growth in women and rats, In: *Current Topics in Experimental Endocrinology* (Martini L, James VHT, eds.), Academic Press, New York, pp. 75–92.
30. Manni A, Boucher AE, Demers LM, Harvey HA, Lipton A, Simmonds MA, et al. (1989) Endocrine effects of combined somatostatin analog and bromocriptine therapy in women with advanced breast cancer. Breast Cancer Res Treat 14:289–298.
31. Anderson E, Ferguson JE, Morten H, Shalet SM, Robinson EL, Howell A (1993) Serum immunoreactive and bioactive lactogenic hormones in advanced breast cancer patients treated with bromocriptine and octeotide. Eur J Cancer 29A:209–217.
32. Salih H, Brander W, Flax H, Hobbs JR (1972) Prolactin dependence in human breast cancers. Lancet 2:1103–1105.
33. Welsch CW, Iturri GC, Brennan MJ (1976) DNA synthesis of human, mouse, and rat mammary carcinomas in vitro: influence of insulin and prolactin. Cancer 38:1272–1281.
34. Peyrat JP, Djiane J, Bonneterre J, Vandewalle B, Vennin P, et al. (1984) Stimulation of DNA synthesis by prolactin in human breast tumor explants. Relation to prolactin receptors. Anticancer Res 4:257–261.
35. Calaf G, Garrido F, Moyano C, Rodriguez R (1986) Influence of hormones on DNA synthesis of breast tumors in culture. Breast Cancer Res Treat 8:223–232.
36. Burke RE, Gaffney EV (1978) Prolactin can stimulate general protein synthesis in human breast cancer cells (MCF-7) in long-term culture. Life Sci 23:901–906.
37. Wilson GD, Woods KL, Walker RA, Howell A (1980) Effect of prolactin on lactalbumin production by normal and malignant breast tissue in organ culture. Cancer Res 40:486–489.
38. Malarkey WB, Kennedy M, Allred LE, Milo G (1983) Physiological concentrations of prolactin can promote the growth of human breast tumor cells in culture. J Clin Endocrinol Metab 56:673–677.
39. Manni A, Wright C, Davis G, Glenn J, Joehl R, Feil P (1986) Promotion by prolactin of the growth of human breast neoplasms cultured in vitro in the soft agar clonogenic assay. Cancer Res 46:1669–1672.
40. Shiu RP, Paterson JA (1984) Alterations of cell shape, adhesion, and lipid accumulation in human breast cancer cells (T-47D) by human prolactin and growth hormone. Cancer Res 44:1178–1186.
41. Shafie SM, Grantham FH (1981) Role of hormones in the growth and regression of human breast cancer cells (MCF-7) transplanted into athymic nude mice. J Natl Cancer Inst 67:51–56.
42. McManus MJ, Welsch CW (1984) The effect of estrogen, progesterone, thyroxine, and human placental lactogen on DNA synthesis of human breast ductal epithelium maintained in athymic nude mice. Cancer 54:1920–1927.
43. Biswas R, Vonderhaar BK (1987) Role of serum in prolactin responsiveness of MCF-7 human breast cancer cells in long term tissue culture. Cancer Res 47:3509–3514.
44. Das R, Ginsburg E, Vonderhaar BK (1994) Tamoxifen as an antilactogen in human breast cancer cells, In: *Proceedings of the International Cancer Congress* (Rao RS, Deo MG, Sanghvi LD, Mittra I, eds.), Monduzzi, Bologna, pp. 1487–1491.
45. Das R, Ginsburg E, Terry-Koroma B, Vonderhaar BK (1997) Tamoxifen and ICI 182780 inhibit PRL-induced growth of ER+ and ER- human breast cancer cells. Submitted.

46. Lemus-Wilson A, Kelly PA, Blask DE (1995) Melatonin blocks the stimulatory effects of prolactin on human breast cancer cell growth in culture. Br J Cancer 72:1435–1440.
47. Lachelin GCL, Yen SSC, Alksne JF (1977) Hormonal changes following hypophysectomy in humans. Obstet Gynecol 50:333–339.
48. Sinha YN (1995) Structural variants of prolactin: occurrence and physiological significance. Endocr Rev 16:354–369.
49. Clevenger CV, Russell DH, Appasamy PM, Prystowsky MB (1990) Regulation of IL-2-driven T-lymphocyte proliferation by prolactin. Proc Natl Acad Sci USA 87:6460–6464.
50. Gellerson B, Kempf R, Teglmann R, DiMattia GE (1994) Nonpituitary human prolactin gene transcription is independent of pit-1 and differentially controlled in lymphocytes and in endometrial stroma. Mol Endocrinol 8:356–373.
51. Richards RG, Hartman SM (1996) Human dermal fibroblast cells express prolactin in vitro. J Invest Dermatol 106:1250–1255.
52. Ginsburg E, Vonderhaar BK (1995) Prolactin synthesis and secretion by human breast cancer cells. Cancer Res 55:2591–2595.
53. Steinmetz RW, Grant AL, Malven PV (1993) Transcription of prolactin gene in milk secretory cells of the rat mammary gland. J Endocrinol 36:271–276.
54. Kurtz A, Bristol LA, Toth BE, Lazar-Wesley E, Takacs L, Kacsoh B (1993) Mammary epithelial cells of lactating rats express prolactin messenger ribonucleic acid. Biol Reprod 48:1095–1103.
55. LeProvost F, Leroux C, Martin P, Gaye P, Djiane J (1994) Prolactin gene expression in ovine and caprine mammary gland. Neuroendocrinology 60:305–313.
56. Clevenger CV, Chang WP, Ngo W, Pasha TLM, Montone KT, Tomaszewski JE (1995) Expression of prolactin and prolactin receptor in human breast carcinoma. Am J Pathol 146:695–705.
57. Ginsburg E, Das R, Vonderhaar BK (1997) Prolactin: an autocrine growth factor in the mammary gland, In: *Biological Signalling in the Mammary Gland* (Wilde CJ, Peaker M, Taylor E, eds.), Ayr, Scotland, pp 47–58.
58. Ginsburg E, Vonderhaar BK (1997) Prolactin synthesis in human breast cancer cells is irrelevant to ER status. Cancer Res. Submitted.
59. Bancroft FC, Tashjian AH (1971) Growth in suspension culture of rat pituitary cells which produce growth hormone and prolactin. Exp Cell Res 64:125–128.
60. Tanaka T, Shiu RPC, Gout PW, Beer CT, Noble RL, Friesen HG (1980) A new sensitive and specific bioassay for lactogenic hormones: measurement of prolactin and growth hormone in human serum. J Clin Endocrinol Metab 51:1058–1063.
61. Markoff E, Sigel MB, Lacour N, Seavey BK, Friesen HG, Lewis UJ (1988) Glycosylation selectively alters the biological activity of prolactin. Endocrinology 123:1303–1306.
62. Lewis UL, Singh RNP, Lewis LJ (1989) Two forms of glycosylated prolactin have different pigeon crop sac-stimulating activities. Endocrinology 124:1558–1563.
63. Walker AM (1994) Phosphorylated and nonphosphorylated prolactin isoforms. Trends Endocrinol Metab 5:195–200.
64. Wicks JR, Brooks CL (1995) Biological activity of phosphorylated and dephosphorylated bovine prolactin. Mol Cell Endocrinol 112:223–229.
65. Pellegrini I, Lebrun JJ, Ali S, Kelly PA (1992) Expression of prolactin and its receptors in human lymphoid cells. Mol Endocrinol 6:1023–1031.
66. Sinha YN, DePaolo LV, Haro LS, Singh RN P., Jacobsen BP, Scott KE, et al. (1991) Isolation and biochemical properties of four forms of glycosylated porcine prolactin. Mol Cell Endocrinol 80:203–213.
67. Hoffman T, Penel C, Ronin C (1993) Glycosylation of human prolactin regulates hormone bioactivity and metabolic clearance. J Endocrinol Invest 16:807–816.
68. Price AE, Loginenko KB, Higgins EA, Cole ES, Richards S (1995) Studies on the microheterogeneity and in vitro activity of glycosylated and nonglycosylated recombinant human prolactin separated using a novel purification process. Endocrinology 136:4827–4833.
69. Young KH, Buhi WC, Horseman N, Davis J, Kraeling R, Linzer D, et al. (1990) Biological activities of glycosylated and nonglycosylated porcine prolactin. Mol Cell Endocrinol 71:155–162.
70. Shaw-Bruha CM, Pirrucello SJ, Shull JD (1997) Expression of the prolactin gene in normal and neoplastic human breast tissues and human mammary cell lines: promoter usage and alternative mRNA splicing. Breast Cancer Res Treat 4:243–253.
71. Kelly PA, Djiane J, Postel-Vinay MC, Edery M (1991) The prolactin/growth hormone receptor family. Endocr Rev 12:235–251.

72. Kelly PA, Ali S, Rozakis M, Goujon L, Nagano M, Pellegrini I, et al. (1993) The growth hormone/prolactin receptor family. Recent Prog Horm Res 48:123–164.
73. Ali S, Edery M, Pellegrini I, Lesueur L, Paly J, Djiane J, et al. (1992) The Nb2 form of prolactin receptor is able to activate a milk protein gene promoter. Mol Endocrinol 6:1242–1248.
74. Lesueur L, Edery M, Ali S, Paly J, Kelly PA, Djiane J (1991) Comparison of long and short forms of the prolactin receptor on prolactin-induced milk protein gene transcription. Proc Natl Acad Sci USA 88:482–828.
75. O'Neal KD, Yu Lee L (1994) Differential signal transduction of the short, Nb2, and long prolactin receptors. J Biol Chem 269:26076–26082.
76. Das R, Vonderhaar BK (1995) Transduction of prolactin's growth signal through both the long and short forms of the prolactin receptor. Mol Endocrinol 9:1750–1759.
77. Goffin V, Kelly PA (1997) The prolactin/growth hormone receptor family: structure/function relations. J Mammary Gland Biol Neoplasia 2:7–17.
78. Rui H, Kirken RA, Farrar WL (1994) Activation of receptor-associated tyrosine kinase JAK2 by prolactin. J Biol Chem 269:5364–5368.
79. David M, Petricoin EF, Igarashi KI, Feldman GM, Finbloom DS, Larner AC (1994) Prolactin activates the interferon-regulated p91 transcription factor and the JAK2 kinase by tyrosine phosphorylation. Proc Natl Acad Sci USA 91:7174–7178.
80. Campbell GS, Argetsinger LS, Ihle JN, Kelly PA, Rillema JA, Carter-Su C (1994) Activation of JAK (JAK2) tyrosine kinase by prolactin receptors in NB (NB2) cells and mouse mammary gland explants. Proc Natl Acad Sci USA 91:5232–5236.
81. Dusanter-Fourt I, Muller O, Ziemiecki A, Mayeux P, Drucker B, Djiane J, et al. (1994) Identification of JAK protein tyrosine kinases as signaling molecules for prolactin. Functional analysis of prolactin receptor and prolactin-erythropoietin receptor chimera expressed in lymphoid cells. EMBO J 13:2538–2591.
82. Waters MJ, Daniel N, Bignon C, Dijiane J (1995) The rabbit mammary gland prolactin receptor is tyrosine phosphorylated in response to prolactin in vivo and in vitro. J Biol Chem 270:5136–5143.
83. DaSilva L, Rui H, Erwin RA, Howard OMZ, Kirken RA, Malabarba MG, et al. (1996) Prolactin recruits STAT1, STAT3 and STAT5 independent of conserved receptor tyrosine TYR402, TYR479, TYR515 and TYR580. Mol and Cell Endocrinol 117:131–140.
84. Wakao H, Gouilleux F, Groner B (1994) Mammary gland factor (MGF) is a novel member of the cytokine regulated transcription factor gene family and confers the prolactin response. EMBO J 13:2182–2191.
85. Liu X, Robinson GW, Gouilleux F, Groner B, Hennighausen L (1995) Cloning and expression of Stat5 and an additional homologue (Stat5b) involved in prolactin signal transduction in mouse mammary tissue. Proc Natl Acad Sci USA 92:8831–8835.
86. Liu X, Robinson GW, Wagner KU, Garrett L, Wynshaw-Boris A, Hennighausen L (1996) Stat5a is mandatory for adult mammary gland development and lactogenesis. Genes Dev 11:179–186.
87. Das R, Vonderhaar BK (1996) Activation of raf-1, MEK and MAP kinase in prolactin responsive mammary cells. Breast Cancer Res Treat 40:141–149.
88. Darnell Jr JE, Kerr IM, Stark GR (1994) Jak-STAT pathways and transcriptional activation in response to IFNs and other extracellular signaling proteins. Science 264:1415–1421.
89. Berlanga JJ, Vara JAF, Martin-Perez J, Garcia-Ruiz JP (1995) Prolactin receptor is associated with c-src kinase in rat liver. Mol Endocrinol 9:1461–1467.
90. Clevenger CV, Medaglia MV (1994) The protein tyrosine kinase p59fyn is associated with prolactin (PRL) receptor and is activated by PRL stimulation of T-lymphocytes. Mol Endocrinol 8:674–681.
91. Clevenger CV, Ngo W, Sokol DL, Luger SM, Gewirtz AM (1995) Vav is necessary for prolactin-stimulated proliferation and is translocated into the nucleus of a T-cell line. J Biol Chem 270:13246–13253.
92. Ali S, Chen Z, Lebrun J-J, Vogel W, Kharitonenkov A, Kelly P, et al. (1996) PTP1D is a positive regulator of the prolactin signal leading to β-casein promoter activation. EMBO J 15:135–142.
93. Daniel N, Waters MJ, Bignon C, Djiane J (1996) Involvement of a subset of tyrosine kinases and phosphatases in regulation of the β-lactoglobulin gene promoter by prolactin. Mol Cell Endocrinol 118:25–35.
94. Erwin RA, Kirken RA, Malabarba MG, Farrar WL, Rui H (1995) Prolactin activates Ras via signaling proteins SHC, growth factor receptor bound 2 and son of sevenless. Endocrinology 136:3512–3518.
95. Elberg G, Rapoport MJ, Vashdi-Elberg D, Gertler A, Scechter Y (1996) Lactogenic hormones rapidly activate p21 ras/mitogen-activated protein kinase in Nb2-11C rat lymphoma cells. Endocrine 4:65–71.

96. Clevenger CV, Torigoe T, Reed JC (1994) Prolactin induces rapid phosphorylation and activation of prolactin receptor-associated RAF-1 kinase in a T-cell line. J Biol Chem 269:5559–5565.
97. Piccoletti R, Maroni P, Bendinelli P, Bernelli-Zazzera A (1994) Rapid stimulation of mitogen-activated protein kinase of rat liver by prolactin. Biochem J 303:429–433.
98. Buckley AR, Rao YP, Buckley DJ, Gout PW (1994) Prolactin-induced phosphorylation and nuclear translocation of MAP kinase in Nb2 lymphoma cells. Biochem Biophys Res Commun 204:1158–1164.
99. Ganguli S, Hu L, Menke P, Collier RJ, Gertler A (1996) Nuclear accumulation of multiple protein kinases during prolactin-induced proliferation of Nb2 rat lymphoma cells. J Cell Physiol 167:251–260.
100. Carey GB, Liberti JP (1995) Stimulation of receptor-associated kinase, tyrosine kinase, and MAP kinase is required for prolactin-mediated macromolecular biosynthesis and mitogenesis in Nb2 lymphoma. Arch Biochem Biophys 316:179–189.
101. Kiley SC, Welsh J, Narvaez CJ, Jaken S (1996) Protein kinase C isozymes and substrates in mammary carcinogenesis. J Mammary Gland Biol Neoplasia 1:177–187.
102. Rillema JA, Wing LY, Foley KA (1983) Effects of phospholipases on ornithine decarboxylase activity in mammary gland explants from midpregnancy mice. Endocrinology 113:2024–2028.
103. Banerjee R, Vonderhaar BK (1992) Prolactin induced protein kinase C activity in a mouse mammary epithelial cell line NOG-8. Mol Cell Endocrinol 90:61–67.
104. Buckley AR, Crowe PD, Russell DH (1988) Rapid activation of protein kinase C in isolated rat liver nuclei by prolactin, a known hepatic mitogen. Proc Natl Acad Sci USA 85:8649–8653.
105. Rillema JA, Waters SB, Tarrant TM (1989) Studies on the possible role of protein kinase C in the prolactin regulation of cell replication in Nb2 node lymphoma cells. Proc Soc Exp Biol Med 192:140–144.
106. Waters SB, Rillema JA (1989) Role of protein kinase C in the prolactin-induced responses in mouse mammary gland explants. Mol Cell Endocrinol 63:159–166.
107. Fan G, Rillema JA (1993) Prolactin stimulation of protein kinase C in isolated mouse mammary gland nuclei. Horm Metab Res 25:564–568.
108. Alsakkaf KA, Dobson PRM, Brown BL (1996) Activation of phosphatidylinositol 3-kinase by prolactin in Nb2 cells. Biochem Biophys Res Commun 221:779–784.
109. VanderKuur J, Allevato G, Billestrup N, Norstedt G, Carter-Su C (1995) Growth hormone-promoted tyrosyl phosphorylation of SHC proteins and SHC association with Grb2. J Biol Chem 270:7587–7593.
110. Das R, Vonderhaar BK (1996) Involvement of SHC, Grb2, Sos and ras in prolactin signal transduction in mammary cells. Oncogene 13:1139–1145.
111. David M, Petricoin E III, Benjamin C, Pine R, Weber MJ, Larner AC (1995) Requirement for MAP kinase (ERK2) activity in interferon α- and interferon β-stimulated gene expression through STAT proteins. Science 269:1721–1723.
112. Zabala MT, Garcia-Ruiz JP (1989) Regulation of expression of the messenger ribonucleic acid encoding the cytosolic form of phosphoenolpyruvate carboxykinase in liver and small intestine of lactating rats. Endocrinology 125:2587–2593.
113. Buckley AR, Buckley DJ, Leff MA, Hoover DS, Magnuson NS (1995) Rapid induction of pim-1 expression by prolactin and interleukin-2 in rat Nb2 lymphoma cells. Endocrinology 136:5252–5259.
114. Stevens AN, Wang Y, Sieger KA, Lu H-F, Yu-Lee LY (1995) Biphasic transcription regulation of the interferon regulatory factor-1 gene by prolactin: involvement of γ-interferon-activated sequence and stat-related proteins. Mol Endocrinol 9:513–525.
115. Musgrove EA, Hui R, Sweeney KJE, Watts CKW, Sutherland RL (1996) Cyclins and breast cancer. J Mammary Gland Biol Neoplasia 1:153–162.
116. Sicinski P, Donaher JL, Parker SB, Li T, Fazeli A, Gardner H, et al. (1995) Cyclin D1 provides a link between development and oncogenesis in the retina and breast. Cell 82:621–630.
117. Hosokawa Y, Onga T, Nakashima K (1994) Induction of D2 and D3 cyclin-encoding genes during promotion of the G1/S transition by prolactin in rat Nb2 cells. Gene 147:249–252.
118. Fuh G, Cunningham BC, Nagata S, Goeddel DV, Wells JA (1992) Rational design of potent antagonists to the human growth hormone receptor. Science 256:1677–1679.
119. Fuh G, Colosi P, Wood WI, Wells JA (1993) Mechanism-based design of prolactin receptor antagonists. J Biol Chem 268:5376–5381.
120. Fuh G, Wells JA (1995) Prolactin receptor antagonists that inhibit the growth of breast cancer cell lines. J Biol Chem 270:13133–13137.
121. Dattani MT, Hindmarsh PC, Brook GD, Robinson ICAF, Kopchick JJ, Marshall NJ (1995) G120R, a human growth hormone antagonist, shows zinc-dependent agonist and antagonist activity on Nb2 cells. J Biol Chem 270:9222–9226.

122. Mode A, Tollet P, Wells T, Carmignac DF, Clark RG, Chen WY, et al. (1996) The human growth hormone (hGH) antagonist G120RhGH does not antagonize GH in the rat, but has paradoxical agonist activity, probably via the prolactin receptor. Endocrinology 137:447–454.
123. Vonderhaar BK, Banerjee R (1991) Is tamoxifen also an antilactogen? Mol Cell Endocrinol 79:C159–C163.
124. Hawkins RA, Roberts MM, Forest AP M. (1980) Estrogen receptors and breast cancer: current status. Br J Surg 67:153–169.
125. Furr BJA, Jordan VC (1984) The pharmacology and clinical uses of tamoxifen. Pharmacol Ther 25:127–205.
126. Nolvadex Adjuvant Trial Organization (1985) Controlled trial of tamoxifen as single adjuvant agent in management of early breast cancer. Lancet 1: 836–839.
127. Sutherland RL, Watts CK W., Hall RE, Ruenitz PC (1987) Mechanism of growth inhibition by non-steroidal antioestrogens in human breast cancer cells. J Steroid Biochem 27:891–897.
128. Green MD, Whybourne AM, Taylor IW, Sutherland RL (1981) Effects of antioestrogens on the growth and cell cycle kinetics of cultured human mammary carcinoma cells, In: *Non-Steroidal Antiestrogens: Molecular Pharmacology and Antitumor Actions* (Sutherland RL, Jordan VC, eds.), Academic Press, New York, pp. 397–412.
129. Chouvet C, Vicard E, Frappart L, Falette N, Lefebvre MF, Saez S (1988) Growth inhibitory effect of 4-hydroxy-tamoxifen on the BT-20 mammary cancer cell line. J Steroid Biochem 31:655–663.
130. Pollak M, Constantino J, Polychronakas C, Blauer HG, Guyda H, Redmond C, et al. (1990) Effect of tamoxifen on serum insulin-like growth factor I levels of stage I breast cancer patients. J Natl Cancer Inst 82:1693–1697.
131. O'Brian CA, Liskamp RM, Solomon DH, Weinstein IB (1985) Inhibition of protein kinase C by tamoxifen. Cancer Res 45:2462–2465.
132. Das R, Biswas R, Vonderhaar BK (1993) Characteristics of the antilactogen binding site in mammary gland membranes. Mol Cell Endocrinol 98:1–8.
133. Sutherland RL, Foo MS (1979) Differential binding of antiestrogen by rat uterine and chick oviduct cytosol. Biochem Biophys Res Commun 91:183–191.
134. Sutherland RL, Murphy LC, Foo MS, Green MD, Whybourne AM, Krozowski ZS (1980) High-affinity anti-oestrogen binding sites distinct from the oestrogen receptor. Nature 288:273–275.
135. Gulino A, Pasqualini JR (1982) Heterogeneity of binding sites for tamoxifen and tamoxifen derivatives in estrogen target and non-target fetal organs of guinea pig. Cancer Res 42:1913–1921.
136. Mehta RG, Cerny WL, Moon RC (1984) Distribution of antiestrogen-specific binding sites in normal and neoplastic mammary gland. Oncology 41:387–392.
137. Faye JC, Fargin A, Valette A, Bayard F (1987) Antiestrogens, different sites of action than the estrogen receptor? Horm Res. 28:202–211.
138. Das R, Vonderhaar BK (1997) Tamoxifen inhibits prolactin signal transduction in estrogen receptor negative NOG-8 mammary epithelial cells. Cancer Lett 116:41–46.
139. Biswas R, Vonderhaar BK (1991) Tamoxifen inhibition of prolactin action in the mouse mammary gland. Endocrinology 128:532 -538.
140. Biswas R, Vonderhaar BK (1989) Antiestrogen inhibition of prolactin induced growth of the Nb2 rat lymphoma cell line. Cancer Res 49:6295–6299.
141. Wakeling AE, Bowler J (1988) Novel antiestrogens without partial agonist activity. J Steroid Biochem 31:645–653.
142. Wakeling AE, Dukes M, Bowler J (1991) A potent specific pure antiestrogen with clinical potential. Cancer Res 51:3867–3873.
143. Osborne CK, Jarman M, McCague R, Coronade EB, Hilsenbeck SG, Wakeling AE (1994) The importance of tamoxifen metabolism in tamoxifen-stimulated breast tumor growth. Cancer Chemother Pharmacol 34:89–95.
144. Nicholson RI, Gee JM, Manning DL, Wakeling AE, Montano MM, Katzenellenbogen BS (1995) Responses to pure antiestrogens (ICI 164384, ICI 182780) in estrogen-sensitive and -resistant experimental and clinical breast cancer. Ann NY Acad Sci 761:148–163.
145. Knabbe C, Lippman ME, Wakefield LM, Flanders KC, Kasid A, Derynk R, et al. (1987) Evidence that transforming growth factor-β is a hormonally regulated negative growth factor in human breast cancer cells. Cell 48:417–428.
146. Arteaga CL, Tandon AK, VonHoffDD, Osborne CK (1988) Transforming growth factor β: potential autocrine growth inhibitor of estrogen receptor-negative human breast cancer cells. Cancer Res 48:3898–3904.

147. Arrick BA, Korc M, Derynck R (1990) Differential regulation of expression of three transforming growth factor β species in human breast cancer cell lines by estradiol. Cancer Res 50:299–303.
148. Warri A, Huovinen RL, Laine AM, Martikainen PM, Härkönen PL (1993) Apoptosis in toremifene-induced growth inhibition of human breast cancer cells *in vivo* and *in vitro*. J Natl Cancer Inst 85:1412–1418.
149. Chen H, Tritton TR, Kenny N, Absher M, Chiu JF (1996) Tamoxifen induces TGF-β1 activity and apoptosis of human MCF-7 breast cancer cells in vitro. J Cell Biochem 61:9–17.
150. Perry RR, Kang Y, Greaves BR (1995) Relationship between tamoxifen-induced transforming growth factor β1 expression, cytosis and apoptosis in human breast cancer cells. Br J Cancer 72:1441–1446.
151. Lin HY, Wang XF, Ng-Eaton E, Weinberg RA, Lodish HF (1992) Expression cloning of the TGF-beta type II receptor, a functional transmembrane serine/threonine kinase. Cell 68:775–785.
152. Tsuchida K, Lewis KA, Mathews LS, Vale WW (1993) Molecular characterization of rat transforming growth factor-beta type II receptor. Biochem Biophys Res Commun 191:790–795.
153. Terry-Koroma B, Vonderhaar BK (1997) Tamoxifen inhibition of prolactin-induced growth of ER- T47Dco human breast cancer cells does not involve TGF-β. Submitted.
154. Colletta AA, Wakefield LM, Howell FV, vanRoozendaal KE, Danielpour D, Ebbs SR, et al. (1990) Anti-oestrogens induce the secretion of active transforming growth factor beta from human fetal fibroblasts. Br J Cancer 62:405–409.
155. Butta A, MacLennan K, Flanders KC, Sacks NPM, Smith I, McKinna A, et al. (1992) Induction of transforming growth factor β1 in human breast cancer *in vivo* following tamoxifen treatment. Cancer Res 52:4261–4264.

V

Endocrine Therapy of Breast Cancer

19 Pharmacology and Use of Antiestrogens in Treatment and Chemoprevention of Breast Cancer

William J. Gradishar, MD
and V. Craig Jordan, PhD, DSc

INTRODUCTION

Breast cancer represents an enormous public health problem for American women, who have a 1 in 8 chance of developing breast cancer in their lifetime *(1)*. In 1998, 178,700 new cases of breast cancer will be diagnosed in the United States, and breast cancer will account for 43,500 cancer deaths. Although early detection and improved treatments have begun to impact on breast cancer mortality, continued research focusing on the treatment of breast cancer is required to improve the outcome of patients afflicted with this disease *(2)*. Furthermore, new insights into the biology of breast cancer will be translated into chemoprevention strategies that can be applied to women determined to be at a high risk for developing breast cancer.

The prognosis of patients diagnosed with breast cancer is dependent on a number of factors, but stage of disease at diagnosis is the most powerful predictor of outcome. Of those patients diagnosed with breast cancer each year, the distribution of patients by stage of disease has been fairly constant: stage 0 (non-invasive, ductal carcinoma *in situ* [DCIS], 13%; stage I, 41%; stage II, 29%; stage III, 5%; stage IV, 4%; unknown, 8% *(3)*. The corresponding 5-year survival is as follows: stage 0, 98%; stage I, 95%; stage I, 70–85%; stage III, 40–50%; stage IV, <20% *(4)*. For those patients rendered free of disease following surgery (stages I–III), the probability that a given patient will develop recurrent disease and ultimately die from breast cancer corresponds to the likelihood of harboring microscopic disease, which increases with increasing stage of disease.

The current standard of care for treatment of breast cancer dictates that the majority of patients with early stage breast cancer receive adjuvant therapy following completion of local therapy (mastectomy or breast-conserving therapy with lumpectomy followed by radiation therapy) *(5)*. Adjuvant therapy generally takes the form of chemotherapy, endocrine therapy, or a combination of both modalities. The rationale for administering adjuvant therapy is to eradicate microscopic metastatic disease and thereby improve survival. For patients with metastatic disease (stage IV), the goals of treatment are palliative. The

From: *Contemporary Endocrinology: Endocrinology of Breast Cancer*
Edited by: A. Manni

choice of therapy in either the adjuvant or metastatic disease setting is based on clinical and biologic features of the disease.

HISTORICAL BACKGROUND FOR ENDOCRINE THERAPY OF BREAST CANCER

The relationship between endocrine manipulation as a potential therapy for breast cancer was first described over 100 years ago. In 1896 Beatson *(6)* demonstrated that the removal of the ovaries from premenopausal women with metastatic breast cancer would cause tumor regression. A few years later Boyd *(7)* reported that approximately one-third of all premenopausal women with metastatic breast cancer would show objective evidence of tumor regression after undergoing surgical oophorectomy, and these women gained approximately 1 year of additional life. Following the first two decades of the 20th century, interest in removing the ovaries surgically diminished as other methods of ablating the ovaries resulted in similar effects on tumor regression.

In 1922 DeCourmelles *(8)* demonstrated the same effect on metastatic disease by administering radiation to the ovaries, although there was a latent period of a few months before the effect was observed. Block et al. *(9)* later showed that this latent effect of radiation on ovarian function correlated with estrogen production reaching basal levels several months following treatment. Huggins and colleagues *(10)* at the University of Chicago revisited the concept of hormonal castration using surgical oophorectomy as a means of removing endogenous estrogen in premenopausal women with advanced breast cancer.

Once synthetic corticosteroids became clinically available in the 1950s, other forms of endocrine ablation became feasible, including surgical adrenalectomy *(10–12)* and hypophysectomy *(13)*. Multiple investigators reported tumor responses in 30–40% of premenopausal women undergoing these procedures. Regrettably, the morbidity and mortality of these surgical procedures were not insignificant. Ultimately, medical means of inducing an adrenalectomy were identified with drugs such as aminoglutethimide *(14)*. Although the precise mechanism responsible for this effect on tumor growth would not be understood for decades, a principle strategy for treatment of breast cancer evolved that focused on blocking or restricting the action of estradiol in its target tissue, the breast.

Much of the early work on hormonal manipulation of breast cancer focused on depriving the tumor of estrogen. However, in 1944 Haddow *(15)* reported that 4 of 13 patients with advanced disease responded to high-dose estrogen therapy and that tumors in postmenopausal patients were more likely to regress. Although many investigators attempted to discover why some patients responded to hormonal manipulation and others did not, their efforts were unsuccessful until Jensen and Jacobsen *(16)* discovered why estrogen target tissues such as the uterus and the vagina respond to estrogen. They synthesized tritiated estradiol and injected small quantities into immature female rats. Radioactivity was taken up and retained by estrogen-target tissue such as the uterus, vagina, and pituitary gland, whereas the radioactivity taken up by nontarget tissues such as muscle was not retained. They suggested that an estrogen receptor (ER) must be present to regulate estrogen action in estrogen-target tissues *(16)*.

Ultimately, the ER protein was isolated and characterized as an extractable protein from estrogen-target tissues by Toft and co-workers *(17)* in 1967. These findings led to the development of ER assays by Jensen et al. *(18)* that could be used to predict which

Table 1
Antitumor Response to Hormone Therapy by Receptor Status in Patients with Advanced Disease

Receptor status	*% Response*
ER+, PR+	75–80
ER+, PR-	25–30
ER-, PR+	40–45
ER-, PR-	<10

(Data from refs. *26* and *27*.)

patients with metastatic breast cancer would respond to endocrine manipulation. In unselected patients with metastatic breast cancer, 30–35% of cases will respond to hormonal manipulation, whereas 55–60% of patients with tumors known to be ER positive responded to hormonal manipulation *(18,19)*. Initially these observations were most useful for identifying patients most likely to benefit from endocrine ablation treatment strategies; however, once compounds known as antiestrogens were developed, the ER assays became very powerful predictors of treatment response for large numbers of patients. Additional insight into the biology of breast cancer was provided with the identification and characterization of the progesterone receptor (PR), which is an estrogen-regulated protein that can be synthesized only if the ER is functional. In 1975 Horwitz and McGuire *(20,21)* hypothesized that the presence of the PR in breast tumors would be a sensitive predictor of response to hormone therapy.

Most breast cancers express ER or PR or both (Table 1). The ER or PR receptor can be isolated from the primary tumor or a metastatic lesion *(22)* and is measured by a ligand-binding method *(23)* or by monoclonal antibodies used to determine receptors by flow cytometry *(24)*. Alternatively, tissue sections from the tumor can be used to determine cellular heterogeneity using immunohistochemistry, or receptors can be quantitated using an ER or PR immunoassay *(25)*. Cutoff points used to determine whether a given tumor is hormone receptor positive (+) or negative (–) have been the subject of much debate, especially since immunohistochemical methods are subjective, and the results are reported as the fraction of cells staining positive for the ER or PR. In general, assay methods that do quantitate the receptor are considered positive if the result is >10 fmol/mg cytosol protein.

The availability of tools to characterize a given breast tumor for the presence or absence of ER and PR led to the ability to predict the probability that a given patient would respond to hormonal manipulation (Table 1) *(26,27)*. Witliff *(26)* reported that of patients with tumors that are ER+/PR+, 75–80% would respond to hormonal therapy, whereas objective tumor responses would be observed in 25–30% and 40–45% of patients with ER+/PR– and ER–/PR+ tumors, respectively. Fewer than 10% of patients with ER–/PR– tumors will respond to hormonal manipulation *(26,27)*. Both Allegra *(28)* and Witliff *(26)* reported that older patients diagnosed with breast cancer were more likely to express ER compared with their younger counterparts (Table 2). Allegra *(28)* reported that 44% of breast cancer patients in the age group 40–49 years express ER, whereas 69% of those who are 70 years or older express ER. Similarly, Witliff *(26)* showed that 72% of premenopausal and 83% of postmenopausal breast cancer patients expressed the ER and

Table 2
Prevalence of Hormone Receptors in Breast Tumors

Receptors	*Premenopausal, %*	*Postmenopausal, %*
ER+, PR+ or both	72	83
ER+, PR-	12	15
ER-, PR+	15	5
ER-, PR-	28	17

(Data from refs. *26* and *28*.)

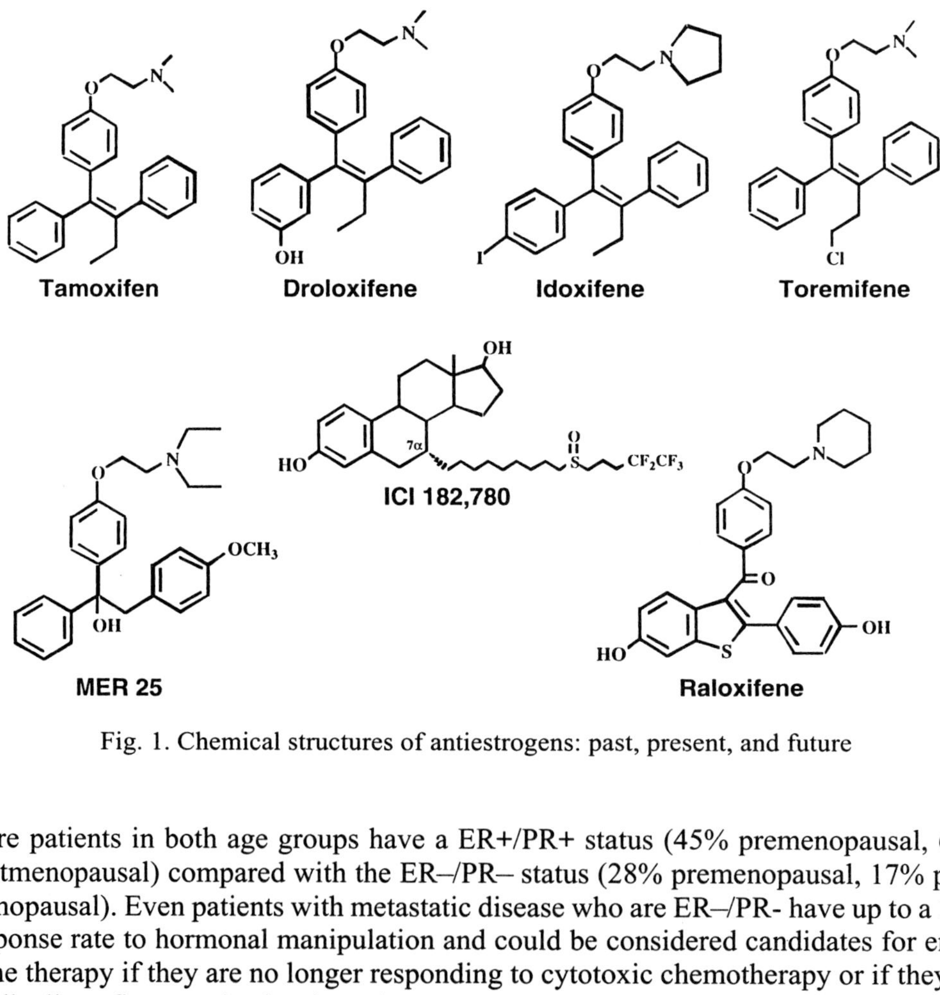

Fig. 1. Chemical structures of antiestrogens: past, present, and future

more patients in both age groups have a ER+/PR+ status (45% premenopausal, 63% postmenopausal) compared with the ER–/PR– status (28% premenopausal, 17% postmenopausal). Even patients with metastatic disease who are ER–/PR- have up to a 10% response rate to hormonal manipulation and could be considered candidates for endocrine therapy if they are no longer responding to cytotoxic chemotherapy or if they are medically unfit to receive it. These data suggest that most patients with metastatic breast cancer are potential candidates for hormonal manipulation at some point in the course of their disease.

In 1958, Lerner and coworkers *(29)* reported the biologic properties of the first nonsteroidal antiestrogen MER-25 (Fig. 1). MER-25 is a structural derivative of the cholesterol-lowering drug triparanol that was initially under evaluation in the 1950s *(30)*. Triparanol causes the accumulation of desmolase *(31,32)*, which has been linked to the development of cataracts; this ultimately led to its withdrawal from the commercial market in 1962 *(33,34)*. MER-25 was found to be an antiestrogen in all species tested and was found to have no other hormonal or antihormonal properties. The discovery was initially thought to be important because MER-25 was found to be a contraceptive in laboratory animals, but its evaluation as a postcoital contraceptive was disappointing because the drug had low potency, and the high doses necessary to achieve the intended effect were associated with unacceptable toxicity on the central nervous system *(35)*. The compound was also evaluated as a means to induce ovulation *(36)* and to treat chronic cystic mastitis and breast and endometrial carcinoma *(37,38)*, but its poor therapeutic index prohibited further clinical development.

Clomiphene was a successor to MER-25 and is an effective antifertility drug in laboratory animals *(39)*, but paradoxically clomiphene induces ovulation in subfertile women *(40)*. Clomiphene had modest activity in patients with metastatic breast cancer *(41,42)*, but its development for this indication was discontinued once tamoxifen entered clinical trials. Clomiphene is now used primarily as a short-term treatment to induce ovulation.

The discovery of tamoxifen, the antiestrogenic, pure *trans* isomer of a substituted triphenylethylene, was made by Harper, Richardson, and Walpole as part of the Fertility Control Program at ICI Pharmaceuticals in the United Kingdom *(43,44)*. The Program was developed to identify a postcoital contraceptive, and tamoxifen had a number of antifertility properties in the rat *(45)*, but it, like clomiphene, induced ovulation in subfertile women *(46)*. Fortunately, preliminary clinical studies conducted in patients with metastatic breast cancer showed tamoxifen to have antitumor activity, leading to its development as the first antiestrogen for the treatment of breast cancer *(47–49)*.

The commitment to develop tamoxifen as a treatment for breast cancer was made on the basis of several factors: (1) higher antitumor potency compared with other compounds being tested at the time *(47)*; (2) a lower reported incidence of side effects for the drug itself *(49)*; (3) a lower incidence of side effects compared with other endocrine therapies available at the time (surgical endocrine ablation or additive therapies such as estrogens or androgens) *(47)*; and (4) no elevation of desmosterol levels, which had been linked to development of cataracts *(48)*.

TAMOXIFEN

Pharmacology and Metabolism of Tamoxifen

The pharmacology and metabolism of tamoxifen have been extensively reviewed elsewhere *(50,51)*. Tamoxifen is able to exert a cytostatic effect on the ER+, MCF-7, human breast cancer cell line at media concentrations of 7.5 µmol/L, above which it has a cytotoxic effect *(52)*. In patients, concentrations above 7.5 µmol/L are unusual; the recommended oral dose is 20 mg/day. After a single oral dose of 10 mg, peak serum concentrations of 20–30 ng/L are detected by 4–7 h *(53)*. Steady-state concentrations of 75–200 ng/L are reached after approximately 4 weeks of treatment *(53)*. After oral administration, elimination of tamoxifen is biphasic, with an initial plasma half-life of 7–14 hours and a terminal half-life of approximately 2 weeks. Tamoxifen and its metabolites are extensively protein bound and undergo enterohepatic recirculation. Tamoxifen is secreted primarily by the biliary system *(54)*. After tamoxifen therapy is discontinued, metabolites can be detected in the serum for 6–8 weeks *(54)*. With oral administration of tamoxifen at 20 mg/d, a significant degree of variability has been demonstrated among

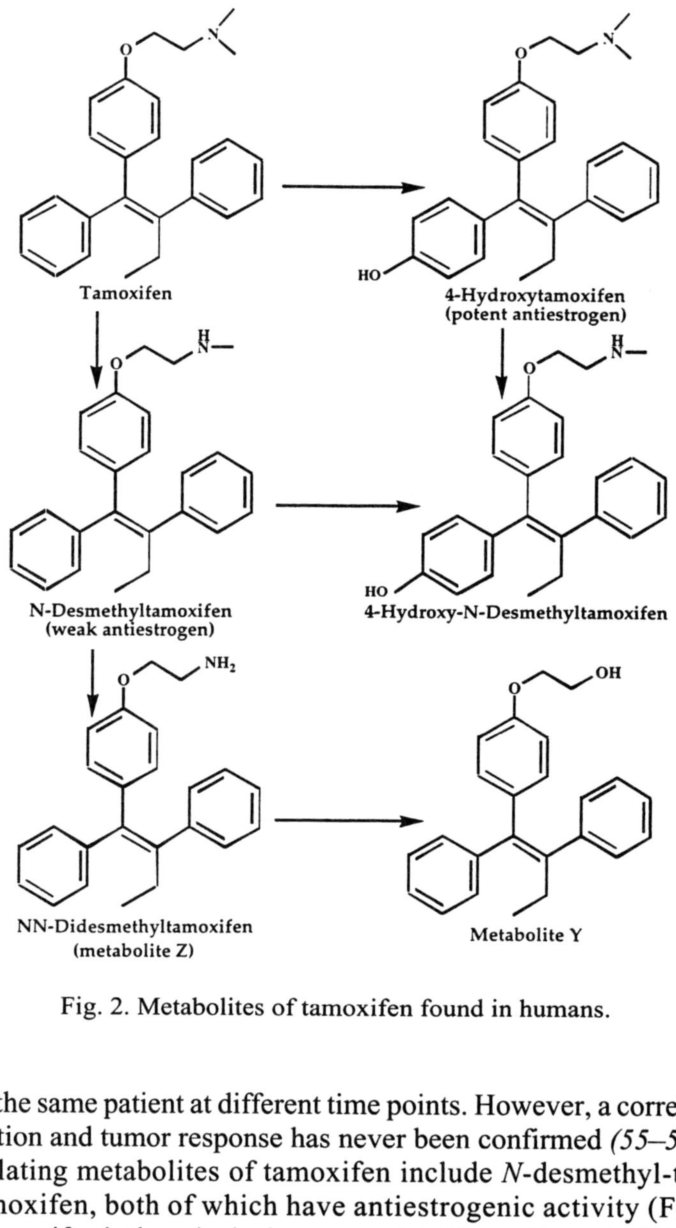

Fig. 2. Metabolites of tamoxifen found in humans.

patients and in the same patient at different time points. However, a correlation between drug concentration and tumor response has never been confirmed *(55–57)*.

Major circulating metabolites of tamoxifen include *N*-desmethyl-tamoxifen and 4-hydroxy-tamoxifen, both of which have antiestrogenic activity (Fig. 2) *(58,59)*. *N*-desmethyl-tamoxifen is the principal serum metabolite and has a half-life twice that of tamoxifen *(58)*; however, it is slightly less potent than the parent compound. 4-Hydroxy-tamoxifen is a minor metabolite with a much shorter half-life, but it has a binding affinity to the ER equivalent to that of estradiol and 20–30 times that of tamoxifen *(58)*.

Mechanism of Action

Tamoxifen's antitumor effect is believed to be mediated primarily through the ER, although other potential effects may contribute to its effect *(60–63)*. The recognition of the ER as a nuclear transcription that binds estrogen or antiestrogens and programs breast cancer cells to replicate or not has focused enormous interest on the mechanism underlying the antitumor effect of antiestrogens *(63)*. Mechanistic models depicting the action

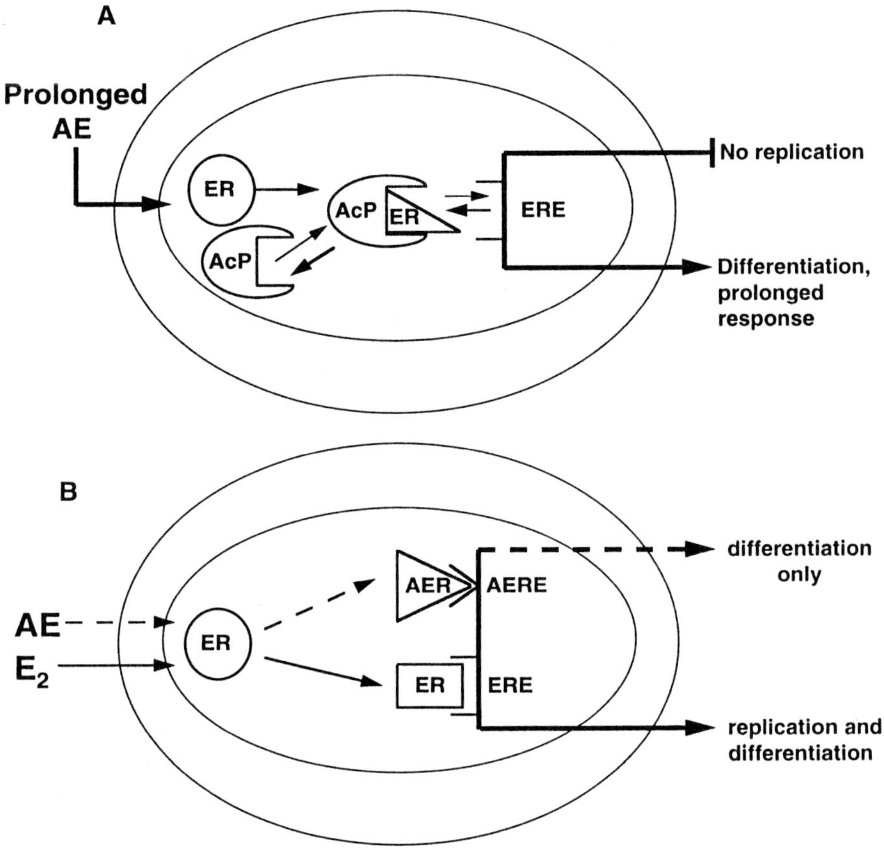

Fig. 3. Possible mechanism of target site-specific action of tamoxifen. **(A)** Interaction of the ER with an antiestrogen (AE) may induce a variety of transcriptional responses, depending on the availability of accessory proteins in a specific cell type. One hypothesis is that the AE-ER complex may induce a conformational change in the ER that does not allow a strong association with a required cell-specific accessory protein (AcP); thus, an attenuated response is induced, with differentiation but no replication. **(B)** A second hypothesis involves specificity at the ERE. The AE-ER complex may interact specifically with distinct DNA sequences, antiestrogen response elements (AERE), to mediate differentiation but not replication. The diagram shows the AE (broken line) and the estradiol (E_2; solid line) going down separate pathways to produce select responses.

of the antiestrogen tamoxifen in an ER+ breast cancer cell is illustrated in Fig. 3. Estradiol or any estrogen binds to the nuclear ER, which produces a change in the shape of the protein complex exposing the DNA binding domain. The activated receptor complex then dimerizes, releases heat shock proteins, and binds to an estrogen response element (ERE) located in the promoter region of the estrogen-responsive genes. Once bound to the ERE, the ER acts an anchor for other transcription factors or associated proteins that, when assembled and associated with RNA polymerase, produce a transcription complex. The estrogen-responsive gene is then transcribed and subsequently translated to proteins that are involved in either growth or differentiation responses, such as progesterone receptor synthesis.

The tamoxifen-ER complex, unlike the estrogen-ER complex, is unable to signal DNA transcription. Presumably the tamoxifen-ER complex is incompletely converted to the fully activated form *(64–69)*. As a result, the complex is only partially active in initiating the programmed series of events necessary to initiate gene activation (Fig. 3) *(64,70)*. Tamoxifen also has other potential actions *(71)* not mediated through the ER that may contribute to its antitumor effect; these include increasing antibody synthesis *(72)*, enhanced natural killer cell activity, inhibition of suppressor T-cell activity *(73)*, inhibition of protein kinase C *(74,75)* and calmodulin-dependent cyclic adenosine monophosphate phosphodiesterase *(76,77)*, inhibition of angiogenesis *(78)*, and decreased synthesis of mitogens that stimulate breast cancer proliferation including insulin growth factor I, transforming growth factor-α (TGF-α), epidermal growth factor, and platelet-derived growth factor *(71,79–81)*. Tamoxifen also modulates inhibitory cytokines such as TGF-β, resulting in increased production in stromal tissue and in ER+ tumor cells *(82)*. TGF-β also seems to inhibit the growth of ER- tumor cells *(82)*. In addition, tamoxifen increases sex hormone binding globulin (SHBG) in postmenopausal patients, further decreasing free estradiol levels that would have the potential to stimulate the tumor *(83)*.

Clinical Uses

The initial trial of tamoxifen in hormonally pretreated, postmenopausal women with metastatic breast cancer revealed a response rate of 22% *(47)*. Subsequent clinical trials with tamoxifen in this patient population have confirmed a response rate of 15–53%, with responses lasting a median of 20 months *(47,49,55,84–96)*. Patient characteristics that predict a response to tamoxifen are similar to those for other endocrine therapies, response to prior endocrine therapy, a long disease-free interval from primary therapy to relapse, older age, disease sites predominantly in soft tissues, bone, and lung, and expression of hormone receptors on the tumor *(84,96)*. ER+ tumors have a 50% probability of responding to tamoxifen compared with <10% if the tumor is ER- (Table 1) *(26)*. In addition, recent data suggest that HER-2/neu-overexpressing breast cancers compared with breast cancers not overexpressing HER-2/neu are less responsive to certain forms of hormonal therapy, particularly tamoxifen *(97,98)*.

Tamoxifen is currently the endocrine treatment of choice for all stages of breast cancer. It was approved for the treatment of breast cancer in 1973 in the United Kingdom and subsequently approved by the Food and Drug Administration in the United States in 1977 for the treatment of metastatic breast cancer in postmenopausal women. Tamoxifen was subsequently approved as a treatment for ER+, metastatic breast cancer in premenopausal women, for metastatic breast cancer in men, and as adjuvant therapy either alone or following chemotherapy in receptor+, pre- or postmenopausal patients with early stage breast cancer.

Tamoxifen as Adjuvant Therapy for Early Stage Breast Cancer

The recent meta-analysis of systemic treatment for all patients with early stage breast cancer confirmed that tamoxifen reduced the annual odds of breast cancer recurrence by 25% and the risk of death due to breast cancer by 16%, compared with patients not treated with tamoxifen. *(99,100)* The benefit produced by tamoxifen was more significant in postmenopausal women, in whom the annual odds of breast cancer recurrence and death due to breast cancer were reduced by 29% and 20%, respectively *(99,100)*. The relative benefit of tamoxifen was the same whether patients were axillary node -positive or negative, but the absolute benefit was greatest in patients with the greatest risk of recurrence (e.g., axillary, node-positive patients). The magnitude of benefit derived from tamoxifen also depended on whether a tumor was ER+ (>10 fmol/mg) or ER-poor (<10 fmol/mg). The annual odds of recurrence were reduced by 13% in

Table 3
Summary of Results from Clinical Trials of Adjuvant Tamoxifen

	Reduction (%) in Annual Odds	
Patient age group (yr)	*Recurrence*	*Mortality*
All	25	16
<50	12	6
≥50	29	20
Premenopausal		
<50	12	6
50–59	33	23
Postmenopausal		
<50	12	—
50–59	28	19
60–69	29	17
>70	28	21

(Data from refs. *99* and *100*.)

patients with ER-poor tumors and by 32% in those with ER+ tumors *(99,100)*. Similarly, the reduction in the annual odds of death was 11% and 21% in patients with ER-poor and ER+ tumors, respectively *(99,100)*. In postmenopausal women whose tumors were ER+, tamoxifen reduced the annual odds of recurrence and death by 36% and 23%, respectively, compared with patients with ER- tumors, in whom the annual odds of recurrence and death were reduced by only 16% *(99,100)*. For ER+ patients under the age of 50 years treated with adjuvant tamoxifen, there is a significant reduction in the odds of death that is comparable to patients over the age of 50 treated with adjuvant tamoxifen and similar to the reduction in the annual odds of death detected in patients under the age of 50 who receive adjuvant chemotherapy. The findings from the Overview are summarized in Table 3.

Tamoxifen in Combination with Chemotherapy

Tamoxifen has also been extensively evaluated in combination with chemotherapy, but the added benefit of one modality plus the other has been difficult to define. Individual studies in pre- and postmenopausal patients have arrived at opposing conclusions as to whether additional benefit is gained by the addition of one modality to the other. The overview analysis indicates that in women over the age of 50, receiving tamoxifen alone vs no treatment, or tamoxifen plus chemotherapy vs chemotherapy alone, tamoxifen adds additional benefit in terms of reducing the annual odds of recurrence (30% and 28%, respectively) and death (19% and 20%, respectively) *(99,100)*. In the same age group analyzed for patients receiving chemotherapy vs chemotherapy and tamoxifen, a significant reduction in the annual odds of recurrence of 26% was detected favoring the addition of tamoxifen, but the reduction in the annual odds of death was statistically insignificant *(10%) (99,100)*. In premenopausal women the role of tamoxifen with chemotherapy is less clear, although there appears to be additional benefit derived from the combination in terms of reducing the odds of recurrence and death *(99,100)*. The results from the 1995 Overview analysis incorporating more mature data from an even greater number of clinical trials are eagerly awaited.

Optimal Duration of Therapy

The optimal duration of adjuvant tamoxifen therapy remains an area of controversy. Five years of adjuvant tamoxifen is currently the accepted standard in clinical trials conducted in the United States; however, in clinical practice tamoxifen is frequently administered for longer duration or until the patient relapses. A critical evaluation of the available clinical data does not allow a definitive statement regarding the optimal duration of tamoxifen therapy. Nevertheless, the National Cancer Institute recently elected to publish a Clinical Alert recommending that tamoxifen should be discontinued after 5 years of treatment *(101)*.

The Overview analysis stratified patients based on tamoxifen therapy administered for <2, 2, and > 2 years *(99)*. Although the Overview does not answer the question regarding the exact duration of tamoxifen therapy, the greatest reduction in the risk of recurrence and death was seen patients receiving >2 years of tamoxifen. The Swedish study compared 2 years vs 5 years of tamoxifen therapy at a dose of 40 mg daily in 3887 node-positive and node-negative postmenopausal patients *(102)*. With >5 years of follow-up, patients receiving 5 years of tamoxifen had a statistically significant improvement in event-free survival and overall survival (80% vs 73% at 10 years) compared with patients receiving 2 years of tamoxifen. In the NSABP B-14 trial, nearly 1200 pre- and postmenopausal, node-negative, receptor-positive patients were randomized to 5 vs 10 years of tamoxifen therapy *(103)*. This trial did not show additional benefit from more than 5 years of tamoxifen therapy, but the number of events in either group was small. Interestingly, the premenopausal women in the National Surgical Adjuvant Breast Project (NSABP) B-14 study had better overall survival compared with the postmenopausal women *(103)*. By contrast, the smaller Eastern Cooperative Oncology Group study suggests that there may be additional benefit from longer therapy with tamoxifen *(104)*. These data seem to suggest that at least 5 years of adjuvant tamoxifen therapy is necessary for receptor-positive patients and that perhaps 5 years is sufficient for receptor-positive, node-negative patients; however, the data are unclear as to whether additional benefit is gained by more than 5 years of therapy, especially in a node-positive patient population *(105)*. Two large studies are under way that will hopefully define the optimal duration of adjuvant tamoxifen therapy. The ATLAS (Adjuvant Tamoxifen Longer Against Shorter) and aTTom (adjuvant Tamoxifen Treatment, offer more?) trials are being coordinated from the United Kingdom *(106)*. Patients with receptor-positive, node-positive or node-negative disease are eligible. Physicians can enter patients regardless of the duration of tamoxifen therapy, and the randomization is between discontinuing therapy after 5 years or continuing treatment beyond 5 years. Both trials seek to accrue approximately 20,000 patients.

Associated Toxicity

Acute toxicity. Tamoxifen is an extremely well-tolerated drug, and only rarely will a patient need to discontinue treatment due to toxicity. It has been previously reported that 5–10% of patients withdraw from clinical trials because of toxicity attributed to tamoxifen; however, it is important to note that a similar fraction of control patients withdraw because of similar toxicities *(107–109)*. The most common adverse effect reported in relation to tamoxifen therapy is vasomotor instability manifested by hot flashes, facial flushing, tachycardia, and sweating. These symptoms are reported in 15–20% of pre- and postmenopausal patients and typically decrease in intensity and frequency over time *(107–109)*. Amenorrhea is the most common gynecologic complaint, occurring in 16–39% of premenopausal women *(89,110,111)*. Other gynecologic adverse effects include vaginal discharge, irregular menses in premenopausal women, and vaginal-vulvar irritation. Other adverse side effects include weight gain and (rarely) nausea and vomiting. Occasionally patients will complain of nonspecific neurologic symptoms (i.e., depression, headache, insomnia, fatigue, irritation, and dizziness), thromboembolic disease, visual disturbances caused by cataract formation, optic neuritis, retinopathy, and macular edema *(107–109)*. Transient thrombocytopenia and mild hypercalcemia are also occasionally observed. Rarely patients with metastatic bone disease will report increased bone pain, with or without associated hypercalcemia, within 1–2 weeks of initiating tamoxifen therapy *(112,113)*. This phenomena is due to the mild estrogenic effect of tamoxifen; it is generally treated with supportive measures (i.e., analgesics) and tends to resolve spontaneously.

Endometrial carcinoma. More recently concerns regarding tamoxifen's long-term safety have been raised. Specifically, the observation that tamoxifen therapy is associated with an increased risk of endometrial cancer has raised the concern that tamoxifen may not be safe for long-term use in the adjuvant or chemopreventive setting. Recent reviews of the medical literature have placed the issue of tamoxifen-associated endometrial carcinoma in perspective *(114–116)*. Approximately 400 cases of tamoxifen-associated endometrial carcinoma have been described, and the disease is found predominantly in postmenopausal women. There *does not* appear to be a strong association between the duration of tamoxifen therapy and likelihood of developing endometrial cancer *(114–116)*. Reanalysis of the Stockholm study that originally concluded that randomization to 2 years of adjuvant tamoxifen did not cause an increase in endometrial cancer whereas 5 years of tamoxifen therapy caused a sixfold increase in the risk of endometrial carcinoma reveals that 12 of 16 patients who developed endometrial carcinoma actually received 2 years of tamoxifen therapy *(117,118)*. Since endometrial carcinoma is known to develop over prolonged preclinical phase, preexisting tumors were most likely detected. Furthermore, uterine samples obtained from tamoxifen-treated patients do not contain DNA adducts *(119)*.

Another concern regarding tamoxifen-associated endometrial carcinoma is whether it represents a more aggressive type of carcinoma compared with the typical *de novo* endometrial carcinoma. This issue was raised by Magriples et al. *(120)* who reported a tumor registry experience and suggested that higher grade lesions and a higher fraction of sarcomatous lesions are detected in tamoxifen-associated endometrial carcinoma. After other reports appeared in the literature, the stage and grade of endometrial cancer associated with tamoxifen therapy appear similar to those described in the Surveillance, Epidemiology, and End Results database for the general population *(121–123)*. For women taking a standard dose of tamoxifen (20 mg/d) for 5 years, the risk of developing endometrial cancer is approximately 2 cases/1000 treated patients/year. Put in perspective, 10 years of tamoxifen therapy will prevent the recurrence of breast cancer in 88/1000 node-positive patients and 51/1000 node-negative patients while causing 20 additional cases of endometrial carcinoma, the majority of which will be cured by hysterectomy *(99)*. As a precautionary measure women should undergo a pelvic examination prior to starting tamoxifen, and any patient who develops abnormal vaginal spotting or bleeding should promptly undergo a thorough gynecologic examination. There is, however, no justification for an extensive screening evaluation to detect endometrial carcinoma in asymptomatic patients receiving adjuvant tamoxifen therapy *(124–127)*.

Hepatocellular carcinoma. Several investigators have reported that tamoxifen is an initiator and promoter of rat liver carcinogenesis *(128–133)*. DNA adduct formation is detected in the liver of rats who have been fed a diet containing high doses of tamoxifen *(129,134)*, whereas DNA adducts are detected much less frequently in the livers of mice fed a similar diet *(134)*. It is reassuring to note that there is no increase in DNA adduct formation in the livers of patients receiving tamoxifen therapy *(135)*. These findings suggest that rat studies are not necessarily relevant to human usage of tamoxifen. Even more instructive is to consider the cumulative dose of drug that rats were exposed to in comparison with the standard regimen recommended to patients. The duration of adjuvant therapy with tamoxifen for postmenopausal women is usually 5 years, which is roughly equivalent to 8% of a woman's life. Thus the animal experiment at the lowest tamoxifen dose to produce tumors *(136)*, 5 mg/kg, is equivalent to a teenage girl (i.e., 14 years old) receiving 20 times the recommended daily dose of tamoxifen (40 pills/day) until she is 40 years old.

Large doses of tamoxifen are required in rat studies to produce therapeutic levels comparable to those in humans because the drug is cleared 10 times faster than in humans *(118)*. As a result, these chronically high doses of drug administered to animals may cause liver carcinogenesis. Clinical trial experience with tamoxifen has not substantiated the concern that there will be an increase in the number of cases of hepatocellular carcinoma. In the Stockholm trial, first reported in 1989 (patients received tamoxifen, 40 mg/day), three cases of hepatocellular carcinoma were detected in the tamoxifen-treated group vs one case in the control group *(117)*. No increase in the incidence of hepatocellular carcinoma has been detected in other clinical trials of tamoxifen *(99)*. Similarly, an isolated report of an increase in colorectal and gastric carcinoma *(122)* has not been substantiated by review of other clinical trials or the Overview analysis *(99)*.

Effects on fertility and pregnancy. As previously noted, tamoxifen was initially considered a potential contraceptive drug, but it actually induces ovulation after a short course of treatment *(137)*. In some countries tamoxifen continues to be used as a therapy for subfertile women. In breast cancer patients, barrier contraception is recommended since hormonal contraception is likely to interfere with the action of tamoxifen. Most of the information regarding tamoxifen's effect on embryonic development is from neonatal animals; here it has been shown to have a number of effects on the developing reproductive tract *(138–140)*. Although there are no data in humans, tamoxifen is not recommended in pregnant women because of concerns regarding its potential teratogenic effects on the developing fetus.

Most premenopausal women continue to menstruate while receiving tamoxifen therapy, but 16–39% of patients experience complete amenorrhea, and the frequency increases with longer use *(89,110,111)*. Long-term or short-term tamoxifen therapy causes an increase in ovarian estrogen and progesterone synthesis *(141–143)*. Serum levels of these hormones often double over those normally observed during a menstrual cycle; however, there is no evidence that elevated hormone levels impact in an adverse way on patient outcome *(89,110,111)*.

Secondary Beneficial Effects

Cardiovascular disease. Tamoxifen is able to lower circulating cholesterol by 15–20%, primarily by reducing low-density lipoprotein (LDL) *(144–147)*. High-density lipoproteins (HDL) are essentially unaffected *(144–147)*. These data suggest that tamoxifen could protect thousands of women from cardiac events if cholesterol is reduced over a long period. In fact, preliminary studies from the Scottish trial demonstrate that 5 years of tamoxifen will reduce the risk of fatal myocardial infarction compared with control patients *(148)*. A recent update from this trial shows a reduced risk of coronary artery disease in ever-users of tamoxifen, but the greatest benefit is in current users *(149)*. Similarly, the Stockholm *(150)* and NSABP B-14 *(151)* trials showed a reduced incidence of hospitalization for any cardiac event in patients receiving tamoxifen compared with controls *(150)*. Potential explanations for the cardioprotective effect of tamoxifen may be (1) reduced circulating cholesterol due to inhibition of the conversion of δ-8-cholestanol to lathosterol in the cholesterol synthesis pathway *(152)*; and (2) an antioxidant effect that protects cardiac membranes from lipid peroxidation *(153)*.

Osteoporosis. Loss of bone density in postmenopausal women can result in fractures, leading to significant morbidity and mortality. Hormone replacement therapy is commonly used to attenuate bone mineral loss after the menopause. Initially there was significant concern that tamoxifen, classified as an antiestrogen, would accelerate osteoporosis in postmenopausal women. Fortuitously, tamoxifen retains an estrogenic effect on bone *(137,152)*. Tamoxifen is capable of inhibiting parathyroid hormone-mediated bone resorption *(153)*, osteoclast activity, and bone loss in the rat *(154)*. Several clinical studies have now confirmed that tamoxifen does not accelerate loss of bone density and that it may actually slow or stop lumbar bone mineral loss *(155–158)*. Some studies in which patients have received tamoxifen for >1 year actually show increases in lumbar bone mineral density.

Effect on contralateral breast cancer. In 1945, Foote and Stewart *(159)* observed that the best predictor of breast cancer in one breast is a prior history of breast cancer in the other breast. Multiple studies have reported that approximately 6–8% of early stage breast cancer patients will develop a second primary breast cancer *(160)* and that patients with *BRCA1*-associated breast cancer have an approximately 50% risk of developing a second primary breast tumor *(161)*. In patients with nonhereditary breast cancer, treatment with tamoxifen reduces the risk of contralateral breast cancer. There is also a correlation between the duration of tamoxifen therapy and the magnitude of risk reduction for developing a second primary breast cancer, such that >2 years of tamoxifen therapy reduces the incidence by 54% compared with a 26% reduction in incidence in patients receiving <2 years of treatment *(99)*. The 1995 Overview, which is expected to be published in early 1998, will provide continuing evidence that tamoxifen given in the adjuvant setting reduces the incidence of contralateral breast cancer and that longer duration of tamoxifen treatment results in greater reductions in incidence *(162)*. On the basis of these observations, three large chemoprevention trials were launched in the United States and Europe for women at high risk of developing breast cancer.

The Royal Marsden has completed recruitment to a pilot, randomized, placebo-controlled trial using tamoxifen, 20 mg/d, for up to 8 years in healthy women at increased risk of developing breast cancer. The trial was initiated in 1986 and enrolled 2012 patients *(163)*. The small size of the trial will not provide the necessary statistical power to determine whether tamoxifen reduces the risk of developing breast cancer in this high-risk population; however, the study is important because it will provide insight into some of tamoxifen's other potential effects. It is also important to recognize that Powles et al. *(164)* reported a 20% decrease in compliance in the study at 5 years, which may further limit the ability of the study to determine if tamoxifen reduces the risk of developing breast cancer.

The NSABP Prevention Trial (P-1) opened in 1992 with an original accrual goal of 16,000 women *(163)*. Those eligible for entry include any woman over the age of 60, or women between ages 35 and 59 who have a 5-year risk of developing breast cancer, as predicted by the Gail model *(165)*, equal to that of a 60-year-old woman. Additionally, any woman over the age of 35 with a diagnosis of lobular carcinoma *in situ* treated by biopsy alone is eligible for entry to the study. A full evaluation of lipid and cholesterol profiles and bone density determinations are incorporated into the study. As of September, 1997 the revised accrual goal of 13,000 women has been reached. Initial results from the study will require several years for the data to mature.

The Italian study is recruiting 20,000 normal women over the age of 45 to be randomized to 20 mg tamoxifen daily or a placebo for 5 years *(163)*. Only women who have undergone a hysterectomy are admitted to the study to avoid issues of pregnancy and endometrial pathology.

NEW ANTIESTROGENS IN DEVELOPMENT

Characteristics of an Ideal Antiestrogen

Drug development of new antiestrogens is an effort to exploit the beneficial effects of tamoxifen while eliminating or diminishing the adverse effects associated with it. An ideal compound would (1) act like an antiestrogen in the breast, thereby reducing the risk of relapse and the development of a new primary tumor; (2) maintain bone density; (3) lower circulating cholesterol and as a result reduce cardiac morbidity; (4) not cause DNA adducts in the liver or uterus, thereby reducing the risk of endometrial or hepatocellular carcinoma; (5) maintain an estrogenic effect in the brain *(166)*, thereby eliminating hot flashes (Fig. 4).

One strategy is to develop compounds that are not crossresistant to tamoxifen and have a safer toxicity profile. Alternatively, some groups are attempting to develop pure antiestrogens that lack any of the estrogen agonist effects in the uterus and that are not associated with the development of premature drug resistance. Such compounds would have potential as first-line therapy in metastatic disease or second-line therapy following tamoxifen. Ultimately, if the features of an ideal antiestrogen can be developed in a drug, it will have enormous potential as long-term adjuvant therapy, a chemopreventive agent, and perhaps a substitute for hormone replacement therapy in healthy postmenopausal women.

Tamoxifen Analogs

TOREMIFENE

Toremifene or chlorotamoxifen (Fig. 1) is approved for the treatment of metastatic breast cancer. The recommended oral dose is 60 mg daily. Laboratory studies show that toremifene is an estrogen antagonist at low concentrations and cytolytic at high concentrations *(167–169)*. Like tamoxifen, toremifene increases the production of TGF-β *(170,171)* and induces apoptotic cell death *(167)*. Toremifene causes modest increases in uterine weight in rats when administered alone *(172,173)*. It is effective in controlling the growth of 7,12-dimethylbenz[a]anthracene (DMBA)-induced rat mammary carcinomas *(173–176)* but appears to be approximately one-third less potent *(177)*. Toremifene will inhibit the growth of ER+ breast cancer cell lines and has been reported to be cytolytic

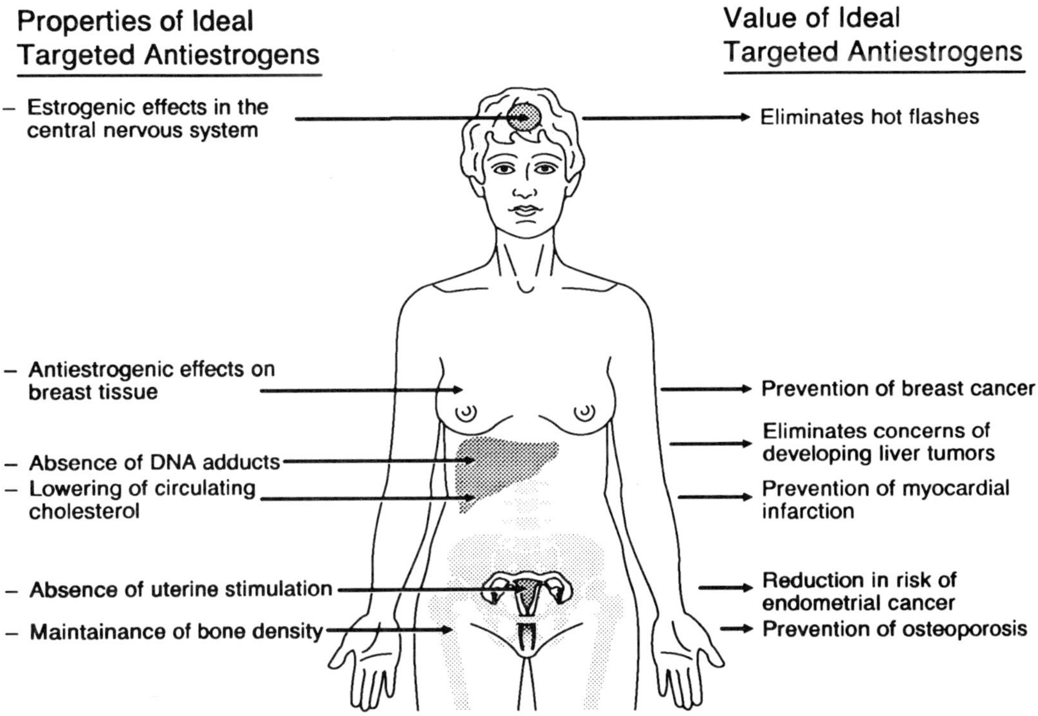

Fig. 4. Properties and beneficial effects of an ideal targeted antiestrogen. The ideal antiestrogen should exhibit estrogenic activity in the liver, bones, and central nervous system and antiestrogenic effects in the breast. It should not induce DNA adducts in the liver. The benefits of a selective estrogen response modifier include prevention of breast and endometrial cancer, prevention of osteoporosis and myocardial infarction, and elimination of hot flashes.

to the ER-, glucocorticoid-sensitive, mouse uterine sarcoma *(178)*. After long-term therapy, toremifene can produce acquired resistance in athymic mice implanted with MCF-7 cells *(179)*. Large daily doses of toremifene (5–20 mg) do not produce DNA adducts in the rat liver, and long-term therapy does not cause hepatocarcinogenesis *(130,180)*; however, recent studies suggest that large doses of toremifene (750 mg toremifene/kg food) can promote rat liver and kidney carcinogenesis *(181)*.

The time to steady state and terminal elimination half-life of toremifene is 2 weeks and 5 days, respectively *(182,183)*. Toremifene and tamoxifen produce the same estrogen-like effects on the histology of the postmenopausal endometrium *(184)*. During treatment with toremifene, luteinizing hormone (LH) and follicle-stimulating hormone (FSH) levels are slightly depressed in postmenopausal women and SHBG is increased *(185–187)*.

Several phase II trials of toremifene in previously untreated, postmenopausal patients with advanced breast cancer have been reported *(188–193)*. With daily, oral doses of toremifene ranging between 20 and 240 mg, overall response rates of 21–68% were observed. Toxicities were generally mild, with hot flashes occurring in 20–30% of patients *(188–193)*. Several randomized trials have compared toremifene to tamoxifen in postmenopausal patients with advanced breast cancer *(194–199)*. The largest trial involved 648 previously untreated, hormone receptor+ or unknown, metastatic breast cancer patients who were randomized to tamoxifen (20 mg/d, orally) or two different doses of toremifene (60 or 200 mg/d, orally) *(199)*. Tamoxifen produced a response rate of 19% and a median survival of 32 months compared with toremifene, which produced a response rate of 21% with the 60-mg dose and 23% with the 200-mg dose. Median survival of toremifene-treated patients was 38 months (60 mg/d) and 30 months (200 mg/d). The median time to disease progression was not statistically different between treatment arms *(199)*. Quality of life assessments were also not different between treatment arms, and toxicity was mild in all patients, although toremifene-treated patients experienced less nausea. The data from this trial support the use of toremifene as an alternative first-line hormonal therapy to tamoxifen for metastatic breast cancer *(199)*.

Several phase II studies of toremifene in advanced breast cancer following disease progression on tamoxifen report low overall response rates *(198–203)*. The largest trial, reported by Vogel et al. *(203)*, involved 102 heavily pretreated, peri- or postmenopausal patients refractory to tamoxifen. Patients received 200 mg/d of toremifene. The overall response rate was 5% with an additional 23% of patients maintaining a stable disease state for a median of 8 months. These data suggest that toremifene has crossresistance to tamoxifen.

Droloxifene

Droloxifene or 3-hydroxytamoxifen (Fig. 1) has been evaluated as a treatment for breast cancer, but it is currently under development as a treatment for osteoporosis in postmenopausal women. Droloxifene acts through the ER, as evidenced by its high binding affinity for ER+, MCF-7 breast cancer cells *(204,205)*. It also induces TGF-β *(171)* and inhibits estrogen-stimulated cell replication *(205–207)* by arresting cells in G_0/G_1 *(208)*. Droloxifene shows antiestrogenic activity in the immature rat uterine weight test, but it also causes a partial increase in uterine wet weight when administered alone *(209,210)*. Droloxifene also maintains bone density in the ovariectomized rat *(211)* and shows significant antitumor activity in several rat and mouse models.

Droloxifene does not produce DNA adducts or hepatocellular carcinomas in male or female rats fed daily doses of 36 mg/kg *(208)*. The same daily dose of tamoxifen fed to rats for 24 months will produce hepatocellular carcinomas in 100% of animals.

Droloxifene is rapidly absorbed and excreted; unlike tamoxifen and toremifene, droloxifene does not appear to accumulate. Steady-state levels of parent drug are achieved within 5 h and under chronic dosing conditions with 40-mg and 100-mg daily doses, the half-lives are 28 and 27 h, respectively *(212)*. There are several metabolites of droloxifene and all are present in serum as both free and glucuronide conjugates *(212)*. This metabolic profile is different from that of tamoxifen, which does not have glucuronide metabolites. Droloxifene causes a dose-dependent decrease in LH and FSH and a dose-dependent increase in SHBG *(213,214)*.

Numerous phase II clinical trials have evaluated droloxifene in advanced breast cancer patients using a dose range of 20–300 mg/d *(215–221)*. Most patients enrolled in these trials were peri-or postmenopausal and had been previously treated with chemotherapy and/or hormone therapy. Response rates ranged from 0 to 70% and most responses were observed in postmenopausal patients. The largest clinical trial was recently updated by Rausching et al. *(220)*. It involved 369 postmenopausal patients who had not received prior hormonal therapy. Patients were randomized among 20-, 40-, and 100-mg daily doses of droloxifene. The response rates were 30% in the 20-mg group, 47% in the 40-mg group, and 44% in the 100-mg group. Responses generally occurred within 2 months, and toxicity was mild at all doses.

Idoxifene

Idoxifene has a binding affinity for the ER that is approximately twice that of tamoxifen (Fig. 1) *(222)*. As a result, idoxifene is slightly more effective at inhibiting ER+, MCF-7 breast cancer cells in culture *(222)*. Since iodoxifene can not be metabolically activated to the 4-hydroxy derivative, it is 10-fold less potent than tamoxifen in immature rat uterine weight tests *(223)*. Idoxifene has less uterotropic activity when administered alone *(222)*. Idoxifene has antitumor properties in the nitrosomethylurea (NMU)-induced rat mammary carcinoma model at a dose somewhat higher (1–2 mg/kg) than observed with tamoxifen *(222)*. This finding is not surprising since the drug can not be metabolically activated.

Idoxifene is designed to be metabolism restricted with a goal of decreasing the liver carcinogenicity produced with tamoxifen *(223)*. *N*-demethylation is the major metabolic route for tamoxifen; therefore, a pyrrolidino group was used to resolve liver toxicity through a reduction in formaldehyde production. Pyrrolidino tamoxifen gives levels of DNA adducts as high as tamoxifen in rat liver *(223)*. Because of the unusual metabolic pathway followed by idoxifene, care must be taken to detect any unusual adverse effects in patients.

Coombes et al. *(224)* reported the only clinical trial with idoxifene. This phase I trial enrolled 20 patients with ER+ or unknown, advanced breast cancer most of whom had received prior tamoxifen, second-line hormone therapy, and chemotherapy. Partial responses were observed in 14% of patients, and an additional 29% of patients had stable disease for 1.4–14 months. Toxicity was mild and not dose related.

PURE ANTIESTROGENS

ICI 182,780

Pure antiestrogens were first described in the 1980s and are currently being developed as a treatment for advanced breast cancer following disease progression while receiving adjuvant tamoxifen *(225)*. Zeneca Pharmaceuticals (UK) is developing the drug, ICI 182,780, which is the pure antiestrogen farthest along in clinical development (Fig. 1).

ICI 182,780 is a competitive inhibitor of estrogen action that blocks estrogen binding to the ER *(226)* and causes destruction of the ER *(227,228)*. ICI 182,780 is a more potent inhibitor of growth in the ER+, MCF-7 cell line compared with tamoxifen *(226)*. The ER-, MDA-MB-231 call line is unaffected by ICI 182,780 *(226)*. It is a potent and complete antiestrogen when administered orally or subcutaneously to immature rats and can also inhibit the partial estrogen-like effects of tamoxifen on the rat uterus *(226)*. In the laboratory, ICI 182,780 will inhibit the growth of tamoxifen-stimulated breast and endometrial tumors *(229,230)*. Although ICI 182,780 can control the growth of tamoxifen-stimulated tumors for prolonged periods, progressive growth eventually develops. There are also preliminary data suggesting that ICI 182,780-resistant tumors can develop *(231)*. Rats with established DMBA-induced tumors have the greatest tumor regression when a pure antiestrogen and the luteinizing hormone-releasing hormone analog, goserelin, are combined compared with treatment with goserelin alone *(232)*. This combination may produce a more complete estrogen blockade, which could be exploited as a treatment strategy for premenopausal women. There have been no reports of carcinogenesis, genotoxicity, or developmental defects in neonatal animals exposed to ICI 182,780.

Studies in both ovariectomized and intact adult female monkeys demonstrate a complete blockade of the uterotrophic effects of estradiol by ICI 182,780 *(233,234)*. These findings suggest that pure antiestrogens may be an effective treatment for endometrial disorders and endometrial carcinoma.

The clinical experience with ICI 182,780 is limited. DeFriend et al. *(235)* assessed the pharmacokinetics, toxicity, and short-term biologic activity of ICI 182,780 in 56 patients with primary breast cancer who received daily intramuscular injections for 7 days (doses 6 mg or 18 mg). Patients treated with ICI 182,780 for a few days prior to definitive primary surgery were noted to have a significant decrease in Ki67, progesterone receptor, and ER in their tumors, whereas no effect on LH, FSH, or SHBG was observed. No significant toxicity was observed. Howell et al. *(236)* reported a 37% response rate in 19 tamoxifen-resistant, advanced breast cancer patients using ICI 182,780 at a dose of 250 mg/month intramuscularly. Soft tissue, bone, and visceral sites of disease responded *(236)*. In addition, 32% of patients maintained a stable disease status. No significant toxicity was observed. The lack of crossresistance with tamoxifen in 69% of patients suggests that ICI 182,780 may be useful as a first-line therapy in advanced disease or as a second-line therapy in advanced disease after progression on tamoxifen. Pure antiestrogens may also be effective in the adjuvant setting.

Targeted Antiestrogens

Raloxifene

Raloxifene, formally called keoxifene, is being developed as a treatment for osteoporosis (Fig. 1). This compound is classified as a selective estrogen response modifier, implying that it retains estrogenic effects on the cardiovascular system and bone while having antiestrogenic actions on the breast and uterus.

Raloxifene has a binding affinity for the ER that is equivalent to estradiol *(237)*. It is a potent inhibitor of ER+, MCF-7 cells. Raloxifene is an antiestrogen in the immature rat uterine weight test, but has little agonist action in the uterus when administered alone. Raloxifene maintains bone density in the ovariectomized rat *(238–240)* and also reduces circulating cholesterol *(239)*. At low doses, raloxifene has weak antitumor activity in the DMBA- *(241)* and NMU-induced *(242)* rat mammary carcinoma models compared with tamoxifen. Raloxifene-stimulated breast tumors have not been described, but raloxifene partially inhibits the tamoxifen-stimulated growth of the human endometrial carcinoma, EnCa101, in athymic mice *(230)*. There have been no reports of DNA adduct formation or hepatocarcinogenesis associated with raloxifene. It causes a decrease in LDL cholesterol, but no change in HDL cholesterol *(243)*.

A phase II trial of raloxifene in patients with metastatic breast cancer who were refractory to tamoxifen was reported in 1988 *(244)*. Fourteen patients received 200 mg/d of oral raloxifene for up to 8 months. The ER status of the patients was not clearly defined. The drug was well tolerated, with no significant clinical or laboratory abnormalities detected, but no objective responses were observed. Preliminary results from a second clinical trial in ER+, metastatic breast cancer patients receiving oral raloxifene, 150 mg twice daily, show a response rate of 14% with an additional 36% of patients maintaining stable disease status for >6 months *(245)*. The ability of raloxifene to maintain bone density in the rat has encouraged the clinical testing of raloxifene as a treatment for osteoporosis. Large international clinical trials of raloxifene as a treatment of osteoporosis have been completed and will be reported in the near future.

SUMMARY AND CONCLUSIONS

The past 20 years have seen a complete revolution in the treatment of breast cancer. In the 1970s there was little value in developing endocrine therapies, but today it is clear that tamoxifen provides benefit to patients with all stages of breast cancer. Most importantly, the low incidence of side effects encouraged the testing of tamoxifen as a preventive in high-risk women. The results of these trials should be available by the turn of the century.

The success of tamoxifen has naturally resulted in the development of new compounds to be used as alternatives to tamoxifen or after the failure of tamoxifen (i.e., pure antiestrogens). Although these drugs may provide some additional benefit, there is little possibility that they will turn out to be of major significance to patients, and conceptually there is reason to believe that they will not be equivalent to tamoxifen or superior to an aromatase inhibitor like anastrozole. The major advance will be made in the prevention of breast cancer with selective estrogen receptor modifiers. Ten years ago, after the discovery that tamoxifen and raloxifene could maintain bone density but block estrogen's action in the uterus, we proposed that these drugs could be used to prevent osteoporosis but at the same time prevent breast and endometrial carcinoma *(246)*. It is now clear, with all the concerns about uterine safety and tamoxifen, that there is little possibility that tamoxifen will be used by postmenopausal women with no breast cancer risk factors. By contrast, raloxifene will soon be available to prevent osteoporosis in postmenopausal women and, for the first time, provide an option for women who are concerned about the risk of breast cancer during hormone replacement. All indications are that the selective estrogen receptor modifiers, which can act like estrogens in bone and on circulating cholesterol and like antiestrogens in the breast and uterus, will revolutionize women's health *(247)*.

REFERENCES

1. Parker SL, Tong T, Bolden S, Wingo, PA (1996) Cancer statistics. CA Cancer J Clin 65:5–27.
2. Anonymous. (1997) Breast cancer mortality tumors by age and race. J Natl Cancer Inst 88:710.
3. Forbes JF (1997) The incidence of breast cancer: the global burden, public health considerations. Semin Oncol 24(suppl. 1):20–35.
4. Nemoto T, Vana J, Bedwani RN, Baker W (1980) Management and survival of female breast cancer. 45:2917–2924.
5. Goldhirsch A, Wood WC, Senn HJ, et al. (1995) Meeting Highlights: International consensus panel on the treatment of primary breast cancer. J Natl Cancer Inst 87:1441–1445.
6. Beatson GT (1986) On the treatment of inoperable cases of carcinoma of the mamma: suggestions for a new method of treatment, with illustrative cases. Lancet 2:104–107, 162–165.
7. Boyd S (1900) An oophorectomy in cancer of the breast. BM J 2:1161–1167.
8. de Courmelles FV (1922) La radiotherapie indirecte, ou dirigée par les correlations organiques. Arch Elect Med 32:264.
9. Block GE, Vial AB, Pullen FW (1958) Estrogen excretion following operative and irradiation castration in cases of mammary cancer. Surgery 43:415–422.
10. Huggins C, Bergenstal DM (1952) Inhibition of human mammary and prostatic cancer by adrenalectomy. Cancer Res 12:134–141.
11. Santen RJ, Worgul TJ, Samojlik E, Interrante A, Boucher AE, Lipton A, et al. (1981) A randomized trial comparing surgical adrenalectomy with aminoglutethimide plus hydrocortisone in women with advanced breast cancer. N Engl J Med 305:545–551.
12. Huggins C, Dao TLY (1953) Adrenalectomy and oophorectomy in the treatment of advanced carcinoma of the breast. JAMA 151:1388–1394.
13. Luft R, Olivecrona H (1953) Hypophysectomy in man. J. Neurosurg 10:301–316.

14. Santen RJ, Worgul TJ, Samojlik E, Interrate A, Boucher AE, Lipton A, et al. (1981) A randomized trial comparing surgical adrenalectomy with aminoglutethimide plus hydrocortisone in women with advanced breast cancer. N Engl J Med 305:545–551.
15. Haddow A (1944) Stilbesterol for advanced breast cancer. BMJ 2:393–398.
16. Jensen EV, Jacobson HI (1962) Basic guides to the mechanism of estrogen action. Recent Prog Horm Res 18:387–414.
17. Toft D, Shyamala G, Gorski J (1967) A receptor molecule for estrogens: studies using cell free system. Proc Natl Acad Sci 57:1740–1743.
18. Jensen EV, Block GE, Smith S, Kyser K, DeSombre ER (1971) Estrogen receptors and breast cancer response to adrenalectomy. NCI Monograph 34:55–70.
19. McGuire WL, Carbone PP, Vollmer EP (Eds): (1975) Estrogen Receptors in Human Breast Cancer. Raven Press, New York.
20. Horwitz KB, McGuire KB (1975) Specific progesterone receptors in human breast cancer. Steroids 25:497–505.
21. Horwitz KB, McGuire WL (1975) Predicting response to endocrine therapy in human breast cancer: a hypothesis. Science 189:726–727.
22. McGuire WL, Clark GM (1989) Prognostic factors for recurrence and survival in axillary node-negative breast cancer. J Steroid Biochem 34:145–148.
23. Witliff J (1987) Steroid hormone receptors, In: *Methods in Clinical Chemistry* (Pesce AJ, Kaplan LA, eds.), Mosby, St. Louis MO, p. 767.
24. Oxenhandler RW, McCune R, Subtelney A, Truelove C, Tyrer HW (1984) Flow cytometry determination of estrogen receptor in intact cells. Cancer Res 44:2516–2523.
25. Jordan VC, Jacobson HI, Keenan EJ (1986) Determination of estrogen receptors in breast cancer using monoclonal antibody technology in the United States. Cancer Res 46:4237S-4240S.
26. Wittliff JL (1984) Steroid-hormone receptors in breast cancer. Cancer 53:630–643.
27. McGuire WL, Chamness GC, Fuqua SAW (1991) Mini-review—estrogen receptor variants in clinical breast cancer. Mol Endocrinol 5:1571–1577.
28. Allegra JC (1984) Role of hormone receptors in determining treatment of breast cancer, In: The Management of Breast Cancer Through Endocrine Therapies. Excerpta Medica, Amsterdam, pp. 1–13.
29. Lerner LJ, Holthaus JF, Thompson CR (1958) A nonsteroidal estrogen antagonist 1-(p-2-diethylaminoethoxyphenyl)-1-phenyl-2-p-methoxyethanol. Endocrinology 63: 295–318.
30. Hollander W, Chobanian AV, Wilkins RW (1960). The effects of triparanol (MER-29) in subjects with and without coronary artery disease. JAMA 174: 87–94.
31. Avigan J, Steinberg D, Vroman HE, Thompson MJ, Hosettig E. (1960) Studies of cholesterol biosynthesis: the identification of desmosterol in serum and tissues of animals and man treated with MER-29. J Biol Chem 235: 3123–3126.
32. Gaylor JL (1963) Biosynthesis of skin sterols II. Reactions of Δ^{24} unsaturated sterols of rat skin. Arch Biochem Biophys 101:108–115.
33. Laughlin RC, Carey TF (1962) Cataracts in patients treated with triparanol. JAMA 181:339–340.
34. von Sallman L, Grimes P, Collins E (1963) Triparanol-induced cataracts in rats. Arch Ophthamol 70,1128–1136.
35. Lerner LJ (1981) The first non-steroidal antioestrogen—MER-25, In: *Non-Steroidal Antioestrogens: Molecular Pharmacology and Antitumour Activity*. (Sutherland RL, Jordan VC, eds), Academic Press, Sydney, pp. 1–16.
36. Tyler ET, Olson HJ, Gotlieb MH (1960) The induction of ovulation with an antiestrogen. Int J Fertil 5:429–431.
37. Kistner RW, Smith OW (1960) Observations on the use of non-steroidal estrogen antagonist—MER-25. Surg Forum 10:725–729.
38. Smith OW, Smith GV, Kistner RW (1963) Action of MER-25 and of clomiphene on the human ovary. JAMA 184:122–130.
39. Holtkamp DE, Greslin SC, Root CA, Lerner LJ (1960) Gonadotropin inhibiting and antifecundity effects of chloramiphene. Proc Soc Expt Biol Med 105,197–201.
40. Kistner RB (1965) Induction of ovulation with clomiphene citrate (Clomid). Obstet Gynecol Surv 20:873–900.
41. Herbst AL, Griffiths CT, Kistner RW (1964) Clomiphene citrate in disseminated mammary carcinoma. Cancer Chemother Rep 43:39–41.
42. Hecker E, Vegh I, Levy CM, Magin CA, Martinez JC, Lovreiro J, et al. (1974) Clinical trial of clomiphene in advanced breast cancer. Eur J Cancer 10:747–749.

43. Harper MJK, Walpole AL (1966) Contrasting endocrine activities of *cis* and *trans* isomers in a series of substituted triphenylethylenes. Nature 212:87.
44. Bedford GR, Richardson DN (1966) Preparation and identification of *cis* and *trans* isomers of a substituted triarylethylene. Nature 212:733–734.
45. Harper MJK, Walpole AL (1967) A new derivative of triphenylethylene: effect on implantation and mode of action in rats. J Reprod Fertil 13:101–119.
46. Williamson JG, Ellis JP (1973) The induction of ovulation by tamoxifen. J Obstet Gynaecol Br Commonwealth 80:844–847.
47. Cole MP, Jones CTA, Todd IDH (1971) A new antioestrogenic agent in late breast cancer: an early clinical appraisal of ICI 46,474. Br J Cancer 25:270–275.
48. Cole MP, Jones CTA, Todd IDH (1972) The treatment of advanced carcinoma of the breast with the antineoplastic agent tamoxifen (ICI 46,474)—a series of 96 patients. Adv Antimicrob Antineoplas Chemotherapy 2:529–531.
49. Ward HWC (1973) Antioestrogen therapy for breast cancer: a trial of tamoxifen at two dose levels. BMJ I:13–14.
50. Catherino WH, Jordan VC (1991) Tamoxifen and derivatives, In: *Handbook of Chemotherapy in Clinical Oncolog* (Cvitkovic E, Vroz JP, Armand JP, Khoury S, eds.), F.I.I.S., Paris, pp. 376–380.
51. Jordan VC, Murphy CS (1990) Endocrine pharmacology of antiestrogens as antitumor agents. Endocr Rev 11:578–610.
52. Sutherland RL, Reddel RR, Murphy LC, Taylor IW (1986) Effects of antiestrogens on cell cycle progression, In: *Estrogen/Antiestrogen Action and Breast Cancer Therapy* (Jordan VC, ed.), University of Wisconsin Press, Madison WI, pp. 265–281.
53. Adams HK, Patterson JS, Kemp JV (1980) Studies on the metabolism and pharmacokinetics of tamoxifen in normal volunteers. Cancer Treat Rep 64:761–764.
54. Langan-Fehey SM, Jordan VC, Fritz NF, Robinson SP, Waters P, Tormey DC (1994) Clinical pharmacology and endocrinology of long-term tamoxifen therapy, In: *Long-term Tamoxifen Treatment for Breast Cancer*. (Jordan VC, ed.), The University of Wisconsin Press, Madison, WI, pp. 27–56.
55. Bratherton DG, Brown CH, Buchanan R, Hall V, Pillers EM, Wheeler TK, et al. (1984) A comparison of two doses of tamoxifen (Nolvadex) in postmenopausal women with advanced breast cancer: 10 mg bd versus 20 mg bd. Br J Cancer 50:199–205.
56. Watkins SM (1988) The value of high dose tamoxifen in postmenopausal breast cancer patients progressing on standard doses: a pilot study. Br J Cancer 57:320–321.
57. Fabian C, Sternson L, El-Serafi M, et al. (1981) Clinical pharmacology of tamoxifen in patients with breast cancer: correlation with clinical data. Cancer 48:876–882.
58. Fromson JMS, Pearson S, Bramah S (1973) The metabolism of tamoxifen (ICI 46:474). Part 2. In female patients. Xenobiotica 3:711–714.
59. Kemp JV, Adams HK, Wakeling AE, Slater, R (1980) Identification and biological activity of tamoxifen and its metabolites. Cancer Treat Rep 64:741–744.
60. Jordan VC, Koerner S (1975) Tamoxifen (ICI 46 474) and the human carcinoma 8S estrogen receptor. Eur J Cancer 11:205–206.
61. JordanVC, Dowse LJ (1976) Tamoxifen as an antitumour agent: effect on oestrogen binding. J Endocrinol 68:297–303.
62. Wolf DM, Fuqua SAW (1995) Mechanisms of action of antiestrogens. Cancer Treat Rev 21:247–271.
63. Green S, Chambon P (1991) The oestrogen receptor: from perception to mechanism, In: *Nuclear Hormone Receptors* (Parker MG, ed.), Academic Press, New York, pp. 15–38.
64. Tate AC, Greene GL, DeSombre ER, Jensen EV, Jordan VC (1984) Differences between estrogen and antiestrogen—estrogen receptor complexes identified with an antibody raised against the estrogen receptor. Cancer Res 44:1012–1018.
65. Martin PM, Berthois Y, Jensen EV (1988) Binding of antiestrogen exposes an occult antigenic determinant in the human estrogen receptor. Proc Natl Acad Sci USA 85:2533–2537.
66. Pham TA, Elliston JF, Nawaz Z, McDonnel DP, Tsai MJ, O'Malley BW (1991) Antiestrogens can establish nonproductive receptor complexes and alter chomatin structure at target enhancers. Proc Natl Acad Sci USA 88:2135–3129.
67. Tzukerman MT, Esty A, Santiso-Mere D, et al. (1994) Human estrogen receptor transactivational capacity is determined by both cellular and promoter context and mediated by two functionally distinct intramolecular regions. Mol Endocrinol 8:21–30.

68. McDonnell DP, Clemm DL, Hermann T, Goldman ME, Pike JW (1995) Analysis of estrogen receptor function reveals three dintinct classes of antiestrogens. Mol Endocrinol 9:659–669.
69. Allan GF, Leng X, Tsai ST, Weigel NL, Edwards DP, Tsai MJ, et al. (1992) Hormone and antihormone induce distinct conformational changes which are central to steroid receptor activation. J Biol Chem 267:19513–19520.
70. Metzger D, White J, Chambon P (1988) The human estrogen receptor functions in yeast. Nature 334:31–36.
71. Colletta AA, Benson JR, Baum M (1994) Alternative mechanisms of action of antiestrogens. Breast Cancer Res Treat 31:5–9.
72. Nagy E, Berczi I (1986) Immunomodulation by tamoxifen and pergolide. Immunopharmacology 12:145–53.
73. Paavonen T, Andersson LC (1985) The oestrogen antagonists, tamoxifen and Fc-1157a, display oestrogen like effects on human lymphocyte functions in vitro. Clin Exp Immunol 61:467–474.
74. O'Brian CA, Liskamp RM, Solomon DH, Weinstein IB (1985) Inhibition of protein kinase C by tamoxifen. Cancer Res 45:2462–2465.
75. Su HD, Mazzei GJ, Vogler WR, Kuo JF (1985) Effect of tamoxifen, a nonsteroidal antiestrogen, on phospholipid/calcium-dependent protein kinase and phosphorylation of its endogenous substrate proteins from the rat brain and ovary. Biochem Pharmacol 34:3649–3653.
76. Gulino A, Barrera G, Vacca A, Farina A, Ferretti C, Screparti I, et al. (1986) Calmodulin antagonism and growth-inhibiting activity of triphenylethylene antiestrogens in MCF-7 human breast cancer cells. Cancer Res 46:6274–6278.
77. Greenberg DA, Carpenter CL, Messing RO (1987) Calcium channel antagonist properties of the antineoplastic antiestrogen tamoxifen in the PC12 neurosecretory cell line. Cancer Res 47:70–74.
78. Gagliardi A, Collins DC (1993) Inhibition of angiogenesis by antiestrogens. Cancer Res 53:533–535.
79. Jordan VC (1993) Growth factor regulation by tamoxifen is demonstrated in patients with breast cancer. Cancer 72:1–2.
80. Murphy LC (1994) Antiestrogen action and growth factor regulation. Breast Cancer Res Treat 31: 61–71.
81. Winston R, Kao PC, Kiang DT (1994) Regulation of insulin-like growth factors by antiestrogen. Breast Cancer Res Treat 31:107–115.
82. Butta A, MacLennan K, Flanders KC, Sacks NP, Smith I, McKinna A, et al. (1992) Induction of transforming growth factor β1 in human breast casncer in vivo following tamoxifen treatment. Cancer Res 52:4261–4264.
83. Jordan VC, Fritz NF, Tormey DC (1987) Endocrine effects of adjuvant chemotherapy and long-term tamoxifen administration on node-positive patients with breast cancer. Cancer Res 47:4517–4518.
84. Hoogstraten B, Fletcher WS, Gad-el-Mawla N, Maloney T, Attman SJ, Vaughn CB et al. (1982) Tamoxifen and oophorectomy in the treatment of recurrent breast cancer. A Southwest Oncology Group study. Cancer Res 42:788–791.
85. Kiang DT, Kennedy BJ (1977) Tamoxifen therapy in advanced breast cancer. Ann Intern Med 87:687–690.
86. Lerner HJ, Band PR, Israel L, Leung BS (1976) Phase II study of tamoxifen. Report of 74 patients with stage IV breast cancer. Cancer Treat Rep 60:1431–1435.
87. Tormey DC, Lippman ME, Edwards BK, Cassidy JG (1983) Evaluation of tamoxifen doses with and without fluoxymestrone in advanced breast cancer. Ann Intern Med 98:139–144.
88. Morgan LR, Schein PS, Wooley V, et al. (1976) Therapeutic use of tamoxifen in advanced breast cancer: correlation with biochemical parameters. Cancer Treat Rep 60:1437–1443.
89. Manni A, Pearson OH (1980) Antiestrogen-induced remissions in premenopausal women with stage IV breast cancer: effects on ovarian function. Cancer Treat Rep 64:779–785.
90. Litherland S, Jackson IM (1988) Anti-estrogens in the management of hormone dependent cancer. Cancer Treat Rev 15:183–94.
91. Rose C, Mouridsen HT (1984) Treatment of advanced breast cancer with tamoxifen. Recent Results Cancer Res 91:230–242.
92. Petru E, Schmahl D (1987) On the role of additive horKlinmone monotherapy with tamoxifen, medroxyprogesterone acetate and aminoglutethimide in advanced breast cancer. Klin Wochenschr 65:959–966.
93. Ingle JN, Malliard JA, Schaid DJ, Krook JE, Gesme DH, Windschitl HE, et al. (1991) A double-blind trial of tamoxifen plus placebo in post menopausal women with metastatic breast cancer. A collaborative trial of the North Central Cancer Treatment Group and Mayo Clinic. Cancer 68: 4–9.

94. Wiggans RG, Woolley PV, Smythe T, Hoth D, McDonald JS, Green L, et al. (1979) Phase-II trial of tamoxifen in advanced breast cancer. Cancer Chemother Pharmacol 3:45–48.
95. Manni A, Trujillo JE, Marshal JS, Brodkey J, Pearson DH (1979) Antihormone treatment of stage IV breast cancer. Cancer 43:444–450.
96. Heuson JC (1976) Current overview of EORTC clinical trials with tamoxifen. Cancer Treat Rep 60:1463–1466.
97. Wright C, Nicholson S, Angus B, Sansbury JR, Farndon J, Cairns J, et al. (1992) Relationship between c-erb B-2 protein product expression and response to endocrine therapy in advanced breast cancer. Br J Cancer 65:118–121.
98. Borg A, Baldetorp B, Ferno M, Killender D, Olsson H, Ryder S, et al. (1994) erb B-2 amplification is associated with tamoxifen resistance in steroid-receptor positive breast cancer. Cancer Lett 81:137–144.
99. Early Breast Cancer Trialists' Collaborative Group. (1992) Systemic treatment of early breast cancer by hormonal, cytotoxic or immune therapy. 133 randomized trials involving 31,000 recrurences and 24,000 deaths among 75,000 women. Lancet 339:1–85.
100. Gelber RD, Goldhirsch A, Coates AS (1993) Adjuvant therapy for breast cancer: understanding the overview. J Clin Oncol 11:580–585.
101. Anonymous (1995) National Cancer Institute Clinical Announcement: Adjuvant therapy of breast cancer—tamoxifen update. National Institutes of Health, Bethesda MD.
102. Swedish Breast Cancer Cooperative Group (1996) Randomized trial of two versus five years of adjuvant tamoxifen for postmenopausal early stage breast cancer. J Natl Cancer Inst 88:1834–1839.
103. Fisher B, Dignam J, Bryant J, DeCillis A, Wickerham DL, Wolmark N, et al. (1996) The worth of five versus more than five years of tamoxifen therapy for breast cancer patients with negative lymph nodes and estrogen-receptor positive tumor. J Natl Cancer Inst 88:1529–1542.
104. Tormey DC, Gray R, Falkson HC (1996) Postchemotherapy adjuvant tamoxifen therapy beyond five years in patients with lymph node positive breast cancer. J Natl Cancer Inst 88:1828–1833.
105. Peto,R. (1996) Five years of tamoxifen—or more? J Natl Cancer Inst 88:1791–1993.
106. Bilimoria MM, Jordan VC, Morrow M (1996) Additional benefits of tamoxifen for postmenopausal patients, In: *Tamoxifen: A Guide for Clinicians and Patients.* PRR, New York, pp. 75–87.
107. Cummings FJ, Gray R, Davis TE, Tormey DC, Harris JE, Filkson G, et al. (1985) Adjuvant tamoxifen treatment of elderly women with stage II breast cancer: a double-blind comparison with placebo. Ann Intern Med 103:324–329.
108. Fisher B, Constantino J, Redmond C, Poisson R, Bowman D, Couture J, et al. (1989) A randomized clinical trial evaluating tamoxifen in the treatment of patients with node negative breast cancer who have estrogen receptor positive tumors. N Engl J Med 320:479–484.
109. Fitsch M, Wolf D (1994) Symptomatic side effects of tamoxifen therapy, In: *Long-Term Tamoxifen Treatment for Breast Cancer* (Jordan VC, ed.), University of Wisconsin Press, Madison WI, pp. 235–256.
110. Margreiter R, Wiegle J (1984) Tamoxifen (Nolvadex) for premenopausal patients with advanced breast cancer. Breast Cancer Res Treat 4:45–84.
111. Planting AST, Alexieva-Figusch J, Blonk-vdWijst J, van Putter WL (1985) Tamoxifen therapy in premenopausal women with metastatic breast cancer. Cancer Treat Rep 69:363–368.
112. Plotkin D, Lechner JJ, Jung WE, Rosen PJ (1978) Tamoxifen flare in advanced breast cancer. JAMA 240:2644–2646.
113. Legault-Poisson S, Jolivet J, Poisson R (1979) Tamoxifen-induced tumour stimulation and withdrawal response. Cancer Treat Rep 63,1839–1841.
114. Assikis VJ, Jordan VC (1995) Gynecological effects of tamoxifen and the association with endometrial cancer. Int J Gynecol Obstet 49:241–257.
115. Assikis VJ, Neven P, Jordan VC, Vergote I (1996) A realistic clinical perspective of tamoxifen and endometrial carcinogenesis. Eur J Cancer 32A:1464–1476.
116. Jordan VC, Assikis VJ (1995) Tamoxifen and endometrial cancer: clearing up a controversy. Clin Cancer Res 1:467–472.
117. Fornander T, Rutqvist LE, Cedermark B, Glas U, Mattson A, Silferswaard C, et al. (1989). Adjuvant tamoxifen in early breast cancer: occurrence of new primary cancers. Lancet I:117–120.
118. Jordan VC, Morrow M (1994) Should clinicians be concerned about the carcinogenic potential of tamoxifen? Eur J Cancer 30A:1714–1721.
119. Carmichael PL, Ugwumadu AHN, Neven P, Herwe AJ, Poon GK, Phillips DH (1996) Lack of genotoxicity of tamoxifen in human endometrium. Cancer Res 56:1475–1479.

120. Magriples U, Naftolin F, Schwartz PE, Carcangui ML (1993) High grade endometrial carcinoma in tamoxifen treated breast cancer patients. J Clin Oncol 11:485–490.
121. Fisher B, Costantino JP, Redmond CK, Fisher ER, Wickerman DL, Clonin WM, et al. (1994) Endometrial cancer in tamoxifen treated breast cancer patients: findings from the National Surgical Adjuvant Breast and Bowel Project (NSABP) B-14. J Natl Cancer Inst 86:527–537.
122. Rutqvist LE, Johansson H, Signomklao T, Johansson U, Fornander T, Wilking N (1995) Adjuvant tamoxifen therapy for early stage breast cancer and second primary malignancies. J Natl Cancer Inst 87:645–651.
123. Barakat RR, Wong G, Curtin JD, Vlamis V, Hoskins WJ (1994) Tamoxifen use in breast cancer patients who subsequently develop corpus cancer is not associated with a higher incidence of adverse histological features. Gynecol Oncol 55:164–168.
124. Barakat RR (1997) Benign and hyperplastic changes associated with tamoxifen use. Oncology 11(suppl):35–37.
125. Kedar RP, Bourne TH, Powles TJ, Collins WP, Ashley SE, Cosgrove DO, et al. (1994) Effects of tamoxifen on uterus and ovaries of postmenopausal women in a randomized breast cancer prevention trial. Lancet 343:1318–1321.
126. Cohen I, Rosen DJ, Shapira J, Cordoba M, Gilboa S, Altares MM, et al. (1993) Endometrial changes in postmenopausal women treated with tamoxifen for breast cancer. Br J Obstet Gynecol 100:567–570.
127. Neven P, De Moylder X, Van Belle Y, Vanderick G, DeMuylder E (1990) Hysteroscopic follow-up during tamoxifen treatment. Eur J Obstet Gynecol Reprod Biol 35:235–238.
128. Williams GM, Iatropoulos MJ, Djordjevic MV, Kaltenberg OP (1993) The triphenylethylene drug tamoxifen is a strong liver carcinogen in the rat. Carcinogenesis 14:315–317.
129. Greaves P, Goonetilleke R, Nunn G, Topham J, Orton T (1993) Two year carcinogenicity study of tamoxifen in Alderley Park Wistar-derived rats. Cancer Res 53:3919–3924.
130. Hard GC, Iatropoulos MJ, Jordan K, Radi L, Kattenberg OP, Imondi AR, et al. (1993) Major differences in the hepatocarcinogenicity and DNA adduct forming ability between toremifene and tamoxifen in female Crl;CD (BR) rats. Cancer Res 53:4534–4541.
131. Dragan YP, Langan-Fahey SM, Street K, Jordan VC, Pitot HC (1994) Studies of tamoxifen as a promoter of hepatocarcinogenesis in female Fisher F344 rats. Breast Cancer Res Treat 31:11–25.
132. Dragan YP, Vaughan J, Jordan VC, Pitot HC (1995) Comparison of tamoxifen and toremifene on liver and kidney tumor promotion in female rats. Carcinogenesis 16:2733–2741.
133. Fahey S, Dragan YP, Nawaysir E, Sattler C, Babcock K, Vaughan J, et al. (1996) Effects of tamoxifen and two fixed ring analogs on multistage rat hepatocarcinogenesis. Carcinogenesis 17:585–594.
134. White INH, deMatteis F, Davies A, Smith LL, Crotton-Sleigh C, Venitt S, et al. (1992) Genotoxic potential of tamoxifen and analogues in female Fischer 344/n rats, DBA/2 and C57BL/6 mice and in human MCL-5 cells. Carcinogenesis 13:2197–2203.
135. Martin EA, Rich KJ, White IN, Woods KL, Powles TJ, Smith LL (1995) 32P-Post labelled DNA adducts in liver obtained from women treated with tamoxifen. Carcinogenesis 16:1651–1654.
136. Jordan VC (1983) Laboratory studies to develop general principles for the adjuvant treatment of breast cancer with antiestrogen: problems and potential for future clinical applications. Breast Cancer Res Treat 3(suppl):573–586.
137. Furr, BJA, Jordan VC (1984) The pharmacology and clinical uses of tamoxifen. Pharmacol Therap 25:127–205.
138. Iguchi T, Hirokawa M, Takasugi N (1986) Occurrence of genital tract abnormalities and bladder hernia in female mice exposed neonatally to tamoxifen. Toxicology 42:1–11.
139. Cunha GR, Taguchi O, Namikawa R, Nishizuka Y, Robboy SG (1987) Teratogenic effects of clomiphene, tamoxifen, and diethyl stilbesterol on the developing human female genital tract. Hum Pathol 8:1132–1143.
140. Chamness GC, Bannayan GA, Landry LA, Sheridan PJ, McGuire WL (1979) Abnormal reproductive development in rats after neonatally administered antiestrogen (tamoxifen). Biol Repro 21:1087–1090.
141. Groom GV, Griffiths K (1976) Effects of the anti-oestrogen tamoxifen on plasma levels of luteinizing hormone, follicle stimulating hormone, prolactin, oestradiol and progesterone in normal pre-menopausal women. J Endocrinol 70:421–428.
142. Jordan VC, Fritz NF, Langan-Fahey S, Thompson M, Tormey DC (1991) Alteration of endocrine parameters in premenopausal women with breast cancer during long-term adjuvant therapy with tamoxifen as the single agent. J Natl Cancer Inst 83:1488–1491.

143. Delrio G, De Placido S, Pagliarulo C, d'Istria M, Fasano S, Marinelli A, et al. (1986) Hypothalamic-pituitary-ovarian axis in women with operable breast cancer treated with adjuvant CMF and tamoxifen. Tumori 72:53–61.
144. Bertelli G, Pronzato P, Amoroso D, Cusmano MP, Conte PF, Montagne G, et al. (1988) Adjuvant tamoxifen in primary breast cancer: influence on plasma lipids and antithrombin III. Breast Cancer Res Treat 12:307–310.
145. Love RR, Weibe DA, Newcomb PA, Cameron L, Leventhal H, Jordan VC, et al. (1991) Effects of tamoxifen on cardiovascular risk factors in postmenopausal women. Ann Intern Med 115:860–864.
146. Love RR, Wiebe DA, Feyzi JM, Newcomb PA, Chappell RJ (1995) Effects of tamoxifen on cardiovascular risk factors in postmenopausal women after 5 years of treatment. J Natl Cancer Inst 86:1534–1539.
147. Bilimoria MM, Assikis VJ, Jordan VC (1996) Should adjuvant tamoxifen treatment be stopped at 5 years? Cancer J from Sci Am 2:140–150.
148. McDonald CC, Stewart HJ (1991) Fatal myocardial infarction in the Scottish tamoxifen trial. BMJ 303:435–437.
149. McDonald CC, Alexander FE, Whyte BW, Forrest AP, McDonald CC, Stewart HJ (1995) Cardiac and vascular morbidity in women receiving adjuvant tamoxifen for breast cancer in a randomized trial. BMJ 311:977–980.
150. Rutqvist LE, Matteson A (1993) Cardiac and thromboembolic morbidity among postmenopausal women with early-stage breast cancer in a randomized trial of tamoxifen. The Stockholm Breast Cancer Study Group. J Natl Cancer Inst 85:1398–1406.
151. Constantino JP, Kuller LH, Ivers PG, et al. (1997) Coronary heart disease mortality and adjuvant tamoxifen therapy. J Natl Cancer Inst 89:776–782.
152. Gylling H, Pyrhonen S, Mantyla E, Maenpaa H, Kangas L, Miettiner TA (1995) Tamoxifen and toremifene lower serum cholesterol by inhibition of Δ 8-cholestenol conversion to lathosterol in women with breast cancer. J Clin Oncol 13:2900–2905.
153. Wiseman H, Cannon M, Astein, HRV, Halliwell B (1993) Tamoxifen inhibits lipid peroxidation in cardiac microsomes. Comparison with liver microsomes and potential relevance to the cardiovascular benefits associated with cancer prevention and treatment by tamoxifen. Biochem Pharmacol 45:1851–1855.
154. Jordan VC, Fritz NF, Tormey DC (1987) Endocrine effects of adjuvant chemotherapy and long term tamoxifen administration on node positive patients with breast cancer. Cancer Res 47:634–630.
155. Love RR, Mazess RB, Barden HS, Epstein S, Newcomb PA, Jordan VC, et al. (1992) Effects of tamoxifen on bone mineral density in postmenopausal women with breast cancer. N Engl J Med 326:852–856.
156. Fornander T, Rutqvist LE, Sjoberg HE, Blomqvist L, Mattson A, Glas U (1990) Long term adjuvant tamoxifen in early breast cancer: effect on bone mineral density in postmenopausal women. J Clin Oncol 8:1019–1024.
157. Ward RL, Morgan G, Dalley D, Kelley PJ (1993) Tamoxifen reduces bone turnover and prevents lumbar spine and proximal femoral bone loss in early postmenopausal women. Bone Min 22:87–94.
158. Kristensen B, Ejlertsen B, Dalgaard P, Larsen L, Holmegaard SN, Transbol I, et al. (1994) Tamoxifen and bone metabolism in postmenopausal low risk breast cancer patients: a randomized study. J Clin Oncol 12:992–997.
159. Foote FW, Stewart FW (1945) Comparative studies of cancerous versus noncancerous breasts. Ann Surg 121:6–53; 197–222.
160. Chaudary MA, Millis RR, Hoskins EO, Halder M, Bulbrook RD, Cuzick J, et al. (1984) Bilateral primary breast cancer: a prospective study of disease incidence. Brit J Surg 71:711–714.
161. Ford D, Easton DF, Bishop DT, Narod SA, Goldsar DE (1994) Risk of cancer in BRCA-1 mutation carriers. Lancet 343:692–695.
162. Henderson IC (1996) Overview of adjuvant tamoxifen therapy, In: *Tamoxifen: A Guide for Clinicians and Patients* (Jordan VC, ed.), PRR, New York, p. 60.
163. Jordan VC (1996) Breast cancer: progress towards the prospects of prevention, In: *Tamoxifen: A Guide for Clinicians and Patients* (Jordan VC, ed.), PRR, New York, pp. 135–145.
164. Powles TJ, Jones AL, Ashley SE, O'Brien ME, Tidy VA, Treleavar J, et al. (1994) The Royal Marsden Hospital pilot tamoxifen chlemoprevention trial. Breast Cancer Res Treat 31:73–82.
165. Gail MH, Brinton LA, Byar DP, Corle DK, Green SB, Schairer C, et al. (1989) Projecting individualized probabilities of developing breast cancer for white females who are being examined annually. J Natl Cancer Inst 81:1879–1886.

166. Tang MX, Jacobs P, Stern Y, Marder K, Schofield P, Garlad B, et al. (1996) Effect of oestrogen during menopause on risk and age at onset of Alzheimers disease. Lancet 348:429–433.
167. Warri AM, Huovinon RL, Laine AM, Martikainen PM, Harkonen PL (1993) Apoptosis in toremifene growth inhibition of human breast cancer cells in vivo and in vitro. J Natl Cancer Inst 85:1412–1418.
168. Grenman RL, Laine KM, Klemi PJ, Grenman S, Hayashida DJ, Joensuu H (1991) Effect of the antiestrogen toremifene on growth of the human mammary carcinoma cell line MCF-7. J Cancer Res Clin Oncol 117:223–226.
169. Robinson SP, Goldstein D, Witt PL, Borden EC, Jordan VC (1990) Inhibition of hormone dependent and independent breast cancer cell growth in vivo and in vitro with the antiestrogen toremifene and recombinant human interferon $\alpha 2$. Breast Cancer Res Treat 15:95–101.
170. Colletta AA, Wakefield LM, Howell FV, Van Roozendaal KE, Danielpour D, Ebbs SR, et al. (1990) Antiestrogens induce the secretion of active transforming growth factor beta from human fetal fibroblasts. Br J Cancer 62:405–409.
171. Knabbe C, Zugmaier G, Schmahl M, Dietel M, Lippman ME, Dickson RB (1991) Induction of transforming growth factor beta by the antiestrogens droloxifene, tamoxifen and toremifene in MCF-7 cells. Am J Clin Oncol 14:15–20.
172. Kangas L (1990) Biochemical and pharmacological effects of toremifene metabolites. Cancer Chemother Pharmacol 27:8–12.
173. DiSalle E, Zaccheo T, Ornati G (1990) Antioestrogenic and antitumour properties of the new triphenylethylene derivative toremifene in the rat. J Steroid Biochem 36:203–206.
174. Huovinen R, Warri A, Collan Y (1993) Mitotic activity, apoptosis and TRPM-2 messenger RNA expression in DMBA-induced rat mammary carcinoma treated with antiestrogen toremifene. Int J Cancer 55:685–691.
175. Huovinen R, Kellokumpu-Lehtinen, P-LI, Collanm Y (1994) Evaluating the response to antiestrogen toremifene treatment in DMBA-induced rat mammary carcinoma. Int J Exp Pathol 75:257–263.
176. Huovinen RL, Alanen KA, Collan Y (1995) Cell proliferation in dimethylbenz(A) anthracene-induced rat mammary carcinoma treated with antiestrogen toremifene. Acta Oncol 34:479–485.
177. Robinson SP, Mauel DA, Jordan VC (1988) Antitumor actions of toremifene in the 7:12 dimethylbenzanthracene (DMBA)-induced rat mammary tumor model. Eur J Cancer 24:1817–1821.
178. Robinson SP, Jordan VC (1989) Antiestrogen action of toremifene on hormone-dependent, independent and heterogeneous breast tumor growth in the athymic mouse. Cancer Res 49:1758–1762.
179. Osborne CK, Jarman M, McCague R, Coronado EB, Hilsenbeck SG, Wakeling AE (1994) The importance of tamoxifen metabolism in tamoxifen-stimulated breast tumor growth. Cancer Chemother Pharmacol 34:89–95.
180. Hirsimaki P, Hirsimaki Y, Nieminen L, Payne BJ (1993) Tamoxifen induces hepatocellular carcinoma in rat liver: a 1 year study with 2 antiestrogens. Arch Toxicol 67:49–59.
181. Dragan YP, Langan-Fahey SM, Street K, Vaughan J, Jorden VC, Pitot HC (1994) Studies of tamoxifen as a promoter of hepatocarcinogenesis in female Fisher F344 rats. Breast Cancer Res Treat 31:11–25.
182. Bishop J, Muray R, Webster L, Pitt P, Stokes K, Fennessy A, et al. (1992) Phase I clinical and pharmacokinetics study of high dose toremifene in postmenopausal patients with advanced breast cancer. Cancer Chemother Pharmacol 30:174–178.
183. Antilla M, Valvaara R, Kivinen S, Maenpaa J (1990) Pharmacokinetics of toremifene. J Steroid Biochem 36:249–252.
184. Tomas E, Kauppila A, Blanco G, Apaja-Serkkinen M, Laatikainen T (1995) Comparison between the effects of tamoxifen and toremifene on the uterus in postmenopausal breast cancer patients. Gynecol Oncol 59:261–266.
185. Szamel I, Hindy I, Vincze B, Eckhardt S, Kangas I, Hajba A (1994) Influence of toremifene on the endocrine regulation in breast cancer patients. Eur J Cancer 30A:154–158.
186. Kivinen S, Maenpaa J (1990) Effect of toremifene on clinical hematological and hormonal parameters at different dose levels in healthy postmenopausal volunteers: phase I study. J Steroid Biochem 36:217–220.
187. Hamm JT, Tormey DC, Kohler PC, Haller D, Green M, Shemano I (1991) Phase I study of toremifene in patients with advanced cancer. J Clin Oncol 9:2036–2041.
188. Valavaara R, Pyrhonen S, Heikkinen M, Rissanen P, Blanco G, Tholiz E, et al. (1988) Toremifene, a new antiestrogenic treatment of advanced breast cancer. Phase II study. Eur J Cancer 24:785–790.
189. Valavaara R, Pyrhonen S (1989) Low-dose toremifene in the treatment of estrogen-receptor-positive advanced breast cancer in postmenopausal women. Curr Ther Res 46:966–973.

190. Gunderson S (1990) Toremifene, a new antiestrogenic compound in the treatment of advanced breast cancer. Phase II study. Eur J Cancer 24:785–790.
191. Hietanen T, Baltina D, Johansson R, Numminen S, Hakala T, Helle L, et al. (1990) High dose toremifene (240 mg daily) is effective as first line hormonal treatment in advanced breast cancer—an ongoing phase-II multicenter Finnish-Latvian cooperatie study. Breast Cancer Res Treat 16(suppl):37–40.
192. Modig H, Borgstrom M, Nilsson I, Westman G (1990) Phase II clinical study of toremifene in patients with metastatic breast cancer. J Steroid Biochem 36:235–236.
193. Valavaara R (1990) Phase II experience with toremifene in the treatment of ER-positive breast cancer of postmenopausal women. Cancer Invest 8:275–276.
194. Konstantinova MM, Gershanovich ML (1990) Results of comparative clinical evaluation of antiestrogens toremifene and tamoxifen in locally advanced and disseminated breast cancer [in Russian]. Vopr. Onkol. 36:1182–1186.
195. Nomura Y, Tominaga T, Abe O, Izuo M, Ogawa N (1993) Clinical evaluation of NK 22 (toremifene citrate) in advanced or recurrent breast cancer—a comparative study by a double blind method with tamoxifen [in Japanese]. Gan to Kagaku Ryoho 20:247–258.
196. Stenbygaard LE, Herrstedt J, Thomsen JF, Svendsen KR, Engelholm SA, Dombernowski P (1993) Toremifene and tamoxifen in advanced breast cancer—a double-blind cross-over trial. Breast Cancer Res Treat 25:57–63.
197. Hayes DF, Van Zyl JA, Hacking A, Goedhals L, Bezwoda WR, Maillard JA, et al. (1995) Randomized comparison of tamoxifen and two separate doses of toremifene in postmenopausal patients with metastic breast cancer. J Clin Oncol 113:2556–2566.
198. Ebbs SR, Roberts J, Baum M (1990) Response to toremifene (Fc-1157a) therapy in tamoxifen failed patients with breast cancer. Preliminary communication. J Steroid Biochem 36:239.
199. Hindy I, Juhos E, Szanto J, Szamel I (1990) Effect of toremifene in breast cancer patients. Preliminary communication. J Steroid Biochem 36:225–226.
200. Jonsson PE, Malmberg M, Bergljung L, Ingvar C, Ericsson M, Ryder S, et al. (1991) Phase II study of high dose toremifene in advanced breast cancer progressing during tamoxifen treatment. AntiCancer Res 11:873–876.
201. Asaishi K, Tominaga T, Abe O, Izuo M, Nomula Y (1993) Efficacy and safety of high dose NK 622 (toremifene citrate) in tamoxifen failed patients with breast cancer [in Japanese] Gan to Kagaku Ryoho 20:91–99.
202. Pyrhönen S, Valavaara R, Vuorinen J, Hajba A (1994) High dose toremifene in advanced breast cancer Resistant to or relapsed during tamoxifen treatment. Breast Cancer Res Treat 29:223–228.
203. Vogel CL, Shemano I, Schoenfelder J, Gams RA, Green MR (1993) Multicenter phase II efficacy trial of toremifene in tamoxifen refractory patients with advanced breast cancer. J Clin Oncol 11:345–350.
204. Roos WK, Oeze L, Loser R, Eppenberger U (1983) Antiestrogen action of 3-hydroxy-tamoxifen in the human breast cancer cell line MCF-7. J Natl Cancer Inst 71:55–59.
205. Loser R, Seibel K, Eppenberger U (1985) No loss of estrogenic and antiestrogenic activity after demethylation of droloxifene (3-OH tamoxifen). Int J Cancer 36:701–703.
206. Eppenberger U, Wosikowski K Kung W (1991) Pharmacologic and biologic properties of Droloxifene, a new antiestrogen. Am J Clin Oncol 14:s5–s14.
207. Kawamura I, Mizota T, Lacey E, Tanaka Y, Morda T, Shimomura K, et al. (1993) Pharmacologic and biologic properties of droloxifene, a new antiestrogen. Jpn J Pharmacol 63:27–34.
208. Hasman M, Rattel B, Loser R (1994) Preclinical data for droloxifene. Cancer Lett 84:101–116.
209. Loser R, Seibel K, Roos W, Eppenberger U (1985) In vivo and in vitro antiestrogenic action of 3-hydroxy-tamoxifen, tamoxifen and 4-hydroxy-tamoxifen. Eur J Cancer Clin Oncol 21: 985–900.
210. Wosikowski K, Kung W, Hasmann M, Loser R, Eppenberger U (1993) Inhibition of growth factor activated proliferation by antiestrogens and effects on early gene expression of MCF-7 cells. Int J Cancer 53:290–297.
211. Ke HZ, Simmons HA, Pirie CM, Crawford DT, Thompson DD (1995) Droloxifene, a new estrogen antagonist/agonist, prevents bone loss in ovariectomized rats. Endocrinology 136:2435–2441.
212. Grill HJ, Pollow K (1991) Pharmacokinetics of droloxifene and its metabolites in breast cancer patients. Am J Clin Oncol 14(suppl 2):s21–s29.
213. Lien EA, Anker G, Lonning PE, Ueland PM (1995) Determination of droloxifene and two metabolites in serum by high pressure liquid chromatography. Ther Drug Monit 17:259–265.
214. Geisler J, Ekse D, Hosch S (1995) Influence of droloxifene (3-hydroxytamoxifen) 40 mg daily on plasma gonadotrophins, sex hormone binding globulin and estrogen levels in postmenopausal breast cancer patients. J Steroid Biochem Mol Biol 55:193–195.

215. Ahlemann L,M., Staab HJ, Loser R, Seibel K, Huber HJ (1988) Inhibition of growth of human cancer by intermittent exposure to the antiestrogen droloxifene. Tumor Diagn Ther 9:41–46.
216. Abe O, Enomote K, Fujiwara K, Izuo M, Iino Y, Tominaga T, et al. (1990) Phase I study of FK 435. Jpn J Cancer Clin 36:903–913.
217. Abe O, Enomote K, Fujiwara K, Izumo M, Iino Y, Tominaga, et al. (1991) Japanese early phase II study of droloxifene in the treatment of advanced breast cancer. Am J Clin Oncol 14:540–451.
218. Bellmunt J, Sole L (1991) European early phase II dose finding study of droloxifene in advanced breast cancer. Am J Clin Oncol 14:536–539.
219. Haarstad H, Gundersen S, Wist E, Raabe N, Mella O, Kuinnsland S (1992) Droloxifene—a new antiestrogen phase II study in advanced breast cancer. Acta Oncol 31:425–428.
220. Raushning W, Pritchard KI (1994) Droloxifene, a new antiestrogen: its role in metastatic breast cancer. Breast Cancer Res Treat 31:83–94.
221. Buzdar AU, Kau S, Hortobagyi GN, Theriault RL, Booser DL, Holmes HA, et al. (1994) Phase I trial of droloxifene in patients with metastatic breast cancer. Cancer Chemother Pharmacol 33:313–316.
222. Chander SK, McCague R, Lugmani Y, Newton C, Dowsett M, Jarmar M, et al. (1991) Pyrrolidino-4-iodotamoxifen and 4-iodotamoxifen, new analogues of the antiestrogen tamoxifen for the treatment of breast cancer. Cancer Res 51:5851–5858.
223. McCague R, Parr IB, Haynes BP (1990) Metabolism of the 4 iodo derivative of tamoxifen by isolated rat hepatocytes. Demonstration that the iodine atom reduces metabolic conversion and identification of four metabolites. Biochem Pharmcol 40:2277–2283.
224. Coombes RC, Haynes BP, Dowsett M, Quigley M, English J, Judson IR, et al. (1995) Idoxifene: report of a phase I study in patients with metastatic breast cancer. Cancer Res 55:1070–1074.
225. Wakeling AE, Bowler J (1987) Steroidal pure antiestrogens. J Endocrinol 112:R7–R10.
226. Wakeling AE, Dukes M, Bowler J (1991) A potent specific pure antiestrogen with clinical potential. Cancer Res 51:3867–3873.
227. Dauvois S, Danielian PS, White R, Parker MG (1992) Antiestrogen ICI 164,384 reduces cellular estrogen receptor by increasing its turnover. Proc Natl Acad Sci USA 89:4037–4041.
228. Gibson MK, Nemmers LA, Beckman WC (1991) The mechanism of ICI 164,384 antiestrogenicity involves rapid loss of estrogen receptor in uterine tissue. Endocrinology 129:2000–2010.
229. Gottardis MM, Jiang SY, Jeng MH, Jordan (1989) Inhibition of tamoxifen stimulated growth of an MCF-7 tumor variant in athymic mice by novel steroidal antiestrogens. Cancer Res 49:4090–4093.
230. Gottardis MM, Ricchio MD, Satyaswaroop PG, Jordan VC (1990) Effect of steroidal and nonsteroidal antiestrogens on the growth of a tamoxifen-stimulated human endometrial carcinoma (EnCa101) in athymic mice. Cancer Res 50:3189–3192.
231. Osborne CK, Coronado-Heinsohn EB, Hilsenbeck SG, McCue BL, Wakeling AE, McClelland RA, et al. (1995) Comparison of the effects of a pure steroidal antiestrogen with those of tamoxifen in a model of human cancer. J Natl Cancer Inst 87:746–750.
232. Nicholson RI, Walker KJ, Bouzukar N, Wills RJ, Gee JM, Rushmere NK et al. (1990) Estrogen deprivation in breast cancer. Clinical, experimental and biological aspects. Ann NY Acad Sci 595:316–327.
233. Dukes M, Miller D, Wakeling AE (1992) Antiuterotrophic effect of a pure antioestrogen ICI 182,780: magnetic resonance imaging of the uterus in ovariectomized monkeys. J Endocrinol 135:239–247.
234. Dukes M, Waterton JC, Wakeling AE (1993) Antiuterotrophic effect of the pure antiestrogen ICI 182,780 in adult female monkeys (*Macaca nemestrina*): quantitative magnetic resonance imaging. J Endocrinol 138:203–210.
235. DeFriend DJ, Howell A, Nicholson RI, Anderson E, Dowsett M, Mansel RE, et al. (1994) Investigation of a pure new antiestrogen (ICI 182,780) in women with primary breast cancer. Cancer Res 54:408–414.
236. Howell A, DeFriend DJ, Robertson JFR, Blamey RW, Anderson L, Anderson E, et al. (1996) Pharmacokinetics, pharmacological and anti-tumour effects of the specific anti-oestrogen ICI 182:780 in women with breast cancer. Br J Cancer 74:300–308.
237. Black LJ, Jones CD, Falcone JF (1983) Antagonism of estrogen action with a new benzothiophene-derived antiestrogen. Life Sci. 32:1031–1036.
238. Evans GL, Bryant HU, Magee D, Sata M, Turner RT (1994) The effects of raloxifene on tibia histomorphometry in ovariectomized rats. Endocrinology 134:2283–2288.
239. Black LJ, Sato M, Rowley ER, Magee DE, Bekele A, Williams DC, et al. (1994) Raloxifene (LY139481 HCl) prevents bone loss and reduces serum cholesterol without causing uterine hypotrophy in ovariectomized rats. J Clin Invest 93:63–69.

240. Sato M, Kim J, Short LL, Slemenda CW, Bryant HV (1995) Longitudinal and cross-sectional analysis of raloxifene effects on tibiae from ovariectomized rats. J Pharmacol Exp Ther 272:1251–1259.
241. Clemens JA, Bennett DR, Black LJ, Jones CD (1983) Effects of a new antiestrogen keoxifene (LY156758) on growth of carcinogen induced mammary tumors and on LH and prolactin levels. Life Sci 32:2869–2875.
242. Gottardis MM, Jordan VC (1987) The antitumor action of keoxifene and tamoxifen in the N-nitrosomethylurea-induced rat mammary carcinoma model. Cancer Res 47:4020–4024.
243. Draper MW, Flowers DE, Hester WJ (1993) Effects of raloxifene (LY 139481 HCL) on biochemical markers of bone and lipid metabolism in healthy postmenopausal women, In: *Proceedinga of the Fourth International Symposium on Osteoporosis, Handelstrykkeriet Aalborg ApS.,* Aalborg, Denmark.
244. Buzdar AU, Marcus C, Holmes F, Hug V, Hortobagyi G (1988) Phase II evaluation of LY156758 in metastatic breast cancer. Oncology 45:344–345.
245. Gradishar WJ, Glussman J, Yili L, Vogel C, Cohen F, Sledge GW (1998) Raloxifene in hormone receptor-positive, metastatic breast cancer. Cancer, submitted.
246. Jordan VC, Phelps E, Lindgren JV (1987) Effect of antiestrogens on bone in castrated and intact female rats. Breast Cancer Res Treat 10:31–35.
247. Jordan VC (1997) Tamoxifen: the herald of new era of preventive therapeutics. J Natl Cancer Inst 89:747–749.

20 LHRH Superagonists and Antagonists in the Treatment of Breast Cancer

P.N. Mainwaring, MBBS, FRACP
and M. Dowsett, PhD

INTRODUCTION

This review aims to summarize the biology of the luteinizing hormone-releasing hormone (LHRH) analogs and to review critically their role in the clinical management of breast cancer.

Ovarian ablation is the oldest form of systemic therapy for the management of breast cancer with surgical oophorectomy for the palliation of premenopausal metastatic breast cancer first described at the end of the last century *(1,2)*. Several methods of ovarian ablation are available and include surgical oophorectomy, radiation ablation, and LHRH analogs. In addition, some adjuvant chemotherapy regimens lead to permanent ovarian ablation. Superactive LHRH agonists have emerged as major new clinical agents in the management of precocious puberty, ovulation induction, prostatic cancer, breast cancer, endometriosis, uterine leiomyoma, and other conditions.

In 1971, LHRH was isolated from hypothalamic extracts, and its amino acid sequence was established by Schally and colleagues *(3)*. Five years later, DeSombre and colleagues *(4)* reported regression of xenograft breast tumors by an LHRH analog, and for the last 16 years, LHRH agonists have been investigated as a treatment modality in both pre- and postmenopausal breast cancer.

About 30–50% of premenopausal women with metastatic breast cancer respond to LHRH agonist therapy, suggesting comparable efficacy with surgical oophorectomy. Women with estrogen receptor (ER)-positive tumors are more likely to respond than those with ER-negative tumors. The predominant mechanism of action in women is estrogen suppression; however, a direct antitumor effect has been proposed, first, because postmenopausal women with metastatic breast cancer occasionally respond to LHRH agonists and second, because clinical responses are seen in premenopausal women with ER-poor tumors. Randomized trials are under way to examine the contribution of LHRH agonists in the adjuvant setting of premenopausal ER-positive women with early breast cancer. The LHRH agonists have

From: *Contemporary Endocrinology: Endocrinology of Breast Cancer*
Edited by: A. Manni © Humana Press Inc., Totowa, NJ

clinical benefits over the other methods of ovarian ablation in premenopausal women. These include (1) reduced morbidity compared with surgical and radiotherapeutic interventions, (2) temporary usage if they prove not to be effective antitumor agents, and (3) their reversibility if preservation of fertility is important to the patient. LHRH antagonists in breast cancer have, until recently, not been clinically applicable because of excessive side effects. New analogs are undergoing clinical testing to demonstrate efficacy, initially in the metastatic setting.

OOPHORECTOMY IN BREAST CANCER

Surgical oophorectomy and ovarian ablation by irradiation produce castration levels of estradiol within 2–7 days and after 6 weeks or more, respectively *(5,6)*.

Response rates following surgical ablation of the ovaries in premenopausal women with metastatic breast cancer are in the range of about 21–37% with a median duration of 10–14 months *(7–10)* in unselected patients and rise to 50% in women with ER-positive disease *(11)*. The response rate for women under the age of 35 is often lower, ranging from 15 to 25%, probably because of a higher incidence of ER-negative tumors *(10,12)*.

The Early Breast Cancer Collaborative Trialists' Group has recently reported their latest 5-yearly systematic overview analysis of ovarian ablation in early breast cancer *(13)*. Among women under 50 years of age, 15-year survival was highly significantly improved among those allocated ovarian ablation (52.4 vs 46.1%, log rank $2p = 0.001$) leading to 6.3% (SD 2.3) fewer deaths per 100 women with a similar benefit in recurrence-free survival (45.0 vs 39.0%; 6.0% [SD 2.3] fewer recurrences per 100 women). Ovarian ablation reduced the recurrence-free event rate by about one-fifth (18.5% [SD 5.5]). Most of the benefit occurred in the first 5 years.

It is important to note that the proportional improvement in recurrence-free survival was 25% (SD 7) in the absence of chemotherapy but only 10% (SD 9) in the presence of chemotherapy. Similarly, the proportional improvement in overall survival was 24% (SD 7) in the absence of chemotherapy but only 8% (SD 10) in the presence of chemotherapy. It seems likely that this reduced effect in the presence of chemotherapy is due to the ovarian ablative effects of the chemotherapy. This will be an important aspect to consider in the interpretation of future data from trials of LHRH agonists in the adjuvant context. It should also be noted that in those studies in which ovariectomy was compared with no adjuvant therapy, patients were not selected according to ER status. (The ER had not been discovered when most of these trials were initiated.) Given that only approx 50% of premenopausal women are ER positive, if treatment was confined to this (now identifiable) subgroup, the degree of benefit for the treated population would be expected to be substantially greater.

Two small randomized trials have compared tamoxifen and oophorectomy for the treatment of metastatic breast cancer in premenopausal women. Neither trial demonstrated a benefit for either therapy in terms of response rates, time to treatment failure, or overall survival; however, both trials accrued slowly and lacked statistical power to detect small, clinically relevant differences *(7,8)*. A recent meta-analysis of four trials, one of which included patients with ER-negative tumors, of tamoxifen vs ovarian ablation as first-line endocrine therapy for premenopausal women with metastatic breast cancer has reported no difference in response rates or mortality *(14)*.

Table 1
Names and Amino Acid Substitutions of LHRH Agonists

Name	*Substitution position 6*	*Substitution position 10*
Buserelin	D-Ser (tBu)	NEt
Deslorelin	D-Trp	NEt
Goserelin	D-Ser (tBu)	aza-Gly
Histrelin	D-His (Bzl)	NEt
Leuprorelin	D-Leu	Gly
Lutrelin[a]	D-Trp	NEt
Meterelin	D-Me-Trp (2)	NEt
Nafarelin	D-Nal (2)	
Triptorelin	D-Trp	

[a]N-Me-Leu substitution at position 7.

LHRH AGONISTS

Structure of LHRH Agonists

The human LHRH receptor gene is localized to chromosome 4q13, contains three exons and two introns, and spans over 20 kb. Receptor cDNAs from humans encode proteins of 328 amino acids putatively containing seven transmembrane domains. The receptors belong to the family of G-protein-coupled receptors and utilize Ca^{2+} as a second messenger. In humans, LHRH receptor mRNA is expressed in the ovary, testes, breast, prostate, and adrenal, and in a number of hormone-dependent tumors and tumor cell lines as well as in the anterior pituitary *(15)*. The functional significance of any receptor in extrapituitary sites is largely unknown. Occupancy by agonist, but not antagonists, has been demonstrated to promote receptor-receptor interactions as an early event *(16)*.

LHRH or gonadotrophin-releasing hormone is a decapeptide (pGlu-His-Trp-Ser-Tyr-Gly-Leu-Arg-Pro-GlyNH-2) that is released in a pulsatile manner from the hypothalamus and acts through specific high-affinity receptors in the anterior pituitary gland stimulating the synthesis and secretion of luteinizing hormone (LH) and follicle-stimulating hormone (FSH) *(17)*. LH is responsible for ovarian androgen production and luteinization of the ruptured graafian follicle with consequent progesterone production. FSH stimulates the conversion of ovarian androgens to estrogens in the follicular granulosa cells. The pituitary can only be prompted to secrete gonadotrophins when it receives repeated stimulation at regular 1–2-hourly intervals. There is now general agreement that the number of pituitary LHRH receptors is increased or decreased by autoregulation. Exposure of the pituitary to supraphysiologic concentrations of LHRH, to continuous administration of LHRH, or to its long-acting analogs suppresses gonadotrophin and consequently gonadal steroid secretion *(18)*. By contrast, LHRH antagonists suppress gonadotrophin secretion immediately by competitive blockade of the LHRH receptor *(19)*.

Over 25 years has passed since the principles for modification of LHRH were described permitting synthesis of superactive LHRH agonists. By substituting amino acids at the 10th position (glycine amide) of the native LHRH sequence with ethylamide or azaglycine and at the 6th position (L-glycine) with other more lipophylic D-amino acids such as D-Phe, D-Leu, or D-Trp, the hormonal activity can be greatly extended (Table 1). Most of these modifications result in more hydrophobic compounds, proportionally increasing receptor affinity and in vitro potency. These alterations also increase resistance to enzymatic degradation, increase plasma protein binding, and prolong the compound's half-life due to decreased renal excretion *(20)*. The binding affinity of LHRH analogues is about 10 times higher than the natural hormone, and the potency may be increased 50–200-fold over native LHRH *(21)*.

Since the decapeptide analogs are sensitive to intestinal peptidases, they are inactivated if given orally. Intranasal and subcutaneous routes of administration have therefore been used. However, intranasal administration requires frequent administration, and consequently is associated with compliance problems. Subcutaneous administration initially also required daily administration but depot formulations were developed allowing monthly, or more recently 3-monthly, injection intervals. All depot LHRH agonists are bound to copolymers in the shape of microcapsules or rods. The analog-copolymer complex is injected subcutaneously or intramuscularly.

Endocrine Effects

Premenopausal Effects

The clinical pharmacology of the large number of agonists when given as depot injections is very similar. Chronic LHRH agonist administration produces a transient (1–2-week) elevation of gonadotrophin and gonadal steroid concentrations, peaking at 2–3, followed by a hypogonadal state with profound reductions in gonadal steroid secretion to castration levels within 3 weeks *(22)*. Suppression of LH release is usually greater than that of FSH, and the pituitary response to exogenous LHRH is also blunted. Amenorrhea normally occurs within 30 days of commencing therapy, and menses usually resume within 80 days of cessation of therapy in premenopausal women *(23)*. LH levels remain low during prolonged treatment, but FSH levels begin to recover after the first month, possibly due to the influence of inhibin *(24)*. There is also a small recovery in estrogen levels after the nadir at month 1, such that the mean estradiol levels are above the mean for castrated women (approx 50 pmol/L vs 30 pmol/L) *(25)*. The higher levels of estradiol result from incomplete folliculogenesis driven by FSH but unsupported by LH. It is unclear whether these marginally higher estrogen levels have therapeutic significance in breast cancer patients treated with medical castration.

Postmenopausal Effects

Estrogen production in postmenopausal women is inhibited to a lesser extent because the ovary in postmenopausal women is devoid of aromatase, and the remaining estrogen production occurs by peripheral aromatization of androgens *(26)*. Two mechanisms have been proposed whereby LHRH agonists may induce responses in postmenopausal breast cancer patients: first, reduction of gonadotrophin levels may result in reduction of ovarian androgens and so indirectly influence peripheral aromatization of androgens to estrogens *(27,28)*, and second, there may be a direct effect on breast cancer cells.

Evidence for Direct Antitumor Effects

Prior to the identification of the LHRH receptor and its tissue distribution, several lines of evidence supported the existence of direct antitumor effects of LHRH analogs: LHRH had been detected in human milk at levels five- to six-fold higher than in plasma measured with a double antibody radioimmunoassay *(29)*. Low-affinity LHRH binding sites have been demonstrated in human breast cells in vitro, and LHRH antagonists competed for binding with an approximately 10-fold higher affinity *(30)*. In addition, in human breast tumor biopsies LHRH immunoreactivity was found more frequently in breast tumors with positive estrogen and progesterone receptors *(31)*. Baumann and colleagues *(32)* analyzed 235 human breast cancer biopsies for LHRH receptor membrane binding using Scatchard analysis of [^{125}I]buserelin binding, with rat pituitary positive controls, revealing low- and high-affinity binding sites. In their study, no significant differences in LHRH agonist binding were reported according to histologic subtypes, menopausal status, estrogen or progesterone receptor status, S-phase index, or tumor stage *(32)*.

In Vitro Evidence

Klijn and colleagues reported that estradiol-stimulated growth of the hormone receptor-positive MCF-7 human breast cancer cells could be inhibited by the LHRH agonist buserelin in a dose-dependent manner *(33)*. Similar antiproliferative effects in MCF-7 cells were reported by Miller and colleagues *(30)*, but no effects were seen in MDA-MB-231 and T-47D cells. In another study in MCF-7 cells, no effect of buserelin on cytoplasmic and nuclear estrogen receptors was demonstrated, whereas the level of estrogen-induced progesterone receptor was decreased. Furthermore, the inhibitory effect of buserelin on growth of MCF-7 cells could partly be abolished by tamoxifen, suggesting a complex interaction at the hormone-receptor level *(34)*. In LHRH-sensitive and -insensitive clonal variants of the MCF-7 cell line, buserelin showed a dose-dependent reduction in cellular proliferation in the sensitive but not insensitive cell lines, and cell cycle analysis of those cells cultured in the presence of LHRH agonist demonstrated a marked increase in the percentage of cells in the G_0/G_1 phase of the cell cycle *(35)*. Clonal variation between phenotypically identical cell lines, different estrogen receptor levels, and variability in culture conditions, especially with respect to serum and insulin concentrations, have been discussed in the reports cited above to explain some of the discrepancies between these findings. Nonetheless there remain several reports of the antiproliferative effects of some LHRH agonists. However, in general, the concentrations required to elicit these effects are 2 logs or more higher than those found in patients, and this throws doubt on their mechanistic relevance in the clinic.

The antiproliferative effects of LHRH agonists and antagonists were compared with 4-hydroxy-tamoxifen in ER-positive breast cancer cell lines *(36)*. None of the compounds inhibited proliferation without estrogen stimulation; however, they all inhibited estradiol-stimulated growth. Unlike 4-hydroxy-tamoxifen, triptorelin had no effect on steroid receptor levels, suggesting different inhibitory mechanisms.

In Vivo Evidence

In the athymic nude mouse, buserelin inhibited estradiol-stimulated MCF-7 tumor formation and produced a 30% regression of mature tumors in intact but not ovariectomized animals, which is consistent with no significant direct inhibitory effect *(37)*. Moreover, high doses of the goserelin depot were required to induce regression of MCF-7 or MDA-MB-231 xenografts *(38)*.

Systemic Effects of LHRH Treatment

Other than infrequent local tolerability problems at the injection site, all adverse effects are induced by the profound gonadal hyposecretion induced by these agents. In most postpubertal women hot flushes are inescapable, and decreased libido is often

Table 2
Response Rates in Premenopausal Women with Advanced Breast Cancer Treated with Single-Agent LHRH Agonist Therapy

Reference	*Year*	*Agonist*	*Median age, (range)*	*No.*	*CR, r/e (%)*	*ORR, r/e (%)*
Harvey *et al. (49)*	1985	Leuprorelin	43 (23–52)	26	0 (0)	11/25 (44)
Höffken *et al.*	1986	Buserelin		15	3/15 (20)	7/15 (47)
Manni *et al.*	1986	Leuprorelin		25	0	11 (44)
Mathé *et al.*	1986	Triptorelin		8	2 (25)	3/8 (38)
Williams *et al. (48)*	1986	Goserelin	45 (29–55)	53	0 (0)	14/45 (31)
Lissoni *et al.*	1988	Buserelin		14	0 (0)	2 (14)
Kaufmann *(47)*	1989	Goserelin	42 (25–55)	134	12/118 (10)	53/118 (45)
Klijn *et al.*	1989	Buserelin		22	9/22 (41)	
Schmidt *et al.*	1989	Goserelin		29	7/29 (24)	11/29 (38)
Dixon et al. *(45)*	1990	Goserelin	44 (31–55)	75	7/75 (9)	25/75 (33)
Dowsett *et al. (46)*	1990	Leuprorelin	40 (33–42)	12	1/6 (17)	5/12 (42)
Bianco *et al. (51)*	1991	Goserelin	41 (28–56)	61	5/53 (9)	16/53 (30)
Brambilla *et al. (52)*	1992	Goserelin	39 (28–52)	22	5/22 (23)	7122 (32)
Neskovic *et al.*	1992	Triptorelin		11	0 (0)	5/11 (45)
Blamey *et al. (44)*	1993	Goserelin	42 (24–55)	333		83/228 (36)
Bajetta *et al. (43)*	1994	Goserelin	43 (27–53)	40	6/38 (16)	17/38 (45)
Taguchi *et al.*	1995	Leuprorelin		106		14/46 (30)
Taguchi *et al.*	1995					12/49 (25)
Garcia *et al.*	1996	Triptorelin	44 (30–52)	27	5/27 (18)	19/27 (70)

Abbreviations: r, number of responders; e, number of evaluable patients; CR, complete clinical response; ORR, overall response rate.

reported. Other common subjective adverse effects include insomnia, mood swings, headaches, and vaginal dryness *(39)*. Nevertheless, the most important clinically relevant long-term complication of therapy is bone mineral loss. In a 3-month period, a bone loss of up to 3% can be expected. Estrogen/progestin combination steroid therapy can prevent this loss with little impact on therapeutic efficacy in some conditions such as endometriosis *(40)*, but this has not been investigated in breast cancer. Partial suppression to minimize adverse effects such as bone mineral loss is not possible because identification of the minimum suppression required for each patient has not been achieved.

Complications or adverse effects have not been reported from overdose with these compounds and, conversely, inadequate gonadal/pituitary suppression may prevent full therapeutic efficacy *(41)*.

Agonists in Breast Cancer Treatment

Premenopausal Women with Advanced Disease

Marked improvement in two of four premenopausal women with metastatic breast cancer using high-dose intravenous and intranasal buserelin was reported by Klijn and de Jong in 1982 *(42)*. Concurrent suppression of pituitary gonadotrophin levels in plasma was noted. Over the last 15 years, a number of clinical trials have examined the role of LHRH agonists for the palliation of metastatic disease in premenopausal women with advanced breast cancer (Tables 2 and 3) under the rationale that these would achieve a

Table 3
Survival of Premenopausal Women with Advanced Breast Cancer Treated with Single-Agent LHRH Agonist Therapy

Reference	*Year*	*Agonist*	*Median time to relapse (range)*	*Median duration of response (range)*	*Median time to progression (range)*	*Median overall survival (range)*
Kaufmann *et al. (53)*	1989	Coserelin	4 months (2–11)	8+ months (2–24+)	7 months (1–30)	
Dixon *et al. (45)*	1990	Goserelin		15 months (7–52)	CR >37 mo	
Bianco *et al. (51)*	1991	Goserelin	12 weeks (8–48)	36 weeks (16–76)	17 weeks (5–76)	93 weeks (5–188)
Brambilla *et al. (52)*	1992	Goserelin		64 weeks (29–77)	23 weeks (8–81)	141 weeks (35–182)
Blamey *et al. (44)*	1993	Goserelin	12 weeks (4–49)	44 weeks (>4–>160)	22 weeks (1->160)	26.5 months (0.8–69)
Bajetta *et al. (45)*	1994	Goserelin		12 months (1–33+)CR	4 months (1–10)	
Garcia *et al.*	1996	Triptorelin		51 months	12 months	72+ months

Abbreviations: CR, complete clinical response.

Table 4
Response Rates in Phase II Trials of Premenopausal Women with Advanced Breast Cancer Treated with LHRH Agonist Therapy in Combination with Other Agents

Reference	*Year*	*Trial treatment*	*No.*	*CR, n/e (%)*	*ORR, n/e (%)*
Nicholson *et al. (57)*	1990	Goserelin	75	7/75 (9)	39/75 (52)
		Goserelin +tamoxifen	50	5/50 (10)	26/50 (52)
Buzzoni *et al. (56)*	1995	Goserelin + tamoxifen	64	7/64 (11)	26/64 (41)
Falkson *et al. (65)*	1992	Buserelin + CAF	66	29/60 (48)	49/60 (82)
Lopez *et al. (64)*	1992	Leuprolide + megestrol acetate	30	1/30 (3)	9/30 (30)

Abbreviations: n, number of patients; e, number of evaluable patients; CR, complete clinical response, ORR, overall response rate; CAF, cyclophosphamide, doxorubicin, and fluorouracil.

steroidal environment similar to surgical oophorectomy, but with less morbidity than surgery and the opportunity for reversibility *(43)*. Comparative review of the reported trials requires caution because of the complexities of different patient inclusion criteria, previous therapeutic maneuvers, hormone-receptor compositions and receptor positivity, different criteria for defining menopause, and different response criteria.

Blamey and colleagues *(44)* in their summary review of 333 patients from 29 clinical trials of goserelin therapy reported an overall response rate of 36% with a median duration of response of 44 weeks (>4–>160), median time to relapse of 12 weeks (range 4–49), and median time to progression of 22 weeks (1–>160).

In general, these trials report higher response rates in ER-positive tumors *(43–48)*; however, several trials have reported responses in ER-negative tumors *(38,47,49)*. Higher response rates were also noted to occur in women with prolonged disease-free intervals *(44,47,50–52)* and locoregional metastases compared with visceral or bone metastases *(45,47,48,51,52)*. In an early report by the Cooperative German Oncology Group, 29% of patients responded to the addition of tamoxifen to continued goserelin after progression on goserelin alone *(53)*. No further responses were seen in patients who had responded initially to LHRH agonists, relapsed, and then proceeded to surgical oophorectomy *(43,48,52)*, supporting the therapeutic equivalence of these two approaches to ovarian ablation.

Combination Therapy Approaches

Early consideration of combinations of tamoxifen with LHRH agonists raised concerns that the potential stimulatory effect of tamoxifen on pituitary-ovarian function might be counteractive to the suppressive effect of LHRH agonist treatment *(54)*. However, combination therapy has been subsequently found to produce essentially the same sex steroid and pituitary hormonal suppression as single-agent LHRH agonist therapy *(55)*.

The Italian Trials in Medical Oncology Group examined combination goserelin and tamoxifen in 64 premenopausal women with advanced breast cancer. Overall 41% of patients responded, especially in soft tissue sites, with a median duration of response of 13 months (range 6–37^{+}) (Table 4) *(56)*. In a series of reports, Blamey's group *(57)* has found similar response rates between premenopausal patients with metastatic breast cancer receiving either goserelin and tamoxifen therapy or goserelin alone (Table 3). In this trial, combination therapy was superior to goserelin alone in a cross-sectional analysis of duration of response ($p = 0.02$), and duration of response was significantly longer in ER-positive patients ($p < 0.0001$) *(58)*. Further analysis of patients in the combination arm revealed increased survival for responding patients, but this is a common feature of responding advanced breast cancer patients to any therapy ($p = 0.002$) *(58)*.

A large, international multicenter study involving 318 pre- and perimenopausal advanced breast cancer patients has examined the role of combination therapy compared with goserelin therapy alone. With a median follow-up of 93 weeks, 31% of goserelin-treated patients had objective responses (Union International contre le cancer criteria) compared with 38% of goserelin plus tamoxifen-treated patients ($p = 0.24$). There was a modest benefit in favor of combination therapy in time to progression ($p = 0.03$) but not in survival ($p = 0.25$; median follow-up for survival 117.5 weeks) (Table 5) *(59)*. A further trial has used a three-arm design in 140 evaluable premenopausal women with advanced breast cancer. Antitumor effect was significantly higher in the combination arm (51%) compared with either arm alone (buserelin 33%, tamoxifen 29%); median progression-free and, most importantly, overall survival were significantly improved in the combination arm *(60,61)*. In all these trials side effects from treatment were comparable.

In a 2 by 2 factorial design, Boccardo and colleagues *(62)* have not found any significant differences in response rates or survival in premenopausal patients with advanced breast cancer receiving ovarian ablation, without and with tamoxifen, goserelin alone, or combined with tamoxifen. However, the power of this trial to detect significant differences was hindered by the low number of patients allocated to each subgroup.

The tamoxifen plus LHRH agonist combination therapy approach has been given under the rationale that tamoxifen may antagonize residual plasma estrogen during ovarian suppression. An alternative approach is to use an aromatase inhibitor in combination with the agonist. Four of six premenopausal women who had previously responded to single-agent goserelin at relapse responded to the addition of the aromatase inhibitor 4-hydroxyandrostenedione to further goserelin *(25,63)*. Future trials may compare LHRH agonists combined with one of the newer, more potent, triazole inhibitors of aromatase with LHRH agonist alone in ER-positive premenopausal women with breast cancer. These studies should include a comparison of *stepwise* estrogen deprivation (i.e., LHRH agonist followed by LHRH agonist plus aromatase inhibitor) with first-line combination treatment.

One group has combined leuprorelin with megestrol acetate in women with advanced disease and reported an overall response rate of 30% with a median duration of response of 19 months (range $7–42^{+}$) *(64)*. Combination cytotoxic and LHRH agonist therapy has also been explored in premenopausal women with resultant high response rates (82%), a median time to treatment failure of 11.5 months, and median survival of 37 months *(65)*.

Adjuvant Therapy in Premenopausal Women

As noted above, it is now well established that oophorectomy yields survival improvements in early premenopausal breast cancer. The role of temporary ovarian ablation using goserelin acetate as adjuvant therapy in the treatment of premenopausal early breast cancer is currently being evaluated in a number of large international multicenter trials *(13)*. Comparisons include randomization against tamoxifen and chemotherapy as well as combinations of these approaches. The results are keenly awaited and will be judged on tolerability as well as efficacy end points.

Table 5
Response Rates and Survival in Randomized Trials of Premenopausal Women with Advanced Breast Cancer Treated with LHRH Agonist Based Therapy

Reference	*Year*	*Trial treatment*	*No.*	*CR, r/e (%)*	*ORR, r/e (%)*	p	*Median PFS*	p	*Median OS*	p
Boccardo *et al.*	1994	Ovarian ablation	18	2/15 (13)	7/15 (47)					
		Goserelin	24	1/22 (5)	6/22 (27)	0.25		n.s.		n.s.
		Ovarian ablation + tamoxifen	19	0/18 (0)	2/18 (11)	0.12		n.s.		n.s.
		Goserelin + tamoxifen	24	4/20 (20)	9/20 (45)	0.66		n.s.		n.s.
Jonat *et al.*	1994	Goserelin	159		50/159 (31)		23 weeks		127 weeks	
		Goserelin + tamoxifen	159		60/159 (38)		28 weeks	$p = 0.03$	140 weeks	0.25
Klijn *et al.*	1996	Buserelin	45		33%	n.s.	8.2 mo		31.4 months	
		Tamoxifen	48		29%	n.s.	10 mo		37.8 months	
		Buserelin + tamoxifen	47		51%	$p = 0.02$	17 mo	0.02	Not reached	0.008

Abbreviations: r, number of responders; e, number of evaluable patients; PFS, progression-free survival; OS, overall survival; CR, complete clinical response; ORR, overall response rate; n.s., not statistically significant.

Table 6
Response Rates in Postmenopausal Women with Advanced Breast Cancer Treated with Single Agent LHRH Agonist Therapy

Reference	*Year*	*Agonist*	*No.*	*CR, n/e (%)*	*ORR, n/e (%)*
Harvey *et al.*	1985	Leuprorelin	31	0/31 (0)	5/31 (16)
Waxman *et al.*	1985	Buserelin	18	0/18 (0)	0/18 (0)
Mathé *et al.*	1986	Triptorelin	15	1/15 (7)	3/15 (20)
Plowman *et al.*	1986	Goserelin	10	0/10 (0)	2/10 (20)
Lissoni *et al.*	1988	Buserelin	14	0/14 (0)	0/14 (0)
Crighton *et al.*	1989	Leuprorelin	15	0/15 (0)	0/15 (0)
Harris *et al.*	1989	Goserelin	28	0/28 (0)	3/ 28 (11)
Saphner *et al.*	1993	Goserelin	54	1/52 (2)	4/52 (8)

Abbreviations: r, number of responders; e, number of evaluable patients; CR, complete clinical response; ORR, overall response rate.

Neoadjuvant Therapy

Two trials have addressed the role of primary LHRH agonist therapy in human breast cancer. Recent reports have demonstrated a reduction in the need for mastectomy with primary medical therapy, also known as neoadjuvant chemohormonal therapy *(66,67)*. The Edinburgh group treated 13 premenopausal women with goserelin *(68)*. The mean ER content in the population was low (30 fmol/mg cytosolic protein), and all of the five responding patients had an ER content >20 fmol/mg cytosolic protein. The group from St. George's Hospital, London, examined the role of leuprorelin in premenopausal women with ER-positive large, operable breast cancer, with 58% of women responding *(69)*. These two pilot studies are encouraging for the future use of LHRH therapy in hormone receptor-positive disease for reduction of tumor size presurgery, in particular for women who refuse chemotherapy.

Prevention

Early menopause reduces a woman's lifetime risk of developing breast cancer *(70)*. Accordingly, LHRH agonist treatment in association with low-dose estrogen replacement therapy to manage the adverse effects of estrogen deprivation has been proposed as a chemopreventive agent for premenopausal women at high risk of breast cancer *(71)*. In support of this concept, normal women on this combination show decreased mammographic density, which may be a surrogate measure of breast cancer risk *(72)*.

Postmenopausal Women

Several trials have assessed the role of LHRH agonists in postmenopausal women with advanced breast cancer (Table 6). Response rates are substantially lower than with conventional antiestrogen therapy *(11)*. In the positive trials, responses were noted in soft tissue sites more frequently than other sites of disease and were of short duration *(50,73)*. If a direct effect is postulated, responses might be expected to be seen in ER-negative tumors. In the Eastern Cooperative Oncology Group study, no responses were seen in the ER-negative group ($n = 16$), and all four responding patients' tumors had high ER content *(73)*. Despite the absence of aromatase activity in the ovary of postmenopausal women, some reduction in plasma estradiol levels does occur with LHRH agonists *(22,74)*. This appears to be secondary to a reduction in plasma androgen levels, which presumably results from the continued androgen production of the postmenopausal ovary being subject to gonadotrophin stimulation. It may therefore be a reduction in estrogen levels *(50,74)* that is responsible for the few responses seen rather than a direct cytotoxic effect *(75)*.

The low response rate means that LHRH agonists cannot be recommended for the treatment of postmenopausal breast cancer. This view is reinforced by the study by Harris and colleagues *(50)*, in which six of seven postmenopausal patients responded to tamoxifen after disease progression on goserelin.

Male Breast Cancer

Male breast cancer represents approximately 1% of all breast cancer diagnosed, with an annual incidence rate of seven per million. Eleven men with recurrent or progressive carcinoma of the breast have been treated with buserelin and cyproterone acetate with objective responses observed in 7 patients (63%) with a median duration of 11.5 months (range, 9–24+ months) *(76)*. In two other consecutive trials, 15 men with metastatic breast cancer were treated with cyproterone acetate plus buserelin or goserelin. As might be expected, response rates (59% vs 53%), duration of response (14 months vs 8.5 months; $p = 0.42$), and median survival (20 months vs 16 months; $p = 0.26$) were not significantly different *(77)*.

LHRH ANTAGONISTS

Theoretical Advantages

The new LHRH antagonist cetrorelix (SB-75) represents an improvement in therapeutic profile compared with earlier generations of LHRH antagonists *(78)*. In particular, suppression of serum levels of FSH and LH occurs within hours, and there is freedom from anaphylactic side effects due to histamine release *(79)*. These advances have made cetrorelix an exciting compound under investigation in controlled phase II clinical studies in breast cancer.

Cetrorelix produces a rapid and marked downregulation of pituitary receptors for LHRH and not merely an occupancy of binding sites *(80)*. In addition to direct receptor competition, cetrorelix has been reported to inhibit both estrogen- and insulin-like growth factor-II-mediated MCF-7 cell growth, suggesting the inclusion of autocrine pathways in its mode of action *(81)*. Cetrorelix induced rapid, dose-dependent inhibition of murine breast xenograft tumor growth *(82)*. New LHRH antagonist-copolymer conjugates have stronger antitumor activity in ER-positive and -negative cell lines and xenografts than LHRH agonists at equimolar concentrations *(83,84)*.

The excellent clinical results with the LHRH agonists and the relatively similar endocrine profile achieved by antagonists make it difficult to expect a major improvement in efficacy with these newer agents. The occasionally clinically significant early stimulatory effects of the agonists should be avoided with the antagonists, but this tolerability issue is more important in prostate than in breast cancer.

FUTURE APPROACHES

Novel approaches to the management of premenopausal breast cancer include LHRH antibodies, conjugates of LHRH, and cytotoxic and LHRH-chimeric toxins *(85–87)*. The impact of these compounds will depend on their affinity for the LHRH receptor as well as pharmacodynamic and pharmacokinetic variables.

REFERENCES

1. Schinzinger AS (1889) Über Carcinoma mammae. Zbl Chir (Beilage) 16:55–56.
2. Beatson GT (1896) On the treatment of inoperable cases of carcinoma of the mamma: suggestions for a new method of treatment with illustrative cases. Lancet 2:104–107.
3. Schally AV, Kastin AJ, Arimura A (1971) Hypothalamic follicle-stimulating hormone (FSH) and luteinizing hormone (LH)-regulating hormone: structure, physiology, and clinical studies. Fertil Steril 22:703–721.
4. DeSombre ER, Johnson ES, White WF (1976) Regression of rat mammary tumors effected by a gonadoliberin analog. Cancer Res 36:3830–3833.
5. Beksac MS, Kisnisci HA, Cakar AN, Beksac M (1983) The endocrinological evaluation of bilateral and unilateral oophorectomy in premenopausal women. Int J Fertil 28:219–224.
6. Stein JJ (1969) Surgical or irradiation castration for patients with advanced breast cancer. Cancer 24:1350–1354.
7. Buchanan RB, Blamey RW, Durrant KR, Howell A, Paterson AG, Preece PE, et al. (1986) A randomized comparison of tamoxifen with surgical oophorectomy in premenopausal patients with advanced breast cancer. J Clin Oncol 4:1326–1330.
8. Ingle JN, Krook JE, Green SJ, Kubista TP, Everson LK, Ahmann DL, et al. (1986) Randomized trial of bilateral oophorectomy versus tamoxifen in premenopausal women with metastatic breast cancer. J Clin Oncol 4:178–185.
9. Veronesi U, Cascinelli N, Greco M, Di FG, Oriana R, Merson M, et al. (1987) A reappraisal of oophorectomy in carcinoma of the breast. Ann Surg 205:18–21.
10. Fracchia AA, Farrow JH, DePalo AJ, Connolly DP, Huvos AG (1969) Castration for primary inoperable or recurrent breast carcinoma. Surg Gynecol Obstet 128:1226–1234.
11. McGuire WL (1978) Hormone receptors: their role in predicting prognosis and response to endocrine therapy. Semin Oncol 5:428–433.
12. Dao TL (1972) Ablation therapy for hormone-dependent tumours. Annu Rev Med 3:1–18.
13. Early Breast Cancer Collaborative Trialists' Group (1996) Ovarian ablation in early breast cancer: overview of the randomised trials. Lancet 348:1189–1196.
14. Crump M, Sawka CA, DeBoer G, Buchanan RB, Ingle JN, Forbes J, et al. (1997) An individual patient-based meta-analysis of tamoxifen versus ovarian ablation as first line endocrine therapy for premenopausal women with metastatic breast cancer. Breast Cancer Res Treat 44:201–210.
15. Kakar SS, Rahe CH, Jennes L (1996) Gonadotropin releasing hormone (GnRH) receptor: molecular cloning, tissue distribution and regulation of gene expression in pituitary, brain and tumor. Mol Androl 8:1–2.
16. Janovick JA, Conn PM (1996) Gonadotropin releasing hormone agonist provokes homologous receptor microaggregation: an early event in seven-transmembrane receptor mediated signaling. Endocrinology 137:3602–3605.
17. Clayton RN (1982) Gonadotropin-releasing hormone modulation of its own pituitary receptors: evidence for biphasic regulation. Endocrinology 111:152–161.
18. Sandow J (1983) Clinical applications of LHRH and its analogues. Clin Endocrinol 18:571–592.
19. Conn PM, Crowley WJ (1991) Gonadotropin-releasing hormone and its analogues. N Engl J Med 324:93–103.
20. Nestor JJ (1987) Design of LHRH agonist drug candidates. J Androl 8:S4–8.
21. Nicholson RI, Walker KJ, Davies P (1986) Hormone agonists and antagonists in the treatment of hormone sensitive breast and prostate cancer. Cancer Surv 5:463–486.
22. Dowsett M, Cantwell B, Lal A, Jeffcoate SL, Harris AL (1988) Suppression of postmenopausal ovarian steroidogenesis with the luteinizing hormone-releasing hormone agonist goserelin. J Clin Endocrinol Metab 66:672–677.
23. West CP, Baird DT (1987) Suppression of ovarian activity by zoladex depot (ICI 118 630), a long-acting luteinizing hormone releasing agonist analogue. Clin Endocrinol 26:213–220.
24. McCann SM, Marubayashi U, Sun HQ, Yu WH (1993) Control of follicle-stimulating hormone and luteinizing hormone release by hypothalamic peptides. Ann NY Acad Sci 687:55–59.
25. Dowsett M, Stein RC, Coombes RC (1992) Aromatization inhibition alone or in combination with GnRH agonists for the treatment of premenopausal breast cancer patients. J Steroid Biochem Mol Biol 43:1–3.
26. Santen RJ, Santner S, Davis B, Veldhuis J, Samojlik E, Ruby E (1978) Aminoglutethimide inhibits extraglandular estrogen production in postmenopausal women with breast carcinoma. J Clin Endocrinol Metab 47:1257–1265.

27. Dowsett M, Jacobs S, Aherne J, Smith IE (1992) Clinical and endocrine effects of leuprorelin acetate in pre- and postmenopausal patients with advanced breast cancer. Clin Ther 14:97–103.
28. Dowsett M, Cantwell BMJ, Harris AL (1989) Endocrinology of Zoladex in postmenopausal women. Horm Res 32:209–212.
29. Sarda AK, Nair RM (1981) Elevated levels of LRH in human milk. J Clin Endocrinol Metab 52:826–828.
30. Miller WR, Scott WN, Morris R, Fraser HM, Sharpe RM (1985) Growth of human breast cancer cells inhibited by a luteinizing hormone-releasing hormone agonist. Nature 313:231–233.
31. Ciocca DR, Puy LA, Fasoli LC, Tello O, Aznar JC, Gago FE, Papa SI, Sonego R (1990) Corticotropin-releasing hormone, luteinizing hormone-releasing hormone, growth hormone-releasing hormone, and somatostatin-like immunoreactivities in biopsies from breast cancer patients. Breast Cancer Res Treat 15:175–184.
32. Baumann KH, Kiesel L, Kaufmann M, Bastert G, Runnebaum B (1993) Characterization of binding sites for a GnRH-agonist (buserelin) in human breast cancer biopsies and their distribution in relation to tumor parameters. Breast Cancer Res Treat 25:37–46.
33. Blankenstein MA, Henkelman MS, Klijn JG (1985) Direct inhibitory effect of a luteinizing hormone-releasing hormone agonist on MCF-7 human breast cancer cells. Eur J Cancer 21:1493–1499.
34. Foekens JA, Henkelman MS, Fukkink JF, Blankenstein MA, Klijn JG (1986) Combined effects of buserelin, estradiol and tamoxifen on the growth of MCF-7 human breast cancer cells in vitro. Biochem Biophys Res Commun 140:550–556.
35. Mullen P, Scott WN, Miller WR (1991) Growth inhibition observed following administration of an LHRH agonist to a clonal variant of the MCF-7 breast cancer cell line is accompanied by an accumulation of cells in the G0/G1 phase of the cell cycle. Br J Cancer 63:930–932.
36. Neri C, Berthois Y, Schatz B, Drieu K, Martin PM (1990) Compared effects of GnRH analogs and 4-hydroxytamoxifen on growth and steroid receptors in antiestrogen sensitive and resistant MCF-7 breast cancer cell sublines. Breast Cancer Res Treat 15:85–93.
37. Harwood JP and Sharfie SM (1983) Acta Endocrinologica 103:91.
38. Vincze B, Palyi I, Daubner D, Kremmer T, Szamel I, Bodrogi I, et al. (1991) Influence of luteinizing hormone-releasing hormone agonists on human mammary carcinoma cell lines and their xenografts. J Steroid Biochem Mol Biol 38:119–126.
39. Friedman AJ, Juneau Norcross M, Rein MS (1993) Adverse effects of leuprolide acetate depot treatment. Fertil Steril 59:448–450.
40. Friedman AJ, Daly M, Juneau Norcross M, Rein MS, Fine C, Gleason R, et al. (1993) A prospective, randomized trial of gonadotropin-releasing hormone agonist plus estrogen-progestin or progestin "add-back" regimens for women with leiomyomata uteri. J Clin Endocrinol Metab 76:1439–1445.
41. Filicori M (1994) Gonadotrophin-releasing hormone agonists: A guide to use and selection. Drugs 48:41–58.
42. Klijn JG, de Jong FH (1982) Treatment with a luteinising-hormone-releasing-hormone analogue (buserelin) in premenopausal patients with metastatic breast cancer. Lancet 1:1213–1216.
43. Bajetta E, Zilembo N, Buzzoni R, Celio L, Zampino MG, Colleoni M, et al. (1994) Goserelin in premenopausal advanced breast cancer: clinical and endocrine evaluation of responsive patients. Oncology 51:262–269.
44. Blamey RW, Jonat W, Kaufmann M, Bianco AR, Namer M (1993) Survival data relating to the use of goserelin depot in the treatment of premenopausal advanced breast cancer. Eur J Cancer 29A:1498.
45. Dixon AR, Robertson JF, Jackson L, Nicholson RI, Walker KJ, Blamey RW (1990) Goserelin (Zoladex) in premenopausal advanced breast cancer: duration of response and survival. Br J Cancer 62:868–870.
46. Dowsett M, Mehta A, Mansi J, Smith IE (1990) A dose-comparative endocrine-critical study of leuprorelin in premenopausal breast cancer patients. Br J Cancer 62:834–837.
47. Kaufmann M (1989) Zoladex in the treatment of premenopausal metastatic breast cancer patients. Horm Res 1:202–205.
48. Williams MR, Walker KJ, Turkes A, Blamey RW, Nicholson RI (1986) The use of an LH-RH agonist (ICI 118630, Zoladex) in advanced premenopausal breast cancer. Br J Cancer 53:629–636.
49. Harvey HA, Lipton A, Max DT, Pearlman HG, Diaz Perches R, de la Garza J (1985) Medical castration produced by the GnRH analogue leuprolide to treat metastatic breast cancer. J Clin Oncol 3:1068–1072.
50. Harris AL, Carmichael J, Cantwell B, Dowsett M (1989) Zoladex: therapeutic effects in postmenopausal breast cancer. Horm Res 1:213–217.
51. Bianco AR, Rosso R, Calabresi F, Fiorentino M, Lopez M, Sismondi PG, et al. (1991) LH-RH analogue Zoladex in the treatment of pre- and perimenopausal women with metastatic breast cancer (results of the Italian Cooperative Study).Eur J Gynaecol Oncol 12:429–437.

52. Brambilla C, Escobedo A, Artioli R, Lechuga MJ, Motta M (1992) Treatment of pre-menopausal advanced breast cancer with goserelin—a long-acting luteinizing hormone releasing hormone agonist. Anticancer Drugs 3:3–8.
53. Kaufmann M, Jonat W, Schachner-Wünschmann E, Bastert G, Maass H (1991) The depot GnRH analogue goserelin in the treatment of premenopausal patients with metastatic breast cancer—a 5 year experience and further endocrine therapies. Onkologie 14:22–30.
54. Klijn JG (1984) Long-term LHRH-agonist treatment in metastatic breast cancer as a single treatment and in combination with other additive endocrine treatments. Med Oncol Tumor Pharmacother 1:123–128.
55. Walker KJ, Walker RF, Turkes A, Robertson JF, Blamey RW, Griffiths K, et al. (1989) Endocrine effects of combination antioestrogen and LH-RH agonist therapy in premenopausal patients with advanced breast cancer. Eur J Cancer Clin Oncol 25:651–654.
56. Buzzoni R, Biganzoli L, Bajetta E, Celio L, Fornasiero A, Mariani L, et al. (1995) Combination goserelin and tamoxifen therapy in premenopausal advanced breast cancer: a multicentre study by the ITMO group. Br J Cancer 71:1111–1114.
57. Nicholson RI, Walker KJ, McClelland RA, Dixon A, Robertson JFR, Blamey RW (1990) Zoladex plus tamoxifen versus Zoladex alone in pre- and peri-menopausal metastatic breast cancer. J Steroid Biochem Mol Biol 37:989–995.
58. Dixon AR, Jackson L, Robertson JF, Nicholson RI, Blamey RW (1991) Combined goserelin and tamoxifen in premenopausal advanced breast cancer: duration of response and survival. Eur J Cancer 27:806–807.
59. Jonat W, Kaufmann M, Blamey RW, Howell A, Collins JP, Coates A, et al. (1995) A randomised study to compare the effect of the luteinising hormone releasing hormone (LHRH) analogue goserelin with or without tamoxifen in pre- and perimenopausal patients with advanced breast cancer. Eur J Cancer 31:137–142.
60. Klijn JG, Seynaeve C, Beex L, Mauriac L, van Zijl J, Veyret C, et al. (1996) Combined treatment with buserelin (LHRH-A) and tamoxifen (TAM) vs single treatment with each drug alone in premenopausal metastatic breast cancer: preliminary results of EORTC study 10881. Proc Annu Meet Am Soc Clin Oncol 15:117.
61. Klijn JGM, Seynaeve C, Beex L, Mauriac L, van Zijl J, Veyret C, et al. (1996) Combined estrogen suppression and receptor (ER) blockade by buserelin (LHRH-A) and tamoxifen (TAM) in premenopausal metastatic breast cancer: preliminary results of a 3-arm randomized study (EORTC 10881). Eur J Cancer. 32A:49.
62. Boccardo F, Rubagotti A, Perrotta A, Amoroso D, Balestrero M, De MA, et al. (1994) Ovarian ablation versus goserelin with or without tamoxifen in pre-perimenopausal patients with advanced breast cancer: results of a multicentric Italian study. Ann Oncol 5:337–342.
63. Stein RC, Dowsett M, Hedley A, Gazet JC, Ford HT, Coombes RC (1990) The clinical and endocrine effects of 4-hydroxyandrostenedione alone and in combination with goserelin in premenopausal women with advanced breast cancer. Br J Cancer 62:679–683.
64. Lopez CPM, Gonzalez LJ, Alonso MC, Casado A, Dominquez S, Adrover E, et al. (1992) Treatment of advanced breast cancer in premenopausal women with LHRH agonists and megestrol acetate. Ann Oncol 3:78.
65. Falkson CI, Falkson HC, Falkson G (1992) Cyclophosphamide, doxorubicin and fluorouracil (CAF) plus depo-buserelin in the treatment of premenopausal women with metastatic breast cancer. Ann Oncol 3:849–853.
66. Fisher B, Brown A, Mamounas E, Wieand S, Robidoux A, Margolese RG, et al. (1997) Effect of preoperative chemotherapy on local-regional disease in women with operable breast cancer: findings from national surgical adjuvant breast and bowel project B-18. J Clin Oncol 15:2483–2493.
67. Smith IE, Walsh G, Jones A, Prendiville J, Johnston S, Gusterson B, et al. (1995) High complete remission rates with primary neoadjuvant infusional chemotherapy for large early breast cancer. J Clin Oncol 13:424–429.
68. Anderson ED, Forrest AP, Levack PA, Chetty U, Hawkins RA (1989) Response to endocrine manipulation and oestrogen receptor concentration in large operable primary breast cancer. Br J Cancer 60:223–226.
69. Gazet JC, Coombes RC, Ford HT, Griffin M, Corbishley C, Makinde V, et al. (1996) Assesssment of the effect of pretreatment with neoadjuvant therapy on primary breast cancer. Br J Cancer 73:758–762.
70. Spicer DV, Pike MC (1994) Sex steroids and breast cancer prevention. J Natl Cancer Inst Monogr 16:139–147.
71. Sismondi P, Biglia N, Giai M, Defabiani E (1994) GnRH analogs in benign breast disease and breast cancer chemoprevention. A challenge for the year 2000. Eur J Gynaecol Oncol 15:108–114.

72. Spicer DV, Ursin G, Parisky YR, Pearce JG, Shoupe D, Pike A, et al. (1994) Changes in mammographic densities induced by a hormonal contraceptive designed to reduce breast cancer risk. J Natl Cancer Inst 86:431–436.
73. Saphner T, Troxel AB, Tormey DC, Neuberg D, Robert NJ, Pandya KJ, et al. (1993) Phase II study of goserelin for patients with postmenopausal metastatic breast cancer. J Clin Oncol 11:1529–1535.
74. Crighton IL, Dowsett M, Lal A, Man A, Smith IE (1989) Use of luteinising hormone-releasing hormone agonist (leuprorelin) in advanced postmenopausal breast cancer: clinical and endocrine effects. Br J Cancer 60:644–648.
75. Plowman PN, Nicholson RI, Walker KJ (1986) Remission of postmenopausal breast cancer during treatment with the luteinising hormone releasing hormone agonist ICI 118630. Br J Cancer 54:903–909.
76. Lopez M, Natali M, Di LL, Vici P, Pignatti F, Carpano S (1993) Combined treatment with buserelin and cyproterone acetate in metastatic male breast cancer. Cancer 72:502–505.
77. Di Lauro L, Vici P, Carpano S, Santini S, Pignatti F, Lopez M (1994) Cyproterone acetate (CPA) alone or with LHRH analogs in metastatic male breast carcinoma (MBC). Proc Annu Meet Am Soc Clin Oncol 13:A177.
78. Reissmann T, Hilgard P, Harleman JH, Engel J, Comaru SA, Schally AV (1992) Treatment of experimental DMBA induced mammary carcinoma with Cetrorelix (SB-75): a potent antagonist of luteinizing hormone-releasing hormone. J Cancer Res Clin Oncol 118:44–49.
79. Reissmann T, Felberbaum R, Diedrich K, Engel J, Comaru Schally AM, Schally AV (1995) Development and applications of luteinizing hormone-releasing hormone antagonists in the treatment of infertility: an overview. Hum Reprod 10:1974–1981.
80. Halmos G, Schally AV, Pinski J, Vadillo Buenfil M, Groot K (1996) Down-regulation of pituitary receptors for luteinizing hormone-releasing hormone (LH-RH) in rats by LH-RH antagonist Cetrorelix. Proc Natl Acad Sci USA 93:2398–2402.
81. Hershkovitz E, Marbach M, Bosin E, Levy J, Roberts CJ, LeRoith D, Schally AV, Sharoni Y (1993) Luteinizing hormone-releasing hormone antagonists interfere with autocrine and paracrine growth stimulation of MCF-7 mammary cancer cells by insulin- like growth factors. J Clin Endocrinol Metab 77:963–968.
82. Reissmann TH, Klenner TH, Deger W, Hilgard P, McGregor GP, Voigt K, et al. (1996) Pharmacological studies with Cetrorelix (SB-75), a potent antagonist of luteinising hormone-releasing hormone. Eur J Cancer 32:1574–1579.
83. Vincze B, Palyi I, Gaal D, Pato J, Mora M, Mezo I, et al. (1996) In vivo studies of the new gonadotropin-releasing hormone antagonist—copolymer conjugates having antitumor activity. Cancer Detect Prev 20:153–159.
84. Palyi I, Vincze B, Kalnay A, Turi G, Mezo I, Teplan I, et al. (1996) Effect of gonadotropin-releasing hormone analogs and their conjugates on gonadotropin-releasing hormone receptor-positive human cancer cell lines. Cancer Detect Prev 20:146–152.
85. Nagy A, Schally AV, Armatis P, Szepeshazi K, Halmos G, Kovacs M, et al. (1996) Cytotoxic analogs of luteinizing hormone-releasing hormone containing doxorubicin or 2-pyrrolinodoxorubicin, a derivative 500–1,000 times more potent. Proc Natl Acad Sci USA 93:7269–7273.
86. Robertson JF, Jacobs E, Watson SA, Michaeli D (1996) GnRH antibodies inhibit the growth of MCF-7 xenografts. Proc Annu Meet Am Assoc Cancer Res 37.
87. Nechushtan A, Yarkoni S, Marianovsky I, Lorberboum Galski H (1997) Adenocarcinoma cells are targeted by the new GnRH-PE-66 chimeric toxin through specific gonadotropin-releasing hormone binding sites. J Biol Chem 272:11597–11603.

VI Benign Breast Disease

21 Benign Breast Lesions

Pathologic Classification and Risk Potential

Roy A. Jensen

HISTOLOGIC ASSESSMENT OF BREAST CANCER RISK

Histopathologic assessment of breast biopsy and mastectomy specimens has for many decades been recognized as a critical factor in the establishment of prognosis for breast cancer patients *(1)*. In the postHalsteadian era of increasingly conservative surgical approaches for breast cancer, histopathology has also taken on an important new role in helping to guide the selection and tailoring of therapy for individual patients from a range of potential therapeutic options. In fact, despite the advent of numerous molecular markers that attempt to presage the utility of various adjuvant therapy regimens, routinely available histologic indices continue to dominate discussions regarding the selection of therapy for individual patients *(2)*.

In parallel to this new role in malignant breast disease, histopathologic assessment of benign breast biopsies has been increasingly recognized as an important tool in the management and definition of breast cancer risk *(3)*. It has only been within the last 20 years that serious consideration has been given to defining precisely premalignant lesions of the breast in regard to their risk implications for the subsequent development of invasive carcinoma. In large part, defining the clinical implications for specific histologic entities of the breast has been made possible by the recognition that this problem requires the marriage of histopathology and epidemiology. Precise, reproducible, histologic definitions must be coupled with long-term follow-up information on large numbers of women to enable meaningful discussions of the problem. This exercise has taken on greater importance in recent years with the advent of mammographic screening programs and the increased recognition of a variety of premalignant breast lesions, in particular ductal carcinoma *in situ* (DCIS).

It is useful to note that in 1983, prior to the advent of widespread screening mammography, there were <3,000 reported cases of DCIS in the US, and in 1992, there were over 23,000 *(4)*. This increase has engendered a tremendous interest in DCIS, and challenged the medical community to deal with a problem that was largely of its own making. The rationale for much of our response has been based on retrospective histologic analyses of the natural history of DCIS published in 1978 *(5)* and 1982 *(6)*. These pioneering

From: *Contemporary Endocrinology: Endocrinology of Breast Cancer*
Edited by: A. Manni © Humana Press Inc., Totowa, NJ

studies establishred the risk attributable to a diagnosis of DCIS, and have been a major influence on efforts to fine-tune the classification and treatment of these entities, as will be discussed in the section entitled High-Risk Lesions.

This discussion of breast histology and risk assessment will emphasize commonly encountered lesions, particularly those that have the greatest impact clinically and those that cont;inue to represent diagnostic challenges.

NO-RISK LESIONS

Fibrocystic disease of the breast was a commonly accepted diagnosis in the early 1980s, since it was widely held that women with clinically lumpy breasts were at an increased risk for breast cancer. The myth of this assumption was exposed in 1985 with the publication by Dupont and Page of "Risk factors for breast cancer in women with proliferative breast disease," and with the subsequent consensus conference convened in 1986 by the College of American Pathologists and the American College of Surgeons *(7,8)*. This conference fostered the assignment of histologic lesions of the breast to categories of risk and recognized the official demise of the term "fibrocystic disease." The reason was that it was believed to be inappropriate to term this condition a disease, when in fact the majority of women have these changes and no increased risk of breast cancer could be attributed to them. Thus, the term fibrocystic "change" was believed to be more appropriate.

This change in philosophy regarding fibrocystic alterations was a significant shift in the ruling paradigm, because it affected a large number of women burdened with the mistaken belief that these changes implied an increased risk for breast cancer. Prior to this time, it was assumed that any women who had even had a biopsy was at increased risk for breast cancer. The finding that the risk elevation was solely attributable to a limited number of specific histologic alterations removed this stigma and emphasized the importance of histologic examination of breast tissue.

Cysts

Cysts are one of the more common types of histologic alterations identified within benign breast biopsies. In postpubertal girls and women in their early 20s, the histologic appearance of the breast is typically quite uniform and is characterized by numerous similar-sized lobular units (*see* Fig. 1). The acini comprising these lobular units nearly all have a well-defined, two-cell layer and are surrounded by a specialized loose connective tissue stroma. As women progress through their 20s a variety of histologic alterations impose themselves on this sea of uniformity. The most common of these is the dilatation and expansion of acini to form cysts (Fig. 2). These cysts range in size from a few millimeters to a few centimeters, and are lined by a variety of epithelial types. Most often the cells have a low columnar to cuboidal appearance with a minimal amount of cytoplasm, but also commonly adopt an apocrine appearance (*see* below). There is a tendency for cystic change to involve all acini of a lobule, and this accounts for the frequent clustering of cystic change within the breast. Cysts are thought to form as a result of increased luminal pressure, which expands and unfolds the acini of the lobular unit. Fortunately, cysts do not predict for an increased risk of breast cancer as long as the epithelium that lines them shows no evidence of atypia.

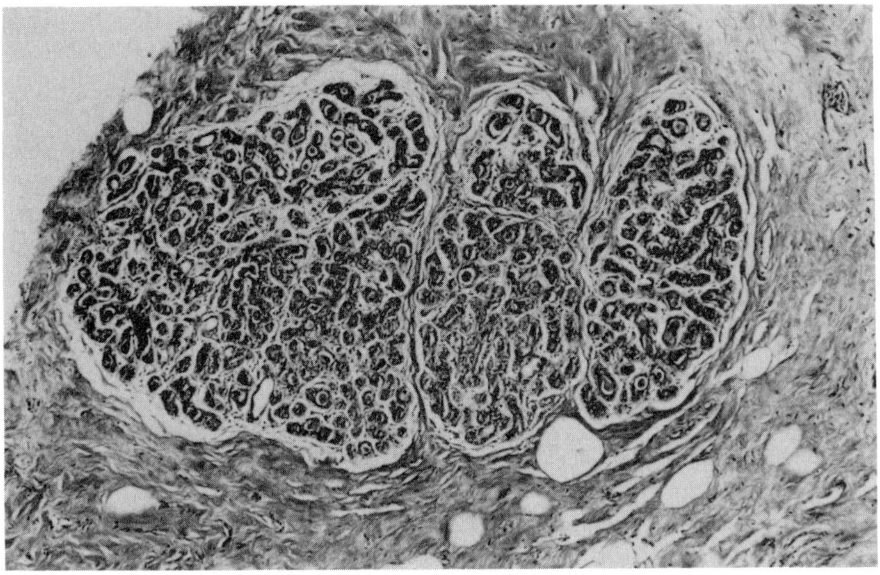

Fig. 1. Normal lobular unit from a 24-yr-old woman (Original magnification 64X).

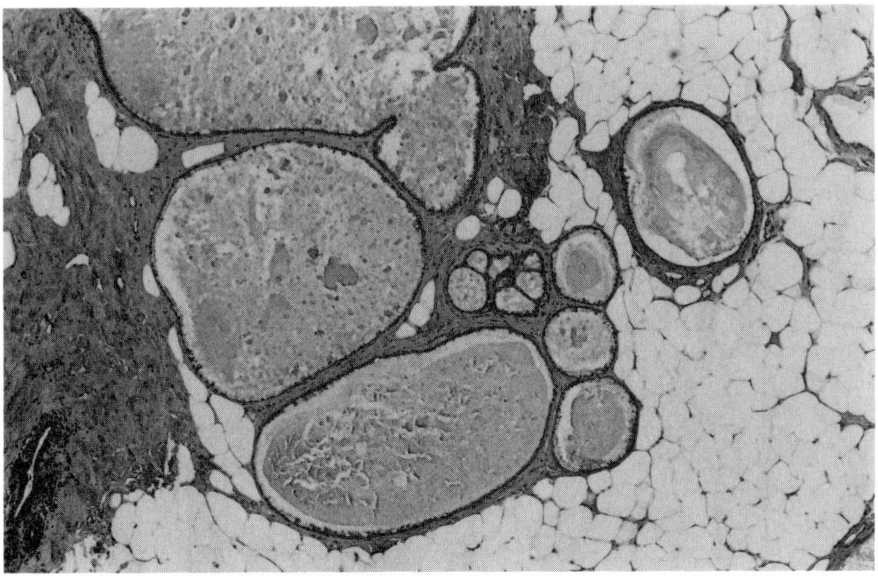

Fig. 2. Cluster of simple benign breast cysts (Original magnification 50X).

Apocrine Change

The term apocrine change encompasses a variety of alterations, including apocrine cysts, apocrine adenosis, and papillary apocrine change. These changes are also relatively common in women past the age of 30–35 and peak in incidence around the time of menopause. Apocrine cysts are simple cysts that are lined by a single layer of characteristic apocrine epithelium. Cytologically, apocrine cells show round, regular nuclei with a single nucleolus and have abundant, pink, slightly grainy cytoplasm (*see* Fig. 3). Apocrine adenosis is diagnosed when apocrine cells are present in the acini of lobular units, but do not otherwise expand or alter the appearance of the lobular unit. Often this change is quite focal in nature.

Papillary apocrine change represents the florid end of the spectrum of this alteration and can be very extensive. The apocrine cells show complex, arcades of papillary structures that can join up and form cribriform spaces. These changes are completely benign in nature, unless they adopt the architectural patterns of carcinoma *in situ* or atypical ductal hyperplasia *(9)*. In this situation, borderline lesions can be very difficult to classify and precise definitions with firm epidemiologic backup can be hard to come by *(10)*. Again, a conservative posture is probably appropriate.

MINIMAL-RISK LESIONS

There are a number of lesions in the breast that indicate a relatively small increase in the relative risk for a subsequent invasive breast carcinoma. These lesions, in general, do not indicate any need for an alteration in the frequency of clinical or mammographic surveillance of the breast, and are associated with about a 1.5- to twofold increase in risk. Specific examples of lesions from this category include usual hyperplasia, sclerosing adenosis, intraductal papilloma, and certain categories of fibroadenoma.

Usual Hyperplasia

Usual or florid hyperplasia is a relatively common alteration seen within benign breast biopsies. In the premammographic era, this change was present in 20–30% of all biopsies and was composed of an epithelial proliferation present within ducts or expanded acini of lobular units *(7)*. This alteration has gone by a wide variety of names, including epitheliosis, papillomatosis, and proliferative disease without atypia. Histologically, usual hyperplasia is characterized by filling of involved spaces or crossing of involved spaces by an increased number of breast epithelial cells. Cytologically, the cells are noted for their variability, both in nuclear size and shape and the overall pattern of cell placement. Quite commonly, usual hyperplasia exhibits small, slit-like, irregular and differently shaped spaces present within the cellular proliferation, which are termed secondary lumina (*see* Fig. 4). Often these slit-like spaces are peripherally arranged, and the cells show characteristic patterns of swirling and/or streaming. The hallmark of this lesion is the profound degree of variability not only from cell to cell, but in how the cells are arranged one to another. Typically, the nucleus from a cell of usual hyperplasia does not have the same shape or size of any cells that are irmmediately adjacent to it. In addition, the secondary lumina that are formed by the cells are also quite irregular in contrast to the secondary lumina formed by ductal carcinoma *in situ*. Usual hyperplasia is quantitated by designating mild hyperplasia as three- to four-cells thick, and with no tendency to cross and enlarge the involved spaces. Moderate and florid hyperplasia cross the involved spaces, enlarge them, and in the case of florid hyperplasia, fill and distend the spaces. Mild hyperplasia carries no significant increased risk for subsequent carcinoma. Moderate and florid hyperplasia each carry an approx 1.5- to 2-fold increased risk for subsequent carcinoma. Usual hyperplasia is somewhat of an exception to the common rule in neoplasia that variability of cell size and placement are indicative of malignancy. In the breast, variability is the hallmark of benignancy, and as discussed below, uniformity is a strong indicator of neoplasia.

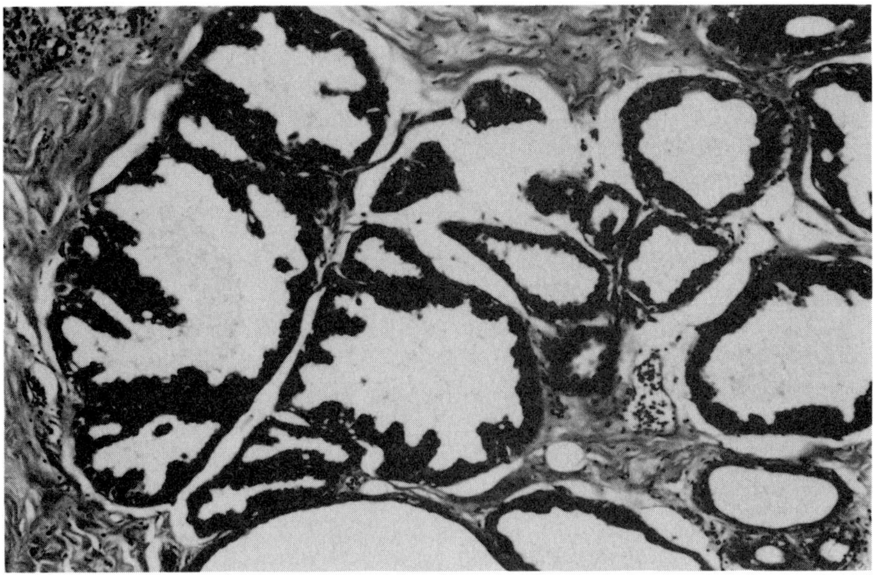

Fig. 3. Papillary apocrine change (Original magnification 80X).

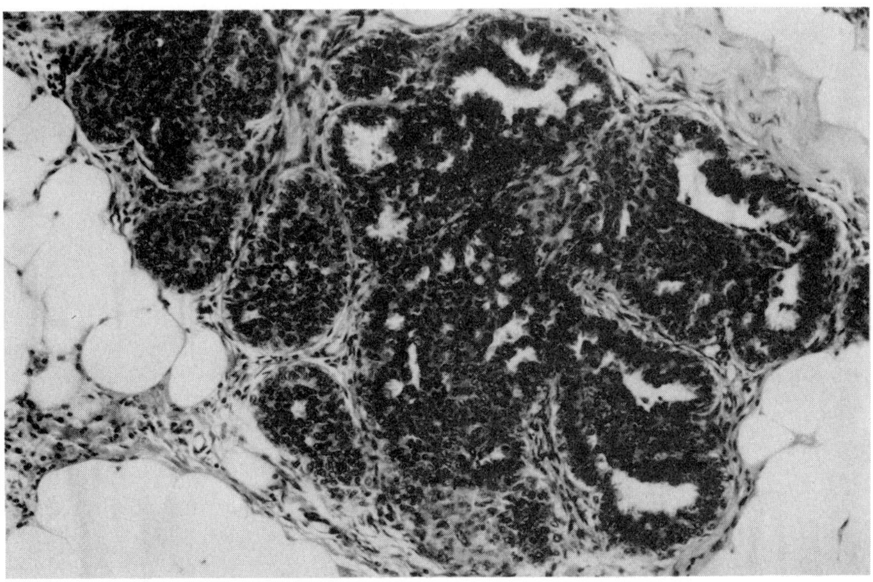

Fig. 4. Florid usual hyperplasia without atypia (Original magnification 128X).

Sclerosing Adenosis

Sclerosing adenosis is a lesion which is found in approx 5–6% of breast biopsies from women in t;he peri-menopausal age group. Following the menopause, the incidence of sclerosing adenosis decreases rapidly, lending credence to the belief that sclerosing adenosis, in fact, represents a proliferative lesion driven by hormonal influences. In the typical setting, sclerosing adenosis is relatively easy to recognize in good histologic preparations, although it can be problematic in frozen section material or suboptimal histologic sections. The defining features are those of an enlarged and disordered lobulocentric process, which consists of elongated acini that are compressed and distorted, and arranged in streaming patterns (*see* Fig. 5). Frequently, there are dilated small microcysts present at the periphery of the lesion, and small foci of microcalcifications present in the epithelial elements.

The risk implications attributable to sclerosing adenosis are relatively low and are in the range of 1.5- to 2.0-fold above the general population. This reassignment to the minimal risk category from the no known risk category was primarily based on the studies of Jensen et al., Tavassoli and Norris, and McDivitt et al. *(11–13)*. Previous to this time, sclerosing adenosis had not been specifically assessed in isolation for its risk potential. This was primarily because sclerosing adenosis often occurred in conjunction with several other histologic alterations within the breast, and it was diffficult to segregate the risk attributable to sclerosing adenosis from these other commonly coincident lesions.

Intraductal Papilloma

Intraductal papillomas are relatively uncommon lesions when all breast biopsies are examined. However, when the subset of biopsies attributable to a nipple discharge is considered, intraductal papillomas account for a relatively large fraction of cases. In contrast to many other lesions within the breast, intraductal papillomas appear to represent true ductal lesions, and are diagnosed when loose fibrovascular connective tissue cores are covered by epithelium and the lesions are present within a duct. The epithelium covering a papilloma can vary widely over the entire spectrum of epithelium changes within the breast, but commonly patterns of usual hyperplasia cover the fibrovascular cores. There is some support in the literature for segregating large intraductal papillomas from multiple small papillomas in regard to risk implications for carcinoma. In general, multiple papillomas tend-to involve segments of the breast and somewhat more frequently the epithelial components contain areas of atypia.

In the study by Page et al., papillomas without coexisting patterns of atypia have a relative risk in the range of two- to threefold above the general population for the subsequent development of carcinoma *(14)*. It is noted, however, that when patterns of atypia hyperplasia were present within papillomas, this risk increased to greater than 10-fold. Because the epithelium covering the papilloma is not contained within the usual confined spaces, the assessment of atypia and carcinoma *in situ* in these lesions can be somewhat problematic. In making these distinctions, we have tried to utilize the same rules that we applied in a more typical situation, and believe that the 2-mm rule proposed by Tavassoli and Norris to distinguish atypical hyperplasia and carcinoma *in situ* lesions is particularly useful *(12)*. Figure 6 shows a rather typical intraductal papilloma covered by epithelium exhibiting florid patterns of usual hyperplasia. There is no evidence of atypia within this lesion, and we would expect the risk attributable to such a papilloma to be in the range of two- to threefold.

Fibroadenoma

Fibroadenomas are particularly common in young women, and by far represent the most common lesion presenting as a mass in women in their teens and 20s. Grossly, these lesions tend to be well circumscribed, and on cut surface, they can have a quite myxoid appearance. Fibroadenomas are recognized by their relatively sharp circumscription from surrounding breast parenchyma, and the characteristic expansion of stromal areas

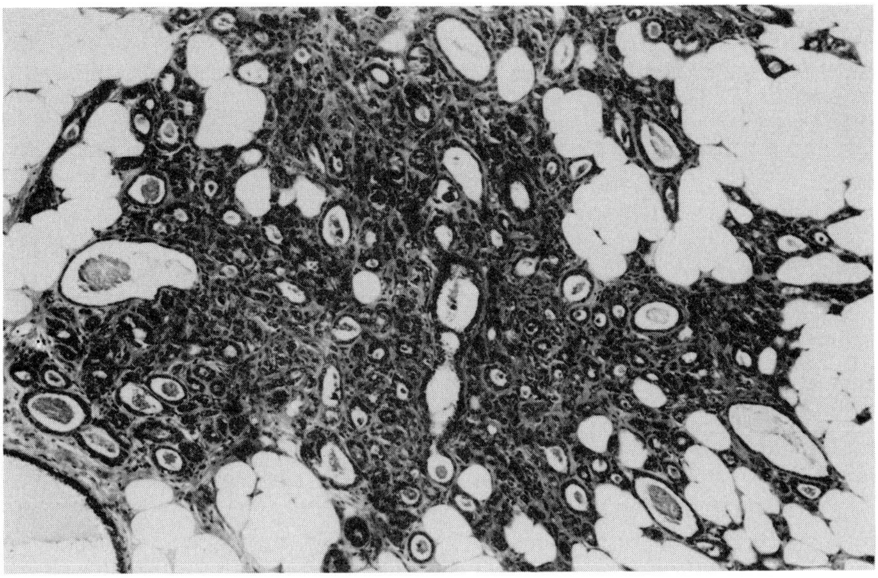

Fig. 5. Sclerosing adenosis (Original magnification 80X).

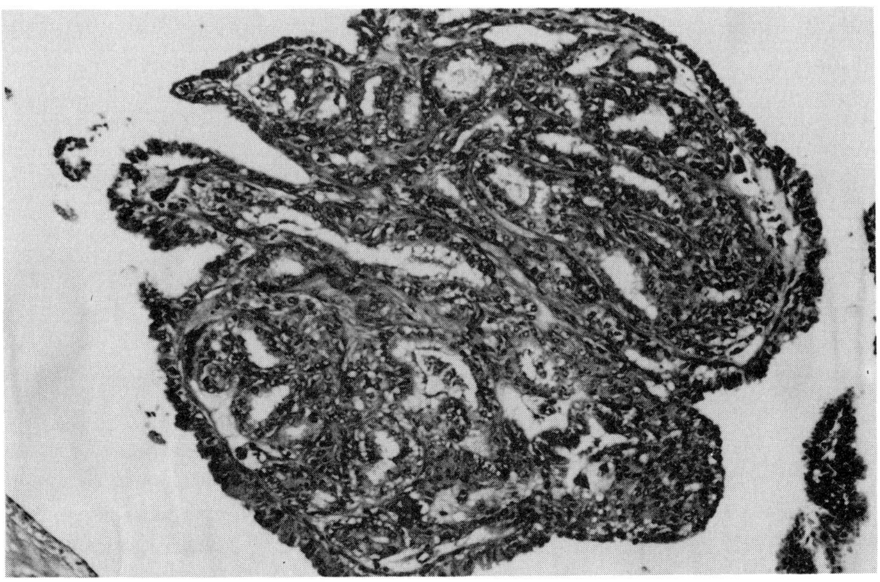

Fig. 6. Intraductal papilloma (Original magnification 128X).

and compression of ductal structures. There can be considerable variation in the microscopic appearance of fibroadenomas, and they often contain cysts, epithelial hyperplasia, apocrine change, and rarely atypical hyperplasia and carcinoma *in situ*. The stroma can vary from an edematous, myxoid appearance to a fairly cellular one with occasional mitoses. Any degree of cellular atypia or increased numbers of mitoses would suggest that the lesion represents an example of the related phyllodes tumor.

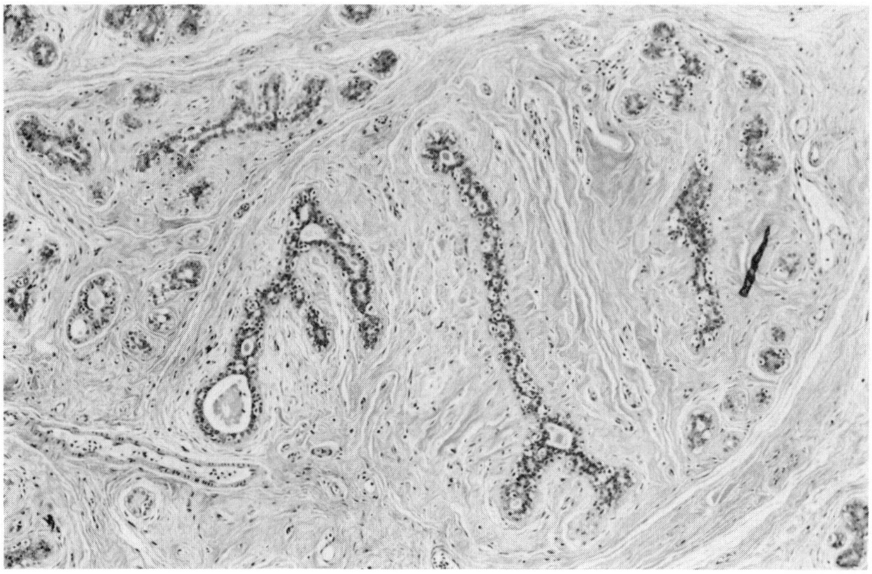

Fig. 7. Fibroadenoma (Original magnification 32X).

Figure 7 shows a typical example of a benign fibroadenoma with a characteristic relationship of the stromal and epithelial elements. Dupont et al., have recently emphasized the possible importance of noting the presence of certain histologic alterations within a fibroadenoma *(15)*. These alterations include the presence of cysts, epithelial calcifications, and sclerosing adenosis. They suggest that these changes imply a slightly greater risk for subsequent breast cancer development, althoug]h no one has yet performed a similar study to confirm these results. Severa l previous studies have suggested that fibroadenomas taken as a group predict for a slightly increased risk of breast cancer, and what is unique about the Dupont et al. study is the suggestion that this risk is primarily limitecl to certain histologic subtypes of fibroadenomas *(15)*. Furthermore, they suggest that the risk for complex fibroadenomas persists over a long period of time at a relatively stable level. As will be discussed below, the risk attributable to the various types of atypical hyperplasia tends to fall with age.

INTERMEDIATE-RISK LESIONS

The Consensus Conference in 1986 *(8)* established the intermediate-risk category primarily to recognize the diagnosis of atypical hyperplasia. These lesions represent not only a histologic intermediate between carcinoma *in situ* and usual hyperplasia, but also an intermediate level of subsequent risk for carcinoma. In most cases, atypical ductal and atypical lobular hyperplasia are relatively easy to distinguish from each other, but in practical terms, the risk level from each lesion closely approximates the other, and there is very little difference in outcome for the diagnosis of lobular vs ductal patterns of atypical hyperplasia.

Atypical Ductal Hyperplasia

Atypical hyperplasia is present in about 10% of breast biopsies in the mammographic era. This represents approximately double the prevalence of this lesion present in the premammographic biopsies and is, no doubt, related to the strong correlation between the likelihood for calcification in these lesions and the ability to be detected by mammography. The diagnosis of atypical ductal hyperplasia is dependent on the pathologist's firm knowledge of the end points of the morphologic spectrum of breast epithelial changes. These end points are usual hyperplasia without atypia and noncomedo ductal carcinoma *in situ*. Atypical hyperplasia represents an intermediate point along this continuum, and the definition of atypical hyperplasia strongly incorporates this idea. The criteria for diagnosis of atypical ductal hyperplasia depends on strong support from three separate components *(16)*. First of all, the architectural pattern of the lesion must be one that strongly suggests a pattern found in noncomedo ductal carcinoma *in situ*. These architectural patterns are comprised of the solid, the cribriform, and micropapillary types. These are all common patterns in noncomedo ductal carcinoma *in situ*, and the analogous atypical hyperplastic lesions of the ductal series may have any of these patterns in isolation or in combination. Second, there must be strong evidence for the presence of cytologic atypia. In general, but not always, this atypia is in the form of hyperchromatic nuclei. The area of concern must comprise the entire bar crossing a space, or at least comprise a population of six or seven cells across. This criterion reduces the likelihood of overdiagnosis of atypical ductal hyperplasia and would represent the lowest level of the definition for that lesion. The final critical component for making the diagnosis of atypical ductal hyperplasia is the assessment regarding the extent of the lesion. Tavassoli and Norris have proposed the useful criteria of measuring the lesion in greatest diameter *(12)*. They have shown that lesions measuring <2 mm in greatest diameter have a risk elevation that is essentially equivalent to the original definition of atypical ductal hyperplasia. Thus, lesions that are quite extensive in the breast, extend out to involve major ducts, or are present on multiple slides are more likely to represent examples of noncomedo cluctal carcinoma *in situ*. In atypical ductal hyperplasia lesions, there is generally a population of evenly spaced uniform cells with similar nuclear features. In contrast to ductal carcinoma in situ, however, this cell population comprises only a portion of the cells present in the involved space. Usually, the second cell population consists of polarized cells that are normally present in the ducts and acini of the breast (*see* Fig. 8). When in doubt regarding the distinction between noncomedo ductal carcinoma *in situ* and atypical ductal hyperplaLsia, it is our philosophy to always go with the more benign diagnosis.

Several groups have utilized the above criteria for atypical ductal hyperplasia, and long-term follow-up studies have confirmed that the relative risk for this lesion is in the range of four- to fivefold greater than that of women in the general population *(7,17,18)*. As a general rule, atypical ductal hyperplasia is a lesion which mects some, but not all, criteria for ductal carcinoma *in situ*. Typically, a lesion will fall short of carcinoma *in situ*, because the neoplastic cells do not; completely involve the acinus or ductal structure under consideration for diagnosis.

Atypical Lobular Hyperplasia

The criteria for the diagnosis of atypical lobular hyperplasia are relatively more straightforward than those for atypical ductal hyperplasia *(19,20)*. First of all, cells with the characteristic lobular neoplasia cytology must be present for the diagnosis to be considcred. Although there is some variation in the classic fried egg appearance of these cells, there is much less variation than is identified in the ductal series of lesions. In

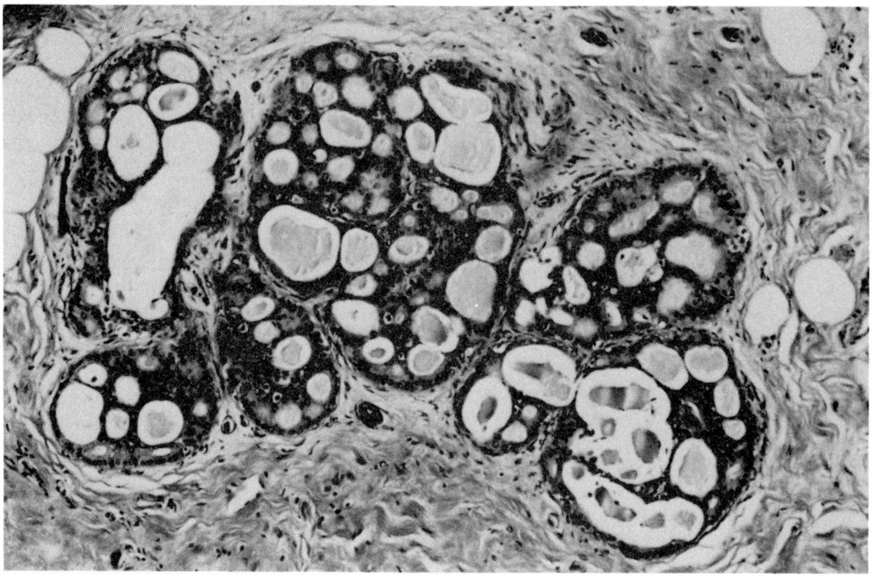

Fig. 8. Atypical ductal hyperplasia, note presence of normal polarized cells present at peripheral aspects of lesion (Original magnification 105X).

atypical lobular hyperplasia, these cells must be present to some extent throughout the lobular unit. Again, the diagnosis of atypical lobular hyperplasia is, in some ways, dependent on reference to lobular carcinoma *in situ*. For atypical lobular hyperplasia, characteristic cells must be present in fewer than half of the acini of a lobular unit, and fewer than half of the acini should be expanded and distorted by these cells. In general, the filling of acini within the lobular unit is incomplete and there are other populations of cells intermixed within the lesion.

Figure 9 shows a classic example of atypical lobular hyperplasia, with the characteristic population of lobular cells present, but there is little or no expansion of the individual acini. When the lobular neoplasia cells not only occupy the acini of the lobular unit, but also extend down ducts, this lesion is termed ductal involvement by atypical lobular hyperplasia. The importance of making this distinction is that this lesion has a somewhat higher risk for subsequent carcinoma than atypical lobular hyperplasia alone, but is less than that of lobular carcinoma *in situ (19)*.

In contrast to atypical ductal hyperplasia, which continues to increase in incidence with age, it is interestingr to note that atypical lobular hyperplasia tends to peak in the premenopausal age group and then fall off with time in a fairly symmetrical curve. Thus, threre is some suggestion that the molecular events driving these two processes may be quite different.

HIGH-RISK LESIONS

The final category of histologic lesions that represent the most worrisome premalignant breast conditions are the carcinomas *in situ*. These lesions represent a very significant elevation of breast cancer risk, and women diagnosed either with ductal carcinoma *in situ* or lobular carcinoma *in situ* have an approx 10- to 11-fold greater chance of

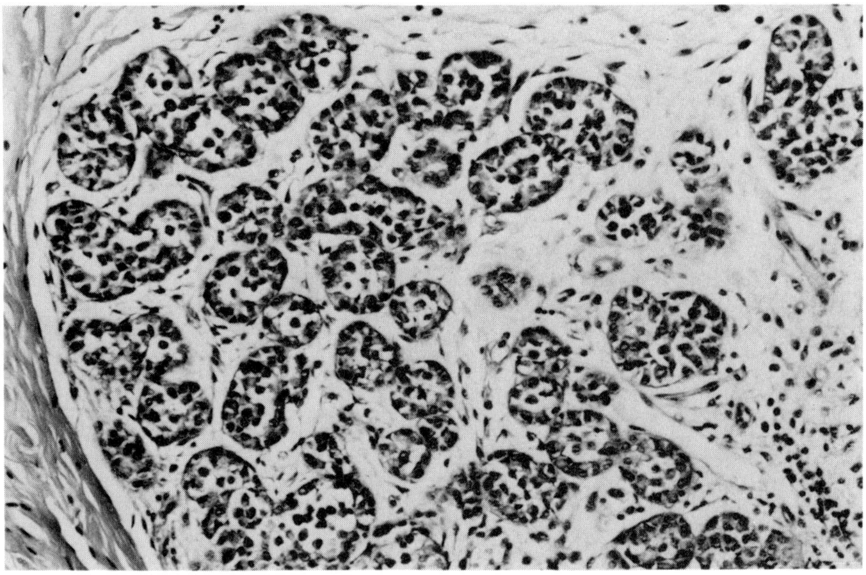

Fig. 9. Atypical lobular hyperplasia (Original magnification 128X).

developing an invasive carcinoma compared to women without these lesions. There has been a great increase in our interest regarding these lesions with the advent of mammography, since we are much better able to detect ductal carcinoma *in situ* owing to its propensity to calcify. This, in turn, has led to a great deal of interest among pathologists regarding the classification of these lesions and the precise definition of their relationship to invasive carcinoma *(21)*.

Ductal Carcinoma In Situ

Prior to the institution of m,ammographic screening programs, ductal carcinoma *in situ* represented no more than 2–5% of breast cancers diagnosed. Since that time, ductal carcinoma *in situ* represents 15–20% of all breast cancers in nearly any screening program examined within the last 15 yr. It has also been noted that there has been a significant shift in the size and histologic pattern of these lesions with a consistent and ongoing decrease in the diameter of these lesions and a shift from the comedo histologic type to the noncomedo histologic type *(22)*.

Ductal carcinoma *in situ* is defined by light microscopic criteria as a lesion consisting of malignant cells present within a basement membrane-lined space for which there is no evidence of invasion. A great deal of effort over the last 10–15 yr has gone into defining the morphologic, and histologic spectrum of these lesions and currently, the classification of ductal carcinoma *in situ* is of great interest in surgical pathology circles *(23–28)*.

Our criteria for ductal carcinoma *in situ* consists of a uniform population of cells forming punched out, rounded spaces or papillary fronds (see Figs. 10A and 10B). A minority of these lesions will consist of a solid sheet of cells completely filling the involved space (*see* Fig. 10C). Furthermore, lesions that qualify as a ductal carcinoma *in situ* must be present in at least two separate basement membrane-lined spaces. Nuclear atypia and monomorphism must be evident and the extent of the disease either measured by involvement of at least two spaces or having a diameter of >2 mm is essential *(29)*.

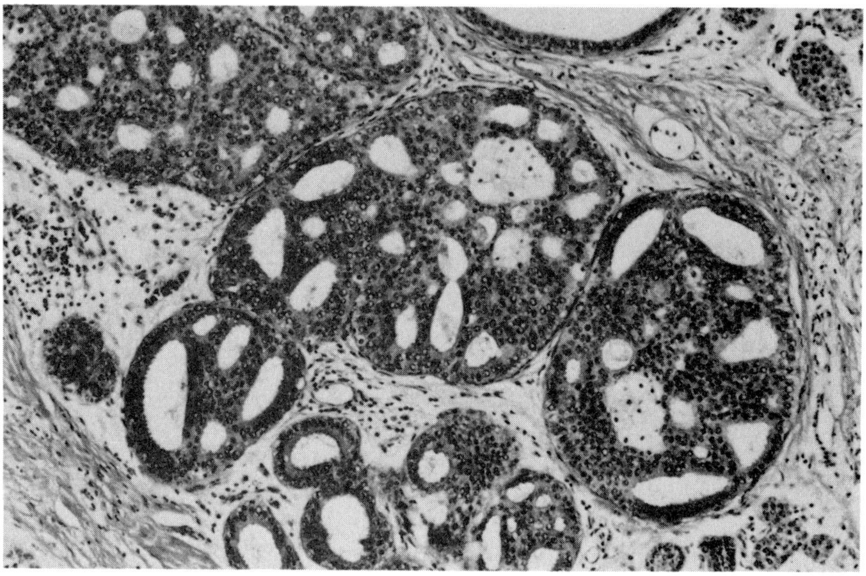

Fig. 10A. Ductal carcinoma *in situ*, cribriform pattern (Original magnification 105X).

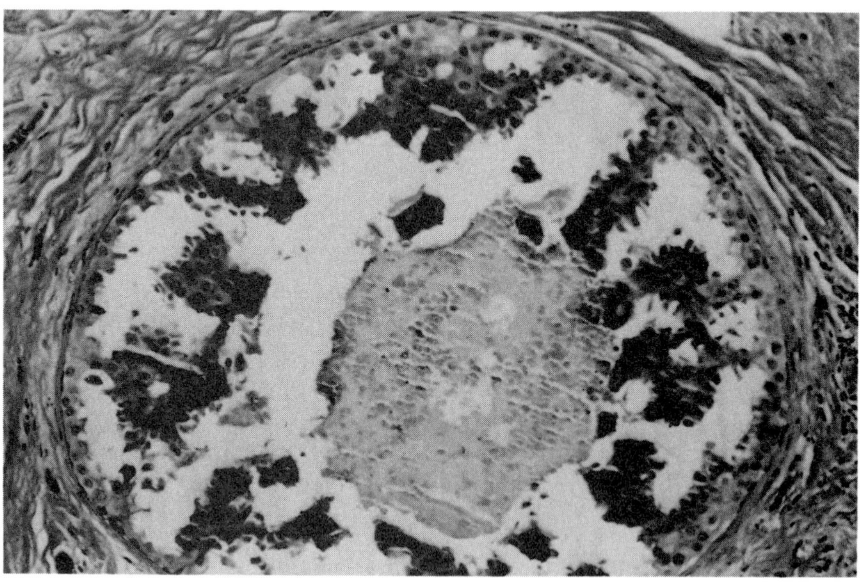

Fig. 10B. Ductal carcinoma *in situ*, micropapillary pattern (Original magnification 256X).

When these criteria are utilized, retrospective analyses have shown that ductal carcinoma *in situ* predicts an approximate 10-fold increased risk for invasive breast cancer in comparison to the general population *(6)*. It should be noted that these risk estimates were developed for relatively small noncomedo ductal carcinomas *in situ,* which had originally been diagnosed as lesser lesions. Therefore, our precise knowledge of the natural history of larger examples of ductal carcinoma in situ, in particular comedo ductal carci-

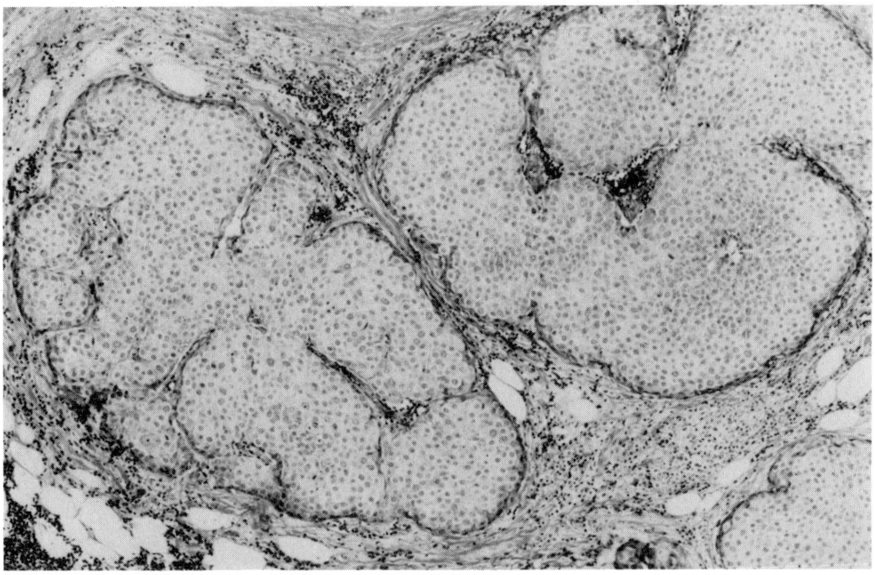

Fig. 10C. Ductal carcinoma *in situ*, solid pattern (Original magnification 80X).

noma *in situ*, is less certain. The breast studies in this regard would suggest that for comedo ductal carcinoma *in situ*, there is an approximate 50% likelihood of developing an invasive cancer within 3 yr of this diagnosis. In contrast, for small examples of noncomedo ductal carcinoma *in situ*, there is an approx 25% chance of developing invasive cancer over a 10-yr period of follow-up *(5,6)*.

Most recent classification st;udies for ductal carcinoma in situ have emphasized the necessity for not only the low-grade and high-grade categories, but also the importance of an intermediate group that has features of both. In general, the high-grade lesions include all comedo carcinomas and are noted for their high nuclear grade and necrosis *(30)*. Noncomedo or low-grade examples show relatively uniform nuclear features and have no evidence of necrosis. Typically, an intermediate lesion will have nuclei that correspond in grade to an intermediate-grade invasive cancer and will also have foci of necrosis that are rather limited in extent.

Lobular Carcinoma In Situ

Lobular carcinoma *in situ*, in contrast to ductal carcinoma *in situ*, is typically a multifocal, multicentric, and often bilateral process. They are often nonpalpable and incidental to mammography, since they have a low propensity to calcify. Analogous to atypical lobular hyperplasia, these lesions also decrease in incidence after menopause.

Lobular carcinoma is defined by the presence of characteristic lobular neoplasia cells present in a uniform population that comprises an entire lobular unit. There must be filling of all acini present in the lobular unit, and there must be expansion and/or distention of at least half of the acini *(29)*. Lesions that fall below this criteria are diagnosed as atypical lobular hyperplasia.

The risk for subsequent invasive cancer with lobular carcinoma *in situ* is nearly identical to ductal carcinoma *in situ*, but in contrast to ductal carcinoma *in situ*, in which the

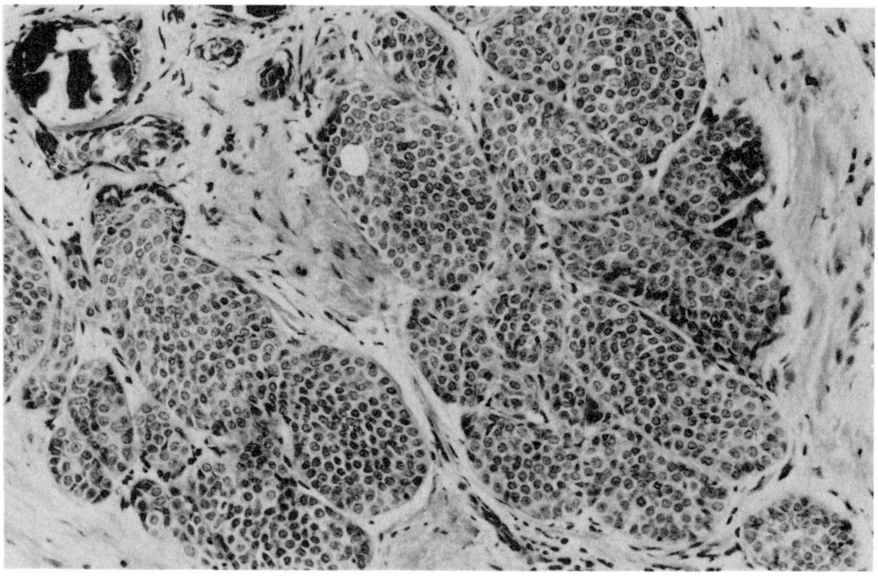

Fig. 11. Lobular carcinoma *in situ* (Original magnification 160x).

risk is almost entirely confined to the area in which the ductal carcinoma *in situ* is located, the risk for lobular carcinoma is nearly equally divided between each breast *(3)*. This has great practical importance in that a unilateral mastectomy becomes an illogical choice for a disease process that may involve either breast equally. Therefore, it becomes appropriate to engage these women in close mammographic surveillance, and there is little or no indication for any further local therapy.

Figure 11 shows a well-developed example of lobular carcinoma *in situ* where over half of the acini are clearly distended and expanded by the lobular neoplasia cells. There is much less, controversy surrounding the diagnosis of atypical lobular hyperplasia vs lobular carcinoma *in situ* because the quantitative criteria for these diagnoses are relatively straightforward, and there is much less variation in the cytologic appearance of lobular neoplasia cells.

SUMMARY

We have reviewed a variety of important lesions that predict a range of subsequent risks of invasive breast cancer. The histologic definitions that recognize these lesions have been evaluated through extensive epidemiologic studies, and are based on patterns that are found within breast biopsies and have been developed to take into account recognizable points of distinction along an admittedly nearly continuous morphological spectrum.

It is important for pathologists and clinicians to recognize that the risk estimates given for these various lesions are intimately tied to these histologic definitions and the criteria for making these diagnoses. Therefore, if one is to use the risk estimates in an meaningful way, they must refer to these specific definitions *(31)*.

Another concept that is important to understand is that risk estimates and the likelihood of developing carcinoma either in the same breast or in both breasts divides these lesions into distinct biological groups *(32)*. The first group is one that represents markers of increased risk, and this includes atypical ductal hyperplasia, atypical lobular hyperplasia, and lobular carcinoma *in situ*. These lesions are only markers of increased risk, because they predict an increased risk that is equally divided between both breasts. The next type of lesion is the determinant lesion represented by noncomedo ductal carcinoma *in situ*. These lesions predict a very strong likelihood of developing breast carcinoma in a very specific region, and, therefore, represent the first lesion with appropriate genetic alterations to qualify as a true precursor lesion. Finally, coinedo ductal carcinoma *in situ* very likely represents a lesion that is largely committed to the neoplastic process and frequently has many genetic alterations. These lesions are comprised of cells that are fully malignant, save one criteria that is the ability to invade a basement membrane.

It is our hope that molecular markers will one day contribute to our precision in defining the potential risks of these lesions *(33)*, but currently the light microscope is shouldering the burden and doing a good job of it.

REFERENCES

1. Fisher, E. R., Gregorio, R. M., and Fisher, B. (1975b) The pathology of invasive breast cancer. A syllabus derived from findings of the national surgical adjuvant breast project (protocol no. 4) *Cancer* **36,** 1–85.
2. Page, D. L. (1994) The epidemiology of tumor markers in breast cancer management: Prognostic Markers. *Cancer Epidemiol., Biomarkers Prev.* **3,** 101–104.
3. Page, D. L., and Dupont, W. D. (1991) Histologic indicators of breast cancer risk. *Bull. Am. Coll. Surg.* **76,** 16–23.
4. Ernster, V. L., Barclay, J., Kerlikowske, K., Grady, D., and Henderson, I. C. (1996) Incidence of and treatment for ductal carcinoma in situ of the breast. *JAMA* **275,** 913–918.
5. Betsill, W. L., Rosen, P. P., Lieberman, P. H., and Robbins, G. F. (1978) Intraductal Carcinoma: Long-term follow-up after treatment by biopsy alone. *JAMA* **239,** 1863–1867.
6. Page, D. L., Dupont, W. D., Rogers, L. W., and Landenberger, M. (1982) Intraductal carcinoma of the breast: follow-up after biopsy. *Cancer* **49,** 751–758.
7. Dupont, W. D., and Page, D. L. (1985) Risk factors for breast cancer in women with proliferative breast disease. *N. Engl. J. Med.* **312,** 146–151.
8. Hutter, R. V. P. (1986) Consensus meeting: Is "fibrocystic disease" of the breast precancerous? *Arch Pathol. Lab. Med.* **110,** 171-173.
9. Page, D. L., Dupont, W. D., and Jensen, R. A. (1996) Papillary apocrine change of the breast: Associations with atypical hyperplasia and risk of breast cancer. *Cancer Epidemiol. Biomarkers Prev.* **5,** 29–32.
10. O'Malley, F. P., Page, D. L., Nelson, E. H., and Dupont, W. D. (1994) Ductal carcinoma in situ of the breast with apocrine cytology: Definition of a borderline category. *Hum. Pathol.* **25,** 164–168.
11. Jensen, R. A., Page, D. L., Dupont, W. D., and Rogers, L. W. (1989) Invasive breast cancer risk in women with sclerosing adenosis. *Cancer* **64,** 1977–1983.
12. Tavassoli, F. A., and Norris, H. J. (1990) A comparison of the results of long-term follow-up for atypical intraductal hyperplasia and intraductal hyperplasia of the breast. *Cancer* **65,** 518–529.
13. McDivitt, R. W., Stevens, J. A., Lee, N. C., Wingo, P. A., and Rubin, G. L. (1992) Histologic types of benign breast disease and the risk for breast cancer. *Cancer* **69,** 1408–1414.
14. Page, D. L., Salhany, K. E., Jensen, R. A., and Dupont, W. D. (1996) Subsequent breast carcinoma risk after biopsy with atypia in a breast papilloma. *Cancer* **78,** 258–266.
15. Dupont, W. D., Page, D. L., Parl, F. F., Vnencak-Jones, C. L., Plummer, W., Jr., Rados, M. S., and Schuyler, P. A. (1994) Long-term risk of breast cancer in women with fibroadenoma. *N. Engl. J. Med.* **331,** 10–15.
16. Page, D. L., and Rogers, L. W. (1992) Combined histologic and cytologic criteria for the diagnosis of mammary atypical ductal hyperplasia. *Hum. Pathol.* **23,** 1095–1097.
17. London, S. J., Connolly, J. L., '3chnitt, S. J., and Colditz, G. A. (1992) A prospective study of benign breast disease and risk of breast cancer. *JAMA* **267,** 941–944.
18. Dupont, W. D., Parl, F. F., Hartrnann, W. H., Brinton, L. A., Winfield, A. C., Worrell, J. A., Schuyler, P. A., and Plummer, W. D. (1993) Breast cancer risk associated with proliferative breast disease and atypical hyperplasia. *Cancer* **71,** 1258–1265.

19. Page, D. L., Kidd, T. E., Duponl, W. D., Simpson, J. F., and Rogers, L. W. (1991) Lobular neoplasia of the breast: Higher risk for subsequent invasive cancer predicted by more extensive disease. *Hum. Pathol.* **22,** 1232–1239.
20. Page, D. L., Dupont, W. D.,]Rogers, L. W., and Rados, M. S. (1985) Atypical hyperplastic lesions of the female breast. A long-term follow-up study. *Cancer* **55,** 2698–2708.
21. Page, D. L., and Lagios, M. D. (1994) Pathology and clinical evolution of ductal carcinoma in situ (DCIS) of the breast. *Cancer Lett.* **86,** 1–4.
22. Frykberg, E. R., Masood, S., Copeland, E., III, and Bland, K. I. (1993) Ductal carcinoma in situ of the brearst. *J. Am. Coll. Surg.* **177,** 425–440.
23. Schnitt, S. J., and Connolly, J. L. (1997) Classification of ductal carcinoma in situ: Striving for clinical relevance in the era of breast conserving therapy. *Hum. Pathol.* **28,** 877–880.
24. Silverstein, M. J. (1997) Ductal carcinoma in situ of the breast. *Br. J. Surg.* **84,** 145–146.
25. Schwartz, G. F., Lagios, M. D., Carter, D., Connolly, J., Ellis, I. O., Eusebi, V., Finkel, G. C., Gorstein, F., Holland, R., Hutter, R. V. P., Masood, S., Millis, R. R., O'Malley, F. P., Palazzo, J. T., Patchefsky, A. S., Rosai, J., Schnitt, S. J., Schwarting, R., Sloane, J. P., Tavassoli, F. A., Feig, S. A., Kopans, D. B., McCormick, B., and Copeland, E. M:., III (1997) Consensus conference on the classification of ductal carcinoma in situ. *Cancer* **80,** 1798–1802.
26. Scott, M. A., Lagios, M. D., Axelsson, K., Rogers, L. W., Anderson, T. J., and Page, D. L. (1997) Ductal carcinoma in situ of the breast: Reproducibility of histological subtype analysis. *Hum. Pathol.* **28,** 967–973.
27. Page, D. L., and Jensen, R. A. (1996) Ductal carcinoma in situ of the breast—Understanding the misunderstood stepchild. *JAMA* **275,** 948,949.
28. Mack, L., Kerkvliet, N., Doig, G-., and O'Malley, F. P. (1997) Relationship of a new histological categorization of ductal carcinoma in situ of the breast with size and the immunohistochemical expression of p53, c-erb B2, bcl-2, and ki-67. *Hum. Pathol.* **28,** 974–979.
29. Page, D. L., and Anderson, T. J. (1987) Diagnostic Histopathology of the Breast (Edinburgh: Churchill Livingstone)
30. Page, D. L., Steel, C. M., and Dixon, J. M. (1995) ABC of breast diseases: Carcinoma in situ and patients at high risk of breast cancer. *Bmj* **310,** 39–42.
31. Jensen, R. A., Dupont, W. D., and Page, D. L. (1993) Diagnostic criteria and cancer risk of proliferative breast lesions. J *Cell Biochem* **53,** 59–64.
32. Page, D. L., and Dupont, W. :D. (1990) Anatomic markers of human premalignancy and risk of breast cancer. *Cancer* **66,** 1326–1335.
33. Holt, J. T., Jensen, R. A., and Page, D. L. (1993) Histopathology-old principles and new methods, in *Cancer Surveys-Advances and Prospects in Clinical, Epidemiological and Laboratory Oncology* (Fentiman, I. and Taylor Papadimitriou, J., eds.), Cold Spring Harbor Laboratory Press, Cold Spring Harbor, New York.

22 Hormonal Treatment of Fibrocystic Disease

Luigi Dogliotti, MD, PhD
and Pasquale Caraci, MD

INTRODUCTION

The term benign breast disease (BBD) has been employed to indicate a wide and heterogeneous group of different morphologic and clinical entities. Many authors have used the term *fibrocystic breast disease* (FCD) to indicate a clinical picture including diffuse nodularity, with or without pain, mainly occurring in the reproductive age; the term is unsatisfactory, but we will refer to FCD because a considerable body of literature stands on this terminology *(1,2)*.

The vast majority of benign breast conditions present with the following symptoms: *lump*, *pain* (cyclical or noncyclical), and *nipple discharge*. They often coexist, but each may occur independently. The clinical manifestations have been linked to a variety of histologic appearance such as fibrosis, lymphocytic infiltration, mycro- and macrocysts, apocrine metaplasia, and atypical hyperplasia with or without atypia *(1,3–5)*. Macrocysts, apocrine metaplasia, and atypical hyperplasia may deserve special attention in relation to breast cancer risk *(3,5–7)*. Sometimes all these histologic findings can be found in asymptomatic patients, leading to the suggestion that FCD is a nondisease *(8)*. However, many patients experience severe discomfort, which supports the concept of real disease.

It is well known that the natural history of FCD is linked to the reproductive events of the woman's life: onset in the reproductive age, menstruation-related clinical course, and postmenopausal improvement *(1,2)*. In fact, structural and functional changes in the breast, associated with clinical symptoms of heaviness and fullness, occur throughout the menstrual cycle *(9,10)*. These observations focus on the central role played by the endocrine system in the pathophysiology of FCD. The endocrine abnormalities are subtle and not easily recognizable with the common laboratory evaluations in individual patients; estrogen excess, progesterone insufficiency with relative hyperestrogenism, and secretory alteration of prolactin (PRL), androgens, and thyroid hormones have all been implicated *(1,2)*. A unifying hypothesis that takes into account proven and supposed mechanisms involved has been proposed by us, as outlined in Fig. 1 *(2)*.

Although rationally designed endocrine protocols for the treatment of FCD have been put forward in the light of its hormonal pathogenesis, the effectiveness of hormonal

From: *Contemporary Endocrinology: Endocrinology of Breast Cancer*
Edited by: A. Manni

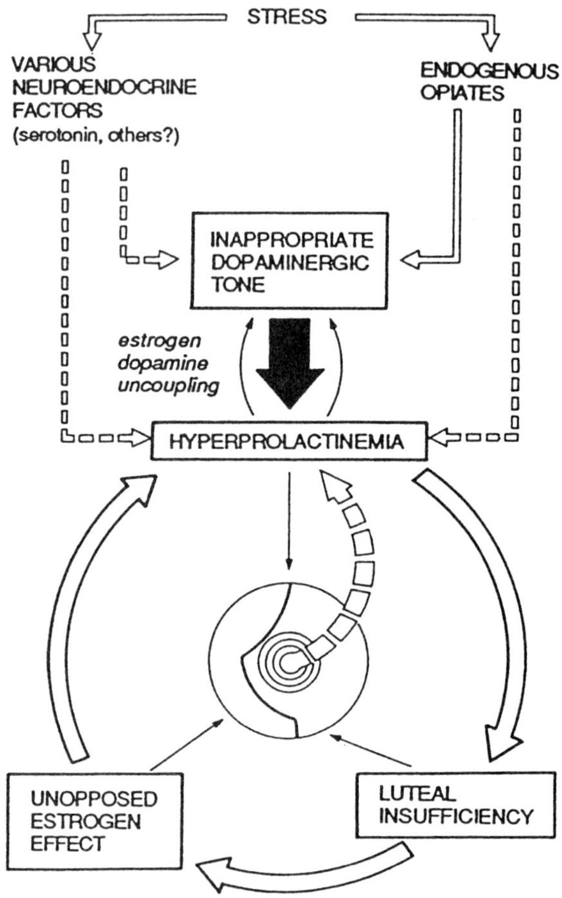

Fig. 1. Endocrine events involved in the pathogenesis of FCD. From Dogliotti et al., 1989 *(2)*, with permission.

agents before their administration is unpredictable. In most individual cases, the treatment remains largely empirical and of varying success.

GENERAL MANAGEMENT PLAN

The management plan of symptomatic FCD should be established in individual patients and may be different in relation to the clinical presentation.

If a *dominant or discrete lump* is present, the management consists primarily in establishing the correct diagnosis and excluding cancer. If a gross breast cyst is found, no treatment other than aspiration is required *(11,12)*. Electrolyte evaluation in the aspirated fluid may be advisable, since a mild increase of later developing cancer risk in patients bearing type I (high K^+/Na^+ intracystic ratio) cysts has been reported *(7)*. As far as hormonal treatment of recurrent gross cysts is concerned, there have been reported encouraging results in the prevention of recurrency using a short course of danazol (100 mg three times daily for 3 months) *(13,14)*. In women who had previously required repeated aspirations of breast cysts, the single short course of danazol resulted in a reduction of cyst formation at 6 months following trial entry, and the effect appeared to be maintained even at three years. Favorable results in reducing cyst recurrency by danazol administration have also been reported by others *(15)*. However, our experience with danazol treatment at 200 mg for 6 months vs observation was unsuccessful (unpublished data).

When *diffuse nodular breasts* are found by clinical examination, further diagnostic evaluation is not generally required. Medical treatment should be considered for patients with associated mastalgia.

Nipple discharge is frequently observed in both benign and malignant breast disease. To be clinically significant, a discharge should be true, spontaneous, persistent and nonlactational *(16)*. Diagnostic approach is aimed at identifying the surgically significant discharges and excluding cancer. Purulent discharge must be treated with an appropriate antibiotic, possibly based on results of cultures. Milky and multicolored discharges are also commonly treated medically *(16)*. In case of hyperprolactinemia, dopamine agonists such as bromocriptine (e.g., 5–7.5 mg daily in refracted doses) are the agents of choice; an imaging study of the sellar region will also be performed to exclude PRL-secreting adenoma. When hyperprolactinemia is not found, a short course of bromocriptine may be tried, since it has been reported to improve milky discharge and to prevent recurrence of nonpuerperal mastitis *(17)*.

Mastalgia is a very common symptom and represents a frequent reason for consultation in general practice. Active treatment is required in only a minority of patients, not exceeding 15–20%. It is generally accepted that moderate and transient cyclical premenstrual pain is a physiologic event and should be managed only by adequate reassurance. Accordingly, some authors have continued to regard mastalgia as a complaint of psychological nature *(18)*. However, the view that these women are neurotic has not been substantiated by formal studies *(19)*. Frequently, simple withdrawal of oral contraceptives or hormone replacement therapy may produce a dramatical response *(20)*. Mastalgia has to be actively treated when breast pain is severe and prolonged (it may last for 2–3 weeks of a monthly cycle), thus interfering with the quality of life, especially in every day activities such as work, sleep, and sexual relationship *(21)*.

Three discrete patterns of breast pain have been recognized: cyclical mastalgia, noncyclical mastalgia, and chest wall pain. Qualitative and quantitative recording of symptoms by the patient herself, using a suitable pain chart according to the model proposed by Maddox and Mansel *(20)*, allows a correct diagnosis and contributes to a decision on the management plan. Severe *cyclic breast pain* is somewhat more amenable to treatment, because of its postulated hormonal etiology *(22)*. *Noncyclic breast pain* has a lower response rate, but differentiation of a subgroup with *chest wall pain* leads to a good response by means of local infiltration with steroids and/or local anaesthetics *(23,24)*. The general management plan for mastalgia is outlined in Fig. 2.

Due to the absence of side effects, the *first-line treatment* may include either placebo-like preparations (i.e., vitamins, topical progesterone gel) or evening primrose oil. The latter is a natural product containing high concentrations of essential unsaturated fatty acids (mainly γ-linolenic acid). A dosage of 3 grams a day for 3 months has been reported to be effective in 40–70% of patients with cyclical mastalgia with moderate or good response *(21)*. It has been suggested that primrose oil may act via prostaglandin pathways, in patients who have been found to be deficient in circulating levels of certain fatty acids *(25)*.

The *second-line treatment* consists of systemic hormonal therapy. Several controlled trials have shown that hormonal treatment will often provide relief for women with breast

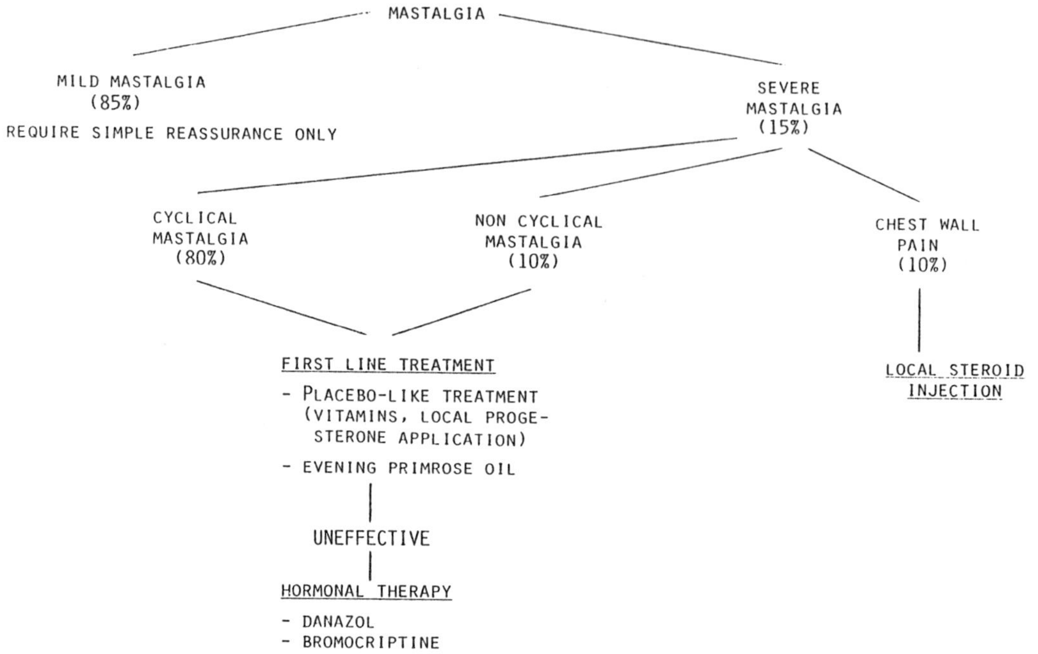

Fig. 2. General management plan of mastalgia. From Maddox et al., 1989, modified. *(20)*

Table 1.
Pharmacological Treatment for Mastalgia and Approximate Response Rate

		Approximate Overall Response, %		
Drug	*Dose*	*CM*	*NCM*	*MSP*
Danazol	200 mg/day	70	31	—
Bromocriptine	5 mg/day	65	20	—
Tamoxifen	10–20 mg/day	70	56	—
Evening primrose oil	3 g/day	45	27	—
Placebo	—	10–40	10–40	?
Steroid injection		—	—	70–90

Abbreviations: CM, cyclical mastalgia; NCM, noncyclical mastalgia; MSP, muscoloskeletal pain.

pain, but the frequent occurrence of side effects should limit this therapy to cases of severe mastalgia. Table 1 lists some drugs employed successfully in FCD, with approximate overall response rates.

HORMONAL TREATMENT OF MASTALGIA

Danazol

Danazol is the 2,3-*d*-isoxazol synthetic derivative of ethisterone (17α-ethinyl-testosterone); it displays mild androgenic/progestogenic effects and antigonadotropinmic activity *(1)*. The efficacy of danazol in feminine disorders was long attributed to the latter property *(26,27)*. Although true suppression of circulating gonadotropins does not really occur during the reproductive age *(28–31)*, interference with pulsatile release of gonadotropins *(32)*, selective inhibition of preovulatory follicle-stimulating hormone and luteinizing hormone peaks *(33)*, and release of higher proportion of biologically inactive gonadotropins have been well documented *(32)*. Danazol may also interfere with ovarian steroidogenesis by direct inhibition of certain enzymes, as shown in experimental animals *(34)*. Therefore, the therapeutic effects of danazol seem to be primarily mediated by decreased concentration of circulating estrogens, as a consequence of both direct and indirect inhibition of ovarian steroidogenesis. Other important mechanisms could be its intrinsic androgenic/progestative action *(27)*, progesterone receptor induction *(35)*, and the postulated reduction of PRL circulating levels *(32,36)*.

Danazol is the most effective hormonal treatment available, with a high response rate of about 75–80%. The use of danazol for mastalgia was first described in 1971 by Greenblatt and co-workers *(37)*, and its activity has since been confirmed in both open *(38–41)* and controlled trials *(42,43)*. Mansel et al. *(42)* carried out a double-blind placebo-controlled study on patients with cyclical mastalgia. At doses as low as 200 mg/d, danazol was beneficial, producing both relief of symptoms and reduction in nodularity.

Treatment dosages reported in literature range from 100 to 800 mg/d *(38–43)*. Side effects are dose related and are mainly caused by gonadotropin interference (e.g., menstrual disturbance/amenorrhea) and androgenic activity (e.g., acne, oily skin, hirsutism, voice change, weight gain). They occur in about 20% of patients on a conventional dosage of 100–200 mg/d *(22)*. Since danazol is potentially teratogenic *(44)*, an effective mechanical means of contraception should be recommended.

In current practice, the treatment should be started with 100 mg daily and continued for at least 2 months *(20,21)*. Individual dosage adjustments are recommended to optimize the therapeutic effects. When a response is obtained, a standard course of therapy should be given for 6 months. After danazol treatment is stopped, the clinical effect can last for 6 months or more *(22)*, possibly because of the induction of progesterone receptors *(34)*, which persists after discontinuation of the drug. A lower maintenance schedule can be used to prevent relapse: it may consist of taking danazol 100 mg on alternate days or simply taking danazol daily on days 14–28 of the menstrual cycle *(45)*.

Bromocriptine

Bromocriptine (2-bromo-α-ergocriptine) is a semisynthetic ergot derivative with long-acting dopaminergic activity. It is the drug of choice for the experimental and clinical suppression of PRL secretion, and its efficacy in both hyper- and normoprolactinemia has been widely demonstrated *(46)*. Due to the postulated role of PRL in the etiopathogenesis of FCD *(1,2)*, bromocriptine has been used to treat symptomatic patients. Schulz et al. *(47)* were the first to use bromocriptine in FCD. Their excellent results in 15 cases of severe breast pain and premenstrual tension with no sign of organic disease have been extensively confirmed in open *(48–50)* and placebo-controlled studies *(41–59)*, using both randomized and sequential protocols. The effectiveness of bromocriptine has been further demonstrated in a large European multicenter randomized controlled trial of nearly 300 patients *(59)*. In this study, which involved 13 European centers, bromocriptine 2.5 mg twice a day was compared with placebo for cyclical mastalgia. The ability of bromocriptine to reduce breast pain was assessed by using a visual analog scale. Alleviation of symptoms occurred with either bromocriptine or placebo, but at each time point evaluated, bromocriptine was significantly better than placebo in improving breast symp-

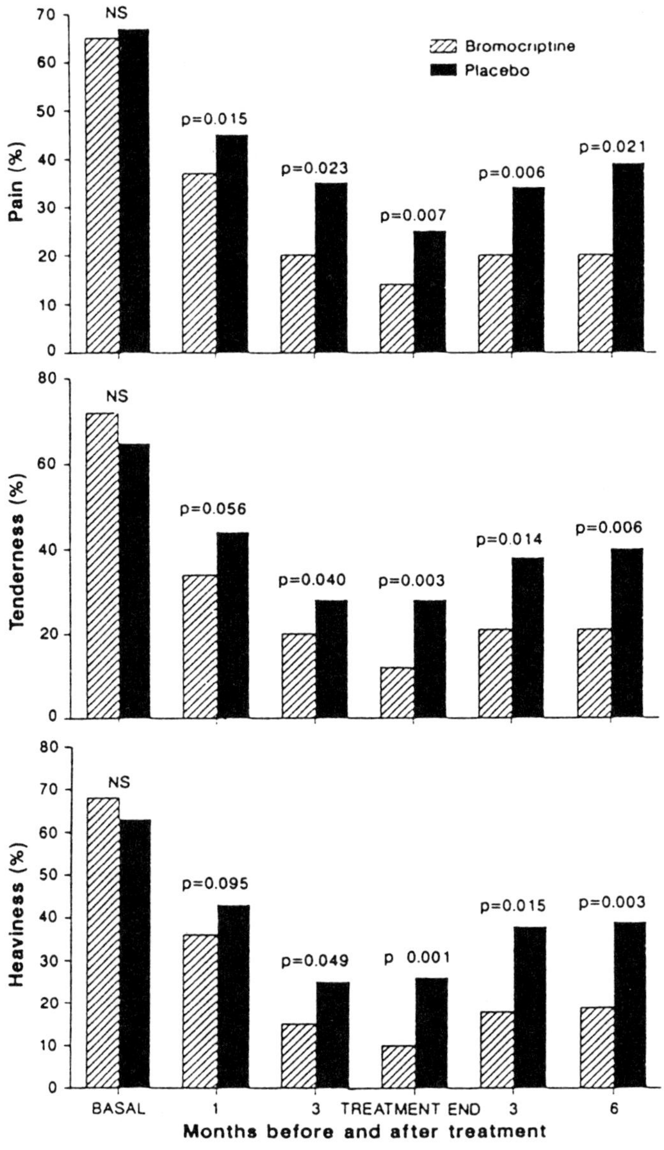

Fig. 3. Effect of bromocriptine therapy: linear visual analog scale scores for pain, tenderness and heaviness. Scores expressed as % of the scale, with maximum at baseline. From Mansel and Dogliotti, 1990 *(59)*, with permission.

toms, as illustrated in Fig. 3. Improvement of symptoms was accompanied by a significant reduction in serum PRL in the bromocriptine-treated group but not in the placebo group (Fig. 4). Interestingly, dynamic PRL secretion, assessed by a preliminary thyrotropin-releasing hormone test, had been previously shown to be a good predictor of response to endocrine therapy *(60)*.

As a whole, a good clinical response can be observed in around 70% of patients, but 25–30% of them experience side effects such as nausea, pyrosis, and dizziness, which commonly tend to improve after 10–15 days of therapy; they can be minimized by starting with a low dose (i.e., 1.25 mg) taken in the evening with a meal, and gradually increasing

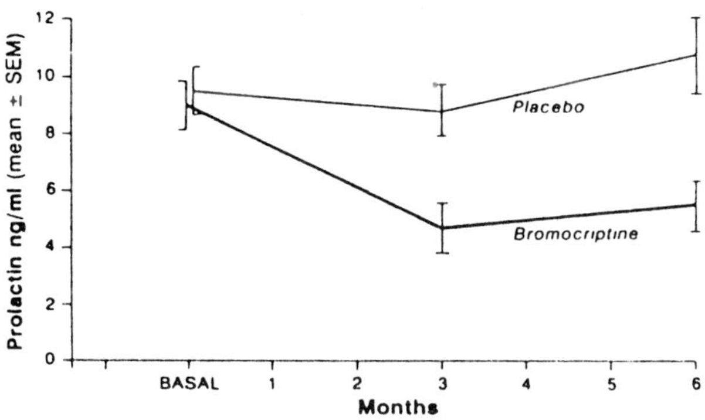

Fig. 4. Effect of bromocriptine therapy on PRL concentrations. From Mansel and Dogliotti, 1990 *(59)*, with permission.

the dosage to 2.5 mg twice a daily. In patients who are responding with good tolerability, the treatment should be continued for about 6 months *(20,21)*.

Progestins

Progesterone and/or its synthetic derivatives have been widely used to treat FCD. The rationale is linked to the luteal deficiency/relative hyperestrogenism hypothesis *(1,2,61)*, which would be open to correction by progestin administration, particularly in the second half of the cycle *(1,61)*. The largest series is that of Mauvais-Jarvis et al. *(62)*, which reported in open studies good results with a combination of oral 10 mg/day lynestrenol (a synthetic norsteroid) and progesterone in hydroalcoholic gel by percutaneous administration. However, a beneficial effect of progestin administration has been reported in open studies *(62–65)*, while the results of clinical randomized trials remain controversial: in controlled double-blind trials, some authors showed significant clinical improvement *(66)*, and others showed only improvement in thermographic appearances and not in clinical findings *(67)*; in further randomized controlled studies, progestogens have not been found to be of any benefit *(20,68)*.

Side effects stem primarily from gonadotropin block. Prolonged administration, particularly when commenced in young subjects, may lead to a fall in estrogen activity, with unpredictable effects on bone mineralization and genital tropism. Other unwanted effects include usually slight, but nevertheless unwelcome, weight increase and a certain degree of hyperandrogenism when nortestosterone derivatives are employed.

Contraceptive Pill

Although most reports from the literature have indicated a generic protective effect in FCD *(69)*, the exact relationship between contraceptive pills and symptomatic mastopathy remains an unsettled question. Whereas some women may experience mastalgia for the first time on starting a new oral contraceptive, others may experience improvement of preexisting symptoms, as in the case of younger women because of the delivery of stable amounts of hormones every month *(11)*. Due to the lack of studies clarifying the issue, an empirical approach to the management of individual patients must be recommended.

Tamoxifen

Tamoxifen is an antiestrogenic agent widely used in the treatment of advanced hormone-dependent breast cancer. It acts through competitive inhibition at the estrogen receptor level and has been occasionally employed in FCD. The first remarkable study was that of Ricciardi and Ianniruberto *(70)*, who observed positive results in 70% of a series of 63 women with various forms of FCD treated with 10 mg of tamoxifen on the 5th to 25th day of three menstrual cycles. Two more recent double-blind controlled trials in Great Britain showed that tamoxifen, 20 mg and 10 mg/d, respectively, significantly improved mastalgia *(71,72)*. Side effects were reported to be minimal with the lower dosage *(72)*.

Administration of tamoxifen in benign breast disease, however, has been extensively criticized and is generally discouraged, especially for long periods. Owing to its antiestrogenic effect at the hypothalamic level, its protracted use prior to the menopause leads to hypersecretion of gonadotropins, followed by enhanced ovarian steroidogenesis with hyperestrogenism *(73)*. Further problems arise because of reported cataracts and hepatocellular carcinoma in rats given high tamoxifen dosage, even though no comparable data have been reported for humans *(74)*.

LHRH Agonists

These hormonal agents have been shown to be effective in improving mastalgia in a controlled trial *(75)*; however, the side effects related to prolonged hypoestrogenism (i.e., effect on bone metabolism) should limit the use of these drugs for mastalgia and at present they are not licensed for benign breast disease.

CONCLUSIONS

Hormonal treatment has been demonstrated to be helpful in management of mastalgia. Only a small percentage of patients, who have severe discomfort not relieved by reassurance, should be considered eligible for endocrine treatment *(1,20,21)*. A better response has been demonstrated for cyclical mastalgia compared with the noncyclical group (Table 1) *(20,21)*, so that patients should be preventively assessed by a pain chart to define the pain pattern before starting therapy.

Only a small number of hormonal drugs have been adequately tested in controlled trials and demonstrated to be effective; these are danazol, bromocriptine, tamoxifen, and LHRH agonists. The choice of treatment will depend on patient characteristics, efficacy, potential side effects, and cost. The most appropriate drug for individual patients will be determined by a process of trial and error, and sometimes several treatments may need to be tried before an optimal response is obtained *(20)*.

REFERENCES

1. Angeli A, Dogliotti L, Faggiuolo R, Orlandi F, Bussolati G, eds. (1984) *Fibrocystic Disease of the Breast. A Revisit and New Perspectives,* Excerpta Medica, Amsterdam.
2. Dogliotti L, Orlandi F, Angeli A (1989) The endocrine basis of benign breast disorders. World J Surg 13:674–679.
3. Haagensen CD, Bodian C, Haagensen DE Jr (1981) *Breast Carcinoma. Risk and Detection.* WB Saunders, Philadelphia.
4. Azzopardi JC (1979) *Problems in Breast Pathology.* WB Saunders, Philadelphia.
5. Dupont WD, Parl FF, Hartmann WH, Brinton LA, Winfield AC, Worrell JA, et al. (1993) Breast cancer risk associated with proliferative breast disease and atypical hyperplasia. Cancer 71:1258–1263.
6. Schuerch C, Rosen PP, Hirota T, Itabashi M, Yamamoto H, Kinnie DW, et al. (1982) A pathologic study of benign breast disease in Tokyo and New York. Cancer 50:1899–1903.

7. Bruzzi P, Dogliotti L, Naldoni C, Bucchi L, Costantini M, Cicognani A, et al. (1997) Cohort study of association of breast cancer with cyst type in women with gross cystic disease of the breast. BMJ 314:925–928.
8. Love SM, Gelman RS, Sile W (1982) Fibrocystic 'disease' of the breast—a non disease? N Engl J Med 307:1010–1014.
9. Osborne MP (1987) Breast development and anatomy, In: *Breast Disease* (Harris JR, Hallman S, Henderson IC, Kinne DW, eds.), JB Lippincott, Philadelphia, pp. 1–14.
10. Russo J, Russo IH (1987) Development of the human mammary gland, In: *The Mammary Gland* (Neville MC, Daniel CW, eds.), Plenum, New York, pp. 67–93.
11. Love SM, Schmitt SJ, Connolly JL, Shirley RL (1987) Benign breast disorders, In: *Breast Disease* (Harris JR, Hellman S, Craig L, Kinne DW, eds.), JB Lippincott, Philadelphia, pp. 15–73.
12. Hughes E, Bundred NJ (1989) Breast macrocysts. World J Surg 13:711–714.
13. Hinton CP, Williams MR, Roebuck CJ, Blamey R (1986) A controlled trial of danazol in the treatment of multiple recurrent breast cysts. Br J Clin Pract 40:3–5.
14. Locker AP, Hinton CP, Roebuck EJ, Blamey RW (1989) Long term follow-up of patients treated with a single course of danazol for recurrent breast cysts. Br J Clin Pract 43(suppl 68):100–101.
15. Rasmussen T, Tobiassen T, Doberl A (1986) Reduction of cysts in fibrocystic breast disease during and after danazol treatment. Ann NY Acad Sci 464:622–625.
16. Leis HP Jr (1989) Management of nipple discharge. Br J Surg 13:736–742.
17. Peters F, Schuth W (1989) Hyperprolactinemia and nonpuerperal mastitis (duct ectasia). JAMA 261,1618–1620.
18. Haagensen CD (1986) The normal physiology of the breast, In: *Disease of the Breast*, 3rd ed. (Haagensen CD, ed.), WB Saunders, Philadelphia, pp 47–55.
19. Preece PE, Mansel RE, Hughes LE (1978) Mastalgia: psychoneurosis or organic disease? BMJ 1:29–34.
20. Maddox ER, Mansel RE (1989) Management of breast pain and nodularity. World J Surg 13:669–705.
21. Mansel RE (1993) Guidelines for referral by general practitioners, In: *Recent Developments in the Study of Benign Breast Disease* (Mansel RE, ed.), Parthenon, London, pp. 25–32.
22. Pye JK, Mansel RE, Hughes LE (1985) Clinical experience of drug treatment for mastalgia. Lancet 2:373–377.
23. Sibbering M, Galea MH, Blamey RW (1993) Chest wall pain in the mastalgia clinic, In: *Recent Progress in the Study of Benign Breast Disease* (Mansel RE, ed.), Parthenon, London, pp. 201–206.
24. Maddox PR, Harrison BJ, Mansel RE, Hughes LE (1989) Non-cyclical mastalgia: an improved classification and treatment. Br J Surg 76:901–907.
25. Gateley CA, Maddox PR, Pritchard GA, Shendan W, Harrison BJ, Pye GK, et al. (1992) Plasma fatty acid profiles in benign breast disorders. Br J Surg 79:407–410.
26. Sherins RJ, Gandy HM, Thorslund TW, Paulsen CA (1971) Pituitary and testicular function studies. I. Experience with a new gonadal inhibitor, danazol. J Clin Endocrinol Metab 32:522–531.
27. Dmowski WP (1979) Endocrine properties and clinical application of danazol. Fertil Steril 31:237–242.
28. Franchimont P, Cramillon C (1977) The effect of danazol on anterior pituitary function. Fertil Steril 28:814–817.
29. Lind T, Cook DB (1976): How does danazol work? Lancet 1:1401–1402.
30. Barbieri RL, Ryan KJ (1981) Danazol: endocrine pharmacology and therapeutic applications. Am J Obstet Gynecol 141:453–463.
31. Bevan JR, Dowsett M, Jeffcoate SL (1984) Endocrine effects of danazol in the treatment of endometriosis. Br J Obstet Gynecol 91:160–166.
32. Rannevik G (1987) Hormonal effects of danazol, In: *Benign breast disease: Is it worth treating?* (Wood C, ed.), The Royal Society of Medicine Service, Roundtable Series no. 6, London, pp. 93–99.
33. Greenblatt RB, Chadda JS, Teran AZ, Lewis A (1984) Fibrocystic breast disease: pathophysiology, hormonology, treatment. Contemp Surg 24:49–60.
34. Menon M, Azhar S, Menon KMJ. (1980) Evidence that danazol inhibits gonadotropin-induced ovarian steroidogenesis at a point distal to gonadotrophin-receptor interaction and cyclical AMP formation. Am J Obstet Gynaecol 136:524–530.
35. Panahy C, Pucklefoot JR,Anderson E, Winson GP, Berry CL, Goode AW (1987) Effect of danazol on the incidence of progesterone and estrogen receptors in benign breast disease. BMJ 295:464–466.
36. Bonhet HG, Hanker JP, Schweppe KW, Schneider HPG (1981) Changes of prolactin secretion following long term danazol application. Fertil Steril 36:725–728.
37. Greenblatt RB, Dmowsky WP, Mahesh VB, Scholler HFL (1971) Clinical studies with an antigonadotropin, danazol Fertil Steril 22:102–112.

38. Lauersen NH, Wilson KH (1976) The effect of danazol in the treatment of chronic cystic mastitis. Obstet Gynecol 48:93–98.
39. Asch RH, Greenblatt RB (1977) The use of an impeded androgen—danazol—in the management of benign breast disorders. Am J Obstet Gynaecol 127:130–134.
40. Brookshaw JD (1980) Danazol treatment of benign breast disease: a survey of USA multicenter study. Postgrad Med J 55(suppl 5):52–58.
41. Greenblatt RB, Nezhat C, Ben Nun I (1980) The treatment of benign breast disease with danazol. Fertil Steril 34:242–245.
42. Mansel RE, Wisbey JR, Hughes LE (1982) Controlled trial of the anti-gonadotropin danazol in painful nodular benign breast disease. Lancet 1:928–930.
43. Hinton CP, Bishop HN, Holliday HW, Doyle PJ, Blamey RW (1986) A double-blind controlled trial of danazol and bromocriptine in the management of severe cyclical brest pain. Br J Clin Pract 40:326–330.
44. Wentz AC (1982) Adverse effects of danazol in pregnancy. Ann Intern Med 96:672–675.
45. Maddox PR, Harrison J, Mansel RE (1989) Low dose danazol for mastalgia. Br J Clin Pract 43(suppl 68):43–47.
46. Thorner MO, Fluckiger E, Kalne DB (1980) *Bromocriptine: A Clinical and Pharmacological Review.* Raven Press, New York.
47. Schulz KD, Del Pozo E, Lose KH (1975) Successful treatment of mastodynia with the prolactin inhibitor bromocriptine (CB-154). Arch Gynaekol 220:83–87.
48. Benedek-Jaszman LJ, Hearn-Sturtevant MD (1976) Premenstrual tension and functional infertility. Aetiology and treatment. Lancet 2:1095–1098.
49. Dalton K (1976) Bromocriptine in premenstrual syndrome, In: Pharmacological and Clinical Aspects of Bromocriptine (Parlodel) (Bayliss RIS, Turner P, McLay WP, eds.), Grange Press, Southwick, pp. 106–110.
50. Andersch B, Hahn L, Wendestruan C (1978) Treatment of premenstrual tension syndrome with bromocriptine. Acta Endocrinol 88(suppl 216):165.
51. Harrisson P, Letchworth AJ (1976) Bromocriptine in the treatment of premenstural tension syndrome, In: *Pharmacological and Clinical Aspects of Bromocriptine (Parlodel)* (Bayliss RIS, Turner P, McLay WP, ed.), Grange Press, Southwick, pp. 103–105.
52. Andersen AN, Larsen JF, Steenstrup OR (1977) Effect of bromocriptine on the premenstrual syndrome. A double-blind clinical trial. Br J Obstet Gynecol 84:370–374.
53. Graham JJ, Harding PE, Wise PH, Berriman H (1978) Prolactin suppression in the treatment of premenstrual syndrome. Med J Aust Supplement:18–20.
54. Elsner CW, Buster JE, Shindel RA (1980) Bromocriptine in the treatment of premenstrual tension syndrome. Obstet Gynaecol 56:723–727.
55. Ylostalo P, Kauppila A, Puolakka J, et al. (1982) Bromocriptine and norethisterone in the treatment of premenstrual syndrome. Obstet Gynecol 59:292–298.
56. Mansel RE, Preece PE, Hughes LE (1978) A double blind trial of the prolactin inhibitor bromocriptine in painful benign breast disease. Br J Surg 65:724–727.
57. Durning P, Sellwood RA (1982) Bromocriptine in severe cyclical breast pain. Br J Surg 69:248–249.
58. Blicher-Toft M, Anderson AN, Henriksen OB, Mygind T (1979) Treatment of mastalgia with bromocriptine: a double blind crossover study. BMJ 1:237.
59. Mansel RE, Dogliotti L (1990) European multicentre trial of bromocriptine in cyclical mastalgia. Lancet 335:190–193.
60. Kumar S, Mansel RE, Hughes LE, Edwards CA, Scanlon MF (1985) Prediction of response to endocrine therapy in pronounced cyclical mastalgia using dynamic tests of prolactin release. Clin Endocrinol 23:669–672.
61. Sitruk-Ware R, Sterkers N, Mowszowicz I, Mauvais-Jarvis P (1977) Inadequate corpus luteus function in women with benign breast diseases. J Clin Endocrinol Metab 44:771–774.
62. Mauvais-Jarvis P, Sterkers N, Kuttenn F, Beauvais J (1978) Traitement des mastopathies benignes par la progesterone, et les progestatifs. J Gynaecol Obstet Biol Reprod 7:477–484.
63. Kuttenn F, Fournier S, Sitruk-Ware R, et al. (1983) Progesterone insufficiency in benign breast disease, In: *Endocrinology of Cystic Breast Disease* (Angeli A, Bradlow HL, Dogliotti L, eds.), Raven Press, New York, pp. 231–233.
64. Vorherr H (1986) Fibrocystic breast disease: pathophysiology, pathomorphology, clinical picture and management. Am J Obstet Gynaecol 154:161–167.
65. Kuttenn F, Mouttarege A, Mauvais-Jarvis P (1978) Bases hormonales de la contraception progestative discontinué. Nouv Press Med 7:3109–3113.

66. Dennerstein L, Spencer-Gardiner C, Gotts G (1985) Progesterone and premenstrual syndrome: a double blind crossover trial. BMJ 290:1617–1621.
67. Colin C, Gaspard U, Lambotte R (1978) Relationship of mastodynia with its endocrine environment and treatment in a double blind trial with lynestrenol. Arch Gynaekol 225:7–13.
68. Day JB (1979) Clinical trials in premenstrual syndrome. Curr Med Res Opin 6(suppl 5):40–45.
69. Ory H, Cole P, MacMahon B (1976) Oral contraceptives and reduced risk of benign breast disease. N Engl J Med 294:419.
70. Ricciardi I, Ianniruberto A (1979) Tamoxifen induced regression of benign breast lesion. Obstet Gynecol 54:80–84.
71. Fentiman IS, Caleffi M, Brame K, Chaudary MA, Hayward JL (1986) Double-blind controlled trial of tamoxifen therapy for mastalgia. Lancet 1:287–288.
72. Fentiman IS, Caleffi M, Hamed H, Chaudary MA (1988) Dosage and duration of tamoxifen treatment for mastalgia: a randomized trial. Br J Surg 75:845–846.
73. Sherman BM, Chapler FK, Crikard K (1979) Endocrine consequences of continuous antiestrogen therapy with tamoxifen in premenopausal women. J Clin Invest 64:398–404.
74. Fentiman IS, Powles TJ (1987) Tamoxifen and benign breast conditions. Lancet 2:1070–1071.
75. Hamed H, Caleffi M, Chaudary MA, Fentiman IS (1990) LHRH analogue for treatment of recurrent and refractory mastalgia: a controlled trial. Br J Surg 75:845–848.

23 Gynecomastia and Galactorrhea

David L. Kleinberg, MD

In the proper hormonal milieu, both male and female breasts are capable of significant development. At puberty, the female breasts normally develop mainly under the influence of estrogen and growth hormone (GH). However, in some clinical settings, abnormal breast development may also occur in males, and abnormal secretion of milk may occur in both males and females. This chapter will focus on the endocrine diseases of the mammary gland, with a particular emphasis on gynecomastia and galactorrhea. In addition, the chapter will discuss the normal development of the female mammary gland so that the pathophysiology of endocrine disorders of the male breast may be put into perspective.

OVERVIEW OF NORMAL MAMMARY DEVELOPMENT

Rodents and humans are born with mammary fat pads that contain small glandular anlagen. At specific stages of life (e.g., puberty), these undergo development and differentiation in response to appropriate stimulation by hormones and growth factors. The glandular elements of the mammary gland are derived from the dermis and extend into mesenchyme. The glandular elements and the mesenchyme together form the structure that will eventually become transformed into a mature mammary gland. At birth, the mammary gland is often prominent in both male and female fetuses as a result of exposure to placental and maternal hormones. Shortly after birth, however, mammary activity recedes and the mammary gland remains relatively quiescent until puberty, or shortly before.

At puberty, a surge of estrogen starts the process of normal mammary development or thelarche. Estrogen acts directly on the mammary gland to induce development *(1)*. Development from immature ductal anlagen to the adult female mammary gland occurs by a process called ductal morphogenesis. This process involves the development of structures called terminal end buds. Terminal end buds are multilayered, club-shaped structures in which active cell division is taking place. Under the influence of hormones, terminal end buds form and subsequently extend and penetrate into the surrounding fat pad. They lead the process of ductal morphogenesis and eventually fill the mammary fat pad with ductal structures *(2)*. Later, these terminal end buds further differentiate into alveolar structures. Alveoli may also arise directly from ducts. During pregnancy, the

From: *Contemporary Endocrinology: Endocrinology of the Breast*
Edited by: A. Manni © Humana Press Inc., Totowa, NJ

development of true single-layered glands capable of milk production takes place, and these structures prepare the mammary gland for lactation.

Although the process of mammary development is dependent on the presence of estrogen, estrogen alone cannot stimulate mammary development unless other hormones, such as GH, are available to interact with it. The presence of a functioning pituitary gland is required, a concept that has been recognized for nearly 60 yr. Although both GH and prolactin were known to participate in mammary development, it was believed by many that prolactin was the active pituitary factor responsible for mammary development because of its established effect on lactogenesis or milk production. In fact, prolactin in combination with estrogen does not stimulate pubertal mammary development in hypophysectomized, oophorectomized rats *(3,4)* or mice, and probably not in monkeys either *(5)*.

Our work has established that GH, working through local GH receptors in the mammary gland *(3,4)*, synergizes with estrogen to induce this critical phase of mammary development. GH permits estrogen to act by a process that is still incompletely understood. Its ability to stimulate estrogen receptors (ER) in the mammary gland could be one of a number of explanations for this interaction. GH appears to act on the stromal compartment of the mammary gland *(6)* to induce mammary development.

The assertion that IGF-1 is the physiological mediator of GH action in mammary development has not yet been fully proven, but is well supported by a number of experimental observations. These include (1) IGF-1 mimics the activity of GH in mammary development in hypophysectomized, gonadectomized animals *(7,8)*, and (2) that GH stimulates IGF-1 mRNA within the mammary gland *(3,6,8)*.

Postpubertal mammary development involves estrogen, progesterone (a stimulator of alveolar development), prolactin, and probably GH. Active further mammary development occurs during pregnancy. It is probable that placental hormones, such as placental lactogen, GH variant, prolactin, and possibly others, in addition to hormones of pituitary origin, participate in mammary gland development in preparation for lactation. In late pregnancy, alveolar elements proliferate in number and begin to produce milk. It is interesting that only a minority of pregnant women have actual expressible milk production during pregnancy. This phenomenon is most likely owing to an inhibitory effect of estradiol on prolactin-induced milk production *(9)*.

After parturition, milk production becomes more pronounced under the influence of suckling. In this setting, circulating levels of estrogen and progesterone are low but prolactin is high. Suckling produces an increase in secretion of prolactin *(10)*, which presumably maintains milk production by a complicated molecular biological process *(11,12)*. Oxytocin affects myoepithelia elements that cause milk ejection and also has other important effects on lactation. As nursing continues, prolactin concentrations fall, but milk production is still active. It is interesting to speculate that increased sensitivity of the mammary gland to prolactin as prolactin levels progressively fall might permit active milk production to continue.

New alveolar structures arise from terminal end buds or similar structures. It is possible that this increase in alveolar number occurs under the influence of GH and estrogen. GH most likely affects the mammary gland after puberty through the actions of IGF-1. Several groups of investigators have observed that transgenic mice overexpressing IGF-1 have hyperplastic glands during lactation. These glands also fail to involute adequately, a phenomenon that is presumed to be the result of inhibition of apoptosis, a known function of IGF-1 *(13,14)*.

GYNECOMASTIA

Gynecomastia is abnormal breast development in men. Testosterone ordinarily prevents mammary development in the male fetus *(15)*, but the male mammary gland contains glandular rests, which under certain hormonal stimuli are capable of developing into palpable subareolar masses or gynecomastia. In fact, for experimentation, male hypophysectomized animals can be employed interchangeably with female animals because their mammary glands respond to hormonal stimulation in an almost identical manner *(3,7,16,17)*.

In many instances, development of gynecomastia reflects an underlying pathological condition (sometimes serious) that should be diagnosed and appropriately treated. For that reason, every man who develops gynecomastia should have a detailed physical examination and perhaps a workup to determine if the condition is caused by one of the underlying disorders known to cause gynecomastia. Another reason for evaluating gynecomastia is to make certain that the patient does not have breast cancer, which can present as gynecomastia. To differentiate between gynecomastia and breast cancer, the combination of physical examination, mammography *(18,19)*, and fine-needle aspiration *(20)* is usually sufficient. In contrast, gynecomastia may not reflect an underlying pathological event, but rather an exaggeration of normal physiology, such as puberty. In that case, gynecomastia is usually a transient event; it disappears as fast as it develops in the majority of boys. The remainder of this section will focus on features of gynecomastia, including a differential diagnosis.

Pathology

The histological features of gynecomastia typically change with time. During the initial stages of gynecomastia, there are many more glandular structures present in the mammary gland compared to later phases of development. Eventually, the gland becomes more fibrous with fewer glandular elements, even though the hormonal abnormalities may still be present. Gynecomastia has been divided into three types by Bannayan and Hajdu *(21)*: florid, fibrous, and intermediate. Florid refers to the active developmental phase, in which multiple budding ducts, marked proliferation of ductal epithelium, periductal edema, and a highly cellular fibroblastic stroma with adipose tissue are present. The fibrous type is characterized by dilated ducts, slight to moderate epithelial proliferation, absence of periductal edema, absence of adipose tissue, and an almost acellular fibrous stroma. The third type is called intermediate with overlapping patterns of the florid and fibrous types. It remains unclear at this time whether all quiescent gynecomastia has at some point in time gone through a florid stage.

Prevalence

Gynecomastia is very common. However, clinically important gynecomastia is not as common as reported in surveys of asymptomatic men. Several investigators, including Nuttall *(22,23)* and Carlson *(24)*, have found that over 30% of military reservists and veterans had gynecomastia, despite normal body weight. These investigators defined gynecomastia as a discrete button of firm subareolar tissue measuring at least 2 cm. At the time of discovery, these patients were mostly asymptomatic.

Signs and Symptoms

Men who are developing gynecomastia typically experience breast tenderness. They often describe a sensitivity to objects they are carrying in their breast pockets or to the shirt material itself. On physical examination, there is a disc of tissue of varying size under the areola that is relatively firm and often quite tender. The nipple may or may not be prominent. Estrogen darkens the areolae, and thus, some patients with gynecomastia notice a change in areolar pigmentation. In contrast to breast cancer, gynecomastia is usually subareolar and not eccentric. There may or may not be significant amounts of fat or connective tissue, making the gland more prominent. The clinician must differentiate between gynecomastia, male breast cancer, or flabby tissue without obvious gynecomastia. Other tumors, such as primary non-Hodgkin's lymphoma, can also present as gynecomastia *(25)*.

Gynecomastia is usually the result of an absolute or relative increase in circulating estrogen levels *(26)*. Therefore, other signs or symptoms of estrogen excess may be present. A large increase in estrogen typically results in a reduction in testosterone secretion (a consequence of inhibition of luteinizing hormone [LH] secretion by estrogen), and patients may therefore experience impotence and loss of libido. In such cases, there may be other signs of feminization, including loss of secondary sex characteristics and testicular atrophy.

Since gynecomastia may be caused by numerous diseases, conditions, or clinical situations (Table 1), one can expect historical facts, or signs and symptoms to be consistent with those of the etiological events. Thus, the best way for a clinician to assess gynecomastia as a presenting symptom or sign is to consider potential etiologies of gynecomastia and proceed accordingly.

Causes of Gynecomastia

Because almost all known forms of gynecomastia can be accounted for by either an actual or relative increase in estrogen (*see* possible exceptions below in the GH and Prolactin section), Frantz and Wilson have classified gynecomastia according to abnormalities in estrogen metabolism *(27)*. They divided the causes into deficiency of testosterone formation or action and increased estrogen production. In normal men, all estrone and most of the estradiol (E_2) are produced as a result of extraglandular conversion from androstenedione and testosterone to estrone and estradiol, respectively. However, the testis produces significant amounts of E_2 in response to human chorionic gonadotropin (hCG) *(28)*. Although estradiol production from the testes is of minor significance in most men, increased E_2 from the testes may account for gynecomastia in patients with elevated LH, such as Klinefelter's syndrome *(29)* or testicular feminization *(30)*. With this in mind, Wilson considers the three principal causes for gynecomastia resulting from actual or relative increased estrogen production to be:

1. Increases in testicular estrogen.
2. Increased substrate for extraglandular aromatase.
3. Increase in extraglandular aromatase.

Physiological Gynecomastia

Neonatal Gynecomastia

Swelling of the breast of the newborn male is likely the result of maternal or placental estrogens. Although not fully established, secretion from the breast of the newborn, which is known as "witch's milk," is likely owing to lactogenic hormones (prolactin, GH variant, GH, or placental lactogen), also of maternal or placental origin. Gynecomastia in the newborn generally disappears shortly after birth.

Table 1

Causes of Cynecomastia

Physiological
Neonatal
Pubertal
Aging
Testicular abnormalities
Testicular feminization
Reifenstein's syndrome
Klinefelter's syndrome
Hermaphroditism
Anorchia
Hemochromatosis
Leprosy
Mumps
Systemic diseases
Thyrotoxicosis
Hepatic failure
Renal failure
Testicular tumors
Adrenal tumors
Congenital adrenal hyperplasia
Nontesticular tumors
Choriocarcinoma
Pineal tumors
Lung cancer
Hepatoblastoma
Breast cancer
Bladder cancer
Stomach cancer
Kidney cancer
Islet-cell tumors
Melanoma
Medications
Trauma
GH
Prolactin

PUBERTAL GYNECOMASTIA

Gynecomastia is very common in adolescent boys. It has been estimated to occur in up to 39–70% of boys *(27)*. Although the exact cause of pubertal gynecomastia is unknown, boys with gynecomastia have been reported to have transient elevations of serum E_2 *(31–33)*, and plasma ratios of testosterone to E_2 tend to be low.

This form of gynecomastia is usually transient. However, it is more severe and long-lasting in a minority of boys. When breast enlargement is severe, it is called pubertal macromastia. Despite detailed investigation of hormonal parameters and ER binding in skin *(34)*, a specific cause for these more serious cases of gynecomastia has yet to be determined. In a single case of severe gynecomastia in an 8-yr-old, very high conversion of androstenedione to estrone was observed *(35)*. Several families have been described in which male members developed significant gynecomastia owing to increased aromatase activity. This in turn results in increased conversion of androstenedione to estrone. In one of the probands, there was increased conversion to estradiol-17β *(36,37)*.

Gynecomastia of Aging

A large number of elderly men have gynecomastia. This could be due to a reduction in testosterone, or to alteration in the testosterone-to-estrogen ratio *(38)*. Onset of gynecomastia in the elderly patient may herald a potentially serious underlying disorder, particularly because of the increased risk of cancer with age. Elderly patients also take many medications and are more likely to develop gynecomastia as a side effect of drug therapy.

Testicular Abnormalities

Patients with testicular abnormalities develop gynecomastia because of the complete absence of or inadequate secretion of testosterone. *In utero*, testosterone is necessary for development of external genitalia, and this sex steroid partially prevents the mammary gland development. In the complete absence of testosterone action, such as in the testicular resistance syndrome called testicular feminization, these patients are phenotypically female and develop breasts at puberty.

Syndromes with testicular abnormalities causing gynecomastia are relatively infrequent compared to the overall prevalence of gynecomastia, but nevertheless should be considered as part of a differential diagnosis. Testicular abnormalities include Klinefelter's syndrome *(29,39)*, testicular feminization, an incomplete form of testicular feminization called Reifenstein's syndrome *(40)*, hermaphroditism *(41)*, and congenital anorchia. Primary testicular failure of any etiology, including leprosy *(42)*, hemochromatosis, and mumps, may cause gynecomastia. Patients with seminepherous tubule failure may also develop gynecomastia. In each of these disorders, gynecomastia is thought to occur because of absolute or relative increases in estrogen owing to high LH. Interestingly, testoterone production has been found to persist in the spermatic vein of patients with bilateral anorchia *(43)*.

Hyperthyroidism

Approximately one-third of male patients with hyperthyroidism have clinically apparent gynecomastia, which recedes once the thyrotoxicosis is treated. Up to 80% of patients with thyrotoxicosis have been noted to have histological evidence of gynecomastia. The etiology of gynecomastia in men with hyperthyroidism is believed to involve an increase in serum E_2. The increased estrogen production is thought to result from elevated rates of peripheral conversion of androgens to estrogens *(27,44,45,47)*. Additionally, testosterone is effectively lower and estrogen higher in hyperthyroidism due to increased production of sex steroid binding globulin. Estrogen is bound less avidly to this protein than is testosterone, which leads to this relative increase in the estrogen-to-testosterone ratio.

Hepatic Failure

Patients with hepatic failure, often from cirrhosis, develop gynecomastia with regularity. Cavanaugh et al. found gynecomastia in 44% of cirrhotics *(47)*. The etiology of gynecomastia in cirrhosis is elevated levels of estrogen thought to be due to increased peripheral conversion of testosterone to E_2 *(48–50)*. These patients have other signs of estrogen increase, including spider nevi and areolar pigmentation. Patients with liver disease also have gonadal insufficiency.

Renal Failure

Nagel and colleagues found that gynecomastia occurred in 11 of 19 patients undergoing hemodialysis *(51)*. Although the etiology of gynecomastia in renal failure or renal failure in patients undergoing dialysis is uncertain, it is likely a multifactorial process involving several endocrine abnormalities. Renal failure patients have primary testicular failure *(52),* low serum testosterone, and high prolactin levels *(53)*. The possibility that the hyperprolactinemia of renal insufficiency is a cause of gynecomastia is discussed below.

Testicular Tumors

Gynecomastia may be the only clinical indication of a testesticular tumor. Therefore, careful examination of the testicles is of utmost importance in patients with gynecomastia. Testicular tumors are much more prevalent in relatively young men, the peak incidence of seminomas occurring between the ages of 35 and 40 yr old *(54)*. In fact, testicular tumors are the most common malignancies in men between the ages of 15 and 34 yr old *(27)*. A distinct mass is usually palpable in testicular tumor patients, but tumors may occasionally be too small to palpate and require high-resolution ultrasonography for detection *(55,56)*. Gynecomastia in patients with testicular tumors results from a net increase in estrogen levels. Increased estrogen levels may be due to direct production of estradiol or testosterone, which subsequently is converted to estradiol. Estradiol may arise from tumors, such as Leydig cell *(57–59)*, Sertoli cell *(60)*, or more usually germ-cell tumors, including seminomas. Germinomas often produce hCG. The hCG directly stimulates testicular production of testosterone and sometimes estradiol. Conversion of testosterone to estradiol by tumor aromatase activity is also a prominent cause of estradiol elevation *(61,62)*. This conversion may occur in the interstitial tissue of the testis *(63)*.

Scully has classified testicular tumors that cause gynecomastia as listed in Table 2 . The reader is referred to the textbook chapter by Scully for further description *(54)*. Most common among these are seminomas and other germ-cell neoplasms.

The treatment of gynecomastia caused by testicular tumors is treatment of the tumor itself.

Adrenal Tumors

Adrenal tissue, like testicular tissue, is capable of producing estrogens. Very occasionally, an adrenal cortical carcinoma will present with feminizing features *(64,65)*. In such patients the tumors usually coproduce high concentrations of other steroids. Thus, measurement of 17-ketosteroids, in addition to serum or urine estrogens and radiologic procedures, might be diagnostically useful if such a tumor is suspected. Pure estrogen-secreting adrenal cancers have been reported as have feminizing adrenal adenomas *(66)*.

Nontesticular Tumors

A variety of nonadrenal and nontesticular tumors cause gynecomastia because of production of hCG rather than direct production of steroid hormones *(67–69)*. These tumors can be either nontrophoblastic or trophoblastic. The mechanism of the gynecomastia, increased estrogen production, is the same as with other hCG-related gynecomastias *(70)*. The tumors include lung cancers *(67,71,72)*, hepatoblastomas *(73)*, pineal gland

Table 2

Classification of Testicular Tumors (1585)

Germ-cell tumors
Seminomas
Teratomas
Embryonal cell carcinoma
Choriocarcinoma
Yolk sac tumor
Gonadoblastomas
Leydig cell tumors
Tumors of adrenocortical type
Sex-cord stromal tumors

tumors, tumors of the mediastinum, breast, bladder, stomach, and kidney, islet cell tumors, and melanomas *(74)*.

Choriocarcinomas and germ-cell tumors can occur in the lung *(75)*, brain, and elsewhere in the absence of a testicular tumor. Pineal germinomas may or may not produce hCG *(76)*. In addition, some of these pineal germ-cell tumors produce carcinoembryonic antigen and α-fetoprotein *(77)*. Measurement of these markers may be useful not only to help in the diagnosis of these tumors, but also to follow the clinical responses to treatment *(68,69)*.

β-hCG (specific tumor marker assay) should be measured in patients with gynecomastia if the etiology is unclear. This may help in the discovery of an otherwise undiagnosed tumor. In addition to high levels of β-hCG, these patients may have unexpectedly high serum testosterone values as well as high serum estrogen *(78)*. Normal individuals may also produce very small amounts of hCG from various tissue sources not related to cancer. However, serum concentrations in normals are not highly elevated and usually below 5 mIU/mL.

Another product of trophoblasts, human chorionic sommatomammotropin or human placental lactogen, has been found to be ectopically produced by many trophoblastic and nontrophoblastic cancers *(79)*. Weintraub and Rosen detected this substance in 11 of 128 patients with malignancies. The role of this hormone in gynecomastia is not clear, however.

Medications

Perhaps the most common cause of nonphysiological gynecomastia is related to drug therapy. The mechanisms by which medications give rise to gynecomastia is varied. Categories of drugs capable of inducing gynecomastia include estrogens and estrogen mimetics, which bind to the ER because of structural similarities (e.g., digitalis) *(80,81)*, antagonists of androgen receptors (e.g., spironolactone) *(82–84)*, and inhibitors of steroidogenesis (e.g., ketoconazole) *(85)*. As with other causes of gynecomastia, medications that cause gynecomastia usually do so by changing the effective activity of steroids, thereby favoring estrogenic over androgenic activity. A partial list of medications and other drugs that cause gynecomastia is presented in Table 3. Gynecomastia is listed as a side effect of hundreds of drugs. Only prominent ones are listed in this table. As part of a workup for gynecomastia, all drugs and exogenous substances to which the patient is exposed should be considered potential candidates for causing the gynecomastia, whether listed in the table or not. There have been a number of epidemics of gynecomastia in men unknowingly taking products contaminated with estrogen. These include exposure to

Table 3

Medications That Cause Gynecomastia

Steroids
Estrogen
Testosterone
Anaboloic steroids
Protein hormones
hCG
GH
? Prolactin
? Placental lactogen
Imidazole derivatives
Ketoconozole
Cimetidine
Thiobendazole
Metronidazole
Etomidate
Drugs that bind to steroid receptors
Digitalis
Spironolactone
Cimetidine
Flutamide
Cyproterone acetate
Chemotherapeutic agents
cis-Platin-containing combinations
Vinblastine
Procarbazine
Prednisone
Chlorambucil
Doxorubicin
Bleomycin
Calcium channel blockers
Neuroleptics
Antiihypertensives
Other drugs
D-Penicillamine
Marijuana
Methadone
Clomiphene citrate withdrawal
Heroin
Phenytoin
Minocycline

estrogen-containing vaginal cream *(86)*, dermal ointment *(87,88)*, and hair cream *(89)*. There have been outbreaks of gynecomastia in employees of a pharmaceutical company that formulated oral contraceptives *(90)* and in schools *(91)*. The possibility of environmental estrogens should always be taken into consideration when working up a patient with gynecomastia.

Treatment with testosterone commonly causes gynecomastia because of aromatization of testosterone to estradiol. Onset of symptoms and signs of gynecomastia are dose-dependent, and can usually be reversed by lowering the dose and/or altering the dose frequency. Similarly, treatment of testosterone deficiency with hCG can cause gynecomastia and elevated levels of serum estradiol. These should be measured routinely in patients receiving this drug to avoid untoward effects.

Administration of GH can also cause gynecomastia in humans *(92)* and in subhuman primates *(93)*. This is not surprising in view of the importance of GH and IGF-1 in mammary development. Medications that raise endogenous prolactin, such as neuroleptics, are also included on the list of drugs that cause gynecomastia. A discussion of GH and PRL in gynecomastia is found below.

Men who use marijuana are at risk for developing gynecomastia *(94)*. In addition, heroin and methodone users have abnornal testicular function, which may, in turn, lead to gynecomastia.

Weight lifters who take anabolic steroids develop gynecomastia with some frequency, in addition to acne and striae *(95)*. Whether the latter is owing to alteration in body composition and distribution or to anabolic steroids is unclear. Some weight lifters also take GH, which can cause gynecomastia. Some also medicate themselves with tamoxifen if the gynecomastia is painful.

Adrenal Hyperplasia

Gynecomastia has been reported in patients with 11-β-hydroxylase deficiency *(96)*, 21-hydroxylase deficiency *(97)*, 17-ketosteroid reductase deficiency, and benign nodular adrenal hyperplasia with hyperprolactinemia *(98)*.

Trauma

Trauma to the chest has long been known to cause gynecomastia. It has been known to occur following thoracotomy *(99)* and after herpes zoster of the chest wall *(100)*.

GH and Prolactin

Although no detailed analysis of the prevalence of gynecomastia in patients with hyperprolactinemia has been carried out, gynecomastia is thought not to be a feature of hyperprolactinemia. Nevertheless, men with hyperprolactinemia frequently have galactorrhea *(101)*. It is possible, therefore, that a prospective study employing careful radiological analysis of the chest would uncover evidence of glandular tissue in the mammary glands of these patients. Despite present dogma, the author occasionally encounters men with gynecomastia who have elevated prolactin, and in whom prolactin inhibition with dopamine agonists improves their condition.

As noted above, GH administration may induce gynecomastia. This is not surprising in light of the role of GH in normal mammary gland development. Gynecomastia is not a very common feature of acromegaly, although it has been reported to occur. Galactorrhea is a common feature in these patients *(101)*.

Treatment of Gynecomastia

It is important to determine the underlying cause of gynecomastia whenever possible. Treating the underlying disorder, if known, may lead to almost complete resolution of the gynecomastia. For example, treatment of thyrotoxicosis will usually reverse the gynecomastia associated with this disease. However, once gynecomastia reaches a certain mass, only surgical extirpation will reduce excessive mammary tissue. Surgery has been considered the only definitive treatment for gynecomastia, particularly when it becomes a cosmetic problem for the patient.

Both clomiphene citrate *(102,103)* and tamoxifen *(104–106)* have been used to treat gynecomastia with generally positive results. However, size reduction is difficult to assess without an objective means of analysis, such as ultrasonography. None of the studies carried out to date have employed such methodology. Clomiphene citrate and tamoxifen do, however, reduce symptoms. If these drugs are employed, they should not take the place of determining the underlying cause of the gynecomastia and initiating appropriate treatment.

Painful gynecomastia is a frequent complication of estrogen treatment for carcinoma of the prostate. Breast irradiation has been employed in some centers to avoid this side effect *(107)*.

GALACTORRHEA

Physicians were aware of the clinical condition of galactorrhea as far back as biblical times, but it was Chiari who first focused our attention on this condition a little over a century ago *(18)*. Prior to 1970, galactorrhea was thought to be an uncommon condition. The true prevalence of galactorrhea did not become apparent until 1970 when investigators finally recognized that prolactin in man was a distinct hormone from GH and were able to develop a sensitive assay that could readily measure prolactin in serum *(109–111)*. We studied 235 patients with galactorrhea in the early 1970s and published our results in 1977 *(101)*. Much of the remainder of this discussion of galactorrhea is based on that experience.

Galactorrhea can be defined as a milky substance that is expressed either bilaterally or unilaterally from the nipple in nonnursing women or in men. The fluid contains milk proteins, such as casein and α-lactalbumin *(113,114)*, and fat. Although usually white, the discharge may be yellowish, cream-colored, or greenish. A black, brown, or reddish discoloration suggests the presence of blood, which may herald the presence of an underlying neoplasm.

Galactorrhea is frequently an indication of an underlying pathological condition. When it occurs together with amenorrhea, the presence of a pituitary tumor is likely. Our study on galactorrhea was carried out before development of magnetic resonance imaging (MRI) and during the early days of computerized tomography. Therefore, our figure indicating that only 32% of women with concomitant galactorrhea and amenorrhea had a pituitary tumor was a gross underestimate, because microprolactinomas were not included.

The majority of patients with pathological forms of galactorrhea have high serum prolactin levels. Therefore, a differential diagnosis of conditions that cause elevated prolactin should be considered in each patient presenting with galactorrhea. A list of conditions that can produce galactorrhea is presented in Table 4 and in Fig. 1.

Pituitary Tumors

With the advent of MRI, the prevalence of pituitary tumors in patients with galactorrhea owing to hyperprolactinemia has risen considerably. The actual percentage of patients with galactorrhea caused by prolactinomas has not been ascertained. However,

Table 4
Underlying Causes of Galactorrhea

Pituitary tumors
Microprolactinomas
Macroprolactinomas
GH-secreting tumors
Other pituitary macroadenomas with elevated prolactin
Nonpituitary tumors
Craniopharyngiomas
Meningiomas
Gliomas
Metastatic tumors
Granulomas
Sarcoid
Eosinophilic granuloma
Idiopathic galactorhea with regular menses
Idiopathic galactorrhea with amenorrhea
Polycystic ovarian disease
Chiari-Frommel syndrome
Medications
Neuroleptics
Benzodiazepines
Oral contraceptives
Isoniazid
Reserpine
Estrogen
Androgen
Cimetidine
Hypothyroidism
Hyperthyroidism
Cushing's disease
Empty sella syndrome

it is higher than our 1977 estimate showing that 20% of all patients with galactorrhea and 34% of patients with galactorrhea and amenorrhea had pituitary tumors. Any patient presenting with galactorrhea should thus be carefully worked up to exclude the presence of a pituitary tumor.

The majority of prolactinomas are small tumors of <1 cm diameter (microadenoma). These tumors usually do not cause space-occupying problems, such as visual field disturbances, although they frequently cause headache. The etiology of prolactinomas is unclear, but most tumors tend to be monoclonal in nature *(115)*. Prolactin concentrations generally correlate with the size of the tumor—lower serum prolactin concentrations generally occur in patients with microprolactinomas than in patients with macroprolactinomas. A serum prolactin concentration of <200 ng/mL is commonplace in patients with small tumors, with many having prolactin concentrations <100 ng/mL. Sexual dysfunction, due mainly to short feedback inhibition of gonadotropin pulsatility, is a common prolactin-associated problem *(116,117)*. Sexual dysfunction may involve amenorrhea, oligomenorrhea, a shortened luteal phase, and hypoestrogenemia in women,

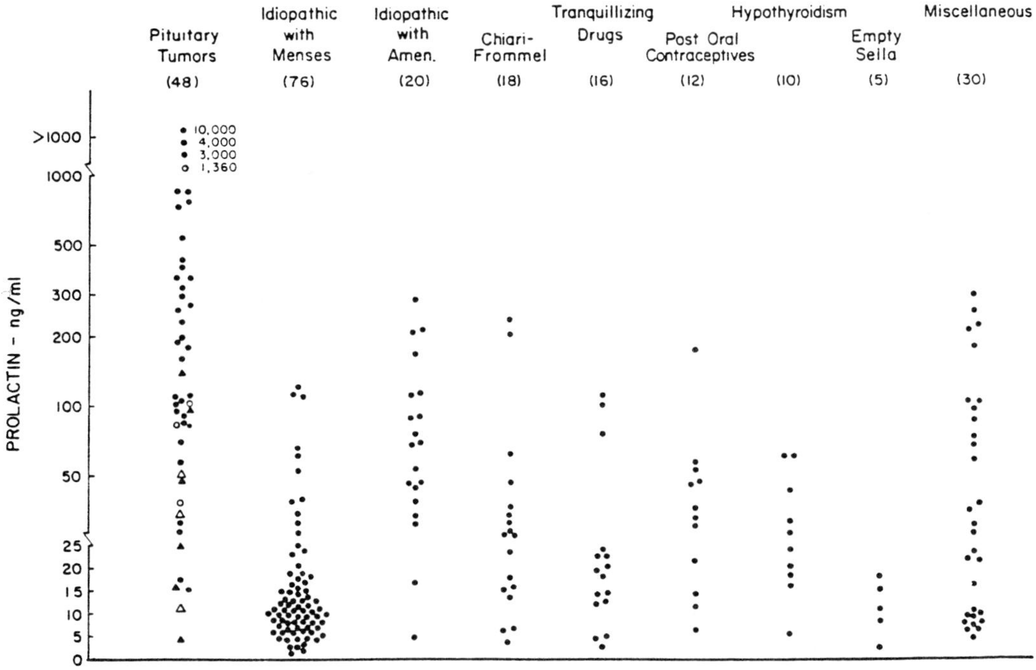

Fig. 1. Plasma prolactin in 235 patients with galactorrhea of various causes. Among the patients with tumors, triangles denote patients with acromegaly. Open circles or triangles denote patients studied only after radiotherapy or operation. (Reprinted from Kleinberg et al., N Engl J Med, 1977;296:589–600.)

and impotence, erectile dysfunction, premature ejaculation, low testosterone, and rarely infertility in men. Osteoporosis is a common feature in patients with hyperprolactinemia and appears to be the result of reduced sex steroid production rather than a direct inhibitory effect of prolactin on bone turnover *(118–120)*. The third part of the triad of clinical sequelae of hyperprolactinemia is galactorrhea.

Tumors larger than 1 cm in size that also produce prolactin are called macroprolactinomas. They typically produce enough prolactin to raise the concentration in serum to above 200 ng/mL—often much higher serum prolactin concentrations (many thousands of ng/mL) are encountered. When levels reach these high concentrations, the likelihood of there being a large tumor is strikingly high. Patients with large tumors sometimes have deficiencies in other pituitary hormones such as GH, TSH, and ACTH, in addition to gonadotropins. In addition to the clinical effects of elevated serum prolactin levels, these patients may have visual field problems and other space-related problems owing to tumor extension or invasion.

GH possesses intrinsic lactogenicity equaling that of prolactin *(121)*. Therefore, it is not surprising that patients with acromegaly develop galactorrhea with a relatively high frequency. However, acromegalics often have less sexual dysfunction than do patients with prolactinomas. This finding is not surprising, since serum GH in patients with acromegaly is not usually >100 ng/mL. Of course, acromegalics have striking clinical features, which should be ascertained during a workup for galactorrhea. Interestingly, approx 50% of patients with acromegaly have elevated prolactin in addition to elevated GH *(101)*. Both men and women develop galactorrhea due to GH-producing and prolactin-producing pituitary tumors. However, galactorrhea is more common in women than in men. A workup for acromegaly should include measurement of IGF-1, which is almost always elevated in these patients. If IGF-1 levels are suspicious, a glucose tolerance test during which GH and glucose are measured should be carried out. Measurement of a single or random GH level is usually of limited clinical diagnostic value unless it is drawn in relation to glucose intake.

Serum prolactin is frequently elevated in patients with pituitary tumors because of interruption of the connections between the hypothalamus and the pituitary, rather than the tumor itself secreting prolactin. Normally, prolactin production from the pituitary is under tonic inhibitory control by dopamine from the hypothalamus. Thus, moderate elevations of prolactin can be encountered in patients with large pituitary tumors that themselves do not secrete prolactin. In this situation, prolactin is usually < 100 ng/mL, but may be as high as 150–200 ng/mL. Therefore, it should not be assumed that a large pituitary tumor is prolactin-secreting in nature unless the serum prolactin concentration is over 200 ng/mL. It is important to distinguish these conditions to ensure that the appropriate treatment is initiated. The appropriate treatment for a prolactinoma is a dopamine agonist drug, whereas the appropriate treatment for a large pituitary tumor that does not secrete prolactin is surgery, radiotherapy, or a combination.

Nonpituitary Tumors

Any tumor in the area of the pituitary that disturbs the connections between the pituitary and hypothalamus can cause an elevated prolactin and, therefore, galactorrhea. In this situation, galactorrhea may be the harbinger of an underlying tumor, such as a craniopharyngioma, glioma, meningioma, or metastatic tumor either from breast cancer or lung cancer. However, these are rare occurrences, and clinical signs other than galactorrhea would be more usual.

Granulomas

Sarcoidosis rarely presents as a pituitary tumor. More frequently, sarcoid is present in the hypothalamus to produce sexual dysfunction or diabetes insipidus. Nevertheless, sarcoidosis as well as Schuller-Christian disease may be associated with galactorrhea due to elevated prolactin. Patients with sarcoidosis of the hypothalamus and pituitary may have extensive disease elsewhere, but occassionaly it is limited to the pituitary area.

Idiopathic Galactorrhea with Regular Menses

Idiopathic galactorrhea with regular menses is perhaps the most common form of galactorrhea. Currently, however, uncertainty exists concerning whether idiopathic galactorrhea represents a benign disease or an appropriate physiological event. Although an elevation of prolactin levels in all patients with galactorrhea might be expected, our early studies using a bioassay for prolactin showed a subset of patients who did not have elevated prolactin. Further investigation of these patients revealed that the majority of these patients had been pregnant at least once and continued to have regular menses.

To determine whether an underlying problem existed in these patients, we subsequently tested their prolactin response to various secretagogues, including chlorpromazine, TRH, and L-DOPA, As a control, similar studies were performed on patients with other forms of galactorrhea. We found that patients with idiopathic galactorrhea with regular menses had responses to secretagogues that were similar to those seen in normal women—the only exception was that 57% of these patients had inadequate responses to chlorpromazine. This abnormality suggests that these patients indeed have an underlying physiological abnormality. The results of these tests are presented in Table 5 and Fig. 2 as reprinted from our original article.

Idiopathic Galactorrhea with Amenorrhea

Despite sensitive tools to detect pituitary tumors, there remain rare patients with high prolactin, no evidence of a pituitary tumor, and no evidence of other known causes of galactorrhea. These patients are considered to fall under this rubric of idiopathic.

Polycystic Ovarian (PCO) Disease

Hyperprolactinemia is a relatively common finding in patients with PCO syndrome. Its cause is unknown. When present, the prolactin is only moderately elevated. Nevertheless, it is necessary to differentiate between PCO and a microadenoma as the cause of the hyperprolactinemia.

Chiari-Frommel Syndrome

In the mid-1800s, Chiari and in 1882 Frommel described the syndrome of postpartum galactorrhea, amenorrhea, and utero-ovarian atrophy *(108)*. In our series performed in 1977, 18 patients had were diagnosed with this disorder. These patients had experienced galactorrhea and amenorrhea for periods ranging from 6 mo to 11 yr (mean 3.5 yr). Levels of serum prolactin ranged from 4.6 to 285 ng/mL, the mean for the entire group being 45.5 ng/mL. Seven of the patients had prolactin concentrations of <25 ng/mL. Gonadotropins were in the normal range, but considered abnormal because the patients were amenorrheic. With improved radiological techniques, at least some of this group would likely have had microadenomas that were not detected by conventional radiological techniques of the time. That some of these patients had pituitary tumors is supported by the fact that Chiari-Frommel syndrome is infrequently diagnosed now that MRI is so readily available. However, the fact that postpartum galactorrhea and amenorrhea are reversible and self-limited lends support to the existence of this disorder.

Surgery and Trauma

Stress temporarily elevates serum prolactin levels to values similar to those seen during major surgical procedures. Rarely, galactorrhea occurs several days to weeks after surgery and may last for periods of weeks to years. Menses are typically not affected. Inappropriate lactation has been reported after thoracoplasty *(101)*, hysterectomy and oophorectomy *(101)*, and cholecystectomy. During surgery prolactin rises to between 100 and 200 ng/mL *(122)*.

Prolactin elevations are somewhat common in patients who have sustained serious head trauma. One of our patients had a prolactin level of 67 ng/mL after an airplane accident. Other endocrine abnormalities, including diabetes insipidus, SIADH, and amenorrhea, have also been noted after head trauma.

Medications

Various medications can produce galactorrhea. The most common of those are dopamine antagonists, which raise prolactin levels by a direct action on lactotropes. In our series, prolactin concentrations in patients who experienced galactorrhea during treatment with

Table 5

Prolactin Function Tests in Patients with Galactorrhea of Various Etiologies

Diagnosis	*No. of patients*[a]	*Chlorpromazine*[c]	*Thyrotropin-releasing hormone*[c]	*L-DOPA*[b]	*Water load*[b]	*Breast stimulation*[c]
Pituitary tumor	19	0/9(0)[d]	1/16 (6)	14/9 (44)	0/3	0/2
Idiopathic with amenorrhea	6	1/5 (20)	2/6 (33)	2/3	0/1	—
Idiopathic with menses	25	8/14 (57)	10/11 (91)	16/19 (84)	1/7 (14)	0/4
Empty sella syndrome	5	1/4	4/5 (80)	5/5 (100)	0/1	—
Chiari-Frommel syndrome	8	3/5 (60)	1/2	2/3	0/2	0/1
Oral conctraceptive-related	9	3/5 (60)	2/2	8/9 (89)	1/3	—
Hypothyroidism	4	1/2	4/4	2/2	0/3	0/2
Hyperthyroidism	2	1/1	1/1	2/2	—	—
Totals	78	17/45 (38)	25/47 (53)	41/52 (79	2/20 (10)	0/9 (0)
Normal		14/14 (100)	16/16 (100)	33/33 (100)	0/22 (0)	6/18 (33)

[a]Total no of patients studied ≥1 test.
[b]Positive response: fall <1/2 of baseline value.
[c]Positive response: rise to >twice baseline value.
[d]Figures in parenthesis denote %.

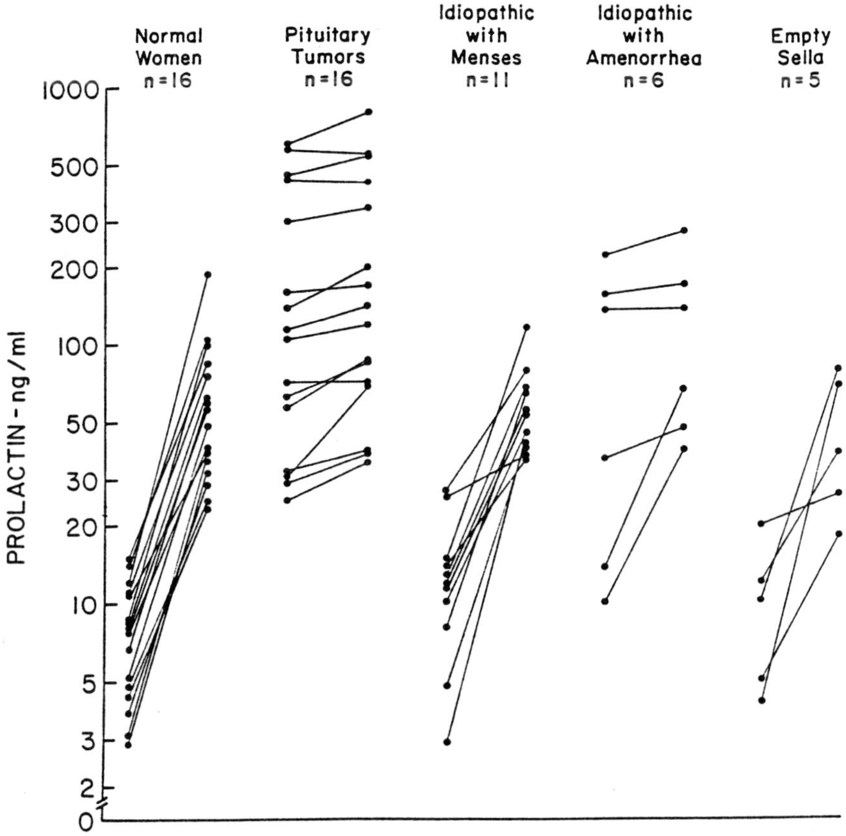

Fig. 2. Serum prolactin concentrations before (left-hand dots) and after (right-hand dots) thyrptrooin-releasing hormone, 500 μg intravenously, in patients with galactorrhea and normal subjects. (Reprinted from Kleinberg et al., N Engl J Med, 1977; 296:589–600.)

neuroleptics ranged from 12.4 to 110 ng/mL (mean 43.6 ng/mL). Only two of nine patients taking phenothiazines had amenorrhea, but menses were irregular in most of the patients. A management dilemma exists in how best to approach the patient on neuroleptics who develops galactorrhea with or without menstrual irregularities. Hyperprolactinemia can obscure the diagnosis of a concomitant pituitary tumor or other disorder. Thus, when prolactin is very high (> 100 ng/mL), an MRI should be performed. In patients with smaller elevations in serum prolactin concentrations, physicians should rely on a pretreatment prolactin level or clinical judgment and proceed accordingly.

A partial list of other drugs that cause galactorrhea can be found in Table 4. They include both administration and withdrawal of oral contraceptives, certain antihypertensives, and isoniazid.

Hypothyroidism

Galactorrhea in hypothyroidism was first described in children with precocious puberty and an enlargement of the sella turcicas *(123)*. Hypothyroidism as a cause of galactorrhea

Table 6

Administration and Duration of Dopaime Agonists

Drug	*Duration of action*	*Dose*	*Frequency of dose*
Bromocriptine	8 h	2.5 mg	BID–TID
Pergolide	>24 h	0.5–2.0 mg	Daily
Cabergoline	7 d	0.25–3.0 mg	Once or twice weekly

is frequently seen in women postpartum, and the disorder has been confused with the Chiari-Frommel syndrome *(124–126)*. In our series, 10 patients with primary hypothyroidism also had galactorrhea. Only three patients had amenorrhea in addition to galactorrhea. All of the 10 patients were women and had previous pregnancies, suggesting that their mammary glands were previously primed to produce milk. The onset of galactorrhea occurred postpartum in four patients and persisted until a diagnosis of hypothyroidism was made. Prolactin was elevated in 50% of the patients with a mean value of 29.3 ng/mL (range 12.1–55 ng/mL). Five patients who were treated with thyroid medication experienced a decrease in the mean prolactin level from 31.1 to 10 ng/mL.

The reason that prolactin may be moderately elevated in patients with hypothyroidism is unclear. However, it should be pointed out that prolactin concentrations >75 ng/mL are unusual if hypothyroidism is the only cause. In my view, patients with elevated prolactin and primary hypothyroidism should have pituitary MRIs performed, because the presentation may mask a pituitary tumor; prolonged primary hypothyroidism may also cause pituitary hyperplasia severe enough to cause visual field deficits *(101)*. Not all endocrinologists agree with this approach, some preferring to determine if treatment with thyroid hormone will normalize prolactin before doing an MRI.

The treatment for galactorrhea caused by hypothyroidism is thyroid hormone.

Empty Sella Syndrome

In our series, we found five patients who had galactorrhea, normal serum prolactin concentrations, and enlarged and empty sella turcicae as determined by pneumoencephalography. Two patients had amenorrhea, and two patients responded inadequately to chlorpromazine stimulation. Thus, it is unclear whether the presence of an empty sella tucicae was associated with their galactorrhea.

Treatment of Galactorrhea

The treatment of galactorrhea should be aimed at treating the underlying disorder. Thus, if hypothyroidism is causing galactorrhea, this disease should be managed with thyroid hormone administration. Since most patients with galactorrhea also have hyperprolactinemia, dopamine agonist therapy is the most common form of therapy. There are three dopamine agonists that are generally available and are presently employed to either lower prolactin or simultaneously lower prolactin and shrink the prolactinoma. Bromocriptine has been available since the early 1970s; pergolide was developed in the early 1980s *(127)*. In the last several years, cabergoline has also come into general use *(128)*. All the dopamine agonists bind more avidly to dopamine type 2 receptors than dopamine itself. A number of similarities exist among these agents, including the ability to lower prolactin production by normal or tumor lactotropes and the propensity to shrink prolactinomas. However, differences among the agents are also apparent particularly with respect to duration of action and side effects. A summary of the durations of action and appropriate doses of these agents are listed in Table 6.

Cabergoline appears to be generally better tolerated than bromocriptine but some patients may sometimes tolerate bromocriptine better than cabergoline. Pergolide is used infrequently because of the lack of studies demonstrating its effectiveness in hyperprolactinemia *(127,129)*. Intolerance of one drug does not necessarily mean intolerance to the others. This author recommends always starting patients off at the lowest possible effective dose and titrating upward as necessary to reduce the occurrence of side effects.

Galactorrhea in the absence of hyperprolactinemia or similar treatable disorder does not require treatment, unless the galactorrhea makes the patient uncomfortable or the benefits of treatment outweigh the risks. If desired, dopamine agonists may be effective in reducing milk production, but do not necessarily stop it.

REFERENCES

1. Silberstein G. B., K. Van Horn, G. Shyamala and C. W. Daniel. Essential role of endogenous estrogen in directly stimulating mammary growth demonstrated by implants containing pure antiestrogens. *Endocrinology* 1994;134:84–90.
2. Daniel C. W. and G. B. Silberstein. Postnatal development of the rodent mammary gland. In: Neville M. C. and C. W. Daniel, eds. *The Mammary Gland.* New York, Plenum Press, 1987; pp. 3–36.
3. Kleinberg D. L., W. F. Ruan, V. Catanese, C. B. Newman and M. Feldman. Non-lactogenic effects of growth hormone on growth and insulin-like growth factor-I messenger ribonucleic acid of rat mammary gland. *Endocrinol* 1990;126:3274–3276.
4. Feldman M., W. Ruan, B. C. Cunningham, J. A. Wells and D. L. Kleinberg. Evidence that the growth hormone receptor mediates differentiation and development of the mammary gland. *Endocrinol* 1993;133:1602–1608.
5. Kleinberg D. L., W. Niemann, E. Flamm, P. Cooper, G. Babitsky and Q. Valensi. Primate mammary development: Effects of hypophysectomy, prolactin inhibition and growth hormone administration. *J. Clin. Invest.* 1985;75:1943–1950.
6. Walden P. D., W. F. Ruan, M. Feldman and D. L. Kleinberg. Evidence that the mammary gland fat pad mediates the action of growth hormone in mammary gland development. *Endocrinology* 1998; in press.
7. Ruan W., C. B. Newman and D. L. Kleinberg. Intact and aminoterminally shortened forms of insulin-like growth factor I induce mammary gland differentiation and development. *Proc. Natl. Acad. Sci. USA* 1992;89:10872–10876.
8. Ruan W., V. Catanese, R. Wieczorek, M. Feldman and D. L. Kleinberg. Estradiol enhances the stimulatory effect of insulin-like growth factor-I (IGF-I) on mammary development and growth hormone-induced IGF-I messenger ribonucleic acid. *Endocrinology* 1995;136:1296–1302.
9. Kleinberg D. L., J. Todd and G. Babitsky. Inhibition by estradiol of the lactogenic effect of prolactin in primate mammary tissue: Reversal by antiestrogens (LY 15678 and tamoxifen). *Proc Natl Acad Sci USA* 1983;80:4144–4148.
10. Noel G. L., H. K. Suh and A. G. Frantz. Prolactin release during nursing and breast stimulation in postpartum and nonpostpartum subjects. *J Clin Endocrinol Metab* 1974;38:413–423.
11. Rosen J. M., S. L. C. Woo and J. P. Comstock. Regulation of casein messenger RNA during the development of the rat mammary gland. *Biochem* 1975;14:2895–2903.
12. Lee K. F., S. H. Atiee, S. J. Henning and J. M. Rosen. Relative contribution of promoter and intragenic sequences in the hormonal regulation of rat-casein transgenes. *Mol Endocrinology* 1989;3:447–453.
13. Hadsell D. L., N. M. Greenberg, J. M. Fligger, C. R. Baumrucker and J. M. Rosen. Targeted expression of des(1-3) human insulin-like growth factor I (IGF-I) in transgenic mice influences mammary gland development and IGF-binding protein expression. *Endocrinology* 1996;136:in press.
14. Neuenschwander S., A. Schwartz, T. L. Wood, C. T. J. Roberts, L. Henninghausen and D. LeRoith. Involution of the lactating mammary gland is inhibited by the IGF system in a transgenic mouse model. *J Clin Invest* 1996;97:2225–2232.
15. Sakakura T. The Mammary Gland-Development, Regulation and Function. In: Neville M. C. and C. W. Daniel, eds. *Mammary Embryogenesis.* New York, Plenum Press, 1987; pp. 37–66.

16. Lyons W. R., R. E. johnson, R. D. Cole and C. H. Li. Mammary growth and lactation in male rats. In: Smith R. W., O. H. gaebler and C. N. H. Long, eds. *The Hypophyseal Growth Hormone, Nature and Actions.* New York, McGraw Hill, 1955; pp. 461–472.
17. Lyons W. R. Hormonal synergism in mammary growth. *Proc Royal Soc (London)* 1993;149:303–325.
18. Jackson V. P. and R. L. Gilmor. Male breast carcinoma and gynecomastia: comparison of mammography with sonography. *Radiololgy* 1983;149:533–536.
19. Stewart R. A., D. C. Howlett and F. J. Hearn. Pictorial review: the imaging features of male breast disease. *Clin Radiol* 1997;52:739–744.
20. Das D. K., T. A. Junaid, S. B. Mathews, T. G. Ajrawi, M. S. Ahmed, J. P. Madda and K. Mirza. Fine needle aspiration cytology diagnosis of male breast lesions. A study of 185 cases. *Acta Cytol* 1995;39:870–876.
21. Bannayan G. A. and S. I. Hajdu. Gynecomastia: clinicopathologic study of 351 cases. *Am J Clin Pathol* 1972;57:431–437.
22. Nuttall F. Q. Gynecomastia as a physical finding in normal men. *J Clin Endocrinol* 1979;48:338–340.
23. Niewoehner C. B. and F. Q. Nuttall. Gynecomastia in a hospitalized male population. *Am J Med* 1984;77:633–638.
24. Carlson H. E. Medical intelligence: current concepts- gynecomastia. *N Engl J Med* 1980;303:795–799.
25. Murata T., H. Kuroda, T. Nakahama, H. Goshima, T. Shiraishi and R. Yatani. Primary non-Hodgkin malignant lymphoma of the male breast. *Jpn J Clin Oncol* 1996;26:243–247.
26. Wilson J. D., J. Aiman and P. C. MacDonald. The pathogenesis of gynecomastia. *Advances in Int Med* 1980;25:1–32.
27. Frantz A. G. and J. D. Wilson. Endocrine disorders of the breast. In: Wilson J. D. and D. W. Foster, eds. *Williams Textbook of Endocrinology.* W. B. Saunders, 1992; pp. 953–975.
28. Weinstein R. L., R. P. Kelch, M. R. Jenner, S. L. Kaplan and M. M. Grumbach. Secretion of unconjugated androgens and estrogens by the normal and abnormal human testis before and after human chorionic gonadotropin. *J Clin Invest* 1974;53:1–6.
29. Wang C., H. W. G. Baker, H. G. Burger, D. M. de Kretser and B. Hudson. Hormonal studies in Klinefelter's syndrome. *Clin Endocrinol* 1974;4:399–411.
30. Kelch R. P., M. R. Jenner, R. L. Weinstein, S. L. Kaplan and M. M. Grumbach. Estradiol and testosterone secretion by human, simian, and canine tests, in males with hypoganodism and in male pseudohermaphrodites with the feminizing testes syndrome. *J Clin Invest* 1972;51:824–829.
31. Biro F. M., A. W. Lucky, G. A. Huster and J. A. Morrison. Hormonal studies and physical maturation in adolescent gynecomastia. *J Pediatr* 1990;116:450–455.
32. Lee P. A. The relationship of concentrations of serum hormones to pubertal gynecomastia. *J Pediatr* 1975;86:212–215.
33. Moore D. C., L. V. Schlaepfer, L. Paunier and P. C. Sizonenko. Hormonal changes during puberty: v. transient pubertal gynecomastia: abnormal androgen-estrogen ratios. *J Clin Endocrinol* 1984;58:492–499.
34. Eil C., M. E. Lippman, E. V. De Moss and D. L. Loriaux. Androgen receptor characteristics in skin fibroblasts from men with pubertal macromastia. *Clin Endocrinol* 1983;19:223–230.
35. Hemsell D. L., C. D. Edman, J. F. Marks, P. K. Siiteri and P. C. MacDonald. Massive extraglandular aromatization of plasma androstenedione resulting in feminization of a prepubertal boy. *J Clin Invest* 1977;60:455–464.
36. Berkovitz G. D., A. Guerami, T. R. Brown, P. C. MacDonald and C. J. Migeon. Familial gynecomastia with increased extraglandular aromatization of plasma carbon19-steroids. *J Clin Invest* 1985;75:1763–1769.
37. Slabaugh M. B., M. E. Lieberman, J. J. Rutledge and J. Gorski. growth hormone and prolactin synthesis in normal and homozygous Snell and Ames dwarf mice. *Endocrinol* 1981;109:1040–1046.
38. Aiman J., P. F. Brenner and P. C. MacDonald. Androgen and estrogen production in elderly men with gynecomastia and testicular atrophy after mumps orchitis. *J Clin Endocrinol Metab* 1980;50:380–386.
39. Gabrilove J. L., E. K. Freiberg, J. C. Thornton and G. L. Nicolis. Effect of age on testicular function in patients with Kleinefelter's syndrome. *Clin Endocrinol* 1979;11:343–347.
40. Griffin J. E. and J. D. Wilson. The androgen resistance syndromes: 5a reductase deficiency, testicular feminization, and related disorders. In: Scriver C. R., A. L. Beaudet and W. S. Sly, eds. *Metabolic Basis of Inherited Disease.* New York, McGraw-Hill, 1989; pp. 1919–1944.
41. Aiman J., D. L. Hemsell and P. C. MacDonald. Production and origin of estrogen in two true hermaphrodites. *Am J Obstet Gynecol* 1978;132:401–409.
42. Morley J. E., L. A. Distiller, J. Sagel, S. H. Kok, G. Kay, P. Carr and M. Katz. Hormonal changes associated with testicular atrophy and gynecomastia in patients with leprosy. *Clin Endocrinol* 1977;6:29–03.

43. Kirschner M. A., J. B. Jacobs and E. E. Fraley. Bilateral anorchia with persistent testosterone production. *N Eng J Med* 1970;282:240–244.
44. Southren A. L., J. Olivo, G. G. Gordon, J. Vittek, J. Brener and F. Rafii. The conversion of androgens to estrogens in hyperthyroidism. *J Clin Endocrinol Metab* 1973;38:207–214.
45. Becker K. L., J. L. Winnacker, M. J. Matthews and G. A. Higgins. Gynecomastia and hyperthyroidism; an endocrine and histological investigation. *J Clin Endocrinol* 1968;28:277–285.
47. Chopra I. J. and D. Tulchinsky. Status of estrogen-androgen balance in hyperthyroid men with Grave's disease. *J Clin Endocrinol Metab* 1974;38:269–277.
48. Cavanaugh J., C. B. Niewoehner and F. Q. Nuttall. Gynecomastia and cirrhosis of the liver. *Arch Intern Med* 1990;150:563–565.
49. Baker H. W. G., H. G. Burger, D. M. Kretser, A. Dulmanis, B. Hudson, S. O'Connor, C. A. Paulsen, N. Purcell, G. C. Rennie, C. S. Seah, H. P. Taft and B. S. Wang. A study of the endocrine manifestations of hepatic cirrhosis. *Quart J Med* 1976;177:145–178.
50. Gordon G. G., J. Olivo, F. Rafii and A. L. Southren. Conversions of androgens to estrogens in cirrhosis of the liver. *J Clin Endocrinol Metab* 1975;40:1018–1026.
51. Edman C. D., P. C. MacDonald and B. Combes. extraglandular production of estrogen in subjects with liver disease. *Gastroenterology* 1975;69:819
52. Nagel T. C., N. Freinkel, R. H. Bell, H. Friesen, J. F. Wilber and B. E. Metzger. Gynecomastia, prolactin, and other peptide hormones in patients undergoing chronic hemodialysis. *J Clin Endocrinol Metab* 1973;36:428–432.
53. Holdsworth S., R. C. Atkins and D. M. de Kretser. The pituitary-testicular axis in men with chronic renal failure. *N Engl J Med* 1977;296:1245–1249.
54. Emmanouel D. S., M. D. Lindheimer and A. I. Katz. Pathogenesis of endocrine abnormalities in uremia. *Endo Rev* 1980;1:28–44.
55. Scully R. E. Testicular tumors with endocrine manifestations. In: DeGroot L. J. ed. *Endocrinology*. Philadelphia, W. B. Saunders, 1995; pp. 2442–2448.
56. Carroll B. Ultrasonography of the scrorum. In: Sarti D. A. ed. *Ultrasound: Text and Cases*. Year Book Medical Publishers, 1997; pp. 570–602.
57. Hendry W. S., W. H. H. Garvie, A. K. Ah-See and A. P. Bayliss. Ultrasonic detection of occult testicular neoplasms in patients with gynecomastia. *Br J Radiology* 1984;57:571–572.
58. Mineur P., S. De Cooman, J. Hustin, G. Verhoeven and R. De Hertogh. Feminizing testicular leyig cell tumor: hormonal profile before and after unilateral orchidectomy. *J Clin Endocrinol Metab* 1987;64:686–691.
59. Bercovici J., K. Nahoul, D. Tater, J. Charles and R. Scholler. Hormonal profile of leydig cell tumors with gynecomastia. *J Clin Endocrinol Metab* 1984;59:625–630.
60. Caine M., S. Perlberg and R. Gordon. The treatment of benign prostatic hypertrophy with flutamide (sch 13521): a placebo-controlled study. *J Urol* 1975;114:564–568.
61. Gabrilove J. L., E. K. Freiberg, E. Leiter and G. L. Nicolis. Feminizing and non-feminizing sertoli cell tumors. *J Urol* 1980;124:757–767.
62. Javadpour N. Value of tumor markers in testicular cancer. In: Talerman A. and L. M. Roth, eds. *Pathology of the Testis and its Adnexa*. New York, Churchill Livingstone. 1986; pp. 221–230.
63. Stepanas A. V., N. A. Samaan, P. N. Schultz and P. Y. Holoye. Endocrine studies in testicular tumor patients with and without gynecomastia. *Cancer* 1978;41:369–376.
64. Payne A. H., R. P. Kelch, S. S. Musich and M. E. Halpern. Intratesticular site of aromatization in the human. *J Clin Endocrinol Metab* 1976;42:1081–1087.
65. Gabrilove J. L., G. L. Nicolis, R. U. Hausknecht and H. H. Wotiz. Feminizing adrenocortical carcinoma in a man. *Cancer* 1970;25:153–160.
66. Desai M. B. and S. N. Kapadia. Feminizing adrenocortical tumors in male patients: adenoma versus carcinoma. *J Urol* 1988;139:101–03.
67. Bhettay E. and F. Bonnici. Pure estrogen-secreting feminizing adrenocortical adenoma. *Arch Dis Child* 1977;52:241–243.
68. Faiman C., J. A. Colwell, R. J. Ryan, J. M. Hershman and T. W. Shields. Gonadotropin secretion from a bronchogenic carcinoma. *N Eng J Med* 1967;277:1395–1399.
70. Vaitukaitis J. L. Immunologic and physical characterization of human chorionic gonadotropin (hCG) secreted by tumors. *J Clin Endocrinol Metab* 1973;37:505–514.
71. Goldenberg D. M., E. E. Kim, F. H. DeLand, J. R. J. van Nagel and N. Javadpour. Clinical radioimmunodetection of cancer with radioactive antibodies to human chorionic gonadotropin. *Science* 1980;208:1284–1286.

72. Kirschner M. A., F. B. Cohen and D. Jespersen. Estrogen production and its origin in men with gonadotropin-producing neoplasms. *J Clin Endocrinol Metab* 1974;39:112–118.
73. Charles M. A., R. Claypool, M. Schaaf, S. W. Rosen and B. D. Weintraub. Lung carcinoma associated with production of three placental proteins. *Arch Intern Med* 1973;132:427–431.
74. Metz S. A., B. Weintraub, S. Rosen, W., J. Singer and R. P. Robertson. Ectopic secretion of chorionic gonadotropin by a lung carcinoma. *Am J Med* 1978;65:325–333.
75. McArthur J. W., G. D. Toll, A. B. Russfield, A. M. Reiss, W. C. Quinby and W. H. Baker. Sexual precocity attributable to ectopic gonadotropin secretion by hepatoblastoma. *Am J Med* 1973;54:390–403.
76. Sherwood L. M. Paraneoplastic endocrine disorders (ectopic hormone syndromes). *Endocrinol* 1995;3:2754–2802.
77. Moran C. A. and S. Suster. Primary mediastinal choriocarcinomas: a clinicopathologic and immunohistochemical study of eight cases. *Am J Surg Pathol* 1997;21:1007–1012.
78. Kubo O., N. Yamasaki and Y. Kamijo. Human chorionic gonadotropin produced by ectopic pinealoma in a girl with precocious puberty. *J Neurosurg* 1977;47:101–105.
79. Lee S. H., N. Sundaresan, B. Jereb and J. H. Galicich. Endodermal sinus tumor of the pineal region: a case report. *Neurosurgery* 1978;3:407–411.
80. Whitcomb R. W., R. N. Schimke, J. L. Kyner, B. P. Lukert and D. C. Johnson. Endocrine studies in a male patient with choriocarcinoma and gynecomastia. *Am J Med* 1986;81:917–920.
81. Weintraub B. D. and S. Rosen, W. Ectopic production of human chorionic somatomammotropin by nontrophoblastic cancers. *J Clin Endocrinol Metab* 1971;32:94–101.
82. Rifka S. M., J. C. Pita, R. A. Vigersky, Y. A. Wilson and D. L. Loriaux. Interaction of digitalis and spironolactone with human sex steroid receptors. *J Clin Endocrinol Metab* 1978;46:338–344.
83. Katzenellenbogen B. S., J. A. Katzenellenbogen and D. Mordecai. Zearalenones: characterization of the estrogenic potencies and receptor interactions of a series of fungal b-resorcylic acid lactones. *Endocrinol* 1979;105:33–40.
84. Loriaux D. L., R. Menard, A. Taylor, J. C. Pita and R. Santen. Spironolactone and endocrine dysfunction. *Ann Int Med* 1976;85:630–636.
85. Caminos-Torres R., L. Ma and P. J. Snyder. Gynecomastia and semen abnormalities induced by spironolactone in normal men. *J Clin Endocrinol Metab* 1997;45:255–260.
86. Doppman J. L., E. H. Oldfield and L. K. Nieman. Bilateral sampling of the internal jugular vein to distinguish between mechanisms of adrenocorticotropic hormone-dependent Cushing syndrome. *Ann Intern Med* 1998;128:33–36.
87. Feldman D. Ketoconazole and other imidazole derivatives as inhibitors of steroidogenesis. *Endo Rev* 1986;7:409–420.
88. DiRaimondo C. V., A. C. Roach and C. K. Meador. Gynecomastia from exposure to vaginal estrogen cream. *N Engl J Med* 1980;302:1089–1090.
89. Beas F., L. Vargas, R. P. Spada and N. Merchak. Pseudoprecocious puberty in infants caused by a dermal ointment containing estrogens. *J Pediatr* 1969;75:127–130.
90. Beas F., L. Vargas, R. P. Spada and N. Merchak. Pseudoprecocious puberty in infants caused by a dermal ointment containing estrogens. *J Pediatr* 1969;July:127–130.
91. Edidin D. V. and L. L. Levitsky. Prepubertal gynecomastia associated with estrogen-containing hair cream. *Am J Dis Child* 1982;136:587–588.
92. Harrington J. M., R. O. Rivera and A. V. de Morales. The occupation hazards of formulating oral contraceptives- a survey of plant employees. *Archives of Environmental Health* 1978;Jan/Feb:12–15.
93. Fara G. M., G. Del Corvo, S. Bernuzzi, A. Bigatello, C. Di Pietro, S. Scaglioni and Chiumello. Epidemic of breast enlargement in an italian school. *Lancet* 1978;11:295–297.
94. Malozowski S. and B. V. Stadel. Prepubertal gynecomastia during growth hormone therapy. *J Pediatr* 1995;126:659–661.
95. Zhou J., O. O. Adesanya, J. Wang, D. LeRoith and C. A. Bondy. Growth hormone treatment induces mammary gland hyperplasia in aging primates. *Nat Med* 1997;10:1141–1144.
96. Harmon J. W. and M. A. Aliapoulios. Marijuana-induced gynecomastia: clinical and laboratory experience. *Surgical Forum* 1974;25:423–425.
97. Evans N. A. Gym and tonic: a profile of 100 male steroid users. *Br J Sports Med* 1997;31:54–58.
98. Maclaren N. K., C. J. Migeon and S. Raiti. Gynecomastia with congenital virilizing adrenal hyperplastia (11-b-hydroxylase deficiency. *J Pediatr* 1973;86:579–581.
99. Kadair R. G., M. B. Block, F. H. Katz and F. D. Hofeldt. "Masked" 21-hydroxylase deficiency of the adrenal presenting with gynecomastia and bilateral testicular masses. *Am J Med* 1977;62:278–282.

100. Boyar R. M. and L. Hellman. Syndrome of benign nodular adrenal hyperplasia associated with feminization and hyperprolactinemia. *Ann Intern Med* 1974;80:389–394.
101. Field J. B., R. T. Solis and W. E. Dear. Case report: unilateral gynecomastia associated with thoracotomy following resection of carcinoma of the lung. *Am J Med Sci* 1989;298:402–406.
102. Epstein S. Herpes zoster of the chest wall and gynecomastia. *S Afr Med J* 1984;54:368–369.
103. Kleinberg D. L., G. L. Noel and A. G. Frantz. Galactorrhea: A study of 235 cases including 48 with pituitary tumors. *N Engl J Med* 1977;296:589–600.
104. LeRoith D., R. Sobel and S. M. Glick. The effect of clomiphene citrate on pubertal gynecomastia. *Acta Endocrinol* 1980;95:177–180.
105. Stepanas A. V., R. B. Burnet, P. E. Harding and P. H. Wise. Clomiphene in the treatment of pubertal-adolescent gynecomastia: A preliminary report. *J Pediatrics* 1977;90:651–653.
106. Jefferys D. B. Painful gynecomastia treated with tamoxifen. *Br Med J* 1979;1119–1120.
107. McDermott M. T., F. D. Hofeldt and G. S. Kidd. Tamoxifen therapy for painful idiopathic gynecomastia. *So Med J* 1990;83:1283–1285.
108. Parker L. N., D. R. Gray, M. K. Lai and E. R. Levin. Treatment of gynecomastia with tamoxifen: A double-blind crossover study. *Metab* 1986;35:705–708.
109. Gagnon J. D., W. T. Moss and K. R. Stevens. Pre-estrogen breast irradiation for patients with carcinoma of the prostate: a critical review. *J Urol* 1979;121:182–184.
110. Sharp E. A. Historical review of a syndrome embracing utero-ovarian atrophy with persistent lactation (Frommel's disease). *Am J Obstet Gynecol* 1935;30:411–414.
111. Frantz A. G. and D. L. Kleinberg. Prolactin: Evidence that it is separate from growth hormone in human blood. *Science* 1970;170:745–747.
112. Kleinberg D. L. and A. G. Frantz. Human prolactin: Measurement in plasma by in vitro bioassay. *J Clin Invest* 1971;50:1557–1568.
113. Friesen H. G. The discovery of human prolactin: a very personal account. *Clin Invest Med* 1995;18:66–72.
114. Hwang P., H. Guyda and H. Friesen. A radioimmunoassay for human prolactin. *Proc Natl Acad Sci USA* 1971;68:1902–1906.
115. Kleinberg D. L. Human -lactalbumin: Measurement in serum and in breast cancer organ culture by radioimmunoassay. *Science* 1995;190:276–278.
116. Kleinberg D. L., J. Todd and M. L. Groves. Studies on human -lactabumin: Radioimmunoassay measurements in normal human breast and breast cancer. *J Clin Endocrinol Metab* 1977; 45:1238–1250.
117. Landis C. A., S. B. Masters, A. Spada, A. M. Pace, H. R. Bourne and L. Vallar. GTPase inhibiting mutations activate the a chain of G_s and stimulate adenylyl cyclase in human pituitary tumours. *Nature* 1989;340:692–696.
118. Sauder S. E., M. Frager, G. A. Case, R. P. Kelch and J. C. Marshall. Abnormal patterns of pulsatile luteinizing hormone secretion in women with hyperprolactinemia and amenorrhea: responses to bromocriptine. *J Clin Endocrinol* Metab 1984;59:941–948.
119. Garcia A., L. Herbon, A. Barkan, S. Papavasiliou and J. C. Marshall. Gonadotropin-releasing hormone (GnRH) stimulation of the number of the number of pituitary GnRH receptors. *Endocrinol* 1985;117:954–959.
120. Schlechte J., L. Walkner and M. Kathol. A longitudinal analysis of premenopausal bone loss in healthy women and women with hyperprolactinemia. *J Clin Endocrinol Metab* 1992;75:698–703.
121. Klibanski A., B. M. K. Biller, D. I. Rosenthal and V. Saxe. Effects of prolactin and estrogen deficiency in amenorrheic bone loss. *J Clin Endocrinol Metab* 1988;67:124–130.
122. Klibanski A. and S. L. Greenspan. Increase in bone mass after treatment of hyperprolactinemic amenorrhea. *N Eng J Med* 1986;315:542–546.
123. Kleinberg D. L. and J. Todd. Evidence that human growth hormone is a potent lactogen in primates. *J Clin Endocrinol Metab* 1980;51:1009–1015.
124. Noel G. L., H. K. Suh, J. G. Stone and A. G. Frantz. Human prolactin and growth hormone release during surgery and other conditions of stress. *J Clin Endocrinol Metab* 1972;35:67–77.
125. Van Wyk J. J. and M. M. Grumbach. Syndrome of precocious menstruation and galactorrhea in juvenile hypothyroidism: An example of hormonal overlap in pituitary feedback. *J Pediatr* 1960;57:416–435.
126. Jackson W. P. U. Post-thyroidectomy hypothyroidism, hypoparathyroidism, exophthalmos and galactorrhea with normal menstruation. *J Clin Endocrinol Metab* 11956;6:1245–1250.
127. Kinch R. A. H., E. R. Plunkett and M. C. Devlin. Postpartum amenorrhea-galactorrhea of hypothyroidism. *Am J Obstet Gynecol* 1969;105:766–773.

128. Ross F. and M. L. Nusynowitz. A syndrome of primary hypothyroidism, amenorrhea and galactorrhea. *J Clin Endocrinol Metab* 1968;28:591–595.
129. Kleinberg D. L., A. E. I. Boyd, S. Wardlaw, A. G. Frantz, A. George, N. Bryan, S. Hilal, J. Greising, D. Hamilton, T. Seltzer and C. J. Sommers. Pergolide for the treatment of pituitary tumors secreting prolactin or growth hormone. *N Engl J Med* 1983;309:704–709.
130. Kleinberg D. L. Pharmacologic therapies and surgical options in the treatment of hyperprolactinemia. *Endocrinologist* 1989;7 Supplement:379–384.
131. Lamberts S. W. J. and R. F. P. Quik. A comparison of the efficacy and safety of pergolide and bromocriptine in the treatment of hyperprolactinemia. *J Clin Endocrinol Metab* 1991;72:635–641.

INDEX

C

D

E

F

G

R

S

T

U

V

W

Z

ABOUT THE EDITOR

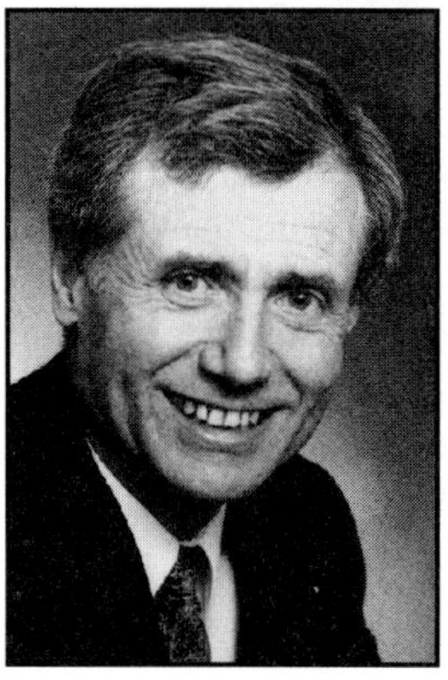

Dr. Andrea Manni is Professor of Medicine at the Pennsylvania State University in the Section of Endocrinology, Diabetes and Metabolism. He has made contributions to basic and clinical breast cancer research since completing his fellowship in Endocrinology at Case Western Reserve University. His major contributions relate to the optimal use of various modalities of endocrine therapy in women with metastatic breast cancer and to the investigation of basic mechanisms of hormonal control of tumor growth in experimental breast cancer systems. A major focus of his current research is on the role of polyamines in breast cancer cell proliferation, mammary carcinogenesis and tumor progression. He has served on numerous NIH review panels, is an editor of *The Journal of Clinical Endocrinology and Metabolism* and an associate editor of *Endocrine-Related Cancer*.